NURSING CARE PLANS FOR NEWBORNS AND CHILDREN:

ACUTE AND CRITICAL CARE

Meg Gulanick, RN, PhD
Clinical Nurse Specialist
Department of Cardiology

Michele Knoll Puzas, RNC, MHPE
Nurse Clinician
Department of Pediatric Nursing

Cynthia R. Wilson, RN, BSN
Assistant Nurse Manager
Special Care Nursery

Humana Hospital-Michael Reese
Chicago, Illinois

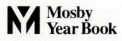 **Mosby Year Book**

St. Louis Baltimore Boston Chicago London Philadelphia Sydney Toronto

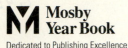

Mosby
Year Book
Dedicated to Publishing Excellence

Editor: Terry Van Schaik
Developmental Editor: Janet R. Livingston
Project Manager: Karen Edwards
Production: Ginny Douglas
Designer: David Zielinski

Printed in the United States of America

Mosby—Year Book, Inc.
11830 Westline Industrial Drive
St. Louis, Missouri 63146

Library of Congress Cataloging in Publication Data

Gulanick, Meg.
    Nursing care plans for newborns and children : acute and critical
care / Meg Gulanick, Michele Knoll Puzas, Cynthia R. Wilson.
       p.   cm.
    Include index.
    ISBN 0-8016-6388-1
    1.   Neonatal intensive care.   2.   Pediatric intensive care.
3.   Nursing care plans.   I.   Title.
    [DNLM: 1.   Acute Disease—in infancy & childhood—nurses
instruction.   2.   Critical Care—in infancy & childhood—nurses'
instruction.   3.   Nursing Diagnosis.   4.   Patient Care Planning—
nurses' instruction.   WY   159 N973943]
RJ253.5.G855   1992
618.92—dc20
DNLM/DLC
for Library of Congress
                                       92-1213
                                         CIP

92 93 94 95 96 GW/VH 9 8 7 6 5 4 3 2 1

Contributors

Kathy Alexander, RN
Linda Arsenault, RN, MSN, CNRN
Eileen Banker, RNC
Margaret Bell, RN
Racquel Gabriel-Bennewitz, RN, BSN, CCRN
Caramen E. Billheimer, RN, BSN
Rhonda Blender, RN, MSN
Carol Boyd, RN, BSN
Catherine Brown, RN, BAN
Ursula M. Brozek, RN, MSN
Marian D. Cachero, RN, BSN
Ruby Rotor-Cajindos, RN, BSN
Mary Leslie Caldwell, RN
Mary Lawson-Carney, RN
Mary Kay Chathas, RN, MSN
Jan Colip, RN, MSN, CCRN
Suzanne M. DeFabiis, RN, MS
Margaret J. Dewey, RN, MSN
Reneé Zubay Fife, RN, MSN
Joan Marie Fogata, RN, BSN
Rosa Fuentes, RN, BSN
Susan Galanes, RN, MS, CCRN
Susan Geoghegan, RN, BSN
Deidra Gradishar, RNC, BA
Terry Griffin, RN, MS
Meg Gulanick, RN, PhD
Frankie Harper, RN
Marilyn Samson-Hinton, RN, BSN
Frank Hohn, DDS
Wilma J. Hunter, RN, MS, CPNP, CNN
Herminia Inawat, RN
Kathleen Jaffrey, RN
Kim Johnson, RN, BSN
Vivian Jones, RN
Linda M. Kamenjarin, RN, BSN, CCRN
Phyllis Lawlor-Klean, RN, MS
Patricia Kling, RNC, MSN, NNP
Audrey Klopp, RN, PhD, CS, ET

Vanida Komutanon, RN
Olga A. Lazala, RN, BSN
Digna S. Limjoco, RN
Tracy Lin, RN, MS
Evelyn M. Lyons, RN, BSN, TNS
Marilyn R. Magafas, RN, MBA
Victoria Malone, RN, BSN, FNP
Susan P. Maloney, RN, BSN
Janet L. McCants, RN, BSN
Michelle McGhee, RN, BSN
Doris McNear, RN, BSN
Anita D. Morris, RN, TNS
Mary Muse, RN, MS
Linda Ehrlich Muzio, RN, MSN, CS
Mary Ann Naccarato, RN, BSN
Dinah Parmuth, RN, BSN
Agnes Jones-Perry, RN, BSN
Michele Knoll Puzas, RNC, MHPE
Charlotte Razvi, RN, MSN, PhD
Deborah Rickard, RN, BSN
Sandra N. Roberts, RN, MSN
Terri L. Russell, RN
Laura L. Rybicki, RN, BSN
Linda M. St. Julien, RN, MS
Rosetonia G. Sapaula, RN, BSN
Carol Sarmiento, RN, BSN
Ruth E. Schumacher, RNC, MSN
Nedra Skale, RN, MS, CNA
Kimberly P. Souder, RN, BSN
Sophia A. Spencer, RN, BSN
Gina Stevens, RN, BSN
Jacqueline Santiago-Tan, RN, BSN
Gail Tipp, RN
Christine Todd, RN, BS, BGS
Linda Walsh, RN, BSN
Sandra P. Wilks, RN, BSN
Cynthia R. Wilson, RN, BSN
Jeff Zurlinden, RN, MS

Preface

Today, hospitals are facing a tremendous challenge to provide quality patient care amidst intensive cost containment efforts and a diminishing supply of nurses. This challenge demands that nurses be creative and efficient in planning for their patients' needs. The use of comprehensive care plan guides that serve as reference standards from which nurses can individualize patient care is now recognized as a valuable solution to this problem. Pediatric patients requiring acute and critical care are seen in many settings: in combined adult and pediatric medical/surgical units, pediatric units in medical centers, and in pediatric intensive care units. Premature and low-birth-weight infants are surviving with the specialized care provided in neonatal intensive care units. Nurses practicing in any of these settings, as well as student nurses, will find this book valuable for its presentation of acute and critical care nursing for children of all ages.

Beginning in 1986, with the publication of the first edition of *Nursing Care Plans: Nursing Diagnosis & Intervention,* Michael Reese Hospital and Medical Center became a leader in the development of such care plan guides. The second edition (1990) contains over 225 "state-of-the-art" care plan guides, developed by practitioners and nursing experts. Although these initial books met the needs of a large acute care patient population, they did *not* address the physical, psychological, and nurturing needs of the infant and child who requires acute and critical care. The nature of intensive care and acute care nursing obviously demands special skill and understanding. Therefore this book was written to provide the practitioner with care plan guides for the clinical problems and treatments encountered by this special population.

This newest text includes a blend of both nursing diagnoses and medical problems. Chapter 1 addresses 33 NANDA-approved nursing diagnoses. This chapter allows a "pure" approach to nursing diagnosis and ensures that the reader can address any patient care issue. Chapter 2 addresses the psychosocial concerns of the hospitalized child. The subsequent chapters are organized by body system or clinical specialty and include the latest trends in nursing and medical practice. Some examples of the range of topics are organ donation, grieving for the terminally ill neonate, high–frequency jet ventilation, substance abuse withdrawal, breastfeeding the infant requiring special care, kidney transplantation, and AIDS. Except for Chapter 1, each chapter is divided into a pediatric and a neonatal care plan section. This book's format aids both the student and the practitioner in deriving the appropriate nursing diagnoses and formulating the plan of care. A concerted effort was made to maintain a strict separation of the components of nursing process. Ongoing assessments and defining characteristics are clearly separated from therapeutic interventions and expected outcomes. Likewise, defining characteristics are separated from related factors.

Moreover, an exciting feature of this book is the inclusion of rationales for particular nursing interventions. These explanations serve as helpful teaching aids and may eliminate the need for an additional reference book. Finally, an introductory section has been included to provide clarification of the various components of care plans and suggestions on how to use these guides.

Nursing Care Plans for Newborns and Children: Acute and Critical Care reflects the evolution of nursing practice and nursing diagnosis. The care plan guides simultaneously incorporate both independent and collaborative nursing interventions according to priority need, depicting nursing practice in the "real world." Nurses of all levels of expertise will find this book helpful. Its content serves as a self-contained teaching guide and source of support for the novice nurse, while serving as a review or organizational tool for the experienced nurse.

ACKNOWLEDGMENTS

This book could not have been written without the support and contributions of many people. A special thanks goes to the 72 talented nurse authors who shared their clinical expertise with us. Further appreciation goes to Thelma Anderson, Diane Talarek, and the nursing department of Humana Hospital-Michael Reese for their ongoing support for this project. We also wish to acknowledge our Nurse Specialist colleagues who provided the necessary encouragement and assistance to see this project to fruition. And finally, we are forever grateful to Emma Glover and Rosalie Clay for their quality work in preparing the manuscript materials for this book.

Meg Gulanick
Michele Knoll Puzas
Cynthia R. Wilson

Preface

vi

Contents

5 Neurological Care Plans, *172*

6 Gastrointestinal Care Plans, *221*

7 Integumentary/Musculoskeletal Care Plans, *276*

8 Renal/Endocrine/Metabolic Care Plans, *331*

9 Hematologic/Oncologic/Immunologic Care Plans, *381*

Introduction:

How to Individualize Nursing Care Plans

Nursing is defined as the diagnosis and treatment of human responses to actual or high-risk health problems. Gordon* defines nursing diagnoses as "actual or potential health problems which nurses by virtue of their education and experience are capable and licensed to treat." Inherent in these definitions is the nurse's ability to identify actual or high-risk problems, and to identify methods of assisting the patient to a resolution of those problems.

Nurses care for large numbers of patients, many or all of whom have complex care needs. Some nursing activities are independent interventions, such as teaching and comfort measures. The nursing process (assessment, diagnosis, planning, implementation, and evaluation) is the organizing framework for these activities. Other activities represent interdependent activities, in which nurses carry out the physician's plan of care and address the patient's response to those interventions. Medication administration is an example of an interdependent activity. Both independent and interdependent activities take place in a complex health care environment, where nurses function as coordinators, arranging the various aspects of health care delivery in a way that best meets patients' needs. Tremendous amounts of information for large numbers of patients must be available to the nurse in a concise, well-organized format.

Although nursing diagnosis is clearly an exciting development for nursing, nurses at the bedside are often acutely reminded that the state-of-the-nursing-diagnosis-art is still very much in a state of evolution. Most research related to nursing diagnosis has addressed only the label, etiologic factors, and defining characteristics; the interventional strategies have not yet been widely addressed. This situation leaves the bedside nurse with a label (or diagnosis), possible related factors, and defining characteristics but without the plan of care related to the diagnoses that pertain to the patient's needs. The nursing care plan guides

in this book have recognized both the independent and interdependent role of the nurse, have clustered groups of nursing diagnoses in such a manner as to facilitate the nurse's coordinative role in today's health care environment, and provide structure and substance for the set of behaviors known as the nursing process. Most importantly, these nursing care plan guides assist the nurse in planning comprehensive, individualized care.

COMPONENTS OF THE CARE PLAN

Each care plan guide throughout this book includes the following information: actual or high-risk nursing diagnoses, related factors, defining characteristics, expected outcomes, and nursing interventions with rationales.

NURSING DIAGNOSIS

The nursing diagnosis is the summary judgment that the professional nurse makes about the data gathered during the nursing assessment. Almost all nursing diagnoses used throughout this book have been approved by NANDA (North American Nursing Diagnosis Association), an organization charged with the responsibility of classifying and developing nursing diagnoses, and are expressed in NANDA's nomenclature. This standardization assists nurses in developing a common language to improve professional communication. However, some original diagnostic labels have been incorporated into the care plan guides formulated for medical diagnoses at the discretion of the clinical nurse. Definitions of the NANDA diagnoses are included with each care plan guide in Chapter 1. Some definitions were developed by NANDA; others were created by the clinical nurse authors based on review of the literature and their clinical expertise.

RELATED FACTORS

Before developing a treatment plan for a nursing diagnosis, the nurse must evaluate those factors thought to be related to or the probable cause of the disorder. Such factors may be physical, psychological, environmental, so-

*From Gordon M: Nursing diagnosis and the diagnostic process, *American Journal of Nursing* 76:1298-1300, 1976.

cial, or spiritual. Each diagnosis in this book lists several contributing factors that may be related to the diagnosis. These related factors serve to direct the selection of subsequent nursing interventions.

DEFINING CHARACTERISTICS

Each nursing diagnosis in this book lists observable signs and symptoms that are usually present when the health problem exists; these descriptive signs are known as the *defining characteristics* for that diagnosis. Some characteristics are quite specific, must be present before a diagnosis can be made, and are considered critical data. Other characteristics are less precise, appear in several diagnoses, and are considered supportive data. The defining characteristics are gathered during the nursing assessment. A valid diagnosis must be based on actual assessment, not assumptions, regarding defining characteristics. Accuracy of a diagnosis can be verified by comparing the assessed defining characteristics with those listed for the standard care plan.

The defining characteristics in this book are a representative, although not an exhaustive, listing of the common characteristics associated with a nursing problem. Many of the identified characteristics were modified from NANDA's listing for each diagnosis.

EXPECTED OUTCOMES

Expected outcomes are concise statements that should identify a specific, observable, realistic, and measurable goal. An example is: "In 24 hours, the child will have relief or reduction of pain, as evidenced by comfortable appearance and verbalization of comfort." Although it would be possible to write such a specific outcome for each nursing diagnosis identified throughout this book, the editors felt that the repetition of the observable, measurable criteria for each goal, namely a listing of the defining characteristics, was unnecessarily repetitious. Therefore the expected outcome section simply includes one broad outcome statement per nursing diagnosis, such as: "Pain will be reduced or relieved," or "Optimal physical mobility will be achieved." Because these care plans serve as guides for actual nursing practice, nurses can individualize outcomes for patients using absence of each defining characteristic as a criterion for achievement.

Expected outcomes must be evaluated within a specific time frame to assist in determining whether the plan of care needs revision or resolution. Because of the individuality and complexities of patient care, no standard time frames were identified in these guides. The readers will have to make this adaptation based on professional judgment.

NURSING INTERVENTIONS

Nursing interventions are those actions or prescriptions that assist in meeting the defined goal or outcome. They include two components of the nursing process: assessments and planned interventions. The *ongoing assessments* listed for each diagnosis are related to the defining characteristics. Because the presence of a specific cluster of characteristics represents an actual problem, ongoing assessments are needed both to validate actual presence of the problem and to measure or document progress in

treating or alleviating the problem. *Therapeutic interventions* are those measures required to accomplish the desired outcome. Because these are orders, they begin with a verb and clearly direct the nurse's actions. They include actual nursing therapies, documentation of actions and results, and consultation and communication with other health professionals. Most interventions reflect treatments that nurses can perform independently. However, the editors did include collaborative (interdependent) practice measures commonly observed in practice (e.g., "Insert Foley catheter as needed"; "Give atropine per protocol"). Many of these therapeutic interventions reflect changing national trends in nurses' professional responsibilities, and, in some practice areas, nurses already perform them independently. This is nursing practice in the "real world."

Not every suggested intervention is appropriate for all children throughout their hospitalization or illness. A broad range of nursing actions is presented here to provide the practitioner with options when adapting the care plan to specific patient needs. As a child's condition changes, some of the interventions for a specific nursing diagnosis will assume higher priority than others. For example, during the acute phase of "Ineffective Airway Clearance," immediate physical therapies supersede follow-up care concerns.

The nursing intervention section also includes patient/family education. These actions are presented in several different formats throughout the book. In the generic nursing diagnosis section in Chapter 1, patient/parent education interventions are listed under a separate heading. In the chapters that contain medical diagnoses and procedures, some teaching interventions are included in many of the subcategories of nursing diagnoses found in that standard care plan.

RATIONALES

Rationales are incorporated into the nursing interventions to explain the purpose for or necessity of particular nursing actions; these rationales serve as learning tools for both the novice and experienced practitioner. Inclusion of such rationales may eliminate the need for an additional reference book.

GENERAL VS. SPECIFIC CARE PLAN GUIDES

Chapter 1 includes general, comprehensive care plan guides for the NANDA-approved nursing diagnoses most commonly used in clinical practice. These guides provide a framework for designing an individual child's care plan. Children may present with one or several nursing diagnoses; careful initial nursing assessment is required for selection of the most appropriate diagnoses. The nursing interventions for these general care plan guides are comprehensive, reflecting several approaches to treating the health problem. Not all interventions may be appropriate for a specific patient. An extensive listing of possible related or risk factors is provided to direct selection of appropriate nursing activities.

Although these general guides allow almost any patient care issue to be addressed, Humana Hospital-Michael Reese nurses identified the need to develop specific guides for those medical problems and treatments most commonly encountered in their intensive care and acute care units. Although recognizing that all patients are individuals with unique health needs, the nurses also realized that most patients share common concerns and problems. These specific care plans focus on similarity among patients, and their use can therefore optimize efficient delivery of nursing care. Specific care plan guides are found in Chapters 2 through 9. These guides include clustering of the common nursing diagnoses most frequently assessed with each medical problem.

In these guides, nursing diagnoses are presented according to priority needs. For example, airway problems or preoperative teaching needs tend to be first. Actual problems are presented before high-risk problems; discharge teaching and planning concerns are usually addressed last or not at all because often the focus is limited to critical care needs. Since the nursing diagnosis is now related to a more specific etiology, the nursing interventions are more specific and concise.

USE OF THE CARE PLAN GUIDES

These care plans were written to be used both as guides for nursing practice and as tools to assist nurses and institutions in meeting the state and local requirements of the Joint Commission on Accreditation of Healthcare Organizations (JCAHO). Although expectations that individualized plans of care be developed and used for each patient exist, other responsibilities and time constraints often limit care planning efforts.

Nursing Care Plans for Newborns and Children: Acute and Critical Care can be used in a variety of ways both individually by nurses and collectively by institutions. Uses include clinical practice, teaching/education, quality assurance, and research. On the clinical units, standardized care plans can be used to write a plan of care for a particular patient, or they can serve as a guide to the care of a patient population in general. Nurses can use the care plan guides as quick references, especially when caring for new or infrequently encountered types of patients. Using these care plans increases efficiency by allowing nurses to spend their scarce time individualizing and adapting care plans rather than creating new ones. Highlighting applicable information, lining out inappropriate information, or writing in parameters and dates particular to one patient are quick methods of individualization.

The care plan guides in this book are educational tools; each guide encapsulates the plan of care in a logical, rational manner. Establishing the care plan guides as standards for a unit or a specific population of patients allows for assessment of staff learning needs, and they may be used with students, new staff members, and other health care team members as instructional guides to patient care. The guides can also be used to evaluate individual nursing practice or to address deficiencies noted in nursing care following quality assurance activities.

These care plan guides are also unique quality assurance tools. Quality assurance activities are based on locally, regionally, and nationally accepted standards of care and practice; this collection of care plan guides reflects the expertise of practicing staff nurses as well as nationally recognized advanced practice nurses who served as resources in the development of these guides. Individual guides can be used to identify and define standards so that nurses involved in quality assurance activities, as well as nurse managers, can identify problem areas in specific aspects of care. Documentation issues, often the focus of quality assurance activities, may be addressed using the care plan guides as the basis for evaluating care given. The importance of such monitoring activities is increasing as third-party payers and certifying/surveying agencies require increasing amounts of evidence of the plan of care, as well as care provided.

The care plan guides also provide a framework for research. The development, refinement, and validation of nursing diagnoses, efficacy of therapeutic interventions, validity of expected outcomes, acuity systems' reliability, and issues of nurse-generated revenue and direct reimbursement for nursing care rendered are applicable topics for research activities.

1

Nursing Diagnosis
Care Plans

Activity intolerance
Airway clearance, ineffective
Anxiety
Aspiration
Body image disturbance
Breathing pattern, ineffective
Cardiac output, decreased
Communication, impaired
Constipation
Coping, family: ineffective
Diarrhea
Diversional activity deficit
Family processes, altered
Fear
Fluid volume deficit
Fluid volume excess
Gas exchange, impaired
Grieving, anticipatory
Growth and development, altered

Hyperthermia
Hypothermia
Infection, high risk for
Mobility, impaired physical
Nutrition, altered: less than body requirements
Nutrition, altered: more than body requirements
Pain
Parenting, altered: actual/high risk for
Skin integrity, impaired: actual/high risk for
Skin integrity, impaired: high risk for (neonate)
Thermoregulation, ineffective
Tissue perfusion, altered: peripheral, cardiopulmonary, cerebral, renal
Urinary incontinence
Urinary retention

Activity intolerance

A state in which a child has insufficient physical or psychological energy to endure or perform desired or required physical activities.

RELATED FACTORS / DEFINING CHARACTERISTICS	NURSING INTERVENTIONS / *RATIONALES*	EXPECTED OUTCOMES

RELATED FACTORS

Generalized weakness

Deconditioned state

Insufficient sleep or rest periods

Lack of motivation/ depression

Prolonged bed rest

Imposed activity restriction

Imbalance between oxygen supply and demand

Pain

DEFINING CHARACTERISTICS

Verbal report of fatigue or weakness

Listlessness

Inability to begin/ perform activity

Abnormal heart rate or BP response to activity

Exertional discomfort or dyspnea

ONGOING ASSESSMENT

- Assess respiratory status before activity:
  - Respiratory quality and quantity
  - Need for oxygen with increased activity
- Assess cardiac function before activity:
  - Pulse: rate, rhythm, volume
  - BP: baseline, orthostatic changes
  - Skin: color, temperature, moisture, perfusion
- Assess child's level of mobility.
- Observe and document response to activity. *Close monitoring serves as a guide for optimal progression of activity.* Report to physician:
  - Rapid pulse (age specific)
  - Palpitations
  - Significant increase in systolic BP (age specific)
  - Significant decrease in systolic BP
  - Dyspnea, labored breathing, wheezing
  - Weakness, fatigue
  - Lightheadedness, dizziness, pallor
  - Frequent cessation of activity/resumed after rest
- Assess nutritional status.
- Assess potential for physical injury with activity.
- Assess need for ambulation aids.

THERAPEUTIC INTERVENTIONS

- Encourage adequate rest periods, especially before ambulation, diagnostic procedures, meals, *to reduce cardiac workload.*
- Assist with ADL as indicated *to reduce energy expenditure.*
- Refrain from performing nonessential procedures *to promote rest.*
- Provide neutral thermal environment *to reduce metabolic needs.*
- Anticipate child's needs (e.g., blanket, toy, bathroom).
- Change the child's position and surroundings if the child is unable to do so.
- Ensure infant/child is receiving adequate nutrition. Provide small, frequent feedings.
- Arrange nursing care activities/routines around the needs and response of the infant/child; *i.e., allow adequate rest before attempting to feed; sucking/eating require some endurance.*
- Encourage active ROM or perform PROM exercises tid *to maintain muscle strength;* if further reconditioning is needed, confer with rehabilitation medicine personnel.
- Provide emotional support while increasing activity. Hold the small child when possible.
- Promote a positive attitude regarding abilities.
- Provide alternatives such as riding in a stroller or wagon. Emphasize "low activity" abilities.

PATIENT/PARENT EDUCATION

- Teach child/parents signs of physical overactivity.
- If age appropriate, involve child/parents in activity, goal-setting, and care planning. *Setting small, attainable goals can increase self-confidence and self-esteem.*
- Teach ROM exercises and activity progression guidelines.

Activity level will be maintained within limits of infant's/ child's ability.

Meg Gulanick, RN, PhD

Airway clearance, ineffective

A state in which the child is unable to clear secretions or obstructions from the respiratory tract to maintain airway patency.

RELATED FACTORS / DEFINING CHARACTERISTICS	NURSING INTERVENTIONS / *RATIONALES*	EXPECTED OUTCOMES

RELATED FACTORS

Decreased energy and fatigue

Tracheobronchial: infection, obstruction (including foreign body aspiration), secretions

Perceptual/cognitive impairment

Trauma

DEFINING CHARACTERISTICS

Abnormal breath sounds (rales, rhonchi, wheezes)

Changes in respiratory rate or depth

Cough

Choking, gagging

Cyanosis

Dyspnea

Fever

ONGOING ASSESSMENT

- Auscultate lungs for presence of breath sounds every shift (or as needed). *Routine assessment of breath sounds allows for early detection and correction of abnormalities.*
- Assess respirations: note quality, rate, pattern, depth, flaring of nostrils, dyspnea on exertion, evidence of splinting, use of accessory muscles, position for breathing.
- Assess changes in orientation and behavior pattern.
- Assess changes in vital signs and temperature.
- Assess child's/parents' present knowledge base of disease process.
- Assess cough:
  Effectiveness
  Productivity
- Note presence of sputum; assess quality, color, consistency.
- Monitor arterial blood gases (ABGs); note changes.

THERAPEUTIC INTERVENTIONS

- Position child with proper body alignment for optimal breathing pattern (if tolerated, head elevated 45 degrees). *This promotes better lung expansion and improved air exchange.* Check the child's positioning frequently so that he or she does not slide down, causing the abdomen to compress the diaphragm, *which would cause respiratory embarrassment.*
- If abnormal breath sounds are present:
  Assist child with coughing:
    Administer pain meds prior to the attempt.
    Splint any incisional/injured area.
    Coach the child through the process; use "games" that are age appropriate *to encourage the child to deep breathe and cough effectively,* e.g., pretending to be a dragon, taking a deep breath before blowing out birthday candles, etc.
  If cough is ineffective, then use oropharyngeal or tracheal suction as needed.
    Explain procedure to child.
    Use soft rubber catheters *to prevent trauma to mucous membranes.*
    Use curved-tip catheters and head positioning (if not contraindicated) *to facilitate secretion removal from a specific side.*
- Provide humidity (when appropriate) via bedside humidifier (positioned near child) and humidified-oxygen therapy *to prevent drying of secretions.*
- Encourage oral intake/fluids within the limits of cardiac reserve *to maintain hydration.*
- Instruct and/or change child's position (e.g., ambulate, turn every 2 hours). *This will facilitate secretion movement and drainage.*
- Administer medications (antibiotics, bronchodilators, diuretics) as ordered, noting effectiveness and side effects.
- Assist with oral hygiene every 4 hours or as needed *to decrease oral flora.*
- Maintain adequate airway. Anticipate the need for an artificial airway (intubation) if secretions cannot be cleared.
- With respiratory therapy department, coordinate optimal time for postural drainage and percussion, i.e., at least 1 hour after eating *to prevent aspiration.*
- Pace activities *to avoid fatigue.*
- Maintain planned rest periods.
- Instruct child to avoid restrictive clothing *that could prevent adequate respiratory excursion.*

Secretions will be mobilized and airway will be maintained free of secretions.

Continued.

Airway clearance, ineffective cont'd

RELATED FACTORS / DEFINING CHARACTERISTICS	NURSING INTERVENTIONS / *RATIONALES*	EXPECTED OUTCOMES

PATIENT/PARENT EDUCATION

- Demonstrate and teach coughing, deep breathing, and splinting techniques *so child/parents will understand the rationale and appropriate techniques to adequately keep the airway clear of secretions.*
- Instruct child/parents on indications for, frequency of, and side effects of medications.
- Teach child/parents about environmental factors that can precipitate respiratory problems.
- Explain effects of smoking, including second-hand smoke.
- Instruct child/parents on warning signs of pending/recurring pulmonary problems.
- Consult with pulmonary clinical nurse specialist as appropriate.

Susan Galanes, RN, MS, CCRN

Anxiety

An apprehensive, uneasy feeling that usually stems from an impending or anticipated circumstance or event. It can be focused on an activity, object, or situation, or unfocused and more generalized. It is believed to be primarily internally motivated, and its source may be nonspecific or unknown to the person experiencing it. The feeling may be experienced as diffuse, and is generally categorized into four levels: mild, moderate, severe, and panic.

RELATED FACTORS / DEFINING CHARACTERISTICS	NURSING INTERVENTIONS / *RATIONALES*	EXPECTED OUTCOMES

RELATED FACTORS

Threat or perceived threat to physical and emotional integrity

Change in health status

Intrusive diagnostic and surgical tests and procedures

Changes in environment and routines

Trauma sustained from assault

Threat or perceived threat to self-esteem

Situational and maturational crises

Intrapersonal conflicts caused by unmet needs and/or emotional fixation at an earlier level of development

Interpersonal conflicts

ONGOING ASSESSMENT

- Assess age and developmental level.
- Assess level of anxiety. *Mild anxiety enhances a child's awareness and ability to identify and solve problems. Moderate anxiety limits awareness of environmental stimuli. Problem solving can occur but may be more difficult, and the child may need help. Severe anxiety decreases the child's ability to integrate information and solve problems. Panic is severe anxiety. The child is unable to follow directions. Hyperactivity, agitation, and immobilization may be observed.*
- Assess coping mechanisms in handling anxiety. *This can be done by interviewing the child and significant others. This assessment helps determine the effectiveness of coping strategies currently used by the child.*
- Assess parents' state of mind, especially if anxious. *A child often reflects the parents' level of apprehension.*

THERAPEUTIC INTERVENTIONS

- Document behavioral and verbal expressions of anxiety. *Symptoms often provide information regarding the degree of anxiety. Physiological symptoms and/or complaints will intensify as the level of anxiety increases.*
- Acknowledge awareness of the child's anxiety. *Acknowledgment of the child's/parent's feelings will validate the feelings and communicate acceptance of those feelings.*
- Reassure child that he or she is safe. Stay with the child if this appears necessary. *The presence of a trusted person assures the child of his or her security and safety during a period of anxiety.*
- Maintain a calm and tolerant manner while interacting with the child/parent. *The staff's anxiety may be easily perceived. The child's/parents' feeling of stability increases in a calm and nonthreatening atmosphere.*

Anxiety will be managed or relieved.

RELATED FACTORS / DEFINING CHARACTERISTICS	NURSING INTERVENTIONS / *RATIONALES*	EXPECTED OUTCOMES

DEFINING CHARACTERISTICS

Autonomic symptoms:
  Increase in blood pressure, pulse, respirations
  Paresthesia in extremities
  Dizziness, light-headedness
  Diaphoresis
  Frequent urination
  Flushing or pallor
  Dyspnea
  Palpitations and/or chest pain
  Frequent vague pains or aches
  Hot or cold flashes
  Dry mouth
  Blurred vision
  Headaches
  Nausea and/or diarrhea

Motor tension:
  Restlessness
  Insomnia, nightmares
  Trembling, shaking
  Muscle tension
  Choking or smothering sensations
  Fatigability
  Jitteriness, sighing respirations

Impairment in cognitive and emotional status:
  Hyperattentiveness
  Excessive worry; impatience
  Feelings of helplessness and discomfort
  Poor impulse control
  Exaggerated startle response
  Rumination and apprehension
  Decreased ability to express feelings as a result of impaired verbal communication or lack of verbal skills
  Uncontrolled crying
  Inconsolable
  Clinging behaviors

THERAPEUTIC INTERVENTIONS cont'd

- Establish a working relationship with the family through continuity of care. *An ongoing relationship establishes a basis for communicating anxious feelings.*
- Orient to the environment as needed. *Orientation and awareness of surroundings promote comfort and a decrease in anxiety.*
- When possible, adjust treatment and care to child's routines. Reduce requests made of the child. *Adjustments in care based on the individual's needs reflect awareness of him or her as an individual with special needs.*
- Assist the parent in recognizing his or her own anxiety and behaviors and how these affect the child's behavior and emotional response.
- Use simple language and brief statements when instructing about diagnostic and surgical tests. If practical, provide this information or wait for the child to review later when intense feelings of anxiety have subsided. *When experiencing moderate to severe anxiety, children are unable to comprehend anything more than simple, clear, and brief instructions.*
- Reduce sensory stimuli by maintaining a quiet environment. *Anxiety may escalate with excessive conversation, noise, and equipment around the child.*
- Encourage the child/parent to notify staff when anxious feelings occur. If possible, plan with child the time of the next staff contact, i.e., "I'll be back after this TV show or after lunch to check on you." *This predictability and consistency will reduce apprehension over being "forgotten about." Staff availability reinforces a feeling of security for the child.*
- Encourage child to talk about his or her anxious feelings and examine the anxiety-provoking situation. Assist the child in assessing the situation realistically and recognizing factors leading to the anxious feelings. Ask structured questions to help work through the situation.
- Avoid false reassurances. As anxiety subsides, encourage the child to explore specific events preceding the onset of the anxious feelings. *Recognition and exploration of factors leading to anxious feelings are important steps in developing alternative responses. Children are often unaware of the relationship between emotional concerns and anxiety.*
- Allow the child to play out feelings that cannot be verbalized. Provide paper and crayons for the older child to *facilitate an emotional outlet and communication tool.*
- Assist the child in developing problem-solving abilities. Provide the child with the knowledge and information needed when identifying a problem and during problem-solving sessions. Emphasize the logical strategies the child can use when experiencing anxious feelings.
- Administer antianxiety medications as ordered.

PATIENT/PARENT EDUCATION

- Assist the child in recognizing symptoms of increasing anxiety; explore alternatives that may be used to prevent the anxiety from immobilizing the child. *The child will be able to use problem-solving abilities more effectively when his or her level of anxiety is low.*
- Assist parents in identifying signs of anxiety in the child and in learning how they can support the child through the experience.
- Remind the parent that anxiety at a mild level can encourage growth and development and is important in mobilizing changes.
- Instruct the child/parent in the proper use of medications and educate the child/parent to recognize adverse reactions. *Medication may be necessary if the child's anxiety continues to escalate and the anxiety becomes disabling.*

Rhonda Blender, RN, MSN; Ursula M. Brozek, RN, MSN

Aspiration

INEFFECTIVE AIRWAY CLEARANCE

The ingestion (drawing in) of harmful substances into the nose, throat, or lungs, which can cause a degree of obstruction and lead to asphyxiation. There are several types of aspiration: foreign body, water intoxication (as occurs in drowning), and meconium.

RELATED FACTORS / DEFINING CHARACTERISTICS	NURSING INTERVENTIONS / *RATIONALES*	EXPECTED OUTCOMES

RELATED FACTORS
Foreign body in airway
Near-drowning
Meconium aspiration at birth
 	
DEFINING CHARACTERISTICS
Dyspnea
Tachypnea
Apnea
Ineffective or asymmetrical chest expansion
Abnormal ABGs
Anxiety
Irritability
Fever
Coughing, gagging
Choking, grunting
Wheezing
Stridor
Radiological evidence
Pneumonia
	ONGOING ASSESSMENT
	• Assess airway for patency, wheezing, stridor, possible aspirant. *Wheezing is indicative of small object aspiration.*
	• Assess respiratory function every 2 hours and prn, including: rate, depth, skin color, chest expansion, and breath sounds. *Asymmetrical chest expansion may indicate bronchial obstruction, usually on the right because of anatomical position.*
	• Monitor temperature, pulse, and blood pressure every 2 hours.
	• Monitor ABGs after ventilator changes and prn.
	• Review x-ray findings for air trapping, hyperexpansion, atelectasis, pneumonia.
	• Assess LOC, neurological function (see Level of consciousness, decreased, p. 173).
	• Assess cardiac output (see Cardiac output, decreased, p. 10).
	
	THERAPEUTIC INTERVENTIONS
	• Suction immediately *to clear and maintain patent airway.*
	• Administer oxygen (humid) therapy.
	• Maintain patent airway. Assist with intubation if necessary.
	• Elevate head of bed *to prevent further aspiration and to maximize lung expansion.*
	• If possible, perform Heimlich maneuver *to attempt to clear foreign bodies from airway* (only on children over 1 year of age).
	• Perform CPR if full arrest occurs.
	• Perform postural drainage and chest PT along with suctioning, as needed.
	• Provide cooling blanket *to maintain body temperature within normal limits.*
	• Obtain blood cultures *to rule out or document sepsis.* Place child in isolation if needed.
	• Administer medications, bronchodilators, and antibiotics, as ordered.
	• Stay with/hold child *to reduce anxiety and promote rest, resulting in decreased oxygen requirements.*
	
	PATIENT/PARENT EDUCATION
	• Provide all parents/significant others with safety and accident prevention information during clinic/well-child visits.
	• Explain all procedures to both parent and child, if possible, before procedures are done.
	• Explain/clarify disorder and ongoing status.
	• Obtain resources if needed:
	    Physician conference
	    Social service
	    Respiratory therapy
		Risks of aspiration will be reduced.

Gina Stevens, RN, BSN

Body image disturbance

A disturbance or alteration in the attitude a child has about the actual or perceived structure or function of all or part of the body; this attitude is dynamic and altered through interaction with other persons and situations and is influenced by age and developmental level.

RELATED FACTORS / DEFINING CHARACTERISTICS	NURSING INTERVENTIONS / *RATIONALES*	EXPECTED OUTCOMES

RELATED FACTORS

Perceived threat to body parts

Situational changes (e.g., temporary presence of visible drain/tube, dressing, attached equipment)

Permanent alterations in structure and/or function (e.g., mutilating surgery, removal of body part [internal or external])

Malodorous lesions

DEFINING CHARACTERISTICS

Verbal identification of feeling about altered structure/ function of body part

Verbal pre-occupation with changed body part or function

Naming changed body part or function

Refusal to discuss/ acknowledge change

Focusing behavior on changed body part and/or function

Actual change in structure/function

Refusal to look at, touch, or care for altered body part

Change in social behavior (withdrawal, isolation, flamboyancy)

Compensatory use of concealing clothing, other devices

ONGOING ASSESSMENT

- Assess age and developmental level.
- Assess perception of change in structure/function of body part (also proposed change). *The perception of a change or the threatened change to a body part is strongly influenced by a child's age and level of development. In early and middle childhood, fantasy and misconception can lead to mistaken fears concerning body image, especially in a hospital setting.*
- Assess perceived impact of change on ADL, social behavior, personal relationships, and school and play activities.
- Note child's behavior regarding actual or perceived changed body part/ function.
- Evaluate parents' perceptions of child.

THERAPEUTIC INTERVENTIONS

- Acknowledge normalcy of emotional response to actual or perceived change in body structure/function.
- Help child identify actual changes.
- Help child identify concerns regarding actual or perceived changes. *This may be accomplished through play therapy; children are not always able to put their fears into words.*
- Encourage verbalization of positive or negative feelings about actual or perceived change.
- Assist child in incorporating actual changes into ADL, social life, interpersonal relationships, school activities.
- Encourage use of support groups if appropriate to age/diagnosis. *Children and adolescents with chronic illnesses (diabetes, sickle cell, lupus) can benefit from peer support.*

PATIENT/PARENT EDUCATION

- Teach child and parent adaptive behaviors to compensate for actual changed body structure/function.
- Help child and parent to identify ways of coping that have been useful for them in the past.

Body image and self-concept will be enhanced through appropriate intervention.

Audrey Klopp, RN, PhD, CS, ET; Michele Knoll Puzas, RNC, MHPE

Breathing pattern, ineffective

A state in which the child's respiratory pattern (cycles of inhalation and/or exhalation) does not enable adequate ventilation.

RELATED FACTORS / DEFINING CHARACTERISTICS	NURSING INTERVENTIONS / *RATIONALES*	EXPECTED OUTCOMES

RELATED FACTORS

Inflammatory process: viral or bacterial

Tracheobronchial obstruction

Hypoxia

Neuromuscular impairment

Pain

Musculoskeletal impairment

Perception or cognitive impairment

Anxiety

Decreased energy and fatigue

Decreased lung expansion

DEFINING CHARACTERISTICS

Dyspnea

Tachypnea

Cough/barky cough

Nasal flaring

Respiratory depth changes

Altered chest excursion

Use of accessory muscles

Pursed-lip breathing or prolonged expiratory phase

Inspiratory stridor

Diminished breath sounds

Substernal and suprasternal retractions

Irritability and restlessness

Cyanosis

ONGOING ASSESSMENT

- Assess respiratory rate and depth by listening to breath sounds at least every shift.
- Assess for dyspnea and quantify; relate dyspnea to precipitating factors.
- Note breathing pattern and monitor for changes. *Respiratory rate and rhythm changes are an early warning sign of impending respiratory difficulties.*
- Note use of muscles used for breathing (i.e., sternocleidomastoid, abdominal, diaphragmatic).
- Note retractions, flaring of nostrils.
- Assess position child assumes for normal/easy breathing.
- Assess for changes in orientation, restlessness.
- Assess skin color, temperature, capillary refill; note central versus peripheral cyanosis.
- Assess for inspiratory stridor at rest. Notify physician if present.
- Monitor ABGs; note differences.
- Note changes in activity tolerance.
- Assess anxiety level.
- Assess presence of sputum for quantity, color, consistency.

THERAPEUTIC INTERVENTIONS

- Position child with proper body alignment for optimal breathing pattern. *If not contraindicated, a sitting position allows good lung excursion and chest expansion.* Maintain head elevation of at least 30 to 45 degrees. Check the child's positioning frequently *so that he or she does not slide down, causing the abdomen to compress the diaphragm, which would cause respiratory embarrassment.*
- Encourage sustained deep breaths by:
  Demonstration (emphasizing slow inhaling, holding end inspiration for a few seconds, and passively exhaling).
  Use of incentive spirometer (place close for convenient patient use).
  Asking child to yawn, *which promotes deep inspiration.*
  Utilizing age-appropriate games to promote taking deep breaths; e.g., deep breaths before blowing out birthday candles, etc.
- Maintain a clear airway by encouraging the child to clear own secretions with effective coughing. If secretions cannot be cleared, suction with caution. Do not deep-suction secretions when inspiratory stridor and barky cough are present. *Suction could result in laryngospasm, leading to partial or complete airway obstruction.*

Optimal respiratory status within the limits of the disease will be achieved.

RELATED FACTORS / DEFINING CHARACTERISTICS	NURSING INTERVENTIONS / *RATIONALES*	EXPECTED OUTCOMES

THERAPEUTIC INTERVENTIONS cont'd

- Pace and schedule the child's activities to provide adequate rest periods *to avoid dyspnea resulting from fatigue.*
- Avoid stimulation of reflexes known to be apnea-producing in infants:
  - Avoid hyperoxia and hyperinflation of lungs *(Hering-Breuer reflex leads to a decrease in respiratory rate).*
  - Use caution with suction technique and with passage of an NG tube. *Stimulation of the posterior pharyngeal vagal receptors may produce apnea and reflex bradycardia.*
  - Avoid cold stress and monitor warming procedures carefully. *Apnea occurrence increases during warming.*
- Closely monitor during feedings *to prevent choking or regurgitation.*
- Use apnea monitor and/or pulse oximetry as ordered.
- Provide reassurance and allay anxiety by staying with child during acute episodes of respiratory distress. *Air hunger can produce an extremely anxious state.*
- Administer cool mist and/or oxygen and ensure that the oxygen delivery system is appropriately applied to the child *so that the appropriate amount of oxygen is continuously delivered and desaturation does not occur.*
- Anticipate need for intubation and mechanical ventilation if the child is unable to maintain adequate gas exchange with the present breathing pattern, or if obstruction to the airway is imminent.

PATIENT/PARENT EDUCATION

- Explain all procedures to child (as age appropriate) and parents *to decrease their anxiety.*
- Explain the use of oxygen therapy to child and parents.
- Explain environmental factors that may worsen child's pulmonary condition (e.g., pollen, second-hand smoke) and discuss possible precipitating factors (e.g., allergens and emotional stress).
- Explain symptoms of a "cold" and impending problems. *A respiratory infection would increase the work of breathing.*
- Teach child/parents appropriate breathing, coughing, and splinting techniques *to facilitate adequate clearance of secretions.*
- Teach parents how to count child's respirations and to relate respiratory rate to activity tolerance.
- Prepare the family for at-home care:
  - Teach parents to recognize signs of respiratory compromise.
  - Schedule parents to participate in basic life support class for CPR, appropriate to child's age.
  - Refer to Social Services or social worker for further counseling and/or support groups related to child's condition.
  - Instruct child/parents about the oxygen therapy to be used at home.
  - Instruct parents about child's medications: indications, dosage, frequency, and potential side effects.
  - Review the use of at home monitoring capabilities, as appropriate, and refer to resources for rental equipment.

Susan Galanes, RN, MS, CCRN

Cardiac output, decreased

A state in which the left and/or right ventricle is unable to maintain a cardiac output sufficient to meet the needs of the body. Common causes of reduced cardiac output include (1) congenital heart defect, (2) acquired heart defect, (3) pulmonary hypertension, (4) cardiomyopathy, (5) arrhythmias, (6) drug effects, (7) fluid overload, (8) decreased fluid volume, and (9) noncardiac diseases (anemia, metabolic/endocrine disorders, respiratory disease).

RELATED FACTORS / DEFINING CHARACTERISTICS	NURSING INTERVENTIONS / *RATIONALES*	EXPECTED OUTCOMES

RELATED FACTORS
 	
Increased/decreased ventricular filling (pre-load)
Impaired contractility
Alteration in heart rate/rhythm/conduction
Decreased oxygenation
Cardiac muscle disease
 	
DEFINING CHARACTERISTICS
 	
Variations in hemodynamic parameters (BP, heart rate, CVP pulmonary artery pressures, cardiac output, neck veins)
Arrhythmias, ECG changes
Rales, tachypnea, dyspnea, orthopnea, cough, abnormal ABGs, frothy sputum
Weight gain, edema, decreased urine output
Restlessness
Extreme irritability
Dizziness
Weakness, fatigue
Feeding difficulty
Abnormal heart sounds
Decreased peripheral pulses; cool, pale skin; poor capillary refill
Confusion, change in mental status
	ONGOING ASSESSMENT
	• Assess age and developmental level.
	• Assess physical status, document and report findings outside of normal parameters for age:
	  Arterial BP, orthostatic changes, pulsus paradoxus
	  Apical heart rate
	  Respirations, breath sounds
	  Heart sounds, murmurs, rubs
	  Jugular venous distention, right atrial pressure, pulmonary artery pressure
	  Peripheral pulses (strength, equality)
	  Skin color, temperature, moisture
	  Capillary refill
	  Fluid balance, presence of peripheral edema
	  I&O; weight (same scale and amount of clothes)
	  Change in mental status
	• Compare vital signs with electronic monitoring devices every shift and prn.
	• Monitor continuous ECG as appropriate. Set alarms for age-specific limits.
	• Monitor ECG for rate, rhythm, ectopy, and change in PR, QRS, and QT intervals. *Tachycardia, bradycardia, and ectopic beats can compromise cardiac output.*
	• Assess child's response to increased activity. *Physical activity increases the demands placed on the heart. Young children seem to be able to self-pace activities; older children and adolescents may try to do what they cannot.*
	• Assess contributing factors *so appropriate plan of care can be initiated.*
	
	THERAPEUTIC INTERVENTIONS
	• Administer medication as ordered, noting response and observing for side effects and toxicity. Clarify with physician parameters for withholding medications. *(Common medications include digitalis therapy, diuretics, vasodilators, and inotropic agents.)*
	• Maintain optimal fluid balance:
	  Administer fluid challenge as ordered, closely monitoring effects.
	  Maintain hemodynamic parameters at prescribed levels.
	  Restrict fluid and Na as ordered. (For infants, use high-calorie formulas.)
	• Maintain adequate ventilation/perfusion:
	  Place child in optimal position (semi-Fowler's) *to reduce preload and ventricular filling;* supine *to increase venous return and promote diuresis.*
	  Administer humidified oxygen as ordered.
	• Maintain physical and emotional rest:
	  Restrict activity *to reduce oxygen demands.*
	  Provide quiet, relaxed environment. *Emotional stress increases cardiac demands.*
	  Provide explanations as appropriate *to allay anxiety.*
	  Organize nursing and medical care *to allow rest periods.*
	  Monitor progressive activity within limits of cardiac function.
		Optimal cardiac output will be maintained.

Cardiac output, decreased cont'd

RELATED FACTORS / DEFINING CHARACTERISTICS	NURSING INTERVENTIONS / *RATIONALES*	EXPECTED OUTCOMES
	THERAPEUTIC INTERVENTIONS cont'd • If arrhythmia occurs, determine child's response; document and report if arrhythmia is significant or symptomatic. *Both tachyarrhythmias and bradyarrhythmias can reduce cardiac output.* • Have antiarrhythmic drugs readily available. • Treat arrhythmias according to medical orders or protocol and evaluate response. **PATIENT/PARENT EDUCATION** • Explain symptoms and interventions for decreased cardiac output related to cause. • Explain drug regimen, purpose, dose, and side effects.	

Meg Gulanick, RN, PhD

Communication, impaired

Either the inability to send information in a manner understandable to others or the inability to receive information sent by others. This can be a very difficult area to assess, especially in the infant or young child.

RELATED FACTORS / DEFINING CHARACTERISTICS	NURSING INTERVENTIONS / *RATIONALES*	EXPECTED OUTCOMES

RELATED FACTORS
Disorders of the senses
Underdeveloped senses
Prematurity
Retardation
Trauma
Illness
Hospitalization
Regressive response
 	
DEFINING CHARACTERISTICS
Infant
Listlessness
No eye contact
No response to sound
No cry
No vocalization, babbling
Toddler
No babbling
No words
No understanding of spoken words
No response to touch/signs
	ONGOING ASSESSMENT
	• Assess age and developmental level.
	• Assess hearing, vision, touch, and speech.
	• Assess for conditions that may inhibit ability to communicate. *The toddler with a speech deficit may actually have a hearing impairment; speech is learned by hearing and repeating.*
	• Assess parents' ability to understand child's communication patterns. *Parents spend time with the child, so they are more likely to understand the differences in their infant's cries or recognize an acute deficit.*
	• Identify means and methods with which to communicate successfully with child.
	
	THERAPEUTIC INTERVENTIONS
	• Communicate with parents if child is unable or too young to understand.
	• Use methods of communication that are successful for the individual child:
	    Sign language
	    Picture board
	    Word board
	    Electronic voice generator
	    Touch
	• Use method of communication as defined by age and needs. *Infants require frequent gentle touch, security, warmth, and pleasant voices and usually communicate in return by the intensity/pitch of their cry and body tension.*
	• Listen attentively *to gain understanding of communication patterns/pronunciation and meaning.* Pay attention to nonverbal cues.
		Optimal methods of communication are facilitated.

Continued.

Communication, impaired cont'd

RELATED FACTORS / DEFINING CHARACTERISTICS	NURSING INTERVENTIONS / *RATIONALES*	EXPECTED OUTCOMES

DEFINING CHARACTERISTICS cont'd
 	
School age/adolescent
  Impaired speech
  Impaired hearing
  Impaired vision
  Absence of proper response to stimulus
	THERAPEUTIC INTERVENTIONS cont'd
	▪ Obtain consults as needed:
	  Speech pathology
	  Hearing
	  Social Service
	  Medical
	▪ Treat underlying cause of deficit.
	
	PATIENT/PARENT EDUCATION
	▪ Explain assessments and findings to parent/child.
	▪ Discuss underlying disorder if applicable.
	▪ Teach child/parent use of alternate method of communication.
	▪ Explain the necessity of follow-up and therapy when applicable.	

Michele Knoll Puzas, RNC, MHPE

Constipation

A change in normal bowel habits characterized by a decrease in the frequency and/or passage of hard, dry stools, or oozing of liquid stool past a collection of hard, dry stool.

RELATED FACTORS / DEFINING CHARACTERISTICS	NURSING INTERVENTIONS / *RATIONALES*	EXPECTED OUTCOMES
RELATED FACTORS Congenital dysfunction (Hirschsprung's) Psychological disorder Purposeful (toilet training) Inadequate fluid intake Low-fiber diet Immobility Fear of pain Medication use Lack of privacy Pain Laxative abuse Tumor or other obstructing mass Surgery/anesthesia	**ONGOING ASSESSMENT** ▪ Assess age and developmental level. ▪ Assess home pattern of elimination; compare with present pattern. Include size, frequency, color, and quality. ▪ Evaluate laxative use, type, and frequency. ▪ Evaluate reliance on enemas for elimination. *Abuse/overuse of cathartics and enemas can result in dependence on them for evacuation.* ▪ Evaluate usual dietary habits, eating habits, eating schedule, and liquid intake; compare with hospital regimen. ▪ Evaluate type of formula/breast milk if infant. ▪ Assess food preferences. ▪ Assess activity level. *Prolonged bed rest and lack of exercise contribute to constipation.* ▪ Auscultate for bowel sounds every shift. ▪ Evaluate current medication usage, *which may contribute to constipation.* ▪ Assess privacy for elimination (i.e., enforced use of bedpan). ▪ Evaluate fear of pain. ▪ Assess degree to which child's procrastination or secondary gain contributes to constipation. ▪ Check for history of bowel obstruction, congenital deformity. ▪ Check for history of paralytic ileus. ·	Constipation/impaction will be relieved.

RELATED FACTORS / DEFINING CHARACTERISTICS	NURSING INTERVENTIONS / *RATIONALES*	EXPECTED OUTCOMES

DEFINING CHARACTERISTICS

Straining at stools

Passage of liquid fecal seepage

No stool in diapers

Flexion of lower extremities

Grunting

Frequent but non-productive desire to defecate

Anorexia

Abdominal distention

Nausea and vomiting

Dull headache, restlessness, and depression

Verbalized pain/fear of pain

THERAPEUTIC INTERVENTIONS

- Encourage and provide daily fluid intake, if not contraindicated medically.
- Encourage increased bulk in diet, e.g., raw fruits, fresh vegetables (if appropriate).
- Consult dietitian if appropriate.
- Encourage child to eat prunes, prune juices, cold cereals, bean products (if appropriate).
- Add a few drops to ½ tsp of prune juice, or corn syrup to each bottle of milk. *An infant being weaned from breast milk to formula or from formula to cow's milk may experience constipation.*
- Show child location of bathroom.
- Increase child's physical activity by planning ambulation periods if possible.
- Assist with ambulation.
- Provide a regular time for elimination, e.g., after breakfast or at child's usual time.
- Offer a bedpan to bedridden child. Assist child to assume a high Fowler's position with knees flexed. *This position best uses gravity and allows for effective bearing down.* Curtain off the area; allow child time to relax.
- Initiate occupational/physical therapy consultation as needed.
- Assist with passive/active ROM exercises.
- Instruct in isometric abdominal and gluteal exercises *to strengthen muscles needed for evacuation* unless contraindicated.
- Encourage as much self-help as possible.
- Use pharmacological agents as appropriate:
  Metamucil: *increases fluid, gaseous, and solid bulk of intestinal contents.*
  Stool softeners, e.g., Colace.
  Chemical irritants, e.g., castor oil, cascara, milk of magnesia. *These irritate the bowel mucosa and cause rapid propulsion of contents of small intestine.*
  Suppositories: *aid in softening stools and stimulate rectal mucosa; best results occur when given 30 min before usual defecation time or after breakfast.*
  Oil: retention enema *to soften stool.*
- Digitally remove fecal impaction.
- Minimize rectal discomfort:
  Warm sitz bath
  Ointments/lotion
- Initiate child/family counseling (psychological) if necessary.

PATIENT/PARENT EDUCATION

- Explain to child/family the importance of the following:
  Balanced diet that contains adequate bulk, fresh fruits, vegetables
  Adequate fluid intake
  Regular meals
  Regular time for evacuation and adequate time for defecation
  Regular exercise
  Privacy for defecation
  Administration of rectal suppositories, enemas, or laxatives when necessary
- Provide instruction concerning normal child development and relationship to toilet training. *Child should not begin toilet training until physically and emotionally ready.*

Audrey Klopp, RN, PhD, CS, ET; Michele Knoll Puzas, RNC, MHPE

Coping, family: ineffective
The stress response seen in family members of a hospitalized patient.

RELATED FACTORS / DEFINING CHARACTERISTICS	NURSING INTERVENTIONS / *RATIONALES*	EXPECTED OUTCOMES

RELATED FACTORS

Unfamiliar environment

Loss of role as primary caretaker

Separation of family members

Knowledge deficit regarding illness, prognosis

Inaccurate, incomplete, or conflicting information

Overwhelming situation

DEFINING CHARACTERISTICS

Expressed concern inappropriate to need

Distortion of reality

Restlessness

Verbalization of problem

Disregard for child's needs

Inappropriate behavior

Limited interaction with child

Statement of misconception

Intolerance

Agitation/depression

Abandonment

ONGOING ASSESSMENT

- Assess age and developmental level of family members.
- Assess family's knowledge and understanding of the need for hospitalization and treatment plan.
- Assess level of family's anxiety.
- Assess normal coping patterns in family.
- Assess support systems available to family.
- Assess family structure.
- Identify other stressors affecting coping abilities.
- Assess for significant psychiatric history.

THERAPEUTIC INTERVENTIONS

- Approach in calm, reassuring manner.
- Encourage questions or expression of concerns. *Coping difficulties vary, depending on developmental level, extent of social contacts outside the family, and former experience with separation.*
- Relay pertinent questions to physician.
- Schedule care conferences to maintain ongoing communication.
- Provide honest, appropriate answers to family members' questions.
- Encourage frequent visitation *to decrease separation anxiety and increase a sense of security.*
- Discuss ways families can continue to be involved in daily care.
- Maintain flexible visiting hours.
- Offer assistance in notifying clergy, other family members, etc., of child's status.
- Obtain necessary consults: social service, clergy, psychiatric, medical.

PATIENT/PARENT EDUCATION

- Orient family to:
    Surroundings (cafeteria, parking, telephone)
    Child's room (call light, TV)
    Equipment
    Health professionals
- Discuss child's condition and care needed. *Distorted ideas, if not clarified, may be more frightening than the reality of the situation.*

Effective family coping will be demonstrated.

Nedra Skale, RN, MS, CNA; Michele Knoll Puzas, RNC, MHPE

Diarrhea

The expulsion of large amounts of fluid along with fecal material. Diarrhea can be a short-term annoyance associated with viral, bacterial, or protozoal infection or can be caused by bowel irritation caused by ingestion of disagreeable foods. In infants and small children, however, diarrhea can be life threatening if GI losses are not continuously or adequately replaced. Diarrhea can cause rapid significant dehydration, electrolyte imbalance, and hypovolemic shock.

RELATED FACTORS / DEFINING CHARACTERISTICS	NURSING INTERVENTIONS / *RATIONALES*	EXPECTED OUTCOMES

RELATED FACTORS

Protozoal infestation, e.g., *Giardia*

Viral infection, e.g., rotavirus, parvovirus

Bacterial infection, e.g., *Salmonella, Shigella*

Feeding intolerance

Food allergy

Irritable bowel syndrome

Crohn's disease

Malrotation of bowel

Ulcerative colitis

DEFINING CHARACTERISTICS

Abdominal pain/ cramping

Abdominal distention

Irritability, inconsolable

Frequent watery stools

Output > intake

Decreased weight

Pallor

Tachycardia

Hypotension

Increased Hct (hemoconcentration)

Increased urine specific gravity

Oliguria

Decreased K⁺

Decreased Ca

Decreased Na

Increased BUN

ONGOING ASSESSMENT

- Assess age and developmental level.
- Obtain baseline vital signs and monitor every 2 hours.
- Monitor I&O.
- Review CBC/electrolytes.
- Assess current weight; compare with most recently known weight.
- Assess LOC.
- Assess skin turgor, mucous membranes, skin color and temperature, capillary refill, eyes and fontanels (in infants, eyes and fontanels will be sunken).
- Assess for thirst.
- Assess recent oral intake, amount and type of food/fluids. Assess for vomiting.
- Assess amount and frequency of stools.
- Observe stools for consistency, color, composition, odor.
- Employ hematest for stools. *Frequent defecation and some infections can cause ulceration and bleeding.*
- Monitor results of stool culture and sensitivity (C&S), ova and parasites (O&P).
- Assess anal area for fissures, and diapered area in infants for skin irritation/loss.

THERAPEUTIC INTERVENTIONS

- Notify physician of symptoms of dehydration.
- Assist child with toileting/hygiene.
- Change infant's diapers frequently. Protect skin from excoriation with ointments/barrier sprays. Clean skin gently.
- If rash or excoriation has occurred, place infant on abdomen and leave area open to air.
- Practice meticulous handwashing when in contact with stool *to prevent cross-contamination.* Isolate patients as necessary.
- Administer medications as ordered:
  Lomotil (limited to patients 2 years old and older), Kaolin, or Cholestyramine *to diminish diarrhea*
  Vitamin K *to replace losses*
  Antibiotics *to treat bacterial infections*
  Antiprotozoals
- Provide oral fluid and electrolyte replacements (therapy of choice) such as Pedialyte.
- Provide IV replacement if oral intake is inadequate or contraindicated. *Electrolyte replacement and fluid rate is based on degree of dehydration, ongoing diarrheal losses, insensible loss, and serum electrolyte levels.*
- Limit solid food intake initially *to allow the intestine to rest.* Progress diet gradually. Avoid foods known to be irritating or to cause an allergic response.

Diarrhea and its effects will be reduced.

Continued.

15

Diarrhea cont'd

RELATED FACTORS / DEFINING CHARACTERISTICS	NURSING INTERVENTIONS / *RATIONALES*	EXPECTED OUTCOMES

PATIENT/PARENT EDUCATION
- Explain all tests/procedures to parent and child.
- Teach good hygiene habits.
- Explain source of infections, if applicable and known.
- Review medications and effects.
- Explain necessity of temporary alteration in diet/formula.
- Discuss home care measures and the need for immediate attention for prolonged diarrhea and dehydration.

Michele Knoll Puzas, RNC, MHPE

Diversional activity deficit

ALTERED SELF-IMAGE; ISOLATION

Lack of physical and mental exercise due to confinement in the hospital. Inability to experience normal play behaviors because of illness or injury.

RELATED FACTORS / DEFINING CHARACTERISTICS	NURSING INTERVENTIONS / *RATIONALES*	EXPECTED OUTCOMES
RELATED FACTORS Prolonged hospitalization Environmental lack of diversional activity Usual play cannot be undertaken in hospital Lack of usual level of socialization Physical inability to perform tasks: isolation, traction, oxygen therapy, IV therapy **DEFINING CHARACTERISTICS** Verbal expression of boredom Preoccupation with illness Frequent use of call light in absence of physical need Excessive complaints Withdrawal Depression	**ONGOING ASSESSMENT** - Assess developmental level and attention span. - Assess for physical limitations. - Inquire about child's interests and hobbies before hospitalization, e.g., art, reading, writing. - Identify in-hospital activities suitable for age/level of development. **THERAPEUTIC INTERVENTIONS** - Provide frequent contact. - Be certain that child is aware of your presence. - Set up a schedule with the child *so he or she will know when to expect contact/activities.* - Provide materials for hobby/interests if possible. - Suggest new interests: crafts, puzzles, etc. - Observe and document response to activities. - Encourage family/friends to visit and bring diversional materials. - Provide dietary changes if possible. *Most hospital menus rotate on a weekly or biweekly basis and soon become repetitive for the long-term patient.* - Obtain consultations as needed: dietary, social work, psychiatric liaison, volunteers, child life therapist or department. - Spend time with child without providing physical care. *Engaging the child in activity or conversation without focusing on illness will divert attention and help pass the time.* - Move child's bed or wheelchair to playroom, solarium, hallway *to change surroundings.* - Provide roommates of similar ages if possible. **PATIENT/PARENT EDUCATION** - Instruct child/family concerning necessity for continued hospitalization. - Obtain instructional materials for new hobbies/interests. - Encourage continuation of formal education while child is hospitalized.	Child's attention will be diverted to interests other than illness and hospitalization.

Michele Knoll Puzas, RNC, MHPE

Family processes, altered

INEFFECTIVE COPING

A situation or event that causes a change in family members' roles or expectations. The inability of one or more members to adjust or perform, resulting in family dysfunction and prevention of the growth and development of the family and members.

RELATED FACTORS / DEFINING CHARACTERISTICS	NURSING INTERVENTIONS / *RATIONALES*	EXPECTED OUTCOMES

RELATED FACTORS

Illness of family member
Change in socioeconomic status
Births and deaths
Conflict between family members
Developmental needs of children

DEFINING CHARACTERISTICS

Inability to meet physical needs of family members
Inability to function in larger society, e.g., no job, no community activity
Inability to meet emotional needs of family members (grief, anxiety, conflict)
Inability to meet developmental needs or foster growth and maturation of children
Ineffective family decision-making process
Rigidity in roles, behaviors, and beliefs

ONGOING ASSESSMENT

- Assess age and developmental level.
- Assess for precipitating events, e.g., divorce, illness.
- Elicit past attempts at problem-solving.
- Assess individual's perceptions of problem.
- Evaluate strengths, coping skills, and current support systems.
- Identify problems with the family.

THERAPEUTIC INTERVENTIONS

- Explore feelings. Identify loneliness, anger, and aggression, *because the feelings of one family member affect others in the family system.*
- Phrase problems as "family" problems, *so they are owned and dealt with by the family.*
- Encourage members to empathize or act out the parts of other family members. *Role-playing allows members to see how they look to others, as well as increasing understanding of others' feelings.*
- Assist family in breaking down problems into manageable parts. Assist with problem-solving process, with delineated responsibilities and follow-through.

PATIENT/PARENT EDUCATION

- Provide information regarding stressful situation, as appropriate.
- Arrange social work or psychological consultations as needed.
- Identify community resources that may be helpful in dealing with particular situations, e.g., hotlines, self-help groups, educational opportunities.

Dysfunction in family process will be reduced.

Michele Knoll Puzas, RNC, MHPE

Fear

A strong and unpleasant emotion caused by the awareness or anticipation of pain or danger. This emotion is primarily externally motivated, and its source is specific. The individual experiencing the fear can identify the person, place, or thing precipitating this feeling. The older child may be able to be specific about fear of hospitalization or death, but the very young child may not be able to articulate or specify the cause of fear. The young child will evidence fear through behaviors, e.g., fear of separation or painful procedure will cause crying, clinging behaviors. The nurse must also recognize and alleviate the parents' fears, because the parents' emotions and behaviors will greatly influence the child's fears and reactions.

RELATED FACTORS / DEFINING CHARACTERISTICS	NURSING INTERVENTIONS / *RATIONALES*	EXPECTED OUTCOMES

RELATED FACTORS

Anticipation of pain

Anticipation or perceived threat of danger

Unfamiliarity with environment

Impairment in comprehension and communication:
Language barrier
Knowledge deficit
Sensory impairment

Specific phobias (see Anxiety, p. 4, for other related factors)

DEFINING CHARACTERISTICS

Increased respirations and heart rate

Dilated pupils

Diaphoresis

Tremors

Crying

Inconsolable

Expression of extreme fearfulness

Denial

Muscle tightness

Fatigue

Urinary frequency

Palpitations

Shortness of breath

Irritability

Difficulty concentrating

Loss of appetite

Nausea, vomiting, diarrhea (see Anxiety, p. 4, for other defining characteristics)

ONGOING ASSESSMENT

- Assess age and developmental level.
- Determine what the child/parent is fearful of by asking questions such as "What are you afraid of?" "What is worrying you?" "What is it that you are afraid will happen?" *This will clarify for the clinician the source of the childs'/parents' fear.*
- Assess the degree of the child's fear and the measures he uses to cope with that fear. As part of this process, inquire about other situations in which the child/parent felt fear: *survival of other situations may lend a helpful perspective on the current one and identify coping mechanisms. This assessment helps determine the effectiveness of coping strategies used currently by the child/parent.*
- Document behavioral and verbal expressions of fear. *Symptoms will provide information about the degree of fear. Physiological symptoms and/or complaints will intensify as the level of fear increases. Note that fear differs from anxiety in that it is a response to a recognized and usually external threat. Manifestations of fear are similar to those of anxiety.*

THERAPEUTIC INTERVENTIONS

- Acknowledge your awareness of the child's or parent's fear. *This will validate the feelings the child/parent is having and communicate an acceptance of those feelings.*
- Reassure the child/parent that he or she is safe. Stay with the child/parent if necessary. *The presence of a trusted person assures the child a sense of security and safety during a period of fear.*
- Maintain a calm and tolerant manner while interacting with the child/parent. *The child's feeling of stability increases in a calm and non-threatening atmosphere.*
- Establish a working relationship through continuity of care. *An ongoing relationship establishes trust and a basis for communicating fearful feelings.*
- Orient to the environment as needed. *This promotes comfort and a decrease in fear.*
- When possible, adjust the child's treatment and care to normal routines. Reduce requests made of the child/parent.
- When practical, allow the child to make choices, such as when to perform a procedure: "before or after bathtime." *The child's fear will lessen as he perceives that he has more control over his surroundings.*
- Use simple language and brief statements when instructing the child/parent regarding diagnostic and surgical procedures. *When experiencing excessive fear or dread, the child may be unable to comprehend more than simple, clear, and brief instructions.*
- Provide diversional activities with regard to level of development and desires.

Fear will be managed or relieved.

Fear cont'd

RELATED FACTORS / DEFINING CHARACTERISTICS	NURSING INTERVENTIONS / *RATIONALES*	EXPECTED OUTCOMES
	THERAPEUTIC INTERVENTIONS cont'd ▪ Encourage child/parent to verbalize fearfulness, and examine the fear-provoking situation. *Magical thinking and misunderstandings, if not clarified, become more frightening than the reality of the situation.* ▪ Allow the child (if able) to play with items that are fearful. ▪ Assist the child/parent in developing problem-solving abilities. Provide pain control before painful events whenever possible. ▪ Emphasize the logical strategies the child/parent can use when fearful. ▪ Inquire of the child what the nurse can do to be helpful by asking, "What is it that you most need from us now?" and "What can we do that would be most helpful?" ▪ Encourage child to interact with others, such as in the playroom. *Self-imposed isolation tends to intensify symptoms.* ▪ Allow child to keep favorite toys/dolls nearby. ▪ Encourage parental participation in child's care. ▪ Ask the parent to bring familiar objects from home: blanket/pillow, bottle, pictures. **PATIENT/PARENT EDUCATION** ▪ Reinforce the idea that fear is a normal and appropriate response to situations when pain, danger, or loss of control are anticipated or experienced. ▪ Provide all information to parent/child in understandable terms as often as possible. *Keeping the parent and child informed will help lessen fears.*	

Rhonda Blender, RN, MSN; Ursula M. Brozek, RN, MSN

Fluid volume deficit   *A state of vascular, cellular, or intracellular dehydration.*

RELATED FACTORS / DEFINING CHARACTERISTICS	NURSING INTERVENTIONS / *RATIONALES*	EXPECTED OUTCOMES
RELATED FACTORS Inadequate fluid intake and differing nutritional needs Active fluid or blood loss (diuresis, abnormal drainage/bleeding, suctioning, vomiting, diarrhea, excessive GI obstruction) Electrolyte/acid-base imbalances Fluid shifts (edema/effusions) Immature urinary system	**ONGOING ASSESSMENT** ▪ Assess age and developmental level. ▪ Assess turgor and mucous membranes for signs of dehydration. ▪ Assess for marked increase or decrease in urination. Assess color of urine. *Concentrated urine denotes deficit.* Report urine output of <2 ml/kg/hr for infant and <1 ml/kg/hr for patients 2 years old and older. ▪ Observe for fever. *Febrile states decrease body fluids through perspiration and increased respiration.* ▪ Assess for sunken fontanels in infant. ▪ Assess for sudden decrease or change in weight. ▪ Monitor for active fluid loss from wound drainage, tubes, diarrhea, bleeding, and vomiting; maintain accurate I&O data collection and recording. ▪ Assess for weakness, apathy, or lethargy. ▪ Document baseline mental status for later comparison.	Adequate fluid volume and electrolyte balance will be maintained.

Continued.

RELATED FACTORS / DEFINING CHARACTERISTICS	NURSING INTERVENTIONS / *RATIONALES*	EXPECTED OUTCOMES

RELATED FACTORS cont'd

Increased metabolic rate (fever, infection)

Difficulty swallowing or feeding self

Dietary problems

Hyperpnea

Climate: excessive dryness; exposure to heat/sun

Decreased fluid reserves

DEFINING CHARACTERISTICS

Mild:

Dry mucous membranes

Decreased urine output

Moderate:

Reduced skin turgor

Sunken eyeballs

Hyperpnea

Orthostatic hypotension

Tachycardia

Severe:

Decreased alertness

Listlessness

Decreased skin perfusion

Decreased skin temperature

Impaired capillary refill (>2 sec)

Pale, blue, mottled appearance

Laboratory:

Urine volume: small/oliguria or anuria

Specific gravity: >1.035

Blood:

BUN—WNL to elevated

pH—WNL to <7.10

ONGOING ASSESSMENT cont'd

- Evaluate whether child has any related heart problems before initiating parenteral therapy. *Cardiac patients often have precarious fluid balance and are prone to develop pulmonary edema.*
- Evaluate specific cause for fluid deficit *to guide intervention.*
- Determine child's fluid preferences: type, temperature of formula or food.
- Monitor serum electrolytes/urine osmolality.
- Monitor and document vital signs.
- Observe for signs of orthostatic hypotension when the child rises from a lying to a standing (or sitting) position. *A decrease in blood pressure of 15 mm Hg or an increase in pulse of 20 beats/min after 2-3 min is considered significant. This indicates reduced circulating fluids.*
- Assess skin perfusion. *Decreased skin perfusion may produce decreased skin temperature, impaired capillary refill (>2 sec) and a pale, blue, or mottled appearance.*

THERAPEUTIC INTERVENTIONS

- Encourage child to drink prescribed fluid amounts if oral fluids are tolerated.
- Be creative in selecting fluid sources (gelatin, popsicles, ice cream, juices).
- Assist child if unable to feed self.
- Oversee daily activities *so child is not too tired at mealtime.*
- Provide oral hygiene *to promote interest in drinking.*
- Administer 20 ml/kg of NS or LR solution by IV over 20 minutes or as ordered. If a poor therapeutic response is noted, repeat the initial infusion over 20-30 min as ordered (assuming normal renal and cardiac function). *Children who are significantly dehydrated require immediate infusion of fluids, particularly if there are abnormal vital signs or altered mental status.*
- Assist physician with insertion of central venous or arterial line as indicated *for more effective fluid administration and monitoring.*
- Advance diet slightly in both volume and composition once ongoing fluid losses have stopped.
- Pick up and hold infant during feedings with head and back supported and a proper positioning of bottle *to ensure effectiveness of feeding.*
- Change feeding techniques, such as feeding with a spoon, cup feedings, allowing infant to assist with feedings *to foster growth and development during feeding time.*

PATIENT/PARENT EDUCATION

- Teach causes of fluid losses or decreased fluid intake.
- Explain/reinforce rationale and intended effect of treatment program.
- Explain importance of maintaining proper nutrition and hydration.
- Teach interventions to prevent future episodes of inadequate intake.
- Identify symptoms to be reported.
- Teach safe use and potential side effects of medications.
- Inform child/parents/significant others of importance of maintaining prescribed fluid intake and special diet considerations involved.

Jacqueline Santiago-Tan, RN, BSN

Fluid volume excess
State of increased fluid retention and edema.

RELATED FACTORS / DEFINING CHARACTERISTICS	NURSING INTERVENTIONS / *RATIONALES*	EXPECTED OUTCOMES

RELATED FACTORS

Excessive fluid intake (IV therapy), especially if given with nonisotonic solutions

Water intake in excess of output

Steroid therapy

Excessive sodium intake (formula, food, or IV)

Low protein intake/malnutrition

Overtransfusion with plasma expanders, blood/packed cells

Head injury

Liver disease: cancer, ascites, cirrhosis

Acute or chronic renal failure

Inflammatory processes

Effusion: pleural, pericardial

Tissue insult: cell wall injury, cellular hypoxia

NGT irrigation with water

Dependent venous pooling/venostasis, immobility

Decreased cardiac output; chronic or acute heart disease, arrhythmia

Hormonal disturbances

Venous pressure points, e.g., tight bandage, cast, or restraints

Repeated tap-water enemas

Inadequate lymphatic drainage

Immature kidneys

Differing nutritional needs of different age-group

Failure to excrete water in presence of normal intake, such as with CHF, renal disease

ONGOING ASSESSMENT

- Assess age and developmental level.
- Assess intake, especially sodium.
- Assess for edema around eyes, on pressure points, extremities, distal to casts and bandages.
- Assess skin turgor and mucous membranes for edema or weeping.
- Monitor for headache, flushed skin.
- Monitor for increased CVP.
- Collect all urine and weigh diapers if more accurate measurement of child's output is necessary.
- Palpate fontanels for fullness.
- Weigh daily with same scale, preferably at the same time of day to evaluate true fluid status.
- Monitor intake and output closely.
- Assess characteristics of sputum.
- Assess lung sounds and breathing patterns, especially shortness of breath, tachypnea, and cough.
- Assess for marked increase or decrease in urination.
- Document baseline mental status for later comparison.
- Evaluate whether patient has any related heart problem before initiating diuretic therapy or fluid restriction.
- Evaluate specific cause for fluid retention *to guide intervention.*
- Monitor serum electrolytes/urine osmolarity.
- Monitor and document vital signs.
- Observe for signs of hypertension and tachycardia.

THERAPEUTIC INTERVENTIONS

- Discontinue or decrease fluid intake or IV infusion as appropriate or as ordered.
- Decrease oral or intravenous salt intake.
- Shift weight/reposition/shift appliances *to change pressure points as able.*
- Elevate edematous extremities (unless contraindicated by heart failure) *to increase venous return.*
- Reduce constriction of vessels (use appropriate garments; avoid crossing of legs or ankles or constrictive clothing) *to prevent venous pooling.*
- Apply antiembolic stockings or bandages as ordered *to help promote venous return.*
- Provide adequate activity/position changes as able *to prevent fluid accumulation in dependent areas.*
- Provide passive or active ROM exercises to all extremities every 4 hours.
- Avoid injections, IVs, BPs using extremities with inadequate lymphatic drainage.
- Prevent dry skin, minimize soap use and rinse well; apply lotions as needed *to protect edematous skin from injury.*
- Provide pacifier *to meet sucking needs.*

Adequate fluid volume and electrolyte balance will be maintained.

Continued.

Fluid volume excess cont'd

RELATED FACTORS / DEFINING CHARACTERISTICS	NURSING INTERVENTIONS / *RATIONALES*	EXPECTED OUTCOMES
DEFINING CHARACTERISTICS Weight gain Change in mental state (lethargy or confusion) Seizures Intake greater than output Malaise, weakness, fatigue Decreased level of activity Edema; puffy eyes Shortness of breath, pulmonary congestion Cough; pinkish or frothy sputum Increased abdominal girth Dilute urine; change in specific gravity Rales or rhonchi Decreased urine output Increased venous filling Increased respiratory rate Arrythmia or tachycardia Orthopnea or dyspnea on exertion Increased blood pressure or pulse volume Pupillary changes Taut, shiny, or weeping skin Jugular vein distention Increased CVP Full bounding pulse Full bulging anterior fontanel Gross muscle strength deficit and/or isolated muscle twitching Decreased or absent tendon reflexes Change in electrolyte, BUN, creatinine, Hgb, and Hct (hemodilution)	**PATIENT/PARENT EDUCATION** • Teach causes of fluid volume excess and/or excess intake to child/family. • Provide information as needed regarding the individual's medical diagnosis (e.g., CHF, renal failure). • Explain/reinforce rationale and intended effect of treatment program. • Identify signs and symptoms of fluid volume excess. • Explain importance of maintaining proper nutrition and hydration, diet modifications. • Teach intervention to prevent future episodes of fluid volume excess. • Identify symptoms to be reported. • Instruct on proper use of equipment and/or assistive devices, as age appropriate.	

Fluid volume excess cont'd

RELATED FACTORS / DEFINING CHARACTERISTICS	NURSING INTERVENTIONS / *RATIONALES*	EXPECTED OUTCOMES
DEFINING CHARACTERISTICS cont'd Generalized edema and distention, e.g., ankles and feet; periorbital, abdominal distention/ascites Signs/symptoms of water intoxication: hyponatremia, hyperirritability, coma, seizures, muscle twitching, vomiting/nausea		

Jacqueline Santiago-Tan, RN, BSN

Gas exchange, impaired

ARDS; PNEUMONIA

A state in which the child experiences an imbalance between oxygen uptake and carbon dioxide elimination at alveolar–capillary membrane gas exchange area.

RELATED FACTORS / DEFINING CHARACTERISTICS	NURSING INTERVENTIONS / *RATIONALES*	EXPECTED OUTCOMES
RELATED FACTORS Altered oxygen supply Alveolar capillary membrane changes Altered blood flow Altered oxygen-carrying capacity of blood **DEFINING CHARACTERISTICS** Confusion Somnolence Restlessness Irritability Listlessness Anxious, frightened expression Inability to move secretions Hypercapnia Hypoxia	**ONGOING ASSESSMENT** • Assess age and developmental level. • Assess respirations: note quality, rate, pattern, depth, flaring of nostrils, dyspnea on exertion, evidence of splinting, use of accessory muscles, position assumed for easy breathing. • Assess breath sounds every shift. • Monitor vital signs, noting any changes. *With initial hypoxia and hypercapnia, BP, heart rate, and respiratory rate all rise. As the hypoxia and/ or hypercapnia becomes more severe, BP may drop, heart rate tends to continue to be rapid with arrhythmias, and respiratory failure may ensue, with the child unable to maintain the rapid respiratory rate.* • Assess for changes in orientation and behavior. • Assess child's ability to cough effectively to clear secretions. Note quantity, color, and consistency of sputum. • Monitor ABGs and note changes. • Assess for presence of central cyanosis. **THERAPEUTIC INTERVENTIONS** • Maintain the prescribed oxygen delivery system at appropriate levels *to prevent hypoxemia.* Note: If the child is allowed to eat, oxygen still needs to be applied, but perhaps in a different manner, e.g., from mask to a nasal cannula. *Eating is an activity, and more oxygen will be consumed than when the child is at rest.* Immediately following the meal, the original oxygen delivery system should be returned.	Optimal gas exchange will be maintained.

Continued.

Gas exchange, impaired cont'd

RELATED FACTORS / DEFINING CHARACTERISTICS	NURSING INTERVENTIONS / *RATIONALES*	EXPECTED OUTCOMES

THERAPEUTIC INTERVENTIONS cont'd

- Use pulse oximetry, as available, *to continuously monitor oxygen saturation and pulse rate.* Keep alarms on at all times. *Pulse oximetry has been found to be a useful tool in the clinical setting to detect changes in oxygenation.*
- Position child with proper body alignment for optimal respiratory excursion (if tolerated, head elevated 45 degrees). *This promotes good lung expansion and improves air exchange.* Check the child's positioning frequently so that he or she does not slide down, causing the abdomen to compress the diaphragm, *which would cause respiratory embarrassment.*
- Use sniffing position for infants *to maintain an open airway* and prop with shoulder rolls.
- Pace activities and schedule rest periods *to avoid fatigue. Even simple activities (such as bathing), while on bed rest, can fatigue a child and cause an increase in oxygen consumption.*
- Change child's position every 2 hours. *This will facilitate secretion movement and drainage.*
- Use "games" that are age appropriate to encourage the child to deep breathe and cough *to clear secretions,* e.g., pretending to be a dragon or taking a deep breath before blowing out birthday candles.
- Suction as needed *to clear secretions.*
- Provide reassurance and allay anxiety:
  Have an agreed-on method for the child to call for assistance, e.g., call light, bell.
  Stay with the child during episodes of respiratory distress.
- Anticipate need for intubation and mechanical ventilation if child is unable to maintain adequate gas exchange.

PATIENT/PARENT EDUCATION

- Explain to child/parents the need to restrict and pace activities *to decrease oxygen consumption during the acute episode.*
- Explain the type of oxygen therapy being used and why its maintenance is important.
- Teach appropriate deep breathing and coughing techniques *to facilitate adequate air exchange and secretion clearance.*

Susan Galanes, RN, MS, CCRN

Grieving, anticipatory

DYING CHILD; NEONATAL LOSS; LOSS OF A BODY PART

A state in which an individual grieves before an actual loss. This may apply to individuals who suffer a perinatal loss or the loss of a body part or who have received a terminal diagnosis for themselves or a loved one.

RELATED FACTORS / DEFINING CHARACTERISTICS	NURSING INTERVENTIONS / *RATIONALES*	EXPECTED OUTCOMES

RELATED FACTORS
Perceived potential loss of child/parent
Perceived potential loss of physical or psychosocial well-being
	ONGOING ASSESSMENT
	- Identify behaviors that are suggestive of the grieving process (see defining characteristics).
	- Assess what stages of grief are being experienced by child or parent:
	  Denial
	  Anger
	  Bargaining
	  Depression
	  Acceptance
		Family will verbalize their feelings and will establish and maintain functional support for each other.

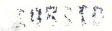

RELATED FACTORS / DEFINING CHARACTERISTICS	NURSING INTERVENTIONS / *RATIONALES*	EXPECTED OUTCOMES

RELATED FACTORS cont'd

Perceived potential loss of personal possessions
Situational crisis
Maturational crisis
Family crisis
Temporary disorganization

DEFINING CHARACTERISTICS

Child or parent shows distress at prospect of loss
Denial of potential loss
Sorrow
Crying
Guilt
Anger/hostility
Bargaining
Depression
Acceptance
Changes in eating habits
Alteration in activity level
Altered libido
Altered communication patterns
Fear
Hopelessness
Distortion of reality

ONGOING ASSESSMENT cont'd

- Assess the influence of the following factors on coping:
   Past problem-solving abilities
   Socioeconomic background
   Educational preparation
   Cultural beliefs
   Spiritual beliefs
- Assess whether child/parents differ in their stage of grieving.
- Identify support systems available:
   Family
   Peer support
   Primary physician
   Consulting physician
   Nursing staff
   Clergy
   Therapist/counselor
   Professional/lay support group
- Identify potential for pathological grieving response.
- Evaluate need for referral to social service representatives, legal consultants, or support groups.
- Observe nonverbal communication. *Body language may communicate a great deal of information.*

THERAPEUTIC INTERVENTIONS

- Establish good rapport with family. Listen, encourage to verbalize feelings. *This opens lines of communication and facilitates successful resolution of grief.*
- During the stage of shock and disbelief:
   Provide as much privacy as possible.
   Allow use of denial and other defense mechanisms.
   Avoid reinforcing denial.
   Avoid judgmental and defensive responses to criticisms of health care providers.
   Do not encourage use of pharmacological interventions.
   Do not force parents to make decisions.
- During the stage of developing awareness of potential loss:
   Provide child/parents with ongoing information, diagnosis, prognosis, progress, and plan of care.
   Encourage parents to assist with child's physical care.
   Facilitate flexible visiting hours and include younger children and extended family when appropriate.
   Help child and family to share mutual fears and concerns, plans and hopes for each other.
   Help parents to understand that child's verbalization of anger should not be perceived as a personal attack.
   Encourage parents to maintain their own self-care needs for rest, sleep, nutrition, leisure activities, and time away from child/hospital.
- During the stage of acceptance of impending loss:
   Facilitate discussion with child/family on "final arrangements," e.g., burial, autopsy, organ donation, funeral (if appropriate for child's age, level of development).
   Provide information about support groups (Compassionate Friends, Candle Lighters Foundation). *Participation in group activities with others who have experienced similar circumstances may help parents successfully work through grief process.*
- If the grief is the result of an imminent death:
   Promote discussion on what to expect when death occurs.
   Encourage family/child to share their wishes in respect to which family members should be present with child at time of death.

Grieving, anticipatory cont'd

RELATED FACTORS / DEFINING CHARACTERISTICS	NURSING INTERVENTIONS / *RATIONALES*	EXPECTED OUTCOMES

THERAPEUTIC INTERVENTIONS cont'd

Help parents to accept that not being present at time of death does not indicate lack of love or caring.

Assure that nurse was with child when needed.

- Use visual method to identify the child's critical status, e.g., color-coded door marker. *This will inform all hospital personnel of the child's status in an effort to ensure that staff do not act or respond inappropriately to crisis situation.*
- Initiate process that provides additional support and resources.
- Refer to other resources: counseling, pastoral support, group therapy. *Parents may need additional help to deal with individual concerns.*
- Provide anticipatory guidance and follow-up as condition continues.

PATIENT/PARENT EDUCATION

- Involve parents in discussions *to help to reinforce understanding of all individuals involved.*
- Orient child/family to hospital procedures, cafeteria, phones, local restaurants, and rest facilities/lounges.

Mary Leslie Caldwell, RN; Charlotte Razvi, RN, MSN, PhD; Michele Knoll Puzas, RNC, MHPE

Growth and development, altered

DEVELOPMENTAL DELAY

Altered growth refers to a disturbance in physical growth, which can be retarded or accelerated, depending on the source of the disorder. Altered development refers to differences in the usual patterns of mental and emotional maturation. While accelerated development can be problematic, the term usually refers to slower than average mental and/or emotional maturation. The admission of a child to a hospital or intensive care unit causes disruption of the normal patterns of growth and development. Efforts should be made to address the individual needs of children in ICUs to prevent developmental delay.

RELATED FACTORS / DEFINING CHARACTERISTICS	NURSING INTERVENTIONS / *RATIONALES*	EXPECTED OUTCOMES

RELATED FACTORS

Genetic disorder:
Physical defects
Brain function defect
Hormonal dysfunction
Trauma:
Birth or prenatal
Accidental
Environmental
Disease

ONGOING ASSESSMENT

- Assess age and developmental level.
- Interview and elicit information concerning:
  Family profile
  Support systems
  Individual profile:
    Past medical history
    Medications
    Perceived current physical status
  Personality before admission as perceived by self and primary care-taker
  Development before admission:
    Language
    Fine and gross motor function
    School performance
- Perform a physical examination and note deviations from expected norms for age. *Abnormalities found in newborn indicate a need for further investigation because some life-threatening disorders are associated with outward physical abnormalities, e.g., cardiac function can be impaired in the infant born with signs of trisomy 21, Down's syndrome.*

Potential abilities will be maximized.

RELATED FACTORS / DEFINING CHARACTERISTICS	NURSING INTERVENTIONS / *RATIONALES*	EXPECTED OUTCOMES

DEFINING CHARACTERISTICS

Physical/biological:
Small stature
Stunted limbs
Malformed extremities
Delayed growth milestones
Motor/self-care:
Poor gross motor function
Poor fine motor function
Lack of coordination
Delayed achievement of skills/competencies
Hyperactive or hypoactive
Sensory:
Sight/hearing deficits
Perceptual deficits
Cognitive/Intellectual:
Short attention span
Poor impulse control
Thought/reasoning deficits
Perceptual deficit
Language:
Poor comprehension of spoken words
Inability to adequately express self
Learning difficulties
Psychosocial:
Delayed achievement of social skills
Learning difficulties
Aberrant behaviors
Psychosexual:
Sexual expression aberrant for age/social situation
Spiritual/moral:
Poor impulse control
Lack of understanding of right from wrong

ONGOING ASSESSMENT cont'd

- Obtain laboratory specimens pursuant to physical findings. *Lack of development or precocious development of secondary sex characteristics indicates the need for hormone studies.*
- Perform a neuromuscular examination and note deviations.
- Evaluate socioeconomic status and environment for adverse conditions that affect growth, development, and behavior. Assess for signs of abuse and neglect, as well as psychiatric or aberrant behaviors in other family members. *Changes in behavior and development, especially in children, are sometimes symptoms of a problem in another close family member.*
- Assess behavior, coping strategies, and family interaction.

THERAPEUTIC INTERVENTIONS

- Listen carefully to comments and concerns of mother/caretaker. *Especially when caring for infants and children, primary caretaker is usually able to identify changes or lack of change in growth and development.*
- Create an environment as near to normal as possible (own clothing, eating utensils, playthings, dining and nap times).
- Provide unrestricted visiting for parents; encourage holding and talking to child. Assist parent in holding infant connected to monitors/IVs, etc. *Parents are often afraid of disturbing tubes and equipment.*
- Use form of communication best suited to individual needs:
  Word board
  Signing
  Personal language
  Electronic talking box
  Infants need close eye-to-eye, face-to-face contact while being held.
- Encourage older child to express desires and fears if able. *Although limits need to be identified, some desires can be met in PICU and fears/misconceptions the child develops can be corrected.*
- Allow child as much freedom of movement as is safe.
- Provide age-appropriate diversional activities. Consult child-life therapist.
- Provide assistive devices as needed:
  Wheelchair
  Infant seat/swing
- Assist with ADL as needed, but allow to perform self-care as much as possible *to foster self-confidence, independence, and success, e.g., do not diaper a toilet-trained toddler unless absolutely necessary.*
- Arrange consults:
  Social worker
  OT/PT
  EENT
  Psychiatric
  Neurological
  Orthopedic
  Clergy; *religious/cultural beliefs may need to be addressed to facilitate/accomplish acceptable outcomes.*
- Refer for genetic screening/testing if genetic abnormality is suspected.
- Refer parents/child for psychological or psychiatric counseling if necessary.
- Refer for neurological follow-up if deficit is identified.

PATIENT/PARENT EDUCATION

- Explain all tests/procedures, including why and how they will be done.
- Explain results of examinations, including information on normal development.
- Provide information concerning disorders or deficits and their treatment and prognosis.
- Explain how parents can have a normalizing effect on their child's development even while the child is in PICU.

Hyperthermia

FEBRILE ILLNESS; MALIGNANT HYPERTHERMIA;
HYPERPYREXIA

A state in which a child's temperature is elevated above normal. Normal temperatures vary from person to person and also within an individual. Variances occur after meals and exercise, after sleep, and as a hormonal response. Hyperthermia is a sustained temperature above the normal variance, usually greater than 38°C (100.4°F). Hyperthermia in children is frequently related to infection but can be metabolic/neurological in origin.

RELATED FACTORS / DEFINING CHARACTERISTICS	NURSING INTERVENTIONS / *RATIONALES*	EXPECTED OUTCOMES
RELATED FACTORS Exposure to hot environment Vigorous activity Medications Anesthesia Increased metabolic rate Illness/trauma Dehydration Inability to perspire **DEFINING CHARACTERISTICS** Body temperature >38° C (100.4° F) Hot, flushed skin Diaphoresis Increased heart rate Increased respiratory rate Irritability Fluid/electrolyte imbalance Convulsions	**ONGOING ASSESSMENT** • Obtain age and weight. *Extremes of age or weight increase the risk for inability to control body temperature.* • Assess vital signs. • Measure I&O. • Monitor serum electrolytes. • Determine precipitating factors. • Monitor cardiac function. **THERAPEUTIC INTERVENTIONS** • Control environmental temperature. • Remove excess clothing and covers. • Provide antipyretic medications as ordered. • Cool with tepid bath. *Do not use alcohol, because it cools the skin too rapidly, causing shivering. Shivering increases metabolic rate and body temperature.* • Provide ample oral or intravenous fluids. • Provide cooling mattress. • Adjust cooling measures based on physical response. *Too-rapid cooling in the infant can cause shock and cardiac changes.* • Apply cardiopulmonary monitor. • Notify physician of significant changes. **PATIENT/PARENT EDUCATION** • Explain temperature measurement and all treatments. • Provide information regarding normal temperature and control. • Provide instruction regarding home care and temperature measurement.	Temperature within normal limits will be attained.

Michele Knoll Puzas, RNC, MHPE

Hypothermia

COLD STRESS

The state in which a child's body temperature is sustained at a significantly lower level than normal, usually lower than 35° C (95° F). Hypothermia in children is frequently related to exposure, whereas hypothermia in infants is often related to hypoglycemia.

RELATED FACTORS / DEFINING CHARACTERISTICS	NURSING INTERVENTIONS / *RATIONALES*	EXPECTED OUTCOMES

RELATED FACTORS

Exposure to cold environment
Illness/trauma
Inability to shiver
Poor nutrition
Inadequate clothing
Medications: vasodilators
Excessive evaporative heat loss from skin
Decreased metabolic rate
Inactivity
Prematurity

DEFINING CHARACTERISTICS

Body temperature <35° C (95° F)
Cool, pale skin
Decreased heart rate
Decreased respiratory rate
Hypoxemia
Hypoglycemia
Fluid/electrolyte imbalance
Irritability
Mental confusion in the older child
Convulsions
Respiratory arrest

ONGOING ASSESSMENT

- Obtain age and weight.
- Assess vital signs.
- Monitor electrolytes.
- Evaluate for drug consumption.
- Determine precipitating event and risk factors.
- Evaluate peripheral perfusion at frequent intervals.

THERAPEUTIC INTERVENTIONS

- Provide extra covering:
    Clothing, including head covering. *Heat loss tends to be greatest from the top of the head.*
    Blankets
- Keep child's linen dry. *Moisture facilitates evaporative heat loss.*
- Control environmental temperature; place infant in isolette.
- Provide extra heat source:
    Heat lamp, radiant warmer
    Heated oxygen
    Warming mattress, pads of blankets
    Warmed IV fluids/lavage fluids
- Regulate heat source according to physical response.

PATIENT/PARENT EDUCATION

- Explain all procedures and treatments.
- Provide information regarding normal temperature.
- Enlist support services as appropriate.

Body temperature within normal limits will be attained.

Michele Knoll Puzas, RNC, MHPE

Infection, high risk for

Any condition in which the child is at risk for being invaded/injured by pathogenic organisms. Infection can be bacterial, viral, or fungal in origin.

RELATED FACTORS / DEFINING CHARACTERISTICS	NURSING INTERVENTIONS / *RATIONALES*	EXPECTED OUTCOMES

RELATED FACTORS

Malnutrition
Trauma
Immunosuppression
Immobility
Invasive therapy
Altered skin integrity
Respiratory disorders, stasis of secretions, or intubation
Drug therapy
Exposure to communicable disease
Chronic disease
Indwelling catheters/drains

DEFINING CHARACTERISTICS

Hyperthermia
Skin flushing or pallor
Tachycardia
Open wounds
Foul smelling drainage from tubes
Cloudy urine
Wound drainage/pus
Weight loss/muscle wasting
Abnormal radiological results
Hypotension or hypertension
Rising WBC count
Tachypnea
Positive wound/blood cultures

ONGOING ASSESSMENT

- Assess age and developmental level.
- Monitor for signs of infection:
    Vital signs (T, P, R, and BP). *Infants and young children do not always exhibit fever because of immature thermoregulatory or immune response systems.*
    Skin color and temperature
    Wound appearance
    Urine appearance
    Appearance and consistency of respiratory secretions
- Monitor CBC with differential count.
- Monitor all culture results.
- Assess for recent exposure to communicable diseases.
- Identify conditions/areas for potential risk:
    Open wounds
    Urinary catheters
    Endotracheal tubes
    Immobility
    Malnutrition
    Venous/arterial access devices
    Peritoneal devices
    Immunosuppression

THERAPEUTIC INTERVENTIONS

- Maintain optimal aseptic environment.
- Use sterile technique during placement/manipulation of invasive lines. Maintain sterile occlusive dressing over access device according to policy.
- Inform physician of signs of infection.
- Administer medications as ordered.
- Use sterile technique when collecting specimens (blood, urine, and wound).
- Dress wounds as ordered or according to policy.
- Isolate child if required.
- Use good handwashing practice.
- Limit visitors if needed; screen siblings for recent illness and up-to-date immunizations.
- Encourage coughing, deep breathing, incentive spirometry; adjust for age: blowing games, chest PT. Obtain respiratory therapy assistance.
- Suction trachea/bronchi using sterile technique.
- Employ universal precautions.

PATIENT/PARENT EDUCATION

- Teach child/family signs and symptoms of infection.
- Teach parent/older child techniques for temperature measurement.
- Explain procedures, especially if gown and mask are required.
- Instruct child in breathing exercises, incentive spirometry.
- Demonstrate and require return demonstration of all high-risk home care procedures:
    Self-injections
    Self-catheterization (may be clean)
    Peritoneal dialysis
    Dressing changes

Risk for infection will be reduced.

Kim Johnson, RN, BSN

Mobility, impaired physical

IMMOBILITY

A state in which a child has limitations of independent physical movement.

RELATED FACTORS / DEFINING CHARACTERISTICS	NURSING INTERVENTIONS / *RATIONALES*	EXPECTED OUTCOMES

RELATED FACTORS

Musculoskeletal impairment
Neuromuscular impairment
Medical restrictions
Prolonged bed rest
Limited strength
Pain

DEFINING CHARACTERISTICS

Inability to move purposefully within physical environment, including bed mobility, transfer, and ambulation
Reluctance to attempt movement
Limited ROM
Decreased muscle strength, control, or mass
Imposed restrictions of movement, including mechanical, medical protocol, and impaired coordination
Inability to perform action as instructed

ONGOING ASSESSMENT

- Assess child's ability to carry out ADL based on age-appropriate developmental milestones.
- Assess child's/parent's knowledge of immobility (what they know, need to know, or understand).
- Assess for developing thrombophlebitis (calf pain, Homans' sign, redness, localized swelling, and rise in temperature).
- Assess skin integrity. Check for signs of redness, tissue ischemia (especially over ear, shoulders, elbows, sacrum, hips, heels, ankles, and toes).
- Monitor I&O record as needed; monitor daily consumption. Assess nutritional needs as they relate to immobility (possible hypocalcemia, negative nitrogen balance). *Pressure sores develop more quickly in children with a nutritional deficit.*
- Assess elimination status (usual pattern, present patterns, signs of constipation).
- Assess emotional response to disability/limitation.
- Evaluate need for home assistance (physical therapy, visiting nurse, assistive device).

THERAPEUTIC INTERVENTIONS

- Encourage and facilitate early ambulation and other ADL when possible. Assist with each initial change—dangling, sitting in chair, ambulation.
- Encourage age-appropriate play activities.
- Obtain adequate assistance when transferring child to bed, chair, or stretcher.
- Encourage appropriate use of assisting devices.
- Provide positive reinforcement during activity.
- Keep side rails up and bed in low position *to promote safe environment.*
- Consult rehabilitation medicine personnel as appropriate for exercise program or necessary assistive devices.
- Turn and position every 2 hours or as needed *to optimize circulation to all tissues and to relieve pressure.*
- Maintain limbs in functional alignment (e.g., with pillows, sandbags, or wedges):
  Support feet in dorsiflexed position *to prevent footdrop.*
  Use bed cradle *to keep heavy bed linens off feet.*
- Assist with passive/active ROM exercise *to increase venous return, prevent stiffness, and maintain muscle strength and endurance.*
- Turn to prone or semiprone position at least once daily, unless contraindicated *to drain bronchial tree.*
- Use prophylactic antipressure devices as appropriate *to prevent tissue breakdown.*
- Clean, dry, and moisturize skin as needed.
- Encourage coughing and deep breathing exercises. Use suction as needed *to prevent buildup of secretions.* Use incentive spirometer *to increase lung expansion.*
- Encourage liquid intake *to optimize hydration status and prevent hardening of stool.*
- Initiate supplemental high-protein, high-calorie feedings as appropriate.

Optimal physical mobility will be maintained.

Continued.

Mobility, impaired physical cont'd

RELATED FACTORS / DEFINING CHARACTERISTICS	NURSING INTERVENTIONS / *RATIONALES*	EXPECTED OUTCOMES
	THERAPEUTIC INTERVENTIONS cont'd ▪ Set up a bowel program as needed (adequate fluid, foods high in bulk, physical activity, stool softeners, mild laxatives). Record bowel activity daily. ▪ Assist child in accepting limitations. Emphasize abilities (see Constipation, p. 12). **PATIENT/PARENT EDUCATION** ▪ Explain progressive physical activity to child. Help child/parents to establish reasonable and obtainable goals. ▪ Instruct child/parent about hazards of immobility. Emphasize importance of position change, ROM, coughing exercises. ▪ Reinforce principles of exercise, emphasizing that joints are to be exercised to the point of pain, not beyond. ▪ Instruct parents regarding need to make home environment safe. ▪ Encourage verbalization of feelings, strengths, and weaknesses. ▪ Encourage visits from family and friends to offer emotional support and opportunities for learning child's care.	

Linda Arsenault, RN, MSN, CNRN; Linda Ehrlich Muzio, RN, MSN, CS

Nutrition, altered: less than body requirements

The state in which the child experiences an intake of nutrients insufficient to meet metabolic and growth needs.

STARVATION; WEIGHT LOSS; ANOREXIA

RELATED FACTORS / DEFINING CHARACTERISTICS	NURSING INTERVENTIONS / *RATIONALES*	EXPECTED OUTCOMES

RELATED FACTORS

Inability to ingest foods

Inability to digest foods

Inability to absorb/ metabolize foods

Inability to procure adequate amounts of food

Knowledge deficit

Pica

Unwillingness to eat

Increased metabolic needs due to disease process or therapy

DEFINING CHARACTERISTICS

Loss of weight with or without adequate caloric intake

>10%-20% below ideal body weight

Documented inadequate caloric intake

Caloric intake inadequate to keep pace with abnormal disease/metabolic state

ONGOING ASSESSMENT

- Assess age and developmental level.
- Document child's actual weight on admission (do not estimate); weigh at-risk children and infants daily.
- Obtain nutritional history from primary caretaker.
- Monitor urine/serum electrolytes, CBC, glucose, and urine sugar/acetone as needed.

THERAPEUTIC INTERVENTIONS

- Consult dietitian when appropriate.
- Document appetite. Record exact I&O (do not estimate). Encourage child's participation (daily log), as appropriate. *Determination of type, amount, and pattern of food/fluid intake is facilitated by accurate documentation by child/nurse as the intake occurs; memory is insufficient.*
- Assist child with meals as needed.
- Encourage frequent oral ingestion of high-calorie/protein foods and fluids.
- Provide higher calorie infant formulas when necessary.
- Implement enteral tube feedings in extreme cases.
- Encourage high-fiber foods; give stool softeners as ordered *to promote regular elimination patterns.*
- Encourage exercise. *Metabolism and utilization of nutrients are enhanced by activity.*
- Encourage family to bring food from home as appropriate.
- Consult lactation specialist for breastfed infants; supplement if needed.

PATIENT/PARENT EDUCATION

- Review and reinforce the following to parent and child:
  Importance of maintaining adequate caloric intake
  Foods high in calories/protein that will promote weight gain and nitrogen balance (e.g., small, frequent meals of foods high in calories and protein)
- Assist parent/child in recognizing regular eating patterns.
- Educate family in necessity of emotional support.
- Explain necessity and purpose of all extraordinary measures.

Optimal caloric intake will be maintained.

Michele Knoll Puzas, RNC, MHPE

Nutrition, altered: more than body requirements

The state in which a child's intake of nutrients exceeds metabolic demands.

OBESITY; OVERWEIGHT

RELATED FACTORS / DEFINING CHARACTERISTICS	NURSING INTERVENTIONS / *RATIONALES*	EXPECTED OUTCOMES

RELATED FACTORS
Lack of knowledge of nutritional needs, food intake, and/or food preparation
Poor dietary habits
Use of food as coping mechanism
Metabolic disorders
Diabetes
Sedentary activity level
 	
DEFINING CHARACTERISTICS
Weight 10%-20% over ideal weight for height and age
Reported or observed dysfunctional eating patterns
	ONGOING ASSESSMENT
	▪ Assess age and developmental level.
	▪ Determine any known diagnoses that may cause or potentiate obesity.
	▪ Perform nutritional assessment.
	▪ Document child's actual weight on admission (do not estimate).
	▪ Monitor urine/serum electrolytes, CBC, glucose, and urine sugar/acetone levels as needed.
	▪ Assess for psychosocial causes/effects of obesity.
	
	THERAPEUTIC INTERVENTIONS
	▪ Consult dietitian when appropriate.
	▪ Assist parent/child with selection of appropriate foods from each food group.
	▪ Encourage child to keep a daily log of food/liquid ingestion and caloric intake, as appropriate. *Memory is inadequate for quantification of intake. A visual record may also help child make more appropriate food choices and serving sizes.*
	▪ Encourage water intake.
	▪ Encourage child to be more aware of nutritional habits:
	    To realize the time needed for eating (encourage putting fork down between bites)
	    To focus on eating and to avoid other diversional activities (e.g., reading, television viewing, telephoning)
	    To observe for cues that lead to eating (e.g., odor, time, depression, boredom)
	    To eat in the same place as often as possible
	    To identify actual need for food
	▪ Encourage exercise.
	▪ Arrange psychosocial counseling.
	
	PATIENT/PARENT EDUCATION
	▪ Review and reinforce dietitian's teaching regarding:
	    Four food groups and proper serving sizes
	    Caloric content of food
	    Methods of preparation
	▪ Include person primarily responsible for grocery shopping and food preparation in education.
	▪ Encourage diabetic children to attend diabetes classes; review and reinforce principles of dietary management of diabetes.
		Nutritional intake will be appropriate to meet metabolic needs.

Michele Knoll Puzas, RNC, MHPE

Pain

A highly subjective state in which a variety of unpleasant sensations and a wide range of distresses may be experienced. Pain may be acute, a symptom of injury or illness, or pain may be chronic, lasting longer than 6 months. Pain may also arise from emotional, psychological, cultural, or spiritual distress. Pain can be very difficult to explain, because it is unique to the individual; pain should be accepted as described by the sufferer.

RELATED FACTORS / DEFINING CHARACTERISTICS	NURSING INTERVENTIONS / *RATIONALES*	EXPECTED OUTCOMES

RELATED FACTORS

Operative pain
Cardiovascular pain
Pain resulting from medical problems
Musculoskeletal pain
Pain resulting from diagnostic procedures or medical treatments
Pain resulting from trauma

DEFINING CHARACTERISTICS

Child/parent report pain
Guarding behavior, protective
Self-focusing, narrowed focus (altered time perception, withdrawal from social or physical contact), depression, loss of appetite
Relief/distraction of behavior; may be culturally influenced (e.g., moaning, crying, pacing, seeking out other people or activities; restlessness, irritability, altered sleep pattern)
Facial mask of pain
Altered muscle tone—flaccid/rigid/tense
Autonomic responses not seen in chronic, stable pain (e.g., diaphoresis; change in BP or pulse rate; pupillary movements)

ONGOING ASSESSMENT

- Determine pain profile:
  P—Place (location)
  A—Amount (use 0-3 scale or "faces" or colors)
  I—Interaction (what makes pain worse)
  N—Neutralizer (what makes pain better)
  Use of the pain scale provides objective data and patient input, giving control to the patient and building trust.
- Assess for probable cause of pain.
- Evaluate child's response to pain and to medications or therapeutic measures aimed at abolishing/relieving pain.
- Assess developmental level when pain is being controlled.
- Assess to what degree cultural, environmental, intrapersonal, and intrapsychic factors might contribute to pain.
- Evaluate what the pain means to the child. *The meaning of the pain will directly influence the child's response to that pain. Pain will influence activity, family role, self-concept, etc.*
- Determine baseline vital signs to evaluate effects or side effects of interventions.
- Assess child's/parent's past coping mechanisms *to determine what measures worked best in the past.*
- Assess expectations for pain relief. *Some children may be content to have pain decreased; others will expect complete elimination of pain. This will affect their perception of the effectiveness of the treatment modality and their willingness to participate in further treatments.*
- Assess willingness/ability to explore a range of techniques aimed at controlling pain.
- Assess for effects of chronic pain:
  Depression
  Guilt
  Hopelessness
  Sleep and nutritional disturbances
  Alterations in interpersonal relationships
- Obtain a chronic-pain profile:
  Coping behaviors
  Identify what makes pain worse
  Identify what makes pain better
  Obtain individual's description of pain

THERAPEUTIC INTERVENTIONS

- Anticipate need for analgesics or additional methods of pain relief. *One can most effectively deal with pain by preventing it. Early intervention may decrease the total amount of analgesic required.*
- Respond immediately to complaint of pain. *While in the midst of painful experiences, the child's perception of time may become distorted. Prompt and positive responses to complaints may result in decreased anxiety. Nursing interventions will be more effective if anxiety has not exaggerated the child's or parent's experience of pain. The child needs to know that the nurse believes the pain is present and has a plan to relieve the suffering.*

Pain will be relieved or reduced, or child will begin to show signs of adaptation.

Continued.

RELATED FACTORS / DEFINING CHARACTERISTICS	NURSING INTERVENTIONS / *RATIONALES*	EXPECTED OUTCOMES

DEFINING CHARACTERISTICS cont'd

Decreased respiratory rate, pallor, nausea; *these are signs of stress in acute pain and have little value in evaluating a patient with pain*

Verbalized concepts of pain:
Discomfort
Displeasure
Hurt
Grief
Misery
Described
physical, emotional, or psychological state
Feelings of lack of control/powerlessness
Fatigue
Decreased appetite/mobility

THERAPEUTIC INTERVENTIONS cont'd

- Reassure child that nurse will continue to assess and provide for pain control. *Reassurance decreases anticipation of pain and anxiety, making the situation more tolerable.*
- Eliminate additional stressors or sources of discomfort whenever possible. *Management of pain is often more difficult in adolescent patients because of their altered self-perceptions and isolation from peers.*
- Give analgesics as ordered, preferably on a fixed schedule (not prn), using both narcotic and nonnarcotic drugs *to affect dual levels of the nervous system and periphery.*
- Notify physician if interventions are unsuccessful or if current complaint is a significant change from child's past experience of pain. *Children who request pain medications at intervals more frequent than prescribed may actually require higher doses of analgesia or a more potent analgesic.*
- Provide rest periods to facilitate comfort, sleep, and relaxation. *The child's experience of pain may become exaggerated as the result of fatigue. In a cyclic fashion, pain may result in fatigue, which may result in exaggerated pain and exhaustion. A quiet environment, a darkened room, and a disconnected phone are all measures that facilitate rest.*
- Whenever possible, reassure child that pain is time limited, and there is more than one approach to easing pain. *When pain is perceived as everlasting and unresolvable, the child may give up trying to cope with it or experience a sense of hopelessness and loss of control.*
- Perform ROM (active or passive) and promote mobility through:
  Position changes
  Proper body alignment
  Supporting the extremities during movement and at rest
  Appropriate exercise
  Self-care whenever possible
  Daily ambulation when appropriate
    Self-care enhances the child's sense of autonomy while encouraging movement and mobility. Mobility will counteract the adverse consequences of disuse. Pain during exercise is an indication to modify the exercise to a more gentle activity.
  Application of:
    Hot, moist compresses
    Cold compresses to affected area when ordered
    Hot, moist compresses have a penetrating effect. The warmth rushes blood to the affected area to promote healing. Cold compresses may reduce local edema and promote some numbing, thereby promoting comfort.
- If the child is developmentally capable, instruct in the use of one or a combination of the following techniques:
  Imagery: *The use of a mental picture or an imagined event that involves the use of the five senses to distract oneself from painful stimuli.*
  Distraction techniques: *Heightening one's concentration on nonpainful stimuli to decrease one's awareness and experience of pain.*
    Breathing modifications
    Nerve stimulation
  Relaxation exercises: *Techniques used to bring about a state of physical and mental awareness and tranquility. The goal of these techniques is to reduce tension, subsequently reducing pain.*
  Massage affected area when appropriate. *Massage decreases muscle tension and can promote comfort.*
- Provide diversional activities as tolerated; consult child life therapist.
- Reassure child/parent concerning physical status. *Both the child's health and self-perceptions are affected by pain and its management.*

Pain cont'd

RELATED FACTORS / DEFINING CHARACTERISTICS	NURSING INTERVENTIONS / *RATIONALES*	EXPECTED OUTCOMES
	PATIENT/PARENT EDUCATION	
	▪ Provide anticipatory instruction on pain causes, appropriate prevention, and relief measures.	
	▪ Explain cause of pain/discomfort, if known.	
	▪ Instruct child/parent to report pain so that relief measures may be instituted.	
	▪ Instruct child/parent to evaluate and to report effectiveness of measures used.	
	▪ Obtain supportive therapies as needed:	
	Social service	
	Support for religious beliefs	
	Physiological intervention	
	Self-help groups	

Mary Muse, RN, MS; Deidra Gradishar, RNC, BA; Linda Ehrlich Muzio, RN, MSN, CS

Parenting, altered: actual/ high risk for

CHILD ABUSE; INEFFECTIVE COPING; ALTERED FAMILY PROCESS

The state in which the ability of the nurturing person is at risk, or the person is unable to create an environment that promotes the optimal growth and development of another human being from infancy through adolescence.

RELATED FACTORS / DEFINING CHARACTERISTICS	NURSING INTERVENTIONS / *RATIONALES*	EXPECTED OUTCOMES
RELATED FACTORS	**ONGOING ASSESSMENT**	More effective parenting behaviors will be demonstrated.
Lack of available role model	▪ Assess parents' strengths, weaknesses, age, marital status, available sources of support, cultural background, and individual response to child-rearing and parenting role.	
Ineffective role model	▪ Evaluate nature of emotional and physical parenting that parents received during their own childhood. *Parenting is learned, and individuals use their own parents as role models.*	
Physical and psychosocial abuse of nurturing figure	▪ Assess parents' interpersonal communication skills and their relationship to each other, friends, and other family members.	
Lack of support	▪ Assess motivation to learn.	
Unmet social, emotional, and maturational needs of parenting figures	▪ Determine degree of insight.	
	▪ Evaluate the significance of nonverbal communication.	
Unrealistic expectations of self and/or partner	▪ Identify disturbing conversational topics.	
	▪ Identify inappropriate emotional responses.	
Extremes of age	▪ Identify parents' significant life values.	
Past experiences	▪ Identify appropriate use of defense mechanisms.	
Culture	▪ Observe parent/partner for excessive stress level.	
Fatigue	▪ Observe for evidence that the parent/partner is reaching out for emotional support.	
Physical discomforts/ impairment		
Social isolation	**THERAPEUTIC INTERVENTIONS**	
Mental or physical illness	▪ Provide an atmosphere of acceptance.	
	▪ Express warmth and friendliness to parent/partner. *This will facilitate their communicating concerns.*	
Family or personal stress (financial, legal, recent crisis)	▪ Encourage acceptance of responsibility for infant/child.	
	▪ Encourage awareness of positive responses from others.	
	▪ Encourage expression of feelings.	
Limited cognitive functioning	▪ Listen attentively and talk with parent. *This will promote trust between caregiver and child/parent.*	

Continued.

Parenting, altered: actual/high risk for cont'd

RELATED FACTORS / DEFINING CHARACTERISTICS	NURSING INTERVENTIONS / *RATIONALES*	EXPECTED OUTCOMES

DEFINING CHARACTERISTICS

Lack of parental attachment behaviors

Inappropriate visual, tactile, auditory stimulation of child

Negative identification with characteristics of infant/child

Negative attachment of meanings to characteristics of infant/child

Verbalization of resentment toward infant/child

Verbalization of role inadequacy

Noncompliance with health appointments for infant/child

Inappropriate or inconsistent discipline practices

Frequent childhood accidents

Frequent illness of infant/child

Growth and developmental lag in child

Verbalizes desire to have child call parent by first name versus traditional name

Child receives care from caretakers without consideration of infant/child needs

Compulsively seeks role approval from others

Inattention to infant/child needs

Verbal disgust at body functions of infant/child

Abandonment of infant/child

Child runs away

THERAPEUTIC INTERVENTIONS cont'd

- Encourage recognition of one's various roles in life.
- Encourage use of normal coping mechanisms.
- Explore with parents evidence of recurring problems.
- Explore with parents the effects of their behavior on their children.
- Introduce to groups/persons who have and are successfully dealing with similar parenting problems. *This will provide group support.*
- Refrain from negatively criticizing parent.
- Maintain and support realistic assessment of the situation.
- Refer parent to other support services as indicated: social service, psychological counseling, etc.
- Advise early correction of problem.
- Emphasize importance of recognition of tension within oneself.

PATIENT/PARENT EDUCATION

- Explain importance of maintaining a positive self-image.
- Explain that parental beliefs/attitudes affect child development.
- Explain that undesirable thoughts and feelings are normal.
- Explain the causes of the health problems that may be present.

Carol Sarmiento, RN, BSN

Skin integrity, impaired: actual/high risk for

A state in which a child's skin is, or may become, adversely altered.

PRESSURE SORES

RELATED FACTORS / DEFINING CHARACTERISTICS	NURSING INTERVENTIONS / *RATIONALES*	EXPECTED OUTCOMES

RELATED FACTORS

Adhesives
Allergic reactions
Intubation
Tracheostomy
IV/central lines
Incision/other wounds
Mechanical forces (pressure, shear, friction)
Pronounced bony prominences
Prematurity
Poor nutrition
Immobility
Incontinence
Altered cutaneous sensation

DEFINING CHARACTERISTICS

No impairment:
Epidermis intact
No discoloration
Capillary refill <4 sec
Stage I:
Redness
Pallor
Poor capillary refill or redness that persists after pressure is removed
Stage II:
Blisters (either intact or broken)
Painful, moist, superficial area, usually round or linear, with interrupted epidermis
Stage III:
Open lesion involving dermis and subcutaneous tissue
May have adherent necrotic material
Drainage usually present

ONGOING ASSESSMENT

- Assess age and developmental level.
- Assess for presence of related factors.
- Observe general condition of skin.
- Specifically check intactness of skin over bony prominences, noting color, temperature.
- Assess IV/central line sites.
- Assess incision sites/wounds for healing.
- Assess sites where tape or other adhesives used.
- Assess tracheostomy site and under tracheostomy ties.
- Assess for tape allergies/diaper (disposable) allergies.
- Assess condition under endotracheal tubes. *Prolonged intubation can cause pressure breakdown.*
- Assess child's ability to be involved in own care/movement.
- Reassess whenever child's condition or treatment plan results in an increased number of related factors. *The incidence of breakdown is directly related to the number of risk factors present.*
- Stage any existing pressure sore(s), using defining characteristics.
- Assess need for debridement. *Debridement must be accomplished to stage pressure sores accurately.*

THERAPEUTIC INTERVENTIONS

- Document findings of assessment.
- If child is restricted to bed, implement and post a turning schedule, limiting time in one position to 2 hours or less, and customize the schedule to child's routine and to nursing care needs. *A schedule that does not interfere with the child's and nurses' activities is likely to be followed.*
- Implement pressure-relieving devices commensurate with degree of risk for skin impairment:
    For *low-risk patients:* good quality (dense, at least 3 inch thick) foam mattress overlay
    For *moderate-risk patients:* water mattress, static or dynamic air mattress
    For *high-risk children* or those with existing stage III or IV pressure sores (or with stage II pressure sores *and* multiple risk factors): low air loss beds (Mediscus, Flexicare, Kinair), or air-fluidized therapy (Clinitron, Skytron) are indicated. *Low air loss beds are constructed to allow elevated head of bed and patient transfer. These should be used when pulmonary concerns necessitate elevating head of bed or when getting child up is feasible. Air-fluidized therapy supports child's weight at well below capillary closing pressure but restricts getting child out of bed.*
- Maintain functional body alignment.
- Limit chair-sitting to 2 hours at any one time.
- Encourage ambulation if child is able.
- Increase tissue perfusion by massaging around affected area. *Massaging reddened area may further damage skin.*
- Clean, dry, and moisturize skin, especially over bony prominences, bid or as indicated by incontinence or sweating.
- Keep incision/wounds clean and dry.
- Use as little tape as necessary to anchor tubings to skin/avoid if possible.
- Use cloth diapers for the infant allergic to disposables.

Skin will remain intact *or* evidence of granulation will be present.

Continued.

Nursing Diagnosis Care Plans

RELATED FACTORS / DEFINING CHARACTERISTICS	NURSING INTERVENTIONS / *RATIONALES*	EXPECTED OUTCOMES

DEFINING CHARACTERISTICS cont'd
 	
Stage IV:
Open lesion involving muscle, bone, joint, and/or body cavity
Usually has adherent necrotic material
Drainage usually present
	THERAPEUTIC INTERVENTIONS cont'd
	• Leave blisters intact by wrapping in gauze or applying a hydrocolloid (Duoderm, Sween-Appeal), or a vapor-permeable membrane dressing (Op-Site, Tegaderm). *Blisters are sterile natural dressings.*
	• Consider options for debridement if eschar is present:
	    Wet-to-dry dressings
	    Collagenase ointments as ordered
	    Assisting with sharp surgical debridement if done at the bedside
	    Arranging for whirlpool as indicated
	• *Promote granulation and epithelialization* through use of principles of moist wound healing:
	    Wet-to-dry dressings
	    Hydrocolloid dressings
	    Vapor-permeable membrane dressings
	• Maintain adequate nutrition and hydration; arrange dietitian consultation as appropriate.
	
	PATIENT/PARENT EDUCATION
	• Explain the cause(s) of pressure sore development and use of special equipment.
	• Reinforce the importance of mobility/turning/ambulation in prevention and management of pressure sores.	

Audrey Klopp, RN, PhD, CS, ET; Michele Knoll Puzas, RNC, MHPE

Skin integrity, impaired: high risk for (neonate)

The newly born infant has an immature integumentary system, leading to fragile and excessively permeable skin that is easily abraded. These potential problems are inversely proportional to gestational age. The interventions necessary for stabilization and management of the newborn may damage the skin.

RELATED FACTORS / DEFINING CHARACTERISTICS	NURSING INTERVENTIONS / *RATIONALES*	EXPECTED OUTCOMES
RELATED FACTORS Disruption of skin surface Destruction of skin layers Prematurity Decreased amount of brown fat *Internal (somatic) factors:* Extremely premature infant Altered nutritional status Altered immunological state (microbial colonization) Generalized edema Gelatinous-transparent skin Hypothermia/hyperthermia Altered skin turgor *External (environmental) factors:* Mechanical factors: Shearing forces from adhesives Pressure Use of restraints Use of extremely warm compresses Use of monitoring devices Chemical factors: Infusion and transfusion infiltrations **DEFINING CHARACTERISTICS** Denuded skin areas Abraded skin areas Erythematous skin Bruised and pale skin areas	**ONGOING ASSESSMENT** ▪ Assess age and developmental level. ▪ Review maternal and fetal history: Gestational age Trauma in delivery, bruising, or hematoma Use of invasive monitoring device ▪ Assess skin for: Color Temperature Texture Turgor Moisture Presence/absence of skin breakdown Edema Perfusion ▪ Assess nutritional status: Monitor daily weight and record. Calculate daily caloric intake. Monitor intake and output. Check specific gravity every 4 to 6 hours *to assess hydration.* ▪ Check IV patency before administering drugs and blood products *to avoid IV infiltrations.* ▪ Monitor and document IV sites every hour. ▪ Monitor and record temperatures of body hoods, oxygen hoods, and ventilators every 2 hours *to ensure administration of safe temperatures that will not cause hyperthermia or burns.* **THERAPEUTIC INTERVENTIONS** ▪ Notify physician of changes in skin color, tissue ischemia, and redness. *Early notification of risk factors facilitates prompt intervention.* ▪ Clean skin according to institution's bath policy and procedure. ▪ Place infant in appropriate neutral thermoregulation (see Thermoregulation, p. 42). ▪ Administer adequate nutritional and hydration requirements as ordered. ▪ Limit use of adhesives: Use water-based gel adhesive electrodes Remove adhesive materials with water-soaked cotton balls. Do not peel off! ▪ Apply warm compress to sites of IV infiltrations if markedly edematous or swollen *to increase blood flow to the affected areas and promote removal of extravasated fluid.* ▪ Change infant's position every 2 hours. ▪ Gently massage around pressure areas. ▪ Perform passive ROM exercises (especially when child is immobile). ▪ Rinse off povidone-iodine (Betadine) solution with water on completion of procedure *to prevent irritation to skin.* ▪ Provide prophylactic use of sheepskin. ▪ Use liquid film barriers on skin or protective skin barriers when securing endotracheal tubes. ▪ Use only wide, soft restraints to immobilize an infant.	Optimal skin integrity will be maintained.

Rosetonia G. Sapaula, RN, BSN

Thermoregulation, ineffective

A state in which a child or newborn is at risk for failure to maintain a normal core temperature with minimum oxygen consumption and calorie expenditure as a result of one or more factors that cause physiological response and a change in body temperature. Infants are at high risk for thermoregulatory dysfunction because of their underdeveloped neural center and the lack of stored fats/glycogen. A child may experience problems as a result of drug or chemical ingestion, anesthesia, cranial surgery, or infection.

RELATED FACTORS / DEFINING CHARACTERISTICS	NURSING INTERVENTIONS / *RATIONALES*	EXPECTED OUTCOMES

RELATED FACTORS
 	
 Risk factors:
 Premature birth
 Extremes of weight or age
 Dehydration
 Illness
 Trauma
 Drugs
 Environmental temperature
 Inappropriate clothing
 	
 DEFINING CHARACTERISTICS
 Vacillating body temperature
 Hypothermia
 Hyperthermia
	ONGOING ASSESSMENT
	 • Assess for presence of risk factors.
	 • Assess for precipitating event.
	 • Measure temperature at frequent intervals. Use the same instrument and method at each interval. If method is changed, e.g., axillary versus rectal, document route. *A change of this type usually causes a variance in the temperature obtained.*
	 • Monitor other physical indicators:
	     Heart and respiratory rate
	     Blood pressure
	     Skin condition
	     Fluid balance
	     Electrolytes
	     Mental status
	 • Monitor other environmental factors, e.g., uninsulated windows and walls.
	
	 THERAPEUTIC INTERVENTIONS
	 • Provide preventive measures as necessary:
	     Control environment with use of warmers, isolettes, etc.
	     Provide appropriate clothing/covering.
	     Provide adequate fluid and dietary intake.
	     Administer medications as ordered.
	 • Notify physician of changes in physical status, especially temperature.
	 • If altered body temperature becomes a problem, refer to appropriate care plan:
	     Hypothermia
	     Hyperthermia
	 • Ensure adequate nutrition.
	
	 PATIENT/PARENT EDUCATION
	 • Explain risk factors and rationale for temperature measurement.
	 • Explain prevention of risk factors and the consequences of temperature alterations.
	 • Teach temperature measurement for home use.
	 • Explain well-child/well-baby care, as needed, including proper clothing and nutrition.
	 • Provide community resources, consults as needed.
		A neutral thermal environment will be maintained.

Gina Stevens, RN, BSN

Tissue perfusion, altered: peripheral, cardiopulmonary, cerebral, renal

Reduced arterial blood flow being delivered to body tissues, causing decreased nutrition and oxygenation at the cellular level. Management is directed at removing vasoconstricting factors, improving peripheral blood flow, and reducing metabolic demands on the body.

RELATED FACTORS / DEFINING CHARACTERISTICS	NURSING INTERVENTIONS / *RATIONALES*	EXPECTED OUTCOMES

RELATED FACTORS

Peripheral:
Indwelling arterial catheters
Constricting cast
Compartment syndrome
Embolism/thrombus
Arterial spasm
Positioning
Cardiopulmonary:
Pulmonary embolism
Cerebral:
Increased ICP
Intracranial bleeding
Renal:
Decreased urine output
Edema
Increased specific gravity
Increased osmolality
Cloudy/rusty urine
Increased BUN, creatinine, K+

DEFINING CHARACTERISTICS

Peripheral:
Weak/absent peripheral pulses
Edema
Numbness, pain, ache in extremity
Cool extremities
Dependent rubor
Clammy skin
Mottling
Hypotension
Differences in BP in opposite extremities
Prolonged capillary refill

ONGOING ASSESSMENT
- Assess for age and developmental level.
- Assess for signs of decreased tissue perfusion (see defining characteristics for each category).
- Assess for possible causative factors related to temporarily impaired arterial blood flow. *Early detection of cause facilitates prompt effective treatment.*

THERAPEUTIC INTERVENTIONS
- Notify physician of signs of decreased perfusion.
- Maintain optimal cardiac output *to ensure adequate perfusion of vital organs.*
- Anticipate need for possible embolectomy, heparinization, vasodilator therapy, thrombolytic therapy, fluid rescue.

SPECIFIC INTERVENTIONS
Peripheral
- Keep cannulated extremity still. Use soft restraints or armboards as needed.
- Do passive ROM exercises to unaffected extremity every 2 to 4 hours *to prevent venous stasis.*
- Anticipate/continue anticoagulation as ordered.
- Prepare for removal of arterial catheter as needed.
- If compartment syndrome is suspected, prepare child for surgical intervention (i.e., fasciotomy).
- If cast causes altered tissue perfusion, anticipate cast removal.

Cardiopulmonary
- Administer oxygen as needed.
- Position child properly *to promote optimal lung ventilation and perfusion.*
- Report changes in ABGs (hypoxemia, metabolic acidosis, hypercapnea).
- Anticipate and institute anticoagulation as ordered.
- Institute continuous pulse oximetry.

Cerebral
- Ensure proper functioning of ICP catheter (if present).
- If increased ICP exists, elevate head of bed 30-45 degrees *to promote venous outflow from brain and help reduce pressure.*
- Administer anticonvulsants as needed.
- Reorient to environment prn (as appropriate to age).

Renal
- Report urine output <1 ml/kg/hr to physician.
- Report changes in urine osmolality and specific gravity.
- Ensure proper urinary catheter function.
- If related to hypovolemia, institute fluid therapy as needed.

Optimal tissue perfusion will be maintained.

Continued.

Tissue perfusion, altered: peripheral, cardiopulmonary, cerebral, renal cont'd

RELATED FACTORS / DEFINING CHARACTERISTICS	NURSING INTERVENTIONS / *RATIONALES*	EXPECTED OUTCOMES
DEFINING CHARACTERISTICS cont'd *Cardiopulmonary:* Tachycardia Dysrhythmias Hypotension Tachypnea Abnormal ABGs *Cerebral:* Restlessness Confusion Lethargy Seizure activity Decreased Glasgow coma scores Pupillary changes Decreased reaction to light *Renal:* Hypovolemia	**PATIENT/PARENT EDUCATION** • Explain all procedures and equipment. • Ask child/parent to inform nurse immediately of any behavior changes, pain, or problems with equipment. • Provide information on normal tissue perfusion and possible causes for impairment.	

Margaret Dewey, RN, MSN

Urinary incontinence

ENURESIS

The involuntary loss of urine caused by trauma, infection, or genetic disorder. Incontinence in a previously "dry" child can be brought on by stress. Most children are not physically or psychologically mature enough to control bladder function until about 3 years of age.

RELATED FACTORS / DEFINING CHARACTERISTICS	NURSING INTERVENTIONS / *RATIONALES*	EXPECTED OUTCOMES

RELATED FACTORS
Myelomeningocele
Trauma
Infection
Renal failure (chronic)
Diabetes mellitus
Sickle cell disease
Exstrophy of bladder
CVA
Psychogenic bladder
 	
DEFINING CHARACTERISTICS
Dribbling
Leakage
Frequency
Inability to delay voiding
Bladder distention
Continual involuntary urine loss
	ONGOING ASSESSMENT
	• Evaluate developmental level.
	• Assess for related factors.
	• Assess bladder control history and age achieved.
	• Obtain current age and weight.
	• Ask parent to describe bladder training in the home and age of child when initiated.
	• Assess for changes or stressors in the home or school environment. *Young children sometimes regress to earlier behaviors due to stress. The older child may use bladder control in a power struggle with the parents.*
	• Assess patterns of incontinence as described by parent/child:
	    Urge felt but cannot reach bathroom in time
	    Involuntary urine loss without urge (cough, sneeze, laugh)
	    Frequent toileting
	• Obtain urine culture.
	• Palpate bladder for distention.
	
	THERAPEUTIC INTERVENTIONS
	• Assist in obtaining urine for culture:
	    Apply sterile U-bag.
	    Perform straight catheter insertion.
	• Prepare child for exams: cystourethrogram, cystoscopy, as needed, *to rule out organic disorder.*
	• Provide emotional support for child and parent.
	• Administer medications as ordered.
	• Facilitate access to bathroom, commode, urinal.
	• Help child stay clean and dry. Use external collection devices, intermittent catheterization, or diapers, depending on cause and overall treatment plan. *Wetting and odors are embarrassing to the child.*
	• Prepare child and parent for surgery if indicated, e.g., urethral dilation, stricture removal, artificial sphincter implant.
	• Limit fluid intake before bedtime and encourage emptying of bladder before sleep.
	
	PATIENT/PARENT EDUCATION
	• Explain all tests and procedures.
	• Explain normal limitations of development and maturation. *Toilet training should not begin until the child is ready: diapers are dry for extended periods of time and child can communicate need.*
	• Explain all medications, dosage, and timing. *Anticholinergics are sometimes used in the treatment of enuresis by causing a lightened sleep, allowing the child to waken more easily in response to urinary urge.*
	• Explain bladder training programs, if applicable.
	• Teach the child and parent intermittent clean catheterization. *In the cases of spinal injury, brain injury, and myelomeningocele, intermittent self-catheterization on a routine basis allows for dryness, odor control, and normalization of activity.*
	• Help the parent use positive reinforcement for positive behaviors and avoid using guilt or disapproval. *Positive encouragement will help establish self-confidence, a positive self-image, and self-control in the child.*
		Urinary continence or management of incontinence will be achieved.

Michele Knoll Puzas, RNC, MHPE

Urinary retention

The state in which an individual experiences incomplete emptying of the bladder.

RELATED FACTORS / DEFINING CHARACTERISTICS	NURSING INTERVENTIONS / *RATIONALES*	EXPECTED OUTCOMES

RELATED FACTORS

General anesthesia
Regional anesthesia
High ureteral pressures caused by disease, injury, or edema
Pain
Infection
Inadequate intake
Ureteral blockage

DEFINING CHARACTERISTICS

Decreased (<30 ml/hr) or absent urinary output for 2 consecutive hours
Frequency
Hesitancy
Urgency
Lower abdominal distention
Abdominal discomfort
Dribbling

ONGOING ASSESSMENT

- Assess age and developmental level.
- Assess for related factors.
- Evaluate previous patterns of voiding.
- Visually inspect lower abdomen for distention.
- Palpate over bladder for distention.
- Evaluate time intervals between voidings.
- Assess amount, frequency, character (color, odor, specific gravity).
- Determine balance between I&O.
- Monitor urinalysis, urine culture, and sensitivity.
- If indwelling catheter is in situ, assess for patency, kinking.
- Monitor BUN and creatinine.
- Culture urine.

THERAPEUTIC INTERVENTIONS

- Initiate methods to facilitate voiding:
  Encourage fluids, provide child-preferred items *to maximize compliance.*
  Position in upright position, on toilet if possible.
  Place bedpan/urinal or bedside commode within reach, assist as needed.
  Provide privacy.
  Encourage child to void every 4 hours.
  Have child listen to sound of running water or place hands in warm water and/or pour warm water over perineum.
  Offer fluids before voiding.
  Perform Credé maneuver over bladder.
  Assist with diagnostic examinations/tests.
- Administer bethanechol chloride (Urecholine) as ordered *to stimulate parasympathetic nervous system to release acetylcholine at nerve endings and to increase tone and amplitude of contractions of smooth muscles of urinary bladder.*
  Side effects: rare, following oral administration of therapeutic dose. In small subcutaneous doses: abdominal cramps, sweating and flushing. In larger doses: malaise, headaches, diarrhea, nausea, vomiting, asthmatic attacks, bradycardia, lowered BP, atrioventricular block, and cardiac arrest.
- Institute intermittent catheterization.
- Insert retention (Foley) catheter as ordered:
  Tape catheter to abdomen (male) *to prevent ureteral fistula.*
  Tape catheter to thigh (female).
  Cleanse insertion site every shift with soap and water, and dry thoroughly.
- Prepare child for surgical intervention.

PATIENT/PARENT EDUCATION

- Explain all tests and treatments before they occur.
- Educate child/significant others about the importance of adequate intake, i.e., 8 to 10 glasses of fluids daily.
- Instruct child/significant others on measures to help voiding (as described above).
- Instruct on signs and symptoms of overdistended bladder (e.g., decreased or absent urine, frequency, hesitancy, urgency, lower abdominal distention, or discomfort).
- Instruct on signs and symptoms of urinary tract infection (e.g., chills and fever, frequent urination or concentrated urine, abdominal or back pain).

Adequate urinary elimination patterns will be established.

Doris McNear, RN, BSN; Michele Knoll Puzas, RNC, MHPE

2

Psychosocial Care Plans

PEDIATRIC PATIENT
Child abuse
Depression
The dying child
Organ donation
Rape trauma syndrome
Suicide attempt/suicidal gesture

NEONATAL PATIENT
Developmental enhancement
Grieving for terminally ill neonate
Parenting in special care nursery

Child abuse

The physical or psychological assault or neglect of a child.

CHILD NEGLECT; BATTERED CHILD

NURSING DIAGNOSES/ DEFINING CHARACTERISTICS	NURSING INTERVENTIONS / *RATIONALES*	EXPECTED OUTCOMES
Actual Injury **RELATED TO** Physical assault Physical neglect Psychological assault or neglect **DEFINING CHARACTERISTICS** Fearful of parents, adults, caretakers Evidence of injury Undernourished Tense Tearful Aggressive Destructive Suspicious Apathetic Depressed Silent	**ONGOING ASSESSMENT** ▪ Assess age and developmental level. ▪ Assess immediately for head injury, fractures, ingestions, and respiratory compromise. ▪ Assess child and family behavior and interpersonal relationship, if possible. ▪ Assess for previous history of injury/neglect. ▪ Assess for contributing factors: Cultural Social Psychological ▪ Inspect every child on admission for evidence of abuse, e.g., bruises, lacerations, cigarette burns, old scars. *Many children are brought to the hospital for reasons other than injury.* ▪ Assess for sexual abuse, e.g.: Blood in urine or stool Pain on urination/defecation Penile or vaginal discharge or bleeding Torn vaginal tissues Excessive masturbation Unusual fears Unusual statements concerning body or sex ▪ Complete a nursing history in a nonthreatening, nonjudgmental manner, including: Sleeping habits Toilet habits Playmates Security objects Names/ages of siblings Previous hospitalizations Frequent family visitors or caretakers Developmental level **THERAPEUTIC INTERVENTIONS** ▪ Provide immediate care for observed injuries. *Preservation of life is the initial focus.* ▪ Document assessments. ▪ Establish relationship based on mutual respect, empathy, and sensitivity. ▪ Notify physician/abuse team of suspicions. *A questionable injury should be evaluated as soon as possible to ensure child's discharge to a safe environment.* ▪ Obtain consultation as necessary (see specific care plans for identified injuries/trauma).	Effects of injury are reduced.
Altered Skin Integrity **RELATED TO** Physical assault **DEFINING CHARACTERISTICS** Burns Bruises Buckle marks Skin lesions/rashes Fractures	**ONGOING ASSESSMENT** ▪ Assess for open wounds, complete fractures. ▪ Assess color, moisture, texture, and temperature of skin. ▪ Observe for signs of tissue ischemia every 4 hours. **THERAPEUTIC INTERVENTIONS** ▪ Apply direct pressure to bleeding sites. ▪ Clean wounds/burns with normal saline and sterile water. Cover with sterile gauze. ▪ Prepare for/assist with suturing or placement of steri-strips.	Impairment of skin integrity will be reduced.

NURSING DIAGNOSES/ DEFINING CHARACTERISTICS	NURSING INTERVENTIONS / *RATIONALES*	EXPECTED OUTCOMES

	THERAPEUTIC INTERVENTIONS cont'd
	▪ Apply ointments as ordered:
	  Silvadene *to protect skin*
	  Hydrocortisone *to promote healing and control itching*
	  Nystatin (Mycostatin) *for treatment of oral/skin candidal infections*
	▪ Maintain functional body alignment.
	▪ Keep wounds clean and dry, especially from urine and stool.
	▪ Maintain adequate hydration.	

Altered Level of Consciousness
Related To
Head injury
 	
Defining Characteristics
Change in LOC
Agitation
Inappropriate affect
Impaired memory
Increased head circumference
Fontanels full and tense
	ONGOING ASSESSMENT
	▪ Assess level of consciousness every 2 hours.
	▪ Assess vital signs every 2 hours.
	▪ Assess for contributing factors:
	  Trauma
	  Medications
	  Anesthesia
	
	THERAPEUTIC INTERVENTIONS
	▪ Notify physician of changes in vital signs or level of consciousness (LOC).
	▪ Keep side rails up.
	▪ Reorient child to environment.
	▪ Provide padded rails, helmet, restraints as needed *to prevent further injury.*
		Optimal state of consciousness will be maintained.

Altered Nutrition: Less Than Body Requirements
Related To
Neglect
Lack of parental skills or knowledge
Environmental or socioeconomic barriers
 	
Defining Characteristics
Poor skin turgor
Sunken eyes/fontanels
Underweight
Dry skin
Developmental delay
Flat affect
	ONGOING ASSESSMENT
	▪ Assess weight on admission. Compare with growth charts.
	▪ Obtain birth weight if patient is an infant.
	▪ Assess for dehydration (see Fluid volume deficit, p. 19).
	▪ Obtain nutritional history:
	  Types of foods
	  Type of formula
	  Amount and frequency of feedings/meals
	  Tolerance
	  Dining environment
	  Caretaker responsible for food preparation/feeding
	▪ Assess for other conditions, e.g., diarrhea, vomiting, allergies.
	
	THERAPEUTIC INTERVENTIONS
	▪ Institute I&O and calorie counts.
	▪ Arrange dietary consultations.
	▪ Provide small, frequent feedings high in calories and protein. *Small feedings are more easily tolerated.*
	▪ Involve caretaker at feeding times. *The nurse can serve as a good role model for caretaker.*
	▪ Offer variety in menu selections.
	▪ Provide supplements as ordered:
	  Polycose
	  Sustacal
	▪ Obtain stool for culture and sensitivity (C&S)/ova and parasites (O&P), if appropriate. *Poor nutrition may have a physiological or biological origin.*
	▪ Initiate IV fluid therapy if necessary.
		Recommended body weight will be achieved.

Continued.

Psychosocial Care Plans (Pediatric)

NURSING DIAGNOSES/ DEFINING CHARACTERISTICS	NURSING INTERVENTIONS / *RATIONALES*	EXPECTED OUTCOMES
Self Concept Disturbance **RELATED TO** Sexual abuse Physical abuse Emotional neglect **DEFINING CHARACTERISTICS** Change in behavior Withdrawal Fearfulness Nonverbal cues Excessive masturbation Refusal of assistance with bathing or toileting	**ONGOING ASSESSMENT** • Assess for physical evidence of abuse (see Injury, p. 48). • Assess child's perception of self and relationships. • Assess behaviors for appropriateness to situations. **THERAPEUTIC INTERVENTIONS** • Acknowledge emotional response. • Encourage verbalization if possible. • Provide other emotional outlets: Drawing materials Dolls Play therapy *A child may not possess the verbal skills necessary to describe an assault or ask for help.* • Facilitate consultations and support systems: Psychiatric Social work Religious • Assist child in identifying and using coping behaviors.	A positive self-concept will be maximized.
Fear/Anxiety **RELATED TO** Physical abuse Emotional neglect **DEFINING CHARACTERISTICS** Restlessness Withdrawal Trembling Poor eye contact Tense/wide-eyed appearance Nonverbal signs	**ONGOING ASSESSMENT** • Assess child and family for level of anxiety. • Assess causes of fears. • Look for verbal and nonverbal signs. • Assess usual coping patterns. **THERAPEUTIC INTERVENTIONS** • Display calm attitude. • Orient child and family to environment. • Provide a quiet atmosphere. • Offer opportunities to verbalize emotions. • Allow significant other to stay with child if helpful. • Provide consistent staff members *to enhance bonding, trust, and continuity.* • Make frequent contact in unhurried manner. • Encourage use of supports: Social worker Division of Children and Family Services Psychiatric liaison • Explain all procedures, especially if they will be painful.	Fears and anxiety will be reduced.

NURSING DIAGNOSES/ DEFINING CHARACTERISTICS	NURSING INTERVENTIONS / *RATIONALES*	EXPECTED OUTCOMES
Altered Parenting: Actual **RELATED TO** Unmet social and emotional maturation needs of parenting figures Unrealistic expectations of child and self **DEFINING CHARACTERISTICS** Lack of parental attachment behaviors Lack of social contact Verbalized lack of control Feelings of role inadequacy Absurd explanations for child's injuries Placing blame on others Indication of neglect, abuse, or unloving atmosphere in parents' childhood	**ONGOING ASSESSMENT** ▪ Assess parents' level of comprehension. ▪ Assess behavior, relationships. ▪ Assess cultural and socioeconomic background. ▪ Assess for existing support systems. **THERAPEUTIC INTERVENTIONS** ▪ Provide all explanations at an appropriate level of understanding. ▪ Explain reason for admission and suspicious injuries. ▪ Explore parents' attitudes and feelings. ▪ Report suspicions of abuse to physician, social worker, abuse team; file Division of Children and Family Services report. *While the child may or may not be a victim, a full investigation is necessary to protect the child and initiate treatment for abuser. It is the nurse's obligation to report suspicions to the appropriate authority if an abuse team or social worker is not available.* ▪ Refer parent to support groups: Parents' groups Church groups Hot lines	Parents/caretakers verbalize understanding of current situation and follow up.
Knowledge Deficit: Parental **RELATED TO** Inability to identify parenting supports Inappropriate role models Lack of awareness of normal child development **DEFINING CHARACTERISTICS** Verbalizes unrealistic expectations of child Uses inappropriate learned parenting behaviors	**ONGOING ASSESSMENT** ▪ Assess parent's developmental level. ▪ Assess knowledge of child development: Age-appropriate expectations Reward systems Methods of discipline ▪ Assess current support systems and appropriateness to level of child care required. **THERAPEUTIC INTERVENTIONS** ▪ Provide explanations at level of understanding of caretaker. ▪ Use a variety of instruction methods, e.g., written information, video tapes, group discussion. ▪ Discuss parent alternatives: Babysitter Child care co-ops Family Clergy Schools ▪ Emphasize the necessity for problem-solving and emotional support for oneself. *Stressors other than parenting may influence the behavior of a potentially abusive parent.* ▪ Make appropriate agency referrals: Counselor: psychological, parenting, family Visiting Nurses' Association (VNA)	Parent/caretaker will verbalize appropriate parenting behaviors and identify personal support systems.

Michele Knoll Puzas, RNC, MHPE

Depression

An affective disorder characterized by feelings of unworthiness, profound sadness, guilt, apathy, and hopelessness. A loss of interest and pleasure in usual activities or play is evident. Behavioral characteristics may include a slowing of physical activity or agitation and alterations in sleeping and eating. Depression differs from sadness in that it is a disease rather than a feeling. Depressive features are seen in chronic illness, premenstrual syndrome, alcohol and/or drug withdrawal, and involutional melancholia. Depression may also be reactive and situational, associated with grief and loss of health, independence, or a significant other. Depressive features can be a component of affective/mood disorders, including bipolar (manic-depressive) illness. Suicidal ideation and/or gestures, as well as psychotic thought processes, may be present.

NURSING DIAGNOSES/ DEFINING CHARACTERISTICS	NURSING INTERVENTIONS / *RATIONALES*	EXPECTED OUTCOMES
Self Care Deficits: Bathing/Hygiene, Dressing/ Grooming, Feeding, Toileting **RELATED TO** Psychomotor retardation/agitation Energy depletion Fatigue Weakness Low self-esteem Apathy Poor appetite **DEFINING CHARACTERISTICS** Excessive sleeping, interrupted sleeping patterns, lack of sleep Excessive eating, interrupted eating patterns, lack of appetite Poor hygiene/ grooming Constipation	**ONGOING ASSESSMENT** <ul><li>Assess age and developmental level.</li><li>Assess current and past sleeping patterns. Determine whether the child has trouble falling asleep, wakes during sleep, experiences difficulty with both, has early morning awakening, or sleeps longer than is usual for that individual, but still feels exhausted. *Degree of psychomotor agitation/retardation affects particular sleeping pattern impairment.*</li><li>Assess the current and past: Eating patterns: Has the child lost or gained >10 lb in the past year? Energy level—ask: Do you have the energy to do what you used to do? Activity level—ask: Have you been able to see your family? Your friends? Have you had many sick days off from school or extracurricular activities?</li><li>Monitor food and fluid intake.</li><li>Monitor weight regularly. Determine whether there has been a recent weight loss/gain.</li><li>Assess bowel and bladder elimination patterns.</li></ul> **THERAPEUTIC INTERVENTIONS** <ul><li>Encourage an adequate balance of rest, sleep, and activity.</li><li>Discourage daytime sleeping, but avoid *coercing* the child to remain up. *Depression is exhausting. As the reasons for the illness become clear, and as the depression lifts, the child will have more energy.*</li><li>Set firm but gentle limits on time spent in bed.</li><li>Use prn medication to promote sleep.</li><li>Assist in performing ADLs. *Depressed patients are unable to define and balance need for sleep, rest, and activity.*</li></ul>	Self-care skills improve.
Impaired Physical Mobility **RELATED TO** Psychomotor retardation/agitation Energy depletion Fatigue Weakness Apathy (arises from low self-esteem)	**ONGOING ASSESSMENT** <ul><li>Assess current and past energy levels.</li><li>Assess current and past activity/exercise levels.</li><li>Assess child's ability to respond to staff contact when he or she is agitated.</li></ul> **THERAPEUTIC INTERVENTIONS** <ul><li>Emphasize importance of exercise/activity, relationship to improved mental and emotional status. *Depressed patient often believes he or she doesn't feel well enough to exercise; needs to understand the importance of exercise and activity. ("Do not wait to exercise until feeling better; exercise to feel better.") Offer to go for walks or play with child; involve younger child in physical play.*</li></ul>	*Mobility is enhanced.*

Depression cont'd

NURSING DIAGNOSES/ DEFINING CHARACTERISTICS	NURSING INTERVENTIONS / *RATIONALES*	EXPECTED OUTCOMES
DEFINING CHARACTERISTICS Feeling of heaviness Feeling of numbness (generalized) Restlessness Pacing Hand wringing Aimless walking Decreased motor activity Decreased energy for purposeful activities	**THERAPEUTIC INTERVENTIONS cont'd** • Structure schedule of exercise/activities, providing time alone and with others. Involve child in development of schedule. *(Reinforces importance of input and degree of control.)* • Continue to expect child to attend unit activities despite his refusal. • Avoid showing anger or disappointment if the child does refuse. *This will only lower the child's self-esteem further as the child believes he or she has failed again.*	
Social Isolation **RELATED TO** Withdrawn and regressive behavior Impaired communication Low self-esteem Disruption in personal relationships Sexual dysfunction Fear of rejection Fear of failure **DEFINING CHARACTERISTICS** Feelings of numbness, emptiness, and hopelessness Verbalizations limited in spontaneity and quantity Depressed, dull affect Rumination and preoccupation with negative thoughts Feelings of unworthiness	**ONGOING ASSESSMENT** • Assess affect. • Assess eye contact. • Assess spontaneity and verbal frequency. • Assess involvement with others. **THERAPEUTIC INTERVENTIONS** • Encourage relationship by spending scheduled time with child, providing supportive contact. *Patient's self-worth is enhanced by consistent, supportive staff presence.* • Encourage participation in group activities as tolerated. Allow child to leave group situations when contact with others is too anxiety provoking. *Child needs to feel some degree of control over environment.* • Provide positive reinforcement when he or she participates in group activities and interacts with others *(supports child's efforts; helps augment feelings of self-worth).* • Acknowledge child's involvement in daily activities *to validate staff's awareness of attempts at self-help.*	Social isolation diminishes.
Potential for Violence: Self-Directed **RELATED TO** Low self-esteem Depressed mood Hopelessness Repeated failures in life activities Reality distortion Feelings of worthlessness Feelings of abandonment Anger Guilt Actual/perceived loss	**ONGOING ASSESSMENT** • Interview child to evaluate potential for self-directed violence. Ask: Have you felt like hurting yourself? *Suicidal ideation is process of thinking about killing oneself.* Did you ever attempt to hurt yourself? *Suicidal gestures are attempts to harm oneself that are not considered lethal. Suicidal attempts are potentially lethal actions.* Do you currently feel like killing yourself? Have you recently attempted suicide? Do you have a plan to hurt yourself? What is your plan? Do you have the means to carry out your plan? *Development of plan and ability to carry it out greatly increase risk of patient's harming self.*	Potential for self-directed violence is reduced.

Continued.

Psychosocial Care Plans (Pediatric)

NURSING DIAGNOSES/ DEFINING CHARACTERISTICS	NURSING INTERVENTIONS / *RATIONALES*	EXPECTED OUTCOMES

DEFINING CHARACTERISTICS

Verbalized desire/ plan to harm/kill self

Self-destructive behavior

Aggressive suicidal acts

History of self-destructive behavior

History of suicidal ideation/gestures

Expression of hopelessness and powerlessness to improve life

Preparation for "impending death," (e.g., giving away significant possession)

ONGOING ASSESSMENT cont'd

- Assess for the presence of risk factors that may increase potential for child to attempt suicide:
  Formulated plan
  Means to make plan reality
  History of suicidal attempts
  Mood/activity level that suddenly changes
  Giving away of personal possessions
  Adolescence
  Early stage of treatment with antidepressant medication, during which child's mood/energy elevates. *Remember that every patient has potential for suicide.*

THERAPEUTIC INTERVENTIONS

- Provide safe environment. *Suicide precautions are interventions taken to create safe environment for the child; protect child from acting on self-destructive impulses.* Remove all potentially harmful objects: electrical appliances, sharp instruments, belts/ties, medication, glass items. *Maintaining child safety is a priority.*
- Provide close supervision. Be aware of facility's policy and procedures on children believed to be suicidal. *Many facilities require constant observation of suicidal patients.*
- Develop verbal/written contract (age appropriate) with the child stating that he or she will not act on impulses to harm self. Review and develop new contracts as needed. *Child needs to verbalize suicidal ideations with trusted staff. Written/verbal agreement also establishes permission to discuss subject.*
- Encourage verbalization of feelings with appropriate limits. *Depressed child needs opportunity to discuss thoughts/intentions to harm self. Verbalization of these feelings may lessen their intensity. Child also needs to see that staff can tolerate discussion of suicidal ideation; be available to cope with struggle.*
- Develop agreement that child will contact staff when experiencing suicidal ideations.
- In addition to providing safe environment and taking suicide precautions, spend time with child *to provide sense of security, reinforce self-worth* (refer to Suicidal attempt/suicidal gestures, p. 64).

Knowledge Deficit

RELATED TO

Lack of information about depression and treatment

Reluctance to explore depression, indicated treatment

DEFINING CHARACTERISTICS

Questions about depression causes, course, treatment

Questions about specific treatment interventions: antidepressant medication, electroconvulsive therapy (ECT), hospitalization for increased protection

ONGOING ASSESSMENT

- Assess child's/family's understanding of depression and treatment.

THERAPEUTIC INTERVENTIONS

- Instruct child, family, and significant others about depression:
  Causes, related factors (emotional/physical)
  Treatment
  Antidepressant medication
  ECT
  Light therapy
  Structured activity/exercise
  Suicide precautions
  Psychotherapy
- Identify support groups in the community.

Child/family will understand depression and its treatment.

Ursula M. Brozek, RN, MSN; Rhonda Blender, RN, MSN

The dying child

The death of a child puts tremendous stress on all involved— the child's parents, siblings, other family members and friends, and the health care workers who come into contact with the child and family. The stress and fears that the child feels are directly related to the child's age, developmental level, and state of consciousness. The nurse must consider the child's level of understanding and individual reactions plus the concerns, wishes, and health of the parents and family. Nurses who work with terminally ill children and their families or in areas in which deaths are frequent (PICUs, ERs) must also work to care for themselves and their colleagues.

NURSING DIAGNOSES/ DEFINING CHARACTERISTICS	NURSING INTERVENTIONS / *RATIONALES*	EXPECTED OUTCOMES
Anticipatory Grieving: Child and Family **RELATED TO** Terminal illness Critical condition **DEFINING CHARACTERISTICS** Denial of potential loss Crying Guilt Anger Bargaining Depression Acceptance Fear Hopelessness	**ONGOING ASSESSMENT** • Assess child's/family's awareness of child's impending death. *Degree of awareness determines reaction.* • Assess child's/family's state of grieving (denial, anger, bargaining, depression, acceptance). *Individual family members may be at different stages.* **THERAPEUTIC INTERVENTIONS** • Encourage open communication (allows the uncertainty to be acknowledged by all, including the child). • Provide as much information as honestly as possible about the child's condition and expected changes. • Facilitate flexible visiting hours and include all family members if possible. • Encourage parents to provide physical care for their child. • Provide support group information. • Facilitate discussion of final arrangements between parents and child if the child is old enough and discussion is culturally/socially acceptable to parents. *Parents often cannot discuss impending death with their child because it then becomes too real for the parent to accept.* • Allow the child to express feelings, thoughts, questions in a manner that he or she chooses. *The young child/toddler may draw, color, or play out questions and frustrations. Ask the child about his drawings or what he is playing/pretending. Answer questions simply and honestly. Honesty facilitates the child's trust in the nurse.*	The child/family will be supported through the stages of grieving.
High Risk for Powerlessness **RELATED TO** Terminal illness Genetic component to illness Absence of treatment modalities Death of child **DEFINING CHARACTERISTICS** Expression of lack of control Reluctance to participate in decisions Diminished interactions with child Withdrawal Anxiety Anger Aggression Hopelessness	**ONGOING ASSESSMENT** • Assess usual coping strategies and support systems. • Assess feelings of family members. • Assess decision-making ability. • Assess for desire to participate in care. **THERAPEUTIC INTERVENTIONS** • Allow family to vent feelings. • Listen. • Accept parents' rage at feeling powerless. *Anger is often directed at staff, who must recognize the roots of the parents' emotion.* • Enhance power by fostering involvement in child's care and decision-making. Assist with setting and achieving goals, e.g., making the child comfortable. • Point out accomplishments, e.g., the child is more at ease/less fearful when the parent soothes the child.	Feelings of powerlessness will be acknowledged and diminished.

Continued.

Psychosocial Care Plans (Pediatric)

NURSING DIAGNOSES/ DEFINING CHARACTERISTICS	NURSING INTERVENTIONS / *RATIONALES*	EXPECTED OUTCOMES
High Risk for Altered Family Process **RELATED TO** Absence of child Absence of resources Long-term hospitalization **DEFINING CHARACTERISTICS** Inability to meet emotional needs of family members Ineffective family decision-making process Rigidity in roles, behavior, beliefs	**ONGOING ASSESSMENT** • Assess family for defining characteristics. • Evaluate family members for their tolerance limits to exposure to the stimulating hospital/PICU environment. • Assess need for social service and/or religious support. • Assess need for physician/family conferences to discuss prognosis, current status, DNR, organ donation, etc. **THERAPEUTIC INTERVENTIONS** • Encourage family to take rest periods every couple of hours away from the critical setting. • Allow family to vent feelings. • Help family to participate in final decisions that need to be made for child. • Encourage family members to take turns staying with the child. • Suggest that family (other than parents) take temporary responsibility for other concerns: home, laundry, bills, groceries, etc. *This may alleviate some of the parents' stress and give other family members a role.* • Allow parents access at all times. Assist them in holding/rocking their child. If the child has died, remove IV tubes, clean, and dress child in clean gown. Allow the family as much time as they need. Provide a private room if possible. • Encourage participation in community or other resources. *An absence of community or other resources can increase the family's vulnerability to other problems.*	Adequate family process will be maintained.
High Risk for Social Isolation: Parental **RELATED TO** Diminished energy Overloaded schedule Lack of support/resources **DEFINING CHARACTERISTICS** Withdrawal from spouse/partner Reluctant participation in usual activities Verbal complaint of decreased energy Verbal expression of guilt over feelings of pleasure	**ONGOING ASSESSMENT** • Assess family members' involvement and support. • Assess for outlets of stress and emotions. • Assess for evidence of isolation from partner, other family members. • Assess usual coping strategies. • Assess the need for social support. **THERAPEUTIC INTERVENTIONS** • Assist parents in recognizing isolation behaviors. • Allow parents to verbalize feelings. • Encourage parents to communicate feelings with each other and use each other for support. *The intense grief that each parent feels as an individual can obscure the fact that the other is also in great pain.* • Let parents know that the pain of grief is normal, as is the guilt over feelings of pleasure. *Parents must work through these feelings in their own way, at their own speed.* • Let parents know that it is normal to need time away. *Parents need to know that a temporary respite from pain and grief will help them cope physically and emotionally in the long term and that temporarily forgetting the pain does not mean they have forgotten their child.*	Risks for social isolation will be reduced.
Knowledge Deficit: Child and Family **RELATED TO** Terminal illness Impending death Actual death	**ONGOING ASSESSMENT** • Assess child and family for extent of knowledge. • Assess developmental level of child and desire for understanding. • Assess parents'/family's readiness for explanations and participation in decision-making. • Assess family's expectations of the nursing/medical staff.	Parents and child will acknowledge situation, allowing time (if possible) for understanding and decision-making.

The dying child cont'd

NURSING DIAGNOSES/ DEFINING CHARACTERISTICS	NURSING INTERVENTIONS / *RATIONALES*	EXPECTED OUTCOMES
DEFINING CHARACTERISTICS Verbalized lack of knowledge/under-standing Isolation behaviors Denial Appearance of confusion Multiple questions	**THERAPEUTIC INTERVENTIONS** • Provide ongoing information about the child's status, as well as what parents may expect as condition deteriorates. Speak in terms that are as simple and honest as possible. • Encourage the family to explain or allow the explanation of death in a manner the child can understand. • If the child is unconscious, encourage the parents to talk to the child anyway. *The child may be able to hear his or her parents' voices.* • Explain all procedures/tests before they are done. • Allow the parents to decide what they expect of the medical/nursing staff when death is imminent. • Obtain clergy if desired to help parents understand the situation and assist in making decisions if necessary.	

Kimberly P. Souder, RN, BSN; Michele Knoll Puzas, RNC, MHPE

Organ donation

Donation and transplantation of vital human organs has become a successful treatment in many cases for patients in end-stage organ failure. Nursing care is directed at identifying candidates for potential donation, assessing and maintaining all vital organs and tissues in functioning condition, and offering the utmost emotional support and information to the family members who are faced with the decision of donating organs from a loved one.

NURSING DIAGNOSES/ DEFINING CHARACTERISTICS	NURSING INTERVENTIONS / *RATIONALES*	EXPECTED OUTCOMES
Decreased Cardiac Output **RELATED TO** Defective vasomotor control Hypovolemia due to: diuretic use in attempt to reduce cerebral edema; hemorrhage; diabetes insipidus **DEFINING CHARACTERISTICS** Bradycardia Hypotension Diminished hemodynamic pressures Decreased peripheral pulses Poor capillary refill Decreased urine output	**ONGOING ASSESSMENT** • Monitor heart rate and blood pressure at least every hour. • Monitor central venous and pulmonary artery pressures at least every hour. • Assess color and body temperature every hour. • Assess presence and quality of peripheral pulses and capillary refill. • Monitor fluid intake and output at least every hour. **THERAPEUTIC INTERVENTIONS** • Administer plasma volume expanders and crystalloid fluids as ordered *to resuscitate fluid status and increase blood pressure.* Document response. • Administer vasopressor agents (e.g., dopamine, dobutamine, epinephrine) as ordered *to maintain or regain systolic BP*, documenting all effects and results of medications. • Assist in obtaining an electrocardiogram. • Send serum cardiac enzymes for study *to help determine cardiac functioning.*	Potential transplantable organs will be free of complication and kept well perfused as evidenced by hemodynamic measurements.

Continued.

Organ donation cont'd

NURSING DIAGNOSES/ DEFINING CHARACTERISTICS	NURSING INTERVENTIONS / *RATIONALES*	EXPECTED OUTCOMES
Impaired Gas Exchange **RELATED TO** Apnea Brain death Aspiration pneumonia **DEFINING CHARACTERISTICS** Peripheral cyanosis Decreased ABGs Diminished pulmonary function	**ONGOING ASSESSMENT** • Assess child's chest expansion and breath sounds. • Monitor ABGs. • Assess child's color, noting any cyanosis to lips, nailbeds, or mucous membranes. • Assess for signs of subcutaneous emphysema. • Assess sputum characteristics and document. • Monitor mechanical ventilation. **THERAPEUTIC INTERVENTIONS** • Assist with intubation or reintubation if necessary. • Obtain chest x-ray film *to determine proper placement of ETT as well as pulmonary status.* • Maintain patency of ETT by suctioning tracheobronchial secretions as needed using sterile technique. • Obtain sputum cultures. • Reposition child at least every 2 hours and perform chest physiotherapy *to facilitate lung expansion.*	Adequate gas exchange will be maintained.
Hish Risk for Fluid Volume Deficit **RELATED TO** Diabetes insipidus **DEFINING CHARACTERISTICS** Increased urine output Decreased specific gravity Increased serum electrolyte levels	**ONGOING ASSESSMENT** • Assess vital signs at least every hour. • Monitor intake/output hourly or more frequently if needed. • Monitor urine characteristics and document. • Monitor urine specific gravity every 2 hours. • Monitor serum and urine electrolytes every 4 hours. • Weigh child daily if possible. **THERAPEUTIC INTERVENTIONS** • Obtain urinalysis and urine culture. • Administer IV fluids as ordered *to prevent hypovolemia.* • Administer vasopressin as ordered *for its antidiuretic effect.* Document results. (See Diabetes insipidus, p. 332.)	Adequate fluid status will be maintained.
Ineffective Thermoregulation **RELATED TO** Loss of hypothalamic function **DEFINING CHARACTERISTICS** Decreasing temperature Poor color Bradycardia	**ONGOING ASSESSMENT** • Monitor body temperature and heart rate hourly. • Monitor skin color. **THERAPEUTIC INTERVENTIONS** • Keep child's room warm; minimize drafts. • Utilize warming devices, e.g., hypothermia blankets, overhead warmers, warm packs *to prevent cardiac and/or renal complications.*	Body core temperature will be maintained above 34° C (93.2° F).
High Risk for Infection **RELATED TO** Tracheobronchial suctioning Indwelling catheters Existing wounds	**ONGOING ASSESSMENT** • Monitor temperature and heart rate every hour. • Monitor tracheobronchial secretion characteristics. • Monitor wound drainage characteristics. • Monitor results of CBC, differential, and blood culture. • Monitor urine for cloudiness.	Child will be free of infection.

NURSING DIAGNOSES/ DEFINING CHARACTERISTICS	NURSING INTERVENTIONS / *RATIONALES*	EXPECTED OUTCOMES
DEFINING CHARACTERISTICS Elevated temperature Redness Pain Purulent drainage or secretions Elevated WBC Cloudy urine	**THERAPEUTIC INTERVENTIONS** • Use sterile technique when suctioning ETT. • Use one-piece ET suction catheter if possible. • Use aseptic technique when performing indwelling Foley catheter care. • Use antibacterial preparation and occlusive sterile dressings over IV insertion sites. • Obtain specimens for sputum, blood, and urine culture. • Administer antibiotics as ordered. • Reposition child every 2 hours and perform chest physiotherapy. • Keep skin clean and dry. • Use good handwashing techniques. *Immune response is significantly depleted; infections complicate organ maintenance and transplantation.*	
High Risk for Impairment of Skin Integrity **RELATED TO** Immobility Decreasing cardiac function Poor perfusion **DEFINING CHARACTERISTICS** Redness Drainage Cool to touch Open wounds/lesions	**ONGOING ASSESSMENT** • Assess skin color, temperature, turgor, elasticity. • Document preexisting lesions. **THERAPEUTIC INTERVENTIONS** • Keep skin clean/dry. • Perform massage to dependent areas. • Apply lotion to skin. • Use appropriate pressure-relieving devices. • Reposition the child every 2 hours.	Integument will be free of impairment.
High Risk for Ineffective Coping (Posttrauma Response) **RELATED TO** Traumatic accident involving child Being informed of child's brain death Being faced with the decision of organ and/or tissue donation **DEFINING CHARACTERISTICS** Emotional outbursts Excessive crying Withdrawal Hostility Aggression Anxiety Sleep pattern disturbance GI irritability Depression	**ONGOING ASSESSMENT** • Assess family members' knowledge of child's condition. • Assess family's knowledge of the concept "Brain death" and its implications. • Assess family members' state of emotion: hysteria vs. calm. • Assess family members' physical needs. **THERAPEUTIC INTERVENTIONS** • Offer emotional support to family members, provide privacy. • Request the assistance of the transplant coordinator if needed. If possible, stay with family during initial discussions with physician and transplant coordinator *so conversations/questions the parent may have later can be clarified.* • Request clergy to visit family if appropriate. • Answer questions family members may have regarding the child's condition and organ donation process. Call physician if needed to clarify or confirm child's status. • Encourage family to express their opinions about organ and tissue donation. • Be supportive and empathetic of the family members' decision. • Document family members' response.	Family members will be adequately informed and supported in making their decision.

Gail Tipp, RN

Rape trauma syndrome

A response to the extreme stress and profound fear of death that almost all survivors experience during a sexual assault. It refers to the acute or immediate phase of disorganization and the long-term process of reorganization that occur as a result of attempted or forcible sexual assault. Although every survivor of sexual assault has unique emotional needs and responses, all experience rape trauma syndrome. Since a large number of child sexual assault cases involve a caretaker or family acquaintance, the emotional trauma incurred is even greater, because the child's trust and sense of personal safety within the family have been betrayed. This is further compounded if the incidences of sexual assault are repeated, occurring multiple times over a period of time. The expression of emotion and the understanding of the sexual assault will depend on the stage of development of the child or adolescent. Current literature now refers to victims of sexual assault as survivors; this term is used throughout this care plan.

NURSING DIAGNOSES/ DEFINING CHARACTERISTICS	NURSING INTERVENTIONS / *RATIONALES*	EXPECTED OUTCOMES

Ineffective Coping: Survivor
RELATED TO
Sexual assault trauma
 	
DEFINING CHARACTERISTICS
Acute:
Increased anxiety
Hostility, aggression
Guilt
Withdrawal
No verbalization of occurrence of rape/ denial
Abrupt changes in relationships with men
Emotional outbursts (excessive crying)
Sense of humiliation
Long-term:
Repetitive nightmares/reliving the assault
Phobias:
  Fear of being indoors
  Fear of being outdoors
  Fear of crowds
  Fear of being alone
  Fear of men/ women
Reactivated life problems (e.g., physical or psychiatric illnesses)
	ONGOING ASSESSMENT
	▪ Assess age and developmental level.
	▪ Assess for signs of ineffective coping (see defining characteristics). *These defining characteristics are actually normal coping mechanisms that occur immediately after sexual assault. However, if they persist and interfere with the child's recovery, they become ineffective.*
	▪ Assess the need for referrals.
	▪ Identify previous coping mechanisms.
	▪ Assess survivor/family interaction.
	
	THERAPEUTIC INTERVENTIONS
	▪ Provide a calm and supportive environment. Reassure the survivor that he or she has done nothing wrong and is now safe.
	▪ Assess child's understanding of what happened. *Talking with the child survivor may mean an age-appropriate discussion concerning sex and sexuality. Older children may need help distinguishing between consensual sex and sexual assault.*
	▪ Encourage the survivor to express feelings about the experience.
	▪ Validate the survivor's feelings and assist in channeling them appropriately.
	▪ Allow the survivor time to cope. Help the survivor identify coping skills he or she has used successfully in the past (may require caretaker input).
	▪ Assist the survivor in contacting family or significant others who could serve as the best support system.
	▪ Help the survivor regain a sense of control over self and his or her life. At each stage of your interaction, explain what you would like to do and why. Ask permission. *Asking for permission helps the survivor feel in control.*
	▪ Explain procedures and examinations.
	▪ Explain to the survivor and caretaker that in the future mood swings, withdrawal or aggressive behavior, and feelings of anger, fear, or sadness may be experienced and that this is a normal reaction.
	▪ Facilitate the survivor's decision-making process, using active listening techniques.
	▪ Ensure that the survivor does not go home alone when discharged. *The local police department and Division of Children and Family Services must always be notified. If no responsible family member is available, these agencies will make arrangements for temporary care.* (See also Coping, p. 14; Fear, p. 18.)
		Coping strength will be maximized.

NURSING DIAGNOSES/ DEFINING CHARACTERISTICS	NURSING INTERVENTIONS / *RATIONALES*	EXPECTED OUTCOMES
DEFINING CHARACTERISTICS cont'd Reliance on alcohol and/or drugs Sleep pattern disturbances Eating pattern disturbances GI irritability Sexual dysfunction Depression/loss of self-esteem		

Ineffective Coping: Family or Significant Other
RELATED TO
Sexual assault trauma
 	
DEFINING CHARACTERISTICS
Family or significant other blames survivor for incident
Expressions of guilt
Inability to talk about incident
Withdrawal
Aggression, hostility
Anger
Embarrassment
Humiliation
Increased anxiety
	ONGOING ASSESSMENT
	- Assess family or significant others for defining characteristics.
	- Assess current knowledge of situation.
	- Observe current actions of family and how they are affecting the survivor.
	- Assess the need for referrals.
	- Identify previous coping mechanisms.
	
	THERAPEUTIC INTERVENTIONS
	- Provide supportive, calm environment.
	- Explain procedures.
	- Encourage family to verbalize their concerns and feelings. Identify importance of support, understanding to recovery. *Parents/family play a major role in child's recovery. Verbalized negative feelings (e.g., blaming survivor for assault) must be addressed. Survivor should not feel responsible for the assault; nothing justifies sexual assault.*
	- Validate family's feelings and help them to channel them appropriately. Acknowledge the stress that they are experiencing.
	- Provide support and counseling referrals.
	- Discuss with family/significant others ways to support survivor:
	    Encouraging survivor to verbalize feelings *(important for family to keep good open lines of communication between themselves and the child)*
	    Helping survivor resume usual life activities
	    Avoiding overprotectiveness
	    Being nonjudgmental
	    Holding, touching survivor so as not to reinforce feelings of being unclean
	    Helping mobilize survivor's anger; directing it at assailant and away from self
	    Studies indicate that the type of emotional support a sexual assault survivor receives initially has a direct bearing on recovery.
		Ineffective family coping will be reduced.

High Risk for Associated Physical Injury **RELATED TO** Sexual assault	**ONGOING ASSESSMENT** - Assess for injury (see Defining Characteristics). - Assess need for medication (for pain, nausea, vomiting, muscle tension). - Identify evidence collection needed. - Identify orifices of sexual assault: oral, rectal/vaginal. *Caretaker or child can provide terminology they use to describe body parts. Anatomically correct dolls, if available, may assist the child is clarifying what occurred.* - Assess for torn vaginal/rectal tissue. - Assess for other signs of child abuse.	Complications from injuries will be reduced.

Continued.

Psychosocial Care Plans (Pediatric)

NURSING DIAGNOSES/ DEFINING CHARACTERISTICS	NURSING INTERVENTIONS / *RATIONALES*	EXPECTED OUTCOMES
DEFINING CHARACTERISTICS Survivor or caretaker states child was raped/molested Bruises/swelling Lacerations/abrasions Itching, burning upon urination/defecation Bloody or stained clothing Pain Nausea/vomiting Muscle tension/general soreness Vaginal/oral/rectal irritation Scratches	**THERAPEUTIC INTERVENTIONS** • Obtain parent's/guardian's written consent for examination and treatment. Check hospital policy concerning consent. • Collect, prepare evidence as required by law. Refer to sexual assault procedure in hospital policy. • Medicate as ordered for pain, nausea or vomiting, muscle tension, prevention of VD, and pregnancy. *Urine pregnancy test should be done on all female sexual assault victims in the childbearing years to identify preexisting pregnancy; will alter type of medication ordered.* • Perform wound care as needed. • Give tetanus toxoid as ordered. • Provide follow-up care *to prevent complications (e.g., gonorrhea culture, Chlamydia culture, VDRL, pregnancy test in 4-6 weeks, and HIV testing).* (See Child abuse, p. 48.)	
Knowledge Deficit RELATED TO New situation/crisis **DEFINING CHARACTERISTICS** Verbalizes lack of adequate knowledge about procedures, follow-up care Confusion Asking questions Inaccurate instruction follow-through Improper performance Inappropriate, exaggerated behaviors (hysterical, apathetic)	**ONGOING ASSESSMENT** • Assess ability to verbalize questions. • Assess current understanding of treatment, follow-up, etc. • Assess knowledge base. **THERAPEUTIC INTERVENTIONS** • Instruct child (as appropriate) and family as needed regarding: Hospital procedures Police procedures Collection of evidence procedures Medications and side effects Possibility of sexually transmitted diseases and pregnancy Follow-up care Support referrals Child's/family's potential emotions and feelings in future days/weeks. *Providing this information allows survivor and family to make informed choices.* • Provide written follow-up instructions. *Sexual assault survivor receives large quantity of information while in emergency room. Printed instruction/information sheets/booklets very helpful for review at home.* • Provide information to special patients. For very young or mentally impaired survivor, adapt instructions and information to level of understanding necessary. In some cases (depending on the child's age and mental capability) all information will need to be relayed directly to the parent/guardian.	Patient and family will verbalize understanding of procedures, treatment modalities, and follow-up care.
Self-Concept/Body Image Disturbance RELATED TO Sexual assault trauma	**ONGOING ASSESSMENT** • Assess current self-image. • Assess reactions and feelings regarding the sexual assault. • Assess the need for referrals. **THERAPEUTIC INTERVENTIONS** • Provide private and supportive environment. • Show interest, respect, warmth, and a nonjudgmental attitude. Avoid accusing, negative questions. *Much shame about sexual assault arises from the mistaken belief that rape is primarily sexual; thus survivor or significant others may believe that he or she must in some way have provoked or enticed the rapist. Sexual assault is a crime of violence—it is not a sexual crime.*	Positive expressions of self-worth are acknowledged.

Rape trauma syndrome cont'd

NURSING DIAGNOSES/ DEFINING CHARACTERISTICS	NURSING INTERVENTIONS / *RATIONALES*	EXPECTED OUTCOMES
DEFINING CHARACTERISTICS Embarrassment, humiliation Fear Anger Powerlessness Guilt Loneliness Mood swings Withdrawal Difficulty relating to males/females Negative feelings about body	**THERAPEUTIC INTERVENTIONS cont'd** • Listen attentively to convey belief in what the survivor is saying. • Acknowledge survivor's feelings. *Many survivors are filled with guilt and self-reproach.* Remind survivor that she or he is in no way responsible for the assault. Encourage survivor to direct negative feelings toward the assailant and away from herself or himself. • Be aware of your own feelings and attitudes and effect on survivor. • Interview the parent or significant other who survivor wants present. • Provide anticipatory guidance to survivor/family. • Determine and address survivor's special concerns/immediate needs (e.g., concerns about physical injury, pregnancy, STDs, AIDS). • Encourage female staff member to stay with female survivor, if possible, as an advocate. • Explain that patient's emotional and physical responses are normal; may continue weeks after sexual assault trauma occurs. *Sexual assault is ultimate invasion of privacy; much time (and usually counseling) needed before the survivor feels safe, secure, in control.* (See Body image disturbance, p. 7; Depression, p. 52.)	
Anxiety **RELATED TO** Sexual assault trauma Examination Hospital environment **DEFINING CHARACTERISTICS** *Mild:* Restlessness Increased awareness Increased questioning Exaggerated startle response *Moderate/severe:* Restlessness Insomnia Glancing about, increased alertness Facial tension, wide-eyed look Focus on self Poor eye contact Increased perspiration Anorexia/GI problems Overexcited, jittery Expressed concern Trembling Constant demands	**ONGOING ASSESSMENT** • Assess for symptoms of anxiety (see defining characteristics). **THERAPEUTIC INTERVENTIONS** • Have support person stay with patient: Contact pediatric social worker. If available, contact sexual assault survivor advocate. *Role of the sexual assault survivor advocate is to provide nonjudgmental support and immediate crisis intervention to sexual assault survivor.* Offer to call significant other. • Complete most of history and treatment before police questioning, if possible. • Send copy of chart to hospital social service department for follow-up of all sexual assault survivors. • Provide a calm and supportive environment. *Predominant emotion experienced by survivor is overwhelming fear/terror of death. Help to ease this fear by assuring survivor of safety.* • Help the survivor to talk through feelings, concerns about assault. (See Anxiety, p. 4.)	Anxiety will be reduced.

Evelyn M. Lyons, RN, BSN, TNS; Anita D. Morris, RN, TNS; Eileen Banker, RNC

Suicide attempt/suicidal gesture

A suicide attempt is an act that is carried out with the intent to end one's own life. A suicidal gesture is considered an act that is potentially self-destructive, but not immediately life-threatening. A gesture may be a precursor to an actual attempt.

NURSING DIAGNOSES/ DEFINING CHARACTERISTICS	NURSING INTERVENTIONS / *RATIONALES*	EXPECTED OUTCOMES
Injury: Actual **RELATED TO** Self-inflicted wound, trauma, or poisoning **DEFINING CHARACTERISTICS** Open wounds Blood loss Altered state of consciousness Burns Cardiac/respiratory/ neurological dysfunction	**ONGOING ASSESSMENT** ▪ Identify/locate injury and its course. ▪ Assess child's physical status. **THERAPEUTIC INTERVENTIONS** ▪ Maintain open airway and air exchange. ▪ Maintain cardiac function. ▪ Treat physical injuries *in order of seriousness to preserve life.* ▪ Refer to appropriate care plans based on physical findings.	Effects of injury will be reduced.
Ineffective Individual Coping **RELATED TO** Low-self esteem Hopelessness Anger Depression Known psychiatric illness **DEFINING CHARACTERISTICS** Withdrawal Tearfulness Anger/hostility Fatigue	**ONGOING ASSESSMENT** ▪ Interview child, if able, and family, school counselors, coaches, school nurse, peers. Assess for: 　Behavior pattern and familiar coping mechanisms 　Recent changes in behavior and relationships 　Substance abuse 　Physical illness 　Social and family history of suicidal behaviors/attempts 　Prior attempts at suicide 　Events surrounding attempts, e.g., a planned or impulsive act 　Recent losses: deaths, precious objects, divorce of parents, change in schools, move, loss of boyfriend or girlfriend ▪ Determine level of risk and precautions necessary *to maintain child's safety.* ▪ Have child evaluated by a psychiatrist *to determine need for transfer to psychiatric facility when physically stable.* **THERAPEUTIC INTERVENTIONS** ▪ Orient child to environment. ▪ Develop primary nurse relationship. ▪ Encourage the child to ventilate feelings when able. ▪ Maintain a quiet, structured, safe environment: 　Explain precautions. 　Remove potentially harmful objects. 　Provide a sitter if necessary. 　Provide a room near nurses' station. 　Maintain contact at irregular intervals *so child cannot identify patterns when he will be left alone.* 　Use physical restraints if needed. 　Check mouth after giving medications. 　Explain safety precautions to visitors or other hospital personnel in contact with the child. ▪ Provide a suitable environment for psychiatric interviews/evaluation. *A quiet, private area with no interruption is most conducive to family/ child interviews. Privacy should be maintained if the interview needs to be conducted with the child in bed.* ▪ Report changes in behavior or mood. ▪ Consult psychiatric liaison or nurse specialist as needed. ▪ Provide assurance to child and family of plan to protect child from suicidal attempts.	Healthy coping skills are developed and used.

NURSING DIAGNOSES/ DEFINING CHARACTERISTICS	NURSING INTERVENTIONS / *RATIONALES*	EXPECTED OUTCOMES
Self-Concept Disturbance **RELATED TO** Low self-esteem Feelings of worthlessness Poor body image Guilt Psychiatric disorder **DEFINING CHARACTERISTICS** Lack of self-care behaviors Self-depreciating remarks Verbalized hopelessness, guilt, worthlessness Suicidal ideation Social withdrawal Truancy	**ONGOING ASSESSMENT** • Assess current behaviors. • Assess expressed feelings and perceptions of self. (See Body image disturbance, p. 7.) **THERAPEUTIC INTERVENTIONS** • Allow expression of feelings. *Do not make judgments about feelings; this may further damage self-concept.* • Provide supportive physical care when necessary. • Encourage positive activities and provide positive feedback when it is warranted. *Only honest expressions of positive accomplishment promote a trusting relationship on which the child can rely.* • Encourage participation in self-care activities. • Reinforce child's and family's strengths. • Use play as a means to encourage the working-out and expression of feelings (especially with very young children).	Positive expressions of self-worth are acknowledged.
Knowledge Deficit: Child and/or Family **RELATED TO** No previous experience with suicide Hospital environment Diagnosis **DEFINING CHARACTERISTICS** Expressed lack of awareness Helplessness Questioning Avoidance/withdrawal Embarrassment Fear Anxiety Denial	**ONGOING ASSESSMENT** • Assess past history. • Assess current understanding of problem, treatment, and prognosis. • Assess current ability to listen and discuss needs. **THERAPEUTIC INTERVENTIONS** • Provide information at appropriate times and at level of comprehension. • Provide referrals as necessary: Social work Psychiatric Hot lines Self-help groups Clergy • Provide information about early warning signs of inability to adapt to loss: Sleep disturbances Weight changes Agitation, excessive irritability, decreased frustration tolerance to stress Guilt Thoughts of death Giving away belongings No future objectives/goals Loss of interest in self-care activities or previously enjoyed activities Excessive fatigue • Discuss suicidal gestures: Frequent accidents Overdoses Inadequate or no food intake • Discuss increased risk with decreased social network: No supportive relationships Changes in number/type of friends Perceived inability to ask for help • Discuss necessity of follow-up care. Provide appointments and phone numbers.	Patient and family will verbalize understanding of signs of potential risk of suicide and treatment approaches available.

Janet L. McCants, RN, BSN; Suzanne M. DeFabiis, RN, MS

Developmental enhancement

Interactions that can be visual, tactile, auditory, vestibular, olfactory, and/or gustatory in nature and that will enhance the development of infants in a neonatal intensive care unit.

NURSING DIAGNOSES/ DEFINING CHARACTERISTICS	NURSING INTERVENTIONS / *RATIONALES*	EXPECTED OUTCOMES
Sensory-Perceptual Alteration: Visual **RELATED TO** Excessive or insufficient environmental stimuli **DEFINING CHARACTERISTICS** No eye-to-eye contact Gazes without focus Unattentive	**ONGOING ASSESSMENT** ▪ Review infant's history for possible neurological deficits. ▪ Assess infant's level of receptiveness: Is infant in an alert state? (e.g., bright eyes, follows voice with head and eyes). Is infant using time-out signals? (e.g., sighs, looks away, yawns, skin color or respiratory rate changes). Is the infant stable? (e.g., stable heart rate, color pink, stable oxygen saturation). **THERAPEUTIC INTERVENTIONS** ▪ Encourage establishment of eye contact when possible. *This enables the infant to develop attachment behavior with caretaker.* ▪ Reduce bright lights when possible. Place blanket over isolette. *Alert periods are enhanced.* ▪ Use appropriate visual tools: Organize visual field. *Linear movement with removal of excess items from the field enhances visual perception.* Create black-and-white visual devices that can be used for term infants and older. *These tools attract infant's attention.* Present a visual mobile, preferably black and white geometric shape. Encourage reaching behavior (extension of toes and fingers) in term and older infants. *Visual abilities are enhanced by these activities.* Make big, funny faces at infants. *Provides motor imitation at term, but not before.*	Optimal ability for infant to benefit from appropriate visual stimulation will be achieved.
Sensory-Perceptual Alteration: Tactile **RELATED TO** Excessive or insufficient environmental stimuli **DEFINING CHARACTERISTICS** Cries inappropriately Responds only when procedures are done Easily stimulated/hyperactive Hypoactive	**ONGOING ASSESSMENT** ▪ Assess for presence or absence of defining characteristics. (See previous assessment for sensory-perceptual alteration: visual.) **THERAPEUTIC INTERVENTIONS** ▪ Lightly stroke the infant's whole body with your warm hands in a head-to-toe and a central-to-distal direction. *Myelinization is enhanced and comfort is provided by skin-to-skin warmth (decreases muscle tone, heart rate, and respiratory rate).* ▪ Provide alternative textures for head-to-toe stroking (e.g., cotton, sheepskin, velvet, smooth/rough, flat/raised, warm/cold, sticky/slick, wet/dry). *Different textures provide new sensations.* (Limit to no more than three textures at a time.) ▪ Provide pacifier for sucking. *Sucking is an important tactile sensation.* ▪ Position hand near mouth to encourage self-comforting.	Optimal ability of infant to benefit from tactile stimulation will be achieved.
Sensory-Perceptual Alteration: Auditory **RELATED TO** Insufficient or excessive environmental stimuli	**ONGOING ASSESSMENT** ▪ Review patient's medication history for possible ototoxic medication usage. (See previous assessment for sensory-perceptual alteration: visual.)	Infant's ability to benefit from appropriate auditory stimulation will be maximized.

NURSING DIAGNOSES/ DEFINING CHARACTERISTICS	NURSING INTERVENTIONS / *RATIONALES*	EXPECTED OUTCOMES

DEFINING CHARACTERISTICS
Does not turn head toward noise stimulus (accurate localization at 3 months)
Lack of body response to noise
Decreased alertness
	THERAPEUTIC INTERVENTIONS
	• Talk to infant. Encourage parents to talk to infant. Use maternal/paternal voices (tape recorded if prolonged hospitalization is necessary) while infant is awake or asleep. Use adult or baby talk conversations, preferably slow speech with many inflections. *Infant begins to recognize parents by voice and displays attachment behavior toward them.*
	• Use items emitting agreeable sounds (e.g., music boxes, radios, ticking clocks). *Encourages vocalization and imitation behavior.*
	• Call infant by name. Speak to infant while handling. *Assists in infant's development of self- and name-recognition.*
	• Hold infant close so your heartbeat can be heard (e.g., carry in a strap-on infant sack). *Encourages attachment behaviors.*
	• Reduce excessive auditory stimulation. *Avoids sensory overload.*
	  Lower monitor noises when possible.
	  Avoid excessive conversation around infant bed (e.g., during reports, rounds).
	  Carefully and quietly handle equipment, cabinet drawers, and doors.
	  Keep water drained out of oxygen tubing.	

Sensory-Perceptual Alteration: Vestibular **RELATED TO** Excessive or insufficient environmental stimuli **DEFINING CHARACTERISTICS** Poor growth and development Absent or decreased grasp reflex	**ONGOING ASSESSMENT** • Review patient's history for possible muscular or neurological deficits. • Plot weight gain along Dancis curve/growth curve for appropriate growth curve. (See previous assessment for Sensory-perceptual alteration: visual.) **THERAPEUTIC INTERVENTIONS** • Use oscillating water bed. Limit oscillations of bed to 10/min with rest period. *Oscillations at intervals improves respiratory function.* • Use front-to-back rocking. Lift infant's head from supine to upright position along with side-to-side body movement. *Linear stimulation improves motor growth.* • Use infant swing or rocker for slow, rocking, rhythmic movement. *This type of stimulation improves motor development.* • Perform passive flexion and extension of hips, arms, and legs several times per day. *Exercise enhances muscle control and growth. In addition, it improves the infant's interaction ability.* • Reposition infant at intervals in side-lying or prone positions; provide boundaries for infant (rolled blankets, egg crates, etc.) *to maintain flexion.* • Place a holdable object (e.g., a ball) in infant's hand; encourage infant to close fist around object (grasp reflex fully developed at 32 weeks' gestation). *Enhanced grasp reflex enables self-stimulation in term or older infant.*	Infant's ability to benefit from appropriate vestibular stimulation will be maximized.
Sensory-Perceptual Alteration: Olfactory and Gustatory **RELATED TO** Excessive or insufficient environmental stimuli **DEFINING CHARACTERISTICS** Unresponsive to feeding needs Lack of hand-mouth contact Poor suck reflex	**ONGOING ASSESSMENT** • Assess for absence or presence of defining characteristics. (See previous assessment for Sensory-perceptual alteration: visual.) **THERAPEUTIC INTERVENTIONS** • Provide mother's milk as often as available. Allow infant to smell breast milk container. *Enhances recognition of mother by smell.* • Place infant's hand or pacifier in mouth. Position it so it cannot fall out when sucking movements are observed. *Initiates olfactory-mediated movements—increases alertness, slight flexion movements of extremities, and facial expression change. Infant's self-regulated sucking and saliva production is increased. Enhances hand-mouth contact.* • Place infant in anatomical position. Swaddle infant. • Offer a taste of milk on pacifier with tube feeding. *Stimulates olfactory and gustatory activity.*	Infant's ability to benefit from appropriate olfactory and gustatory stimulation will be maximized.

Continued.

Psychosocial Care Plans (Neonatal)

NURSING DIAGNOSES/ DEFINING CHARACTERISTICS	NURSING INTERVENTIONS / *RATIONALES*	EXPECTED OUTCOMES

High Risk for Altered Parenting **RELATED TO** Infant's hospitalization Knowledge deficit **DEFINING CHARACTERISTICS** Excessive questions Increased anxiety Failure to name infant Excessive or infrequent telephone-calling patterns Verbal/nonverbal expressions regarding infant's condition	**ONGOING ASSESSMENT**
	• Assess degree of parental understanding.
	• Assess parents' support system:
	  Two-parent family
	  Other family member
	  Friends/peers
	• Assess growth and development of infant.
	• Assess extent of parents' involvement with infant.
	
	THERAPEUTIC INTERVENTIONS
	• Instruct in techniques for visual, tactile, auditory, vestibular, olfactory, and gustatory stimulation. *Instruction promotes parents' participation in infant care and increases confidence in caretaking abilities.*
	• Instruct parents on cues that display that infant is attentive. *An attentive state is the optimal time to provide stimulation:*
	  Slows or stops sucking
	  Face brightens
	  Opens eyes
	  Looks at or turns toward you or object
	  Stretches fingers or toes toward you or object
	  Stops movement or squirming
	• Explain infant's time-out signals (cues that infant has had enough stimulation). *Determination of time-out signals is important:*
	  Begins to move arms and legs
	  Squirms
	  Looks away from you or objects
	  Starts to cry
	  Becomes irritable
	• Explain recognizable signs of effective stimulation. *Encourages awareness of infant's abilities as well as accomplishment:*
	  Consistent weight gain
	  Longer periods of wakefulness following feedings
	  Establishment of regular sleep pattern
	  Infant recognizes parents and smiles sooner
	• Provide parents with handout regarding the previous four interventions for review at their leisure. *Written material supports instruction.*
		Parental ability to demonstrate developmental enhancement techniques will be observed.

Phyllis Lawlor-Klean, RN, MS

Grieving for terminally ill neonate

A state in which an individual grieves before and after the actual loss of an infant.

NURSING DIAGNOSES/ DEFINING CHARACTERISTICS	NURSING INTERVENTIONS / *RATIONALES*	EXPECTED OUTCOMES

Anticipatory Grieving: By the Family **RELATED TO** Infant's moribund condition Perceived potential loss of significant other **DEFINING CHARACTERISTICS** Repetitious and inappropriate questions Inability to comprehend explanations Fear of touching or reluctance to touch infant Infrequent calls and visits Silence Critical about care given to infant Denial of potential loss Altered sleeping pattern Altered communication among family members Crying, sadness, silence	**ONGOING ASSESSMENT**
	• Assess infant's condition.
	• Assess family's condition:
	  Involvement with the infant
	  Response to infant's condition
	  Existing support system
	  History of other losses, including perinatal losses
	  Needs for referral to other services, e.g., social service
	
	THERAPEUTIC INTERVENTIONS
	• Communicate with family daily. Adjust the frequency of these contacts, depending on infant's condition.
	• If the mother remains hospitalized, contact the nurse caring for the mother *to facilitate communication with the family.*
	• Give the parents a picture of the baby.
	• Encourage parents to:
	  Name the infant
	  Visit with siblings and other family members
	  Hold the infant
	  Photograph the infant with or without the family members
	• Allow parents to spend extended periods of uninterrupted time with the infant. *This will help the parents accept the terminal condition and help resolve loss and normal grieving process.*
		Opportunities for anticipatory grieving are provided.

High Risk for Dysfunctional Grieving: Family **RELATED TO** Infant's death Absence of anticipatory grief Lack of resolution of previous grieving response Poor support systems History of multiple losses **DEFINING CHARACTERISTICS** Hostility toward health professionals and themselves	**ONGOING ASSESSMENT**
	• Assess family's:
	  Response to infant's death
	  Way of coping with the loss
	  Existing support systems
	• Assess whether parents are at high risk for dysfunctional grieving:
	  Lack of resolution of previous grieving response
	  Poor support systems
	  History of multiple losses
	
	THERAPEUTIC INTERVENTIONS
	• With physician, inform at least two individuals of the infant's death. When only one parent is present, have one of the professional staff stay with parent. Call a clergyman if parent desires this.
	• Explain what happened. Keep explanations simple.
	• Verbalize your concern by using such statements as:
	  "I don't know how you feel, but I'm sure it must be so painful."
	  "I'm sorry, I know this is a bad time for you."
	  "Is there anything I could do for you?"
	  "Can I call anyone for you?"
	These phrases facilitate the grieving process.
		The potential for family's dysfunctional grieving will be reduced.

Continued.

Grieving for terminally ill neonate cont'd

NURSING DIAGNOSES/ DEFINING CHARACTERISTICS	NURSING INTERVENTIONS / *RATIONALES*	EXPECTED OUTCOMES

DEFINING CHARACTERISTICS cont'd

Anger at God
Guilt
Expression of unresolved issues
Difficulty in expressing loss
Idealization
Crying, rage, depression, fear
Denial of loss
Altered eating habits and sleep pattern
Interference with life functioning
Reliving of past losses

THERAPEUTIC INTERVENTIONS cont'd

- Avoid phrases that will downplay grief, such as:
  "You can have other children."
  "The baby would have been abnormal anyway."
  "The little angel is in heaven."
  "It was for the best."
  "You are lucky you are alive."
  "It wasn't a real baby anyway."
  "God wanted it that way."
- Explain infant's appearance.
- Prepare the infant's body by cleaning and wrapping in a blanket.
- Allow the parents to see the dead infant. *This confirms the reality of their baby's life and death.*
- Provide opportunities for parents to:
  Hold and touch the infant
  Take pictures
  Spend time alone with the infant (stay with the family if so requested)
- Give mementos to the parents:
  Crib card with birth date, time of birth, weight and length of the infant
  Identification bands
  Footprint sheet
  Toys and other personal items
  Lock of hair
- If parents refuse the above items, let them know that they will be kept on file and they can call anytime in the future if they want these items. Then place them in box with name, date of birth, and any other important information.
- Describe burial options. Ask parents if they want a private or a hospital burial:
  Private: Encourage parents to seek assistance from family/friends in planning the type of service. If additional information is needed, refer them to "When an Infant Dies" by Compassionate Friends, Inc. (National Headquarters, P.O. Box 3696, Oak Brook, IL 60522).
  Hospital: Depends on each hospital's protocol. For example, inform parents of the following:
    There is no memorial service.
    The body is buried in a common burial site by the county morgue.
    The city contracts with cemeteries, and the cemetery location may change.
    The parents must go to the Bureau of Vital Statistics to obtain a death certificate, which will have the cemetery location but not the plot number.
    The bodies are in unmarked graves.
- Assist the physician/clinician with autopsy counseling.
- Encourage therapeutic ventilation of feelings.
- Anticipate disturbed behavior.
- Facilitate religious or cultural customs. Be sympathetic and adaptable.
- Demonstrate caring and concern, especially immediately after the loss.
- Use touch *to show support.*
- Send a personalized sympathy card.
- Determine the need for support:
  Call the parents the day after the baby's death.
  Encourage parents to openly discuss and express feelings about the loss. Offer booklets and books to facilitate this.
  Support parents in seeking psychological support from clergy or mental health professional during bereavement, as needed.
  Make a referral to support groups as needed, e.g., Compassionate Friends, The Caring Connection.

NURSING DIAGNOSES/ DEFINING CHARACTERISTICS	NURSING INTERVENTIONS / *RATIONALES*	EXPECTED OUTCOMES
	THERAPEUTIC INTERVENTIONS cont'd Provide anticipatory guidance and support. Let the parents know that they will experience the resurgence of grief on anniversaries, holidays, and other significant dates. Encourage attendance at the autopsy conference in 4 to 6 weeks. *It will help the parents better understand the problems of the baby and will assist them in family planning.*	
High Risk for Dysfunctional Grieving: Siblings **RELATED TO** Infant's death Absence of anticipatory grieving Lack of resolution of previous grieving response **DEFINING CHARACTERISTICS** *Less than 4 years old:* Regressive behavior May have nightmares Fear of separation *4-6 years old:* May think they will die Become more dependent Magical thinking that leads to guilt Unable to comprehend the finality of death *7-11 years old:* Acting-out behavior School problems More sensitive to relationships *11 and older:* Aware of others' feelings Sensitive Understands that death is final	**ONGOING ASSESSMENT** • Assess the chronological and psychological ages of the child. • Assess the parents' knowledge of how to inform the child or children of the death. **THERAPEUTIC INTERVENTIONS** • Reinforce the importance of sibling visitation before the infant's death. • Let the parents offer explanations in words the child can understand. Keep explanations simple. • If it is hard for the parents to tell the children about death, have them use appropriate booklets such as: Coloring book: "The Frog Family's Baby Dies" "Where's Jess?" "Tell Me, Papa" • Tell the parents to avoid phrases that could trigger feelings of fear, such as: "The baby went to sleep." *(This could lead to sleep disturbance.)* "God took the baby to heaven because He loved or needed the baby more than we did." *(This may cause resentment against God or a conflict in the child.)* • Reassure the child that the infant had a problem that the sibling will not acquire. • Explain to the child that no family member could have caused or prevented the death by their actions, thoughts, and wishes. *Children may believe that their wishes or thoughts may have caused the infant's death.* • Help siblings understand what death means by: Relating death to stories, books, miniatures, drawings, etc. Reminding them of a dead animal or fading flowers. Reminding them of what living means (e.g., breathing and walking) and that absence of these signs means death. • Advise the parents to let the child or children go to the funeral. *This will help resolve loss and confirm reality of death.* If they don't want to, don't insist. Explain the ritual. Let an adult close to the child accompany him or her to answer questions and to reassure the child if he or she becomes fearful. • Encourage parents to express emotions with the children.	Potential for siblings' dysfunctional grieving will be reduced.

Digna S. Limjoco, RN

Parenting in special care nursery

Changes in ability of nurturing figure(s) to create an environment that promotes the optimal growth and development of another human being.

NURSING DIAGNOSES/ DEFINING CHARACTERISTICS	NURSING INTERVENTIONS / *RATIONALES*	EXPECTED OUTCOMES

Altered Parenting RELATED TO
 	
Separation/hospitalization of infant
 	
DEFINING CHARACTERISTICS
 	
Expresses verbal/ nonverbal fear/anxiety with intensive care environment
 	
Exhibits reluctance to look at infant or come close to bedside
 	
Verbalizes concern that infant may be in pain
 	
Holds unrealistic view of infant's condition/illness
 	
Blames self for infant's condition
 	
Does not demonstrate parental attachment behaviors
 	
Verbalizes resentment toward infant
 	
Verbalizes guilt feelings for having a "less than perfect" infant
 	
Does not visit or call regularly
 	
Delays naming infant
	ONGOING ASSESSMENT
	
	- Assess parents':
	  Developmental stage
	  Feelings regarding impact of pregnancy on the family
	  Level of anxiety
	  Existing support system
	  Cultural background
	  Knowledge of illness or condition
	  Educational level
	
	THERAPEUTIC INTERVENTIONS
	
	- Determine parents' understanding of why infant is in neonatal intensive care unit. *This provides an opportunity to dispel myths.*
	- Explain to parents:
	  Reasons for admission
	  Equipment used/environment
	  Support facilitator
	  Noise level
	- Familiarize parents with staff of NICU *to increase comfort with unit and begin to develop relationships.*
	- Encourage reading of parent booklet *to clarify questions and to decrease anxiety of the unknown.*
	- Offer additional support systems, such as:
	  Social service department
	  Developmental support services
	  Parent support group or parent-to-parent referral
	- Encourage verbalization of perceptions regarding infant *to clarify concerns and provide support systems as indicated, to afford parents the opportunity to share their assessment, and to increase their value as parents.*
	- Encourage parents to touch, kiss, talk to infant. Allow them to hold infant whenever possible.
	- Encourage parents to take pictures or give them pictures of infant *to promote parent/infant attachment and encourage appropriate parenting behaviors.*
	- Encourage participation in basic caretaking skills: diapering, feeding, giving oral medications, bathing, checking temperature, and applying lotion *to promote parenting skills and initiate discharge teaching.*
	- Promote parents' verbalization of feelings.
	- Show parents movies and written materials *to reinforce information and provide emotional support.*
		Ability to parent will be maximized.

NURSING DIAGNOSES/ DEFINING CHARACTERISTICS	NURSING INTERVENTIONS / *RATIONALES*	EXPECTED OUTCOMES
Altered Parenting RELATED TO Inability of parents to visit **DEFINING CHARACTERISTICS** Mother extremely ill Infant transported from another hospital No visiting/telephone calls 24 hours after admission Transportation difficulties Single parent visiting and/or substitute visiting by relatives	**ONGOING ASSESSMENT** ▪ Assess mother's condition after delivery: Check maternal history and type of delivery Obtain report of course of labor Follow up on mother's condition ▪ Assess where parents live and mode of transportation. ▪ Assess economic situation for financial ability to call/visit. ▪ Assess psychosocial situation. **THERAPEUTIC INTERVENTIONS** ▪ Take infant to see mother if infant's condition allows. ▪ Take infant's pictures to parents if in hospital; otherwise send picture. ▪ Arrange to call parents at scheduled times if they are unable to call. ▪ Encourage calling if visiting is impossible *to maintain open communication and knowledge of infant's status.* ▪ Take parents booklet if in hospital; otherwise send booklet *to provide information about the unit and what they may encounter.*	Parental/infant bonding will be initiated.
Altered Parenting RELATED TO Anxiety regarding impending discharge of infant **DEFINING CHARACTERISTICS** Decrease in telephone contacts Change or decrease in visiting Increased anxiety with impending discharge Parents do not call or return telephone calls or are unable to be reached Lack of interest in learning care required to take infant home	**ONGOING ASSESSMENT** ▪ Assess parental support system. ▪ Determine whether parents' degree of involvement has changed. ▪ Determine parents' plans for integrating infant into family structure. ▪ Assess need for referrals to other support services: Visiting nurse Developmental support services Social service Pediatric follow-up Pediatric subspecialty follow-up Follow-up by visiting nurse Follow-up by primary nurses **THERAPEUTIC INTERVENTIONS** ▪ Begin discharge planning and teaching at admission, using the discharge planning tool. ▪ Incorporate parents into infant's care early after admission *to increase parents' comfort with infant care and establish a parental role.* ▪ Document calls and visits on flow sheets and follow up during interdisciplinary rounds *to establish plans, including social service referral.* ▪ Encourage and facilitate open communication between nurses and parents *to develop a nurse/parent relationship.* ▪ Make referrals for follow-up as needed *to provide support after discharge.* ▪ Encourage participation in discharge classes. ▪ Encourage parents to spend extended periods of time with infant *to increase caretaking skills and comfort level with infant.* ▪ Provide demonstration and explanation of special treatments/medications.	Before infant's discharge, parents will demonstrate parental/infant bonding behavior.

Sandra P. Wilks, RN, BSN; Terry Griffin, RN, MS

3

Cardiovascular Care Plans

PEDIATRIC PATIENT
Cardiac catheterization
Central venous pressure (CVP)
Congenital heart disease: medical management
Congenital heart disease: surgical treatment
Pacemaker, external (temporary)
Pacemaker, implantable (permanent)
Shock syndrome: cardiogenic
Shock syndrome: septic
Supraventricular tachycardia (SVT)

NEONATAL PATIENT
Cardiac catheterization
Cardiac surgery
Congestive heart failure
Patent ductus arteriosus (PDA)

Cardiac catheterization

Cardiac catheterization with angiography is a diagnostic procedure whereby the internal anatomy of the heart can be visualized. In addition, chamber pressures and oxygen levels can be measured to confirm heart defects (both acquired and congenital) and to evaluate the severity of the problem.

NURSING DIAGNOSES/ DEFINING CHARACTERISTICS	NURSING INTERVENTIONS / *RATIONALES*	EXPECTED OUTCOMES

Patient and Family Knowledge Deficit/ Anxiety About Cardiac Catheterization **RELATED TO** New procedure **DEFINING CHARACTERISTICS** Increased anxiety level Asking many questions Expressing hesitancy or nervousness about test Restlessness	**ONGOING ASSESSMENT**
	• Assess age and developmental level.
	• Assess child's and family's level of understanding about heart disease and cardiac catheterization.
	• Assess each family member's willingness to learn.
	
	THERAPEUTIC INTERVENTIONS
	• Use educational materials for teaching child and family about heart anatomy and catheterization *to facilitate learning and retention of information.*
	• Explain the details about cardiac catheterization, including:
	  Precatheterization preparation (chest x-ray examination, ECG, echocardiography, laboratory tests, premedication, need for NPO status)
	  Procedure itself and the possible risks
	  Postcatheterization care (vital signs, checking pulses and dressings, need for bed rest)
	• Orient child (as age appropriate) and family to catheterization laboratory *to reduce fear of room.*
	• Support child/family during precatheterization workup, especially while physician is evaluating child, *to clarify and reinforce information.*
	• Encourage family and child to verbalize feelings *to allay fears and clear up misconceptions.*
	• Spend time with child alone explaining the test and the physical feelings experienced during the test (watch videotape of procedure made especially for children) *to help reduce their fears and increase their understanding.*
	• Support family during test if procedure is taking longer than expected and provide information as needed.
		Child and family will express an understanding of the procedure and demonstrate reduced anxiety level.

High Risk for Altered Tissue Perfusion to Catheterized Extremity **RELATED TO** Arterial or venous spasm Thrombus formation **DEFINING CHARACTERISTICS** Decreased or absent peripheral pulses Decreased temperature of affected extremity Mottling, pallor, or cyanosis of affected extremity Decreased sensation in affected extremity Decreased movement of affected extremity	**ONGOING ASSESSMENT** *Precatheterization:* • Assess and record presence of peripheral pulses; mark pedal pulses with an *X.* • If pulses are markedly decreased, obtain Doppler reading *to check for pulse quality or absence.* • Assess and record skin temperature, color, and capillary refill of all extremities. • Assess and record movement and sensation of all extremities. *Postcatheterization:* • Assess and monitor affected extremities for pulse, skin color, temperature, and sensation every 15 min × 4 hours; every 30 min × 2 hours; then every hour until stable. • Assess catheterization site for swelling. • If bilateral sites are present, mark dressing as venous or arterial site. **THERAPEUTIC INTERVENTIONS** • Notify physician immediately of any decrease or change in the characteristics of affected extremity. • If arterial leg has decreased perfusion, warm contralateral leg. *Heat decreases oxygen consumption and increases flow of blood to opposite extremity.* • If venous leg has decreased perfusion, elevate *to increase venous return.*	Tissue perfusion in affected extremity will be maintained.

Continued.

Cardiac catheterization cont'd

NURSING DIAGNOSES/ DEFINING CHARACTERISTICS	NURSING INTERVENTIONS / *RATIONALES*	EXPECTED OUTCOMES
	THERAPEUTIC INTERVENTIONS cont'd • Maintain child on strict bed rest for 6 hours with lower extremities straight. With neonates and infants, place armboard behind knee to straighten extremity. *This allows circulation to flow freely, thus decreasing thrombus formation.*	
Ineffective Breathing Pattern/ Impaired Gas Exchange **RELATED TO** Sedation **DEFINING CHARACTERISTICS** Increase or decrease in respiratory rate Decreased lung expansion Limpness or unresponsiveness Changes in mental status	**ONGOING ASSESSMENT** *Precatheterization:* • Assess age, weight, and height of patient (as well as any allergies) before administering sedative *so proper amount is given.* • Auscultate lungs for quality of respirations. *Postcatheterization:* • Assess respiratory rate. • Assess aeration bilaterally. • Assess child's responsiveness. **THERAPEUTIC INTERVENTIONS** • Encourage child to breathe deeply and to change position frequently. • Notify physician of any change in respiratory status. • If respiratory effort decreases, begin emergency measures as needed.	Optimal gas exchange will be maintained.
High Risk for Bleeding **RELATED TO** Disruption of vessel integrity Heparin administration during cardiac catheterization **DEFINING CHARACTERISTICS** Bleeding on dressing Increased HR, respiratory rate; decreased BP Hematoma at cannulation site Restlessness	**ONGOING ASSESSMENT** • Assess insertion site and dressing for bleeding every 15 min × 4 hours; every 30 min × 2 hours; then every hour until stable. • Assess vital signs and monitor changes. • If bleeding is excessive, notify physician; obtain hematocrit level *to monitor blood volume status.* **THERAPEUTIC INTERVENTIONS** • Maintain bed rest for 6 hours and keep legs straight *to reduce bleeding.* • Keep child flat with only a pillow behind head for 6 hours. • Apply pressure to dressing if child must cough or sneeze *to maintain pressure to site.* • If excessive bleeding is noted, apply pressure to site and call physician.	Risk of bleeding will be reduced.
Fluid Volume Deficit **RELATED TO** Dye-induced diuresis; decreased intake before procedure	**ONGOING ASSESSMENT** • Assess and monitor hydration status. • Assess hemodynamic status. • Monitor urine output and specific gravity every 4 hours *to monitor presence of contrast in system and/or hypovolemia.* • Assess for evidence of dehydration (depressed fontanels in infants; dry mucous membranes; increased specific gravity; decreased skin turgor).	Potential for dehydration will be reduced.

Cardiac catheterization cont'd

NURSING DIAGNOSES/ DEFINING CHARACTERISTICS	NURSING INTERVENTIONS / *RATIONALES*	EXPECTED OUTCOMES
DEFINING CHARACTERISTICS Decreased urine output Increased specific gravity Hematuria Decreased BP; increased HR Dry mucous membranes Depressed fontanels Decreased skin turgor	**THERAPEUTIC INTERVENTIONS** • Notify physician if urine output is poor despite adequate intake *to identify dehydration early.* • Give oral fluids as tolerated. • Decrease IV flow when oral intake is well tolerated *to avoid fluid overload.*	
Pain/Discomfort RELATED TO Bed rest Incision	**ONGOING ASSESSMENT** • Assess catheterized site. • If child is older than infancy, ask if he or she has pain. • Assess cry and child's position.	Pain/discomfort will be reduced or relieved.
DEFINING CHARACTERISTICS Excessive crying Restlessness Unable to comfort	**THERAPEUTIC INTERVENTIONS** • Reassure and comfort child as needed. • Use comfort measures such as bottle, lunch, or television *to relieve discomfort and provide distraction.* • Bring family to bedside to be with child. *Children are comforted by familiar faces.* • Administer analgesics if ordered. • Notify physician of excessive discomfort.	

Susan P. Maloney, RN, BSN

Central venous pressure (CVP)

RIGHT ATRIAL CATHETER

Pressure within the right atrium or in the great veins within the thorax. The CVP pressure is monitored as a guide to fluid replacement in seriously ill children. This venous site also serves as a central site for the administration of medications and as a route for total parenteral nutrition (TPN).

NURSING DIAGNOSES/ DEFINING CHARACTERISTICS	NURSING INTERVENTIONS / *RATIONALES*	EXPECTED OUTCOMES
High Risk for Infection RELATED TO Indwelling catheter; manipulation of catheter or connecting tubing; prolonged use of catheter	**ONGOING ASSESSMENT** • Assess age and developmental level. • Check insertion site for sign of infection. *A foreign body in vascular system increases the risk of sepsis.* • Assess vital signs, especially temperature.	Risk of infection will be reduced.

Continued.

NURSING DIAGNOSES/ DEFINING CHARACTERISTICS	NURSING INTERVENTIONS / *RATIONALES*	EXPECTED OUTCOMES
DEFINING CHARACTERISTICS Redness at site Swelling Change in local temperature Foul drainage Fever	**THERAPEUTIC INTERVENTIONS** • Change IV tubing per unit policy. • Change IV dressing using sterile technique. • Apply antiseptic ointment to site. • Use caps on all stopcock ports. • If infection occurs, notify physician for removal of catheter and infection culturing.	
High Risk for Injury: Fluid Overload **RELATED TO** Excess parenteral fluid intake Inaccurate CVP readings Overestimation of TPN fluid requirements Malfunctioning infusion pump **DEFINING CHARACTERISTICS** Elevated CVP Jugular venous distention Shortness of breath Rales Intake > output Tachycardia Restlessness Weight gain Peripheral or sacral edema Bulging fontanels in infant	**ONGOING ASSESSMENT** • Assess accuracy of CVP measurements. *False low readings can result in mistakenly prescribed fluid administration.* • Assess for defining characteristics. **THERAPEUTIC INTERVENTIONS** • Deliver parenteral fluids at prescribed rate. • Maintain continuous flow of TPN solution via infusion pump. Do not "catch up" infusion rate if "off schedule." • If signs of IV fluid overload are noted, decrease fluid rate as ordered and anticipate diuretic treatment.	Risk of fluid overload will be reduced.
High Risk for Injury: Impaired Catheter Function **RELATED TO** Mechanical impairment (e.g., clotting of catheter) **DEFINING CHARACTERISTICS** Resistant or sluggish infusion of parenteral solutions and blood products Leakage of fluids from catheter or exit site Inability to obtain blood return	**ONGOING ASSESSMENT** • Check continuity of catheter. • Check for patency. • Flush line; note for leakage or resistance. • Observe gravitational flow. **THERAPEUTIC INTERVENTIONS** • Flush catheter per established policy/procedure *to prevent catheter clotting.* • Use mechanical IV pumps *for accuracy.*	Risk of injury will be reduced.

NURSING DIAGNOSES/ DEFINING CHARACTERISTICS	NURSING INTERVENTIONS / *RATIONALES*	EXPECTED OUTCOMES
Knowledge Deficit: Child/Significant Others RELATED TO New procedure DEFINING CHARACTERISTICS Asking many questions Overly anxious Inability to talk about procedure Asking no questions	**ONGOING ASSESSMENT** • Assess learning capabilities of child and parents. • Assess current level of knowledge. **THERAPEUTIC INTERVENTIONS** • Provide child/significant others with information regarding CVP catheter: Purpose Insertion procedure Complications Ongoing care	Child/significant other will verbalize understanding of rationale for use of catheter as appropriate to age.
High Risk for Injury: Pneumothorax RELATED TO Use of subclavian insertion site Patient movement during insertion DEFINING CHARACTERISTICS Shortness of breath Decreased breath sounds on affected side Unequal thoracic wall movement Shift of trachea toward unaffected side	**ONGOING ASSESSMENT** • Assess breath sounds, respiratory patterns, and chest movement before and immediately after insertion. • When checking for catheter placement on x-ray films, note lung expansion. **THERAPEUTIC INTERVENTIONS** • Keep child still during procedure. *Sudden movements increase risk for pneumothorax.* Provide sedatives, local anesthesia, and reassurances as needed. • Provide optimal positioning of insertion area (back/shoulder/subclavian region). • If symptoms of pneumothorax are noted, notify physician and anticipate chest tube insertion.	Occurrence of pneumothorax will be reduced.
High Risk for Injury: Electrical Shock RELATED TO Direct low-resistance pathway of current through catheter to heart Current leakage Improperly grounded electrical equipment Frayed cords, exposed wires Wet skin or bed area Invasive catheters DEFINING CHARACTERISTICS PACs, atrial tachycardia PVCs, ventricular tachycardia fibrillation produced by microshock	**ONGOING ASSESSMENT** • Assess environment for electrical safety. **THERAPEUTIC INTERVENTIONS** • Maintain electrical safety standards when rendering care to high-risk patients: Use as few electrical devices as needed. Substitute battery-operated machines when possible. Keep bed linen dry. Ground electrical equipment *to reduce risk of microshock.*	Risk of electrical shock will be reduced.

Meg Gulanick, RN, PhD

Congenital heart disease: medical management

CONGESTIVE HEART FAILURE

Defects of the heart that children are born with (that occur in utero while the heart is being formed). Depending on the type of defect, many of these children suffer from congestive heart failure. Congestive heart failure (CHF) is the inability of the heart to maintain an adequate cardiac output to meet the demands of the body. Managing CHF medically for a period of time maximizes the child's condition before surgical intervention is attempted. CHF in congenital heart disease can be related to volume loading, as in left-to-right shunting; pressure loading, as in obstructive lesions; dysrhythmias; and anemia.

NURSING DIAGNOSES/ DEFINING CHARACTERISTICS	NURSING INTERVENTIONS / *RATIONALES*	EXPECTED OUTCOMES
Decreased Cardiac Output **RELATED TO** Ineffective cardiac function **DEFINING CHARACTERISTICS** Tachycardia Tachypnea Decreased BP (late sign) Decreased capillary refill Poor color Diaphoresis Hepatosplenomegaly Cardiomegaly	**ONGOING ASSESSMENT** • Assess age and developmental level. • Assess vital signs, perfusion, and child's overall status. • Monitor urine output closely. • Assess quality of pulses; monitor any changes. • Assess apical pulse for heart tones, gallop, and/or murmur. • Evaluate respiratory effort and effectiveness. • Monitor weight and maintain strict I&O *to watch for fluid retention.* • Monitor HR and BP closely (on cardiac monitor) *to note any change quickly.* **THERAPEUTIC INTERVENTIONS** • Administer medication carefully, especially digoxin and diuretics. • Keep child warm and comfortable *to decrease oxygen demands of the body.* • Administer oxygen as necessary *to comfort child and ease breathing.* • Keep head of bed elevated *to ease breathing by allowing good lung expansion.* • Administer inotropic support as necessary.	Adequate cardiac output will be maintained.
Ineffective Breathing Pattern/ Impaired Gas Exchange **RELATED TO** Increased pulmonary blood flow and/or venous congestion **DEFINING CHARACTERISTICS** Tachypnea Retractions, especially subcostal and intercostal Nasal flaring Head bobbing Pallor or cyanosis Harsh cough Restlessness Irritability Dyspnea Abnormal blood gases Rales/rhonchi	**ONGOING ASSESSMENT** • Assess respiratory status frequently and thoroughly. • Monitor blood gas and oxygen saturation levels closely. • Check body temperature frequently. • Assess lung fields for congestion. **THERAPEUTIC INTERVENTIONS** • Elevate head of bed *to maximize lung expansion.* • Administer oxygen as needed. *Mask or head hood is best if child is comfortable. Oxygen will dilate bronchioles to help ease respirations.* • Change child's position frequently and place neck roll behind shoulders *to maximize air entry.* (Sniffing position for infant.) • Provide quiet environment *to ensure rest and sleep to decrease energy consumption.* (Older children should be on strict bed rest.) • Control temperature *to decrease body's oxygen demands.* • Suction as needed *to decrease congestion and secretions.* • Administer diuretics as ordered *to help decrease congestion.* • Correct acidosis if present *to prevent further deterioration.*	Optimal respiratory status will be maintained.

Congenital heart disease: medical management cont'd

NURSING DIAGNOSES/ DEFINING CHARACTERISTICS	NURSING INTERVENTIONS / *RATIONALES*	EXPECTED OUTCOMES
Fluid Volume Excess **RELATED TO** Increased intake Inadequate cardiac function **DEFINING CHARACTERISTICS** Edema—especially periorbital Ascites (late/severe sign in children) Decreased urine output Electrolyte imbalances Increasing weights Diaphoresis Rales Jugular vein distension	**ONGOING ASSESSMENT** <ul><li>Assess weights twice daily.</li><li>Monitor I&O.</li><li>Check electrolyte levels, especially Na^+ and K^+.</li><li>Assess child frequently for overall change in fluid status, e.g., edema or rales.</li></ul> **THERAPEUTIC INTERVENTIONS** <ul><li>Maintain fluid restriction if child is strictly on IV fluids *to decrease chance of fluid overload.*</li><li>Administer diuretics as ordered *to remove excess fluid.*</li><li>Notify physician of increase in weight or inadequate urine output.</li><li>If Na^+ is increased, consider low Na^+ formula *to decrease fluid retention.*</li><li>If K^+ is low, consider supplements, especially before giving digoxin. *Furosemide (Lasix) is a K^+-wasting diuretic that is often used in children.*</li><li>Encourage child to change position frequently *to help mobilize fluids.*</li></ul>	Optimal fluid balance will be maintained.
High Risk for Dysrhythmias **RELATED TO** Inadequate cardiac function and/or medication therapy (digoxin, diuretics, other) **DEFINING CHARACTERISTICS** Irregular heart rate Frequent PVCs or PACs Bradycardia Tachycardia	**ONGOING ASSESSMENT** <ul><li>Monitor ECG strip frequently (every 1-2 hours).</li><li>Use cardiac monitor throughout medication administration.</li><li>Assess heart rate before medication administration.</li><li>If dysrhythmias occur, assess for signs of decreased cardiac output.</li></ul> **THERAPEUTIC INTERVENTIONS** <ul><li>Notify physician of change in heart rate or presence of dysrhythmias.</li><li>Record ECG strip every 2 hours in charting *to accurately document rhythm.*</li><li>Treat dysrhythmia per protocol or as ordered.</li></ul>	Risk of dysrhythmias will be reduced.
Altered Nutrition: Less Than Body Requirements **RELATED TO** Decreased caloric intake and increased metabolic demands **DEFINING CHARACTERISTICS** Inability to take full feeding Decreased weight and height for age Despite increase in calories, child does not gain weight	**ONGOING ASSESSMENT** <ul><li>Assess weight and height against growth chart.</li><li>Assess feeding schedule and any difficulties.</li><li>Assess respiratory status during feedings.</li></ul> **THERAPEUTIC INTERVENTIONS** <ul><li>Provide small, frequent feedings *to provide adequate rest between feedings.*</li><li>Limit feedings to 40 minutes *to prevent stressing infant.*</li><li>Hold baby at 45-degree angle while feeding *to allow maximum lung expansion while sucking.*</li><li>Give formulas or cereals instead of water *to maximize caloric intake and decrease water.*</li><li>Use patience during feedings *to positively reinforce feeding time.*</li><li>Administer calories by NG tube or parenterally if unable to tolerate oral route *to ensure adequate nutritive balance.*</li></ul>	Optimal nutritional status will be maintained.

Continued.

Congenital heart disease: medical management cont'd

NURSING DIAGNOSES/ DEFINING CHARACTERISTICS	NURSING INTERVENTIONS / *RATIONALES*	EXPECTED OUTCOMES
Anxiety/Fear **RELATED TO** Serious condition Prognosis Disease process **DEFINING CHARACTERISTICS** Many questions Parents subdued and overwhelmed Verbalized fear about child's status Restlessness Worry	**ONGOING ASSESSMENT** • Assess anxiety levels of parents and child. • Assess parents' level of understanding regarding problem. • Assess parents' willingness to learn and listen. **THERAPEUTIC INTERVENTIONS** • Provide emotional support to family members and child as needed *to provide reassurance of child's condition.* • Explain rationale for actions taken *to make child more comfortable and to decrease fear of the unknown.* • Begin teaching family at the time of diagnosis how to care for child *to decrease feelings of helplessness.* • Answer questions if possible and notify physician of questions nurse is unable to answer *to reassure family that their questions are important.* • If child is older, encourage him or her to verbalize discomfort and feelings, *so that staff can more accurately provide comfort measures.*	Anxiety levels will be reduced.
High Risk for Digitalis Toxicity **RELATED TO** Decreased absorption and excretion Decreased K⁺ levels **DEFINING CHARACTERISTICS** Nausea and vomiting Diarrhea Dysrhythmias Bradycardia	**ONGOING ASSESSMENT** • Assess for GI upset. • Assess heart rate for regularity and rhythm. • Monitor K^+ levels. • Monitor digoxin levels. **THERAPEUTIC INTERVENTIONS** • Administer digoxin as ordered. Double-check dose with another RN *to ensure that proper dose is given.* NOTE: IV dose of digoxin is two thirds the oral dosage. • Give digoxin on empty stomach *to ensure absorption.* • If child develops signs of toxicity, notify physician. • If digoxin level is obtained, be aware that normal levels can range from 2.5 to 4 mg/100 ml, depending on the infant's or child's age, weight, and normal heart rate. *Digitalis levels are not useful in children unless the level is unusually high or low. It is also helpful to know when the level was drawn in relation to the dose (peak or trough level).* • Administer Digibind (digoxin antagonist) if toxic levels are suspected.	Risk of digoxin toxicity will be reduced.

Susan P. Maloney, RN, BSN

Congenital heart disease: surgical treatment

Congenital heart defects result from abnormal development of fetal cardiovascular structures. The defect or defects may be simple or complex and can involve the heart and/or great vessels.

Simple Defects

Patent ductus arteriosus (PDA): *Occurs when the ductus does not close normally after birth. This defect occurs more commonly in premature infants. Using a thoracotomy incision, the surgeon repairs the patent ductus by suture ties. Mortality is less than 1%.*

Coarctation of the aorta: *Is characterized by a narrow aortic lumen that produces an obstruction to the flow of blood through the aorta, causing an increase in left ventricular pressure and workload. Repair is made through a left thoracotomy incision.*

Ventricular septal defect: *An abnormal opening between the right and left ventricles.*

Atrial septal defect (ASD): *An abnormal opening between the right and left atria.*

Complex Defects

Tetralogy of Fallot: *The most common malformation responsible for cyanosis in patients older than 1 year of age. It includes four defects: VSD, obstruction of right ventricular outflow tract, overriding of aorta, and right ventricular hypertrophy.*

Single ventricle: *A rare anomaly in which a single ventricle receives blood from two separate AV valves or a common AV valve. This is often associated with other anomalies.*

Transposition of great vessels: *This malformation consists of the aorta arising anteriorly from the right ventricle and the pulmonary artery arising posteriorly from the left ventricle.*

Tricuspid atresia: *Characterized by absence of tricuspid orifice and hypoplasia of the right ventricle and the need for an interatrial communication (ASD).*

Pulmonary atresia: *Congenital closure of the pulmonary valve.*

AV canal: *Congenital anomaly of the heart in which the division of the atrioventricular canal in the embryo fails to occur, causing ASD, VSD, and atrioventricular valve incompetence.*

Extracorporeal circulation (ECC): *Complete correction of simple and complex defects sometimes requires the use of extracorporeal circulation (heart-lung machine). A still heart and bloodless field are required for cardiac surgery. The heart-lung machine is used to divert blood from the heart and lungs, to oxygenate it, and to provide flow to the vital organs while the heart is stopped. The major components of extracorporeal circulation are (1) anticoagulation—heparin is used to prevent clots from forming; (2) hemodilution—the blood is diluted to prevent sludging in the microcirculation; and, (3) hypothermia—the entire body is cooled to decrease the metabolic demands during surgery. These factors facilitate extracorporeal circulation and affect postoperative management. Fluid shifts, bleeding, and electrolyte shifts are common aftereffects of ECC.*

NURSING DIAGNOSES/ DEFINING CHARACTERISTICS	NURSING INTERVENTIONS / *RATIONALES*	EXPECTED OUTCOMES
Decreased Cardiac Output **RELATED TO** Extracorporeal circulation and surgical procedure RV failure, LV failure, or biventricular failure **DEFINING CHARACTERISTICS** *Left ventricular failure:* Increased LAP Increased HR, RR Decreased BP, decreased urinary output	**ONGOING ASSESSMENT** • Assess age and developmental level. • Continuously monitor cardiac rate, BP, CVP/RA, LAP. • Assess pulses in all extremities. • Monitor skin color and capillary refill. *Color should be consistent; nailbeds and mucous membranes should be pink (unless unrepaired cyanotic congenital heart disease is present). Capillary refill should be instantaneous unless the child is hypothermic. Prolongation of capillary refill indicates a compromise in tissue perfusion, which may be associated with inadequate cardiac output.* • Assess skin and rectal temperature. *Skin should be warm and rectal temperature should be near 37° C (98.6° F). Younger infants cannot shiver to generate heat. If a younger infant is subjected to a cold temperature, the infant must break down brown fat to generate heat. This process increases oxygen demand and also increases cardiac and respiratory demand. (Hypothermia after a cardiopulmonary bypass procedure should resolve within 1-2 hours postoperatively.)* • Monitor I&O hourly. *(Urine volume should be 0.5 to 2 ml/kg/hr.)* • Monitor changes in ABGs. *Acidosis is an early sign of decreased cardiac output. Report changes.*	Adequate cardiac output will be obtained to perfuse vital organs.

Continued.

Congenital heart disease: surgical treatment cont'd

NURSING DIAGNOSES/ DEFINING CHARACTERISTICS	NURSING INTERVENTIONS / *RATIONALES*	EXPECTED OUTCOMES
DEFINING CHARACTERISTICS cont'd Pulmonary congestion Decreased perfusion and capillary refill *Right ventricular failure:* Increased CVP/RA Increased HR/RR Jugular venous distention Liver enlargement/ ascites Decreased BP, urinary output, and capillary refill Peripheral edema, especially seen in periorbital and sacral areas	**THERAPEUTIC INTERVENTIONS** • Administer vasopressor drugs as ordered: Use infusion pump *to ensure accuracy.* Administer drugs through central line *to ensure absorption and to avoid vascular irritation.* Keep drug calculations at bedside *to ensure accuracy when changing drip rates: desired amount ($\mu g/kg$) × 60 min/hour, divided by standard concentration.* • Maintain hemodynamics within parameters set by surgeon: HR, BP, CVP/RAP. *Hemodynamic parameters may be maintained by titration of vasoactive drugs, most commonly:* *Dopamine:* Increases contractility; vasopressor; increases renal blood flow in low doses. *Amrinone:* Has inotropic and vasodilator effect (monitor liver function and platelet count). *Epinephrine:* Increases contractility, increases heart rate. *Dobutamine:* Increases contractility; may slightly vasodilate. *Isuprel:* Increases heart rate and contractility; decreases pulmonary resistance; useful for RV failure.	
Hypothermia RELATED TO Hypothermia used in conjunction with ECG **DEFINING CHARACTERISTICS** Rectal temperature <37° C (98.6° F) Skin cool with decreased perfusion Tachycardia or heart block Acidosis	**ONGOING ASSESSMENT** • Monitor and document changes in skin temperature, perfusion, and capillary refill; notify physician of changes. • Monitor rectal temperature continuously. • Continuously monitor ECG and maintain pacemaker on standby. **THERAPEUTIC INTERVENTIONS** • Increase body temperature as ordered. Use extra blankets, warming blankets, or warm packs as needed. • Protect skin against burns by providing a layer of protection between skin and warming apparatus. • Place infants under radiant warmers as needed.	Normal body temperature will be maintained.
Impaired Gas Exchange RELATED TO Hypothermia Surgical procedure that adversely affects pulmonary function Atelectasis, pulmonary vascular congestion, x-ray evidence of pneumothorax, effusion, or chylothorax	**ONGOING ASSESSMENT** • Assess chest expansion, breath sounds, presence of rales, rhonchi, and wheezing. • Assess capillary refill, perfusion, cyanosis, sternal and subcostal retractions. • Check ABGs, chest x-ray films for ET tube placement, presence of pneumothorax, effusion, atelectasis. • Use continuous pulse oximeter *to monitor oxygen saturation.* **THERAPEUTIC INTERVENTIONS** • Maintain ventilator settings as ordered. General guidelines: TV —10-15 ml/kg FiO$_2$ —to keep PO$_2$ greater than 80 Rate —16-20/min PEEP—2-3 cm H$_2$O *(Physiological CPAP for child is 2 cm H$_2$O.)* • Change ventilator settings to maintain adequate ABGs within acceptable limits. *(NOTE: Child with preexisting pulmonary dysfunction will have lower PO$_2$ and high PCO$_2$ values.)*	Adequate gas exchange will be maintained.

NURSING DIAGNOSES/ DEFINING CHARACTERISTICS	NURSING INTERVENTIONS / *RATIONALES*	EXPECTED OUTCOMES

Impaired Gas Exchange cont'd

RELATED TO— cont'd

Toracotomy or sternotomy incision (may be painful, causing child to avoid coughing and deep breathing and may precipitate pulmonary complications)

DEFINING CHARACTERISTICS

Increasing FiO_2 required to maintain adequate PO_2

Diminished breath sounds

Asymmetrical or hypoinflated chest expansion

Rales, rhonchi, wheezing

Decreased perfusion, capillary refill

Peripheral or circumoral cyanosis, sternal retraction, nasal flaring

Increasing PCO_2, decreasing PO_2

Rapid, shallow breathing; weak, ineffective cough for intubated child

THERAPEUTIC INTERVENTIONS cont'd

- Perform tracheal suctioning at least every 2 hours and use saline lavage *to loosen secretions.* (NOTE: *Pediatric ET tubes are smaller in diameter and easily clogged with secretions.)* Document amount, color, consistency of secretions.
- Hyperventilate and hyperoxygenate during suctioning *to avoid desaturation.* Inflate lungs gently. Note chest expansion and allow expiration. Listen to breath sounds after each suctioning.
- Tape ET tube in place. As needed, use soft restraints on extremities or place sandbags on either side of child's head *to prevent accidental ET tube displacement.* (NOTE: *Some pediatric ET tubes are uncuffed and easily dislodged.)*
- Unless child is hypotensive, elevate head of bed slightly *to facilitate diaphragmatic expansion and to promote fluid drainage from chest cavity via chest tube.*
- Maintain NGT placement and patency. *Gastric dilation in children can impair ventilation and can also lead to emesis and aspiration.*
- Keep additional ET tubes of same size along with insertion setup at the bedside *for emergency situations.*
- Sedate child as needed *to facilitate adequate ventilation and minimize possible tracheal damage. (Be aware that an ET tube will move with changes in head position—the tip will be displaced downward when the neck is flexed and will migrate upward when the neck is extended.)*
- Keep all appropriate intubation equipment at bedside during extubation *in case reinsertion is needed.*

Fluid Volume Deficit

RELATED TO

Cardiopulmonary bypass (*can cause destruction to many blood cells, causing "sludging" of kidneys, and can also alter coagulation factors*)

Hemorrhage from suture line

Hypothermia

Insufficient fluid replacement

ONGOING ASSESSMENT

- Assess level of hydration:
  Moistness of mucous membranes
  Condition of fontanels (e.g., sunken, flat, bulging)
  Skin turgor
  Urine specific gravity (normal = 1.000–1.020)
- Assess hemodynamic status.
- Assess perfusion, color, warmth of extremities, presence and quality of peripheral pulses.
- Monitor I&O. Include amount of blood drawn for laboratory work.
- Monitor laboratory values (CBC, PT, PTT).
- Monitor chest tube drainage.

THERAPEUTIC INTERVENTIONS

- Administer ordered fluids to maintain filling pressures within set parameters.
- Gently milk chest tube frequently *to maintain patency. Clotted chest tube may precipitate cardiac tamponade.* (Do not milk chest tubes too vigorously—*this can create negative pressure that can injure the heart or lung.*)

Circulating blood volume will be sufficient to achieve maximum cardiac output.

Continued.

Cardiovascular Care Plans (Pediatric)

NURSING DIAGNOSES/ DEFINING CHARACTERISTICS	NURSING INTERVENTIONS / *RATIONALES*	EXPECTED OUTCOMES
DEFINING CHARACTERISTICS Tachycardia Decreased blood pressure, filling pressures, CVP, LAP, RAP Decreased urine output Decreased perfusion, pulses, capillary refill Dry mucous membranes Sunken fontanels Increased urine specific gravity Increased chest tube drainage If blood loss occurs, decreased Hgb and Hct Alteration in coagulation factors (increased PT/increased PTT)	**THERAPEUTIC INTERVENTIONS cont'd** ▪ Notify physician if chest tube drainage is >5 to 10 ml/kg/hr. ▪ Administer blood products, FFP, or platelets as ordered *to correct deficiency.* ▪ Keep cross-matched blood available *in case of severe bleeding.* ▪ Administer vasoconstrictors as ordered *to increase kidney perfusion.*	
Altered Level of Consciousness RELATED TO Microaggregates, clots, air embolism, or anoxia may occur during aortic cannulation or decannulation, causing increased intracranial pressure or cerebral vascular accident (CVA) **DEFINING CHARACTERISTICS** Unequal pupils Failure to awaken from anesthesia Focal deficit on awakening Agitation Seizures Loss of or unequal movements of extremities	**ONGOING ASSESSMENT** ▪ Once general anesthesia wears off, perform neurological assessment *to rule out postoperative complications.* ▪ Check pupils' size and reaction to light. *Pupil constriction may develop after administration of large doses of opiate analgesics (morphine sulfate). Pupil dilation may develop as a result of hypothermia, large doses of atropine, or large doses of sympathomimetics.* ▪ Check strength and equal movements of extremities. ▪ Assess ability to follow commands. ▪ Assess response to analgesics and muscle relaxants, such as fentanyl citrate and pancuronium bromide if used. ▪ Check electrolytes, calcium, glucose, ABGs. **THERAPEUTIC INTERVENTIONS** ▪ Record serial assessments. ▪ Reorient child to surroundings as needed (for older children). ▪ Notify surgeon of any changes in neurological assessment. ▪ Ensure that filters are placed on all IV lines. *(If the child has a persistent right-to-left intracardiac shunt, air can be shunted into aortic and cerebral circulation, producing a cerebral air embolus.)* ▪ If seizures are observed, treat by correcting metabolic imbalance as needed or administering antiseizure medications.	Optimal state of consciousness will be maintained.

NURSING DIAGNOSES/ DEFINING CHARACTERISTICS	NURSING INTERVENTIONS / *RATIONALES*	EXPECTED OUTCOMES
High Risk for Altered Fluid Composition: Electrolyte Imbalance **RELATED TO** Fluid changes; cardiopulmonary bypass; diuretic therapy; volume replacement; changes in acid-base balance **DEFINING CHARACTERISTICS** Na <130 or >140 mEq/L K <3.5 or >5.0 mEq/L Ca <9 or >11 mg/dl Cl <98 or >115 mEq/L Glucose <70 or >110 mg/dl BUN >20 mg/dl Cr >1.8 mg/dl Mg <1.5 or >2 mg/dl	**ONGOING ASSESSMENT** ▪ Observe and document serial laboratory data. Monitor Na, K, Cl, Mg, glucose, Ca, BUN, creatinine as ordered. Notify physician of abnormalities. ▪ Check serum glucose every 4-6 hours with use of chemstrips. *Hypoglycemia may result in seizure or lethargy.* ▪ Monitor ECG changes. Notify physician. ▪ Observe and document changes in mentation, level of consciousness, or presence of seizure activity. ▪ Determine contributing factors (anesthesia, medication) to any changes. **THERAPEUTIC INTERVENTIONS** ▪ Administer desired electrolytes as ordered. *Hypertonic solutions are used to correct Na and Cl deficiencies. Bypass patients tend to retain Na.* ▪ Administer K only if urine output is adequate. *Dilute K and Ca are given via central line over 1 hour to prevent bradycardia or asystole. Be aware that acidosis will produce an increase in serum K and ionized Ca. Alkalosis will produce a fall in serum K and ionized Ca.*	Electrolyte balance will be maintained.
Pain **RELATED TO** Incision Restricted mobility Presence of catheters and tubes **DEFINING CHARACTERISTICS** Facial mask of pain Restlessness Guarding/protective behavior If extubated, loud crying	**ONGOING ASSESSMENT** ▪ Solicit description of pain, using nonverbal communication as appropriate. ▪ Monitor effectiveness of pain medications. **THERAPEUTIC INTERVENTIONS** ▪ Use holding, touching, and soothing verbal reassurances for calming child before and after painful event. ▪ Give pain medications as needed for any painful procedure or during any episode of pain (morphine sulfate, 0.1 to 0.2 mg/kg). ▪ Provide additional comfort measures (position changes, back rubs, distraction techniques). ▪ Provide quiet environment, rest periods *to facilitate comfort, sleep, and relaxation.* ▪ Inform anesthesiologist when child is due to be medicated by caudal catheter. *A catheter is placed in the caudal space. This regional technique provides analgesia without the respiratory or hemodynamic effects of systemic narcotics. A typical dose administered by the physician would be morphine sulfate (Duramorph) 50 μg/kg every 6-24 hours. The catheter can be left in place for 72 hours postoperatively.*	Comfort will be maximized.

Continued.

Cardiovascular Care Plans (Pediatric)

NURSING DIAGNOSES/ DEFINING CHARACTERISTICS	NURSING INTERVENTIONS / *RATIONALES*	EXPECTED OUTCOMES
High Risk for Decreased Cardiac Output **RELATED TO** Use of extracorporeal circulation, which alters electrolyte balances causing dysrhythmias: Premature atrial contractions Junctional escape beats or rhythm Supraventricular tachycardia Atrioventricular dissociation Heart block *(Children very rarely have ventricular dysrhythmias)* Intracardiac repairs that involve valves and/or the septum may interfere with the conduction system **DEFINING CHARACTERISTICS** Irregular heart rate Tachycardia Bradycardia Variations in hemo-dynamic pa-rameters Abnormal electrolyte values	**ONGOING ASSESSMENT** • Assess baseline rhythm and monitor ECG continuously. Note and doc-ument changes by obtaining rhythm strips. Notify physician of changes. • Assess laboratory values on admission and as needed (Na, K, Ca, Mg). **THERAPEUTIC INTERVENTIONS** • Maintain temporary pacemaker at bedside. *Temporary epicardial pacing wires are often placed prophylactically, since dysrhythmias are com-mon. During the first 24 hours, the wires may be connected to a pulse generator kept on standby.* • Use gloves when handling pacing wires. *Pacing wires are on the epicar-dial surface of the heart and provide a direct path for current conduc-tion, which could lead to dysrhythmias.* • Administer electrolytes as ordered. Ensure normal K⁺ level before administering dose. • Treat specific dysrhythmias as described below: *Bradycardia* (may lead to hypoxia and heart block): If immediate, verify that the child's airway is patent and ventilation is adequate. *The most common cause of bradycardia in children is hypoxia.* Rule out an airway or ventilation problem whenever bradycardia occurs. Anticipate atropine administration if bradycardia is symptomatic. Provide demand pacing if external wires are in place. Ensure proper rate and function. *Tachycardia* Administer digitalis as ordered. Ensure that K⁺ levels are normal. *If the ventricular rate exceeds 180-200, ventricular diastolic filling time and coronary artery perfusion time are likely to be compromised, and stroke volume and cardiac output will fall.* *Heart blocks* (most likely to occur following surgery near the conduction system): Anticipate pacing or administration of chronotropic drugs *(isoproterenol HCl [Isuprel] to treat complete heart block with a slow ventricular rate).* *Ventricular arrhythmias* (Uncommon in children. May progress to ventricular tachycardia and fibrillation; multiformed or coupled premature ventricular contractions are worrisome): Ensure that hypoxemia, hypomagnesemia, hypokalemia, and acidosis are eliminated. Anticipate treatment with lidocaine as necessary.	Optimal cardiac rhythm will be maintained.
High Risk for Altered Nutrition: Less Than Body Requirements **RELATED TO** NPO the first 24 hours Prolonged intubation **DEFINING CHARACTERISTICS** Loss of weight Documented inade-quate caloric intake Caloric intake inade-quate to keep pace with abnormal dis-ease/metabolic state	**ONGOING ASSESSMENT** • Assess the need for early nutritional support. • Assess laboratory values: electrolytes, BUN, creatinine, Ca, Mg, glucose, albumin levels. • Assess I&O daily weights. • Monitor patient for evidence of vomiting and diarrhea. • If NG feeding is used, check residual every 4 hours and notify physician of high residual. • Monitor abdominal girth. **THERAPEUTIC INTERVENTIONS** • Provide maximal caloric intake within fluid allowance. *Caloric content of formulas and breast milk may be increased through addition of caloric supplements.* • Following repair of coarctation, feed child slowly, only after bowel sounds are detected. Perform guaiac test of all stools and gastric drain-age *(ischemic gut can occur).* • Maintain head of bed at least 30 degrees when NG feeding *to prevent aspiration.*	Adequate nutritional support will be ob-tained.

NURSING DIAGNOSES/ DEFINING CHARACTERISTICS	NURSING INTERVENTIONS / *RATIONALES*	EXPECTED OUTCOMES
High Risk for Infection **RELATED TO** Surgical incisions Multiple lines and devices Frequent blood draws **DEFINING CHARACTERISTICS** Temperature >38.5° C (101.3° F) Increased WBC Redness around wounds or IV sites Infiltrates on CXR Wound drainage	**ONGOING ASSESSMENT** • Monitor temperature continuously. • Monitor daily CBC; if WBCs increase, check differential. • Assess incisions for erythema or drainage. • Monitor IV sites. • Monitor ET tube secretions. **THERAPEUTIC INTERVENTIONS** • Maintain aseptic technique when entering lines for blood draws or medication administration. • Cap open stopcocks; change if contaminated. • Maintain occlusive dressings over incision and line sites. *Neck lines and sternotomy incisions are prone to contamination from oral secretions.* • Discontinue all invasive lines and devices (IVs, Foley, central and arterial lines) as soon as possible. • Provide vigorous pulmonary toilet. • Draw blood cultures if temperature is >38.5° C (101.3° F). • Change IV bags/tubing per hospital protocol.	Nosocomial infections will be prevented.
Impaired Physical Mobility **RELATED TO** Bed rest, activity restriction Invasive catheters **DEFINING CHARACTERISTICS** Inability to purposefully move within physical environment Limited ROM	**ONGOING ASSESSMENT** • Assess for signs of respiratory problems. • Assess skin integrity for signs of redness, tissue ischemia. **THERAPEUTIC INTERVENTIONS** • Carefully reposition child to sides with use of pillow support *for proper alignment.* (NOTE: *Pediatric ET tubes are uncuffed and easily dislodged.*) • Perform ROM exercises. • Use prophylactic antipressure devices as appropriate. • Clean, dry, and moisturize skin prn.	Optimal physical mobility will be achieved.
Knowledge Deficit **RELATED TO** New condition and treatment **DEFINING CHARACTERISTICS** Expressed need for more information Lack of questions Apparent confusion about events	**ONGOING ASSESSMENT** • Assess parents' knowledge of surgical procedure, equipment being used, postoperative care, expected outcomes. • Observe parents' reactions to changes in child's condition or treatment. **THERAPEUTIC INTERVENTIONS** • Provide parents with information regarding: Intensive care environment and unit policies Rationale behind procedures Routine postoperative care Expected outcomes • Encourage family members to express feelings. • Encourage family's use of support services. • Show concern for family's feelings. • Allow family to participate in care (bathing, feeding, etc.) when appropriate. • Institute discharge planning and family teaching as soon as possible.	Knowledge deficit will be reduced.

Linda M. Kamenjarin, RN, BSN, CCRN; Marian D. Cachero, RN, BSN

Pacemaker, external (temporary)

A device that delivers an artificial electrical stimulus to the heart either via an epicardial catheter, placed in the right ventricular epicardium, a transvenous catheter, wherein the tip of the electrode lies in the right ventricular apex, or a myocardial catheter, in which the straight wire is directly inserted into the ventricular myocardium. Indications include the immediate and temporary relief of bradyarrhythmias caused by surgically induced complete AV block or sinus node dysfunction, and electrical conduction abnormalities underlying heart disease. Epicardial catheters are routinely and prophylactically applied with cardiac surgery repair (e.g., VSD, ASD, tetralogy of Fallot, transposition of great arteries [mustard procedure]).

NURSING DIAGNOSES/ DEFINING CHARACTERISTICS	NURSING INTERVENTIONS / *RATIONALES*	EXPECTED OUTCOMES
High Risk for Decreased Cardiac Output **RELATED TO** External pacemaker malfunction caused by: Pacemaker lead dislodgement Improper placement of pacemaker lead(s) in the myocardium Broken pacing lead wire Poor electrical connections Inadequate pacemaker parameter settings External generator circuitry malfunction Battery exhaustion Improper technique in changing battery Poor environmental and electrical safety measures Pacemaker-induced dysrhythmia resulting from presence of competitive rhythm Unstable pacing and sensing thresholds resulting from exit block (fibrosis) or lead position Postoperative complications resulting from concomitant cardiac surgery (cardiac tamponade, pericardial effusion, etc.) Spontaneous tachy-dysrhythmias	**ONGOING ASSESSMENT** • Assess age and developmental level. • Assess that prescribed pacemaker parameters are maintained (rate, pacing output in mA, sensitivity). • Observe monitor ECG continuously for appropriate pacemaker function: Sensing Capturing Firing (pacing spikes) • Assess for pacemaker-induced dysrhythmias. • If pacemaker is on standby, evaluate pacemaker capture daily and as needed. • Assess for proper environmental and electrical safety measures, *since the pacemaker lead is directly in contact with the myocardium.* • If signs of pacemaker malfunction/dysrhythmia occur, assess child's hemodynamic status until stable. • Observe for signs of cardiac tamponade and pericardial effusion (see Defining Characteristics). **THERAPEUTIC INTERVENTIONS** • Keep monitor alarm on at all times. • Record rhythm strips: Routinely every _____ hours When changes in pacing parameters are made Presence of spontaneous rhythm • If failure to sense is noted, *the pacemaker is not sensing child's rhythm, which could lead to dysrhythmias:* Check that dial is *not* on "asynchronous" pacing (fixed rate). Check for loose connections. Reposition limb of body if lead insertion is through brachial or femoral vein. Notify physician of need to adjust sensitivity dial. Check position of lead by chest x-ray examination. If problem is not corrected and patient has adequate rhythm, check with physician whether pacemaker should be on "standby." • If loss of capture is noted, *the pacemaker fails to depolarize the myocardium:* Check all possible connections. Turn child on left side (endocardial catheter) *to facilitate optimal lead placement.* Increase pacing output (mA) and evaluate for good capture. • If loss of pacing spikes are noted *the pacemaker fails to emit electrical stimulus:* Check that power switch is ON. Check whether needle gauge on pacemaker box is fluctuating. If needle gauge is not fluctuating, replace batteries in generator. Check all possible connections. Check for electromagnetic interference. Replace generator as needed.	Optimal cardiac output will be maintained.

NURSING DIAGNOSES/ DEFINING CHARACTERISTICS	NURSING INTERVENTIONS / *RATIONALES*	EXPECTED OUTCOMES

DEFINING CHARACTERISTICS
 	
Failure to sense
Loss of pacemaker capture
Loss of pacemaker artifacts
Significant decrease in heart rate
Signs of hemodynamic compromise (e.g., confusion, dizziness, loss of consciousness, restlessness, fatigue, hypotension, decrease in cardiac output, decrease in urine output, cool skin)
Signs of cardiac tamponade (e.g., elevated CVP reading, jugular vein distension, distant heart sounds, faint rapid pulse, pulsus paradoxus, hypotension, cool clammy extremities, anuria, altered consciousness, agitation, and restlessness)
Signs of pericardial effusion (e.g., muffled heart sounds, pulmonary crackles, decreased left basilar breath sounds, chest pain, fever, cough)
Palpitation resulting from dysrhythmias
	THERAPEUTIC INTERVENTIONS cont'd
	• If pacemaker malfunction is noted and not easily corrected by the three preceding steps:
	  Evaluate adequate spontaneous rhythm. *(Unreliable escape rhythm will lead to hemodynamic collapse.)*
	  Monitor vital signs every 15-30 minutes.
	  Prepare atropine sulfate, intravenous isoproterenol, epinephrine for standby.
	  If pacemaker lead dislodgement is noted, do not attempt to manipulate pacing catheter for positioning.
	  Notify physician.
	• Maintain proper environmental and electrical safety measures:
	  All electrical equipment is properly grounded.
	  Child is in nonelectrical bed.
	  Environment is dry.
	  Exposed pacing wire terminals and generator are insulated in rubber glove.
	  Free from overlooped terminal pacing wires.
	  If necessary, place mittens on child's hands *to prevent accidental pulling of wires.*
	  Side rails or crib rails up at all times *to protect the child from falling.*	

Impaired Physical Mobility **RELATED TO** Imposed activity restriction secondary to pacemaker lead insertion and need to guard against any tension Medical restriction resulting from concomitant heart surgery	**ONGOING ASSESSMENT** • Auscultate breath sounds and assess respiratory rate, rhythm. • Assess for signs of restlessness and discomfort. • Assess skin integrity. Check for redness or tissue ischemia. • Observe for signs of pulmonary embolism (e.g., shortness of breath, chest pain, tachycardia, fever, cough, decreased BP). • Assess for developing thrombophlebitis (uncommon) (e.g., increased temperature, redness, swelling, calf pain). **THERAPEUTIC INTERVENTIONS** • Turn and position every 2 hours. Watch terminal pacing leads when turning. Avoid right-side positioning if endocardial catheter is inserted *to prevent pacing wire dislodgement.* • Administer passive ROM to nonaffected extremities *to reduce the risks of immobility.*	Complications of immobility will be absent or reduced.

Continued.

Pacemaker, external (temporary) cont'd

NURSING DIAGNOSES/ DEFINING CHARACTERISTICS	NURSING INTERVENTIONS / *RATIONALES*	EXPECTED OUTCOMES
DEFINING CHARACTERISTICS Limited ROM Crying, irritability, expressed anger, restlessness Helplessness Child verbalizes inability to move freely	**THERAPEUTIC INTERVENTIONS cont'd** • Assist the child to sitting position if pacing wire is through the chest. • Ensure that child is on strict bed rest if pacemaker lead is inserted transvenously. Secure arm with an armboard and wrap with gauze if pacemaker lead is in the antecubital fossa *to prevent lead displacement.* • Provide extra tender loving care. Be playful and attentive. Provide toys or stuffed animals *to keep the child occupied.* • Allow mother or member of the family to stay with child unless strictly prohibited.	

Knowledge Deficit: Individual/Family
RELATED TO
Age of patient
Inability to comprehend and understand
Overprotective parent(s)
Misinterpretation of information
New procedure and pacemaker equipment
 	
DEFINING CHARACTERISTICS
Overwhelmed
Increased questioning
Verbalized misconceptions
Overprotection
	ONGOING ASSESSMENT
	• Assess family's understanding of the child's condition, the electrical conduction system of the heart, and pacemaker function.
	• Assess child's level of understanding about the pacemaker.
	• Determine what teaching methods are most effective for both the child and family.
	
	THERAPEUTIC INTERVENTIONS
	• Provide a quiet environment *to allow the child and family to absorb new information.*
	• Use appropriate materials/methods (e.g., temporary pacemaker flip chart, pacemaker device, the show-and-tell approach).
	• Explain:
	    Anatomy and physiology of the heart
	    Function of the pacemaker
	    Insertion procedure
	    Importance of activity restrictions
	• Document teaching.
		Patient and family will increase their understanding of temporary pacemaker function and follow-up care.

Anxiety/Fear **RELATED TO** Insertion or presence of temporary pacemaker Strange environment Imposed activity restrictions Lack of understanding at child's age **DEFINING CHARACTERISTICS** Restlessness, agitation Irritability Anger Crying Helplessness Bewilderment	**ONGOING ASSESSMENT** • Assess physical and emotional symptoms of distress in young child. • Assess family's acceptance of the child's illness. • Evaluate effectiveness of milieu therapy that is best suited for a child. **THERAPEUTIC INTERVENTIONS** • Adapt care to child's need. • Provide tender loving care (e.g., touch, playful, attentive) *to decrease feelings of helplessness and to provide sense of security and love.* • Provide toys *to allow the child to focus on different subjects. Children can be distracted.* • Allow family member to stay with the child *to provide security and alleviate feelings of loss.* • For older child, orient to environment and pacemaker equipment *to reduce the fear of unknown equipment, thereby alleviating anxiety.* • For older child, encourage ventilation of feelings.	Anxiety will be reduced.

NURSING DIAGNOSES/ DEFINING CHARACTERISTICS	NURSING INTERVENTIONS / *RATIONALES*	EXPECTED OUTCOMES
Pain/Discomfort **RELATED TO** Insertion of temporary pacemaker Imposed activity restrictions Subcutaneous irritation by catheter Lead displacement **DEFINING CHARACTERISTICS** Restlessness, crying, irritability Pallor Hiccupping; intercostal or abdominal muscle twitching	**ONGOING ASSESSMENT** ▪ Observe for objective signs of discomfort (see Defining Characteristics). ▪ Assess level of discomfort, location, and onset. ▪ Assess for hiccups or muscle twitching *that may occur with lead displacement or very high pacing output (mA).* ▪ Evaluate effectiveness of given comfort measures. **THERAPEUTIC INTERVENTIONS** ▪ Anticipate need for comfort measures. ▪ Provide comfort measures (e.g., change in position, back rubs, analgesics) as ordered *to reduce discomforts.* ▪ Secure terminal portion of pacing wires with 4 × 4 dressing *to prevent accidental pulling of leads.* ▪ If hiccups or muscle twitching are noted, call physician to evaluate lead placement. *Inaccurate position of leads can stimulate the diaphragm.* Anticipate need to reposition the lead(s).	Optimal comfort will be maintained.
High Risk for Infection **RELATED TO** Invasive procedure with possible introduction of bacteria Concomitant cardiac surgery **DEFINING CHARACTERISTICS** Fever Tenderness, redness, swelling, drainage from the affected site Elevated WBC Positive blood and fluid cultures	**ONGOING ASSESSMENT** ▪ Assess catheter site for signs of infection (see defining characteristics). ▪ Evaluate amount and characteristics of drainage from catheter site. ▪ Monitor temperature every 4 hours and as needed. ▪ Monitor length of time pacemaker catheter is in place and report to physician after 72 hours. ▪ Follow up on WBC, blood and fluid cultures if infection is suspected. **THERAPEUTIC INTERVENTIONS** ▪ Keep dressing dry and intact *to prevent contamination with bacteria.* ▪ Change dressing routinely or as needed per infection control policy. Use sterile technique *to reduce risk of infection to open wounds.* ▪ Avoid frequent and unnecessary contact with the catheter site. ▪ Notify physician if infection is suspected and report excessive drainage if present. ▪ Administer antibiotics as ordered.	Risk of infection will be reduced.

Marilyn Samson-Hinton, RN, BSN

Pacemaker, implantable (permanent)

A battery-powered electronic device that delivers an electrical stimulus to the heart muscle when needed. Types of pacemakers currently available are as follows: (1) Bradycardia pacemaker— its mode of response is either inhibited, triggered, or asynchronous. Indicated for chronic symptomatic bradydysrhythmias including sinus arrest, sinoatrial block, and sinus bradycardia, or for chronic symptomatic second-degree or third-degree atrioventricular block. A dual-chamber pacemaker is indicated for bradycardia with competent sinus node to provide AV synchrony and rate variability. (2) Rate response pacemaker (physiological or nonphysiological)—indicated for patients who can benefit from an increase in pacing rate, either atrial or ventricular, in response to their body's metabolic needs or to activity for increased cardiac output. Contraindicated for patients who can tolerate only limited increases in heart rate as a result of concomitant disease states. (3) Antitachycardia pacemaker—indicated for pace-terminable conditions: recurrent SVT (e.g., A-V reciprocating tachydysrhythmias [as in WPW], atrial flutter, and other atrioventricular tachydysrhythmias).

NURSING DIAGNOSES/ DEFINING CHARACTERISTICS	NURSING INTERVENTIONS / *RATIONALES*	EXPECTED OUTCOMES
High Risk for Decreased Cardiac Output **RELATED TO** Permanent pacemaker malfunction caused by: Lead dislodgement Faulty connection between lead and pulse generator Faulty lead system (e.g., lead fracture, insulation break) Pulse generator circuitry failure Battery depletion Inadequate parameter settings Inappropriate type of pacemaker Ventricular arrhythmias caused by irritation from pacing electrode, asynchronous pacing resulting from malsensing problem Change in myocardial threshold Competitive rhythms Cardiac tamponade resulting from myocardial perforation Pneumothorax Subclavicular thrombosis Pulmonary embolism	**ONGOING ASSESSMENT** • Assess age and developmental level. • If ECG monitored: Assess for proper pacemaker function: capture, sensing, firing, and configuration of paced QRS (difficult to assess pace artifact on digital ECG). Assess for pacemaker-induced dysrhythmias. • If unmonitored: Assess apical/brachial pulses. Assess child's hemodynamic status. • Immediately after pacemaker implantation: Check implant data for: Type of pacemaker (e.g., AV sequential, single-chamber, demand, programmable, rate response) and programmed parameters. *Certain types of pacemakers have variable functions, which can be difficult to interpret.* Monitor chest x-ray films and ECG studies after child returns from OR and as ordered *to verify correct placement of lead and pacemaker function.* Keep monitor alarms on at all times. Record rhythm strips: Routinely every _____ hours If pacemaker malfunction is suspected When pacemaker parameter adjustments are made • If pacemaker malfunction is suspected: Assess reliability of spontaneous rhythm Obtain 12-lead ECG study *to verify function of pacemaker and lead placement. LBBB-paced QRS configuration suggests good right ventricular lead position.* Monitor for signs of hemocongestive heart failure. • If failure to sense is noted: Monitor chest x-ray films *to check for placement and status of pacemaker electrode.* Observe for phrenic nerve stimulation (hiccups) and intercostal or abdominal muscle twitching. *Dislodged pacemaker lead can cause stimulation of chest wall and diaphragm.* Observe for induced ventricular dysrhythmias caused by pacemaker competition.	Optimal cardiac output will be maintained.

NURSING DIAGNOSES/ DEFINING CHARACTERISTICS	NURSING INTERVENTIONS / *RATIONALES*	EXPECTED OUTCOMES

DEFINING CHARACTERISTICS

Loss of sensing
Loss of capture
Loss of pacemaker artifacts
Change in paced QRS configuration
"Runaway pacemaker" (erratic rapid pacing resulting from pulse generator failure)
Pacemaker-mediated tachycardia (PMT) (continuous pacing at the maximum tracking rate triggered by sensed atrial activity)
Ventricular dysrhythmias
Palpitation
Hiccups resulting from phrenic nerve stimulation
Significant decrease in heart rate
Stokes-Adams syndrome
Signs of hemodynamic compromise (restlessness, confusion, dizziness, LOC, fatigue, hypotension, decrease in cardiac output, decrease in urine output)
Signs of cardiac tamponade (elevated CVP reading, jugular vein distension, faint rapid pulse, distant heart sounds, pulsus paradoxus, hypotension, cool clammy skin, stuporousness, agitation, restlessness, decreased cardiac output, and anuria)
Symptoms of pneumothorax (respiratory distress, absence of breath sounds, sudden chest pain)

ONGOING ASSESSMENT cont'd

- If loss of capture is noted:
  Follow the three steps under "failure to sense," above.
  Assess for factors that increase myocardial threshold (i.e., ischemia, fibrosis around the tip of the electrode, acidosis, electrolyte imbalance, antidysrhythmic drugs). *Threshold is the minimum amount of electrical energy needed to pace and capture the heart.*
- If ventricular dysrhythmias occur:
  Assess child for hemodynamic status and for signs of congestive heart failure (see Defining Characteristics).
- Assess for signs of (see Defining Characteristics):
  Cardiac tamponade
  Superior vena cava syndrome
  Pneumothorax
  Pulmonary embolism
  Pericardial effusion

THERAPEUTIC INTERVENTIONS

- If pacemaker malfunction is suspected:
  Notify physician.
  Call the pacemaker specialist to evaluate further pacemaker function and to make changes in parameters if needed through the use of pacemaker programmer. *This is a noninvasive technique of pacemaker programming via radio frequency signal.*
  Initiate basic life support measures as needed.
  Prepare intravenous isoproterenol for standby. *It stimulates the heart muscle and increases the heart rate.*
  Prepare for temporary pacemaker insertion and other advanced life support measures as needed.
  Anticipate possible return to OR
  If failure to sense and loss of capture is noted:
    Turn patient on left side (for endocardial pacemaker) *to facilitate good ventricular wall contact.*
- Anticipate need for possible pericardiocentesis if myocardial perforation is suspected.
- Anticipate chest tube insertion or thoracentesis for suspected pneumothorax.
- Place child in Trendelenburg position or turn to the left side if air thrombus is suspected.

Continued.

Cardiovascular Care Plans (Pediatric)

NURSING DIAGNOSES/ DEFINING CHARACTERISTICS	NURSING INTERVENTIONS / *RATIONALES*	EXPECTED OUTCOMES
DEFINING CHARACTERISTICS **cont'd** Signs of vena cava syndrome (swelling of head and chest, edema of insertion site) Signs of pulmonary embolism (dyspnea, chest pain, tachycardia, weak pulse, decrease in BP, restlessness, fever, cough)		
Impaired Physical Mobility **RELATED TO** Imposed activity restriction Reluctance to attempt movement because of pain at site of pulse generator **DEFINING CHARACTERISTICS** Restlessness, irritability Crying Helplessness Verbalization of inability to move about Limited ROM Muscle weakness Complaints of shoulder joint stiffness/ pain	**ONGOING ASSESSMENT** ▪ Assess for signs of restlessness and discomfort. ▪ Auscultate breath sounds and assess respiratory status. ▪ Assess skin integrity. Check for redness or tissue ischemia. ▪ Assess for pulmonary embolism (shortness of breath, chest pain, tachycardia, increase in blood pressure). ▪ Assess for signs of thrombophlebitis (uncommon) (e.g., redness, swelling, calf pain, increased temperature). **THERAPEUTIC INTERVENTIONS** ▪ Explain to child and family the importance of imposed activity restriction (24 to 48 hours after implant) *to prevent pacing electrode displacement.* ▪ Assist the child in turning or positioning every 2 hours. For endocardial pacemaker, avoid turning to the right side. ▪ Provide passive ROM exercise to shoulder on operative side *to prevent "frozen" shoulder.* ▪ Assist with active ROM exercises to nonaffected extremities tid. ▪ Provide emotional support. ▪ Encourage an older child to verbalize fear or presence of pain. ▪ Advise an older child to cough and deep breathe every hour while awake *to prevent atelectasis.* ▪ Assist and teach child in using affected extremity carefully (e.g., avoid hyperextension of arms and abdomen, where applicable, overhead stretching, and so on for a month after implant); *these can cause electrode displacement.*	Complications of immobility will be absent or reduced.
Pain/Discomfort **RELATED TO** Insertion of permanent pacemaker Imposed activity restriction Lead displacement High pacing energy output "Frozen" shoulder	**ONGOING ASSESSMENT** ▪ Observe for objective signs of discomfort (e.g., crying, restlessness). ▪ Assess level of discomfort, source, quality, location, onset, precipitating and relieving factors. ▪ Assess for hiccups or muscle twitching. ▪ Palpate affected site for presence of pulse generator pocket stimulation. ▪ Evaluate effectiveness of given comfort measures.	Discomfort will be relieved or reduced.

NURSING DIAGNOSES/ DEFINING CHARACTERISTICS	NURSING INTERVENTIONS / *RATIONALES*	EXPECTED OUTCOMES

DEFINING CHARACTERISTICS
 	
Crying, restlessness, irritability
Verbalized discomfort
Splints wound with hands
Reluctance to move
Pallor, diaphoresis
Limited ROM of shoulder on affected side
Hiccuping (phrenic nerve stimulation); intercostal or pectoral muscle stimulation
Pulse generator pocket stimulation
	THERAPEUTIC INTERVENTIONS
	• Anticipate need for comfort measures.
	• Provide additional comfort measures (e.g., backrubs, change in position, gentle massage of shoulder on operative side) *to reduce discomforts.*
	• Administer pain medication as ordered *to promote pain relief.*
	• For older child, instruct him or her to report pain and effectiveness of interventions.
	• Explain to child and family reasons for activity restriction.
	• If hiccups/muscle twitching/pulse generator pocket stimulation are present:
	   Notify physician.
	   Obtain chest x-ray films and ECG studies *to check for lead status and placement and proper function of pacemaker.*
	   Anticipate return to OR for lead repositioning.	

Knowledge Deficit: Individual/Family
RELATED TO
 	
Age of patient
Inability to comprehend
New procedure/ equipment
Overprotective parent
Misinterpretation of information
 	
DEFINING CHARACTERISTICS
 	
Baffled, overwhelmed
Lack of questions
Inappropriate behavior
Verbalized misconceptions
Questioning
Overprotection
	ONGOING ASSESSMENT
	• Assess child's level of understanding about the pacemaker.
	• Assess family's information regarding child's condition, electrical conduction system of the heart, and pacemaker function.
	• Evaluate family's readiness for learning.
	• Determine what teaching methods are most effective for both child and family.
	
	THERAPEUTIC INTERVENTIONS
	• Provide environment conducive to learning. *It allows the child/family to absorb new information.*
	• Gather all teaching materials:
	   Pacemaker flip chart
	   Pacemaker unit (pulse generator demonstration, lead system)
	   Patient's manual
	   Pacemaker videotape
	• Use show-and-tell approach *(effective for younger patient).*
	• Document teaching.
	• Preoperatively, explain:
	   Anatomy and physiology of the heart
	   Pacemaker function and its advantages
	   Insertion procedure
	• Postoperatively (acute):
	   Stress the importance of complete bed rest 24-48 hours after implant *to prevent lead displacement.*
	   Instruct the child to avoid turning to the right side if endocardial pacemaker was inserted *to provide good ventricular wall contact.*
		Patient and family will increase their understanding about pacemaker and patient will better accept activity limitation.

Continued.

Pacemaker, implantable (permanent) cont'd

NURSING DIAGNOSES/ DEFINING CHARACTERISTICS	NURSING INTERVENTIONS / *RATIONALES*	EXPECTED OUTCOMES

THERAPEUTIC INTERVENTIONS cont'd

Explain the importance of notifying the nurse of:
Any pain, wetness, discoloration, loose dressing
Complaints of headache, dizziness, confusion, chest pain, shortness of breath, hiccups, or muscle twitching *that may suggest pacemaker malfunction*
Explain the need for chest x-ray evaluation and 12-lead ECG.
- Before discharge, teach child and family:
How to take and record pulse as needed
The need for regular follow-up care
Signs and symptoms of pacemaker malfunction
Signs and symptoms of infection
Wound care for insertion site
To discuss with physician type of sports activities the child can participate in (e.g., no backflip, sommersault, or any contact sports)
To avoid over-the-head arm motion or overstretching for 1 month *to prevent lead displacement, because it takes about 1 month for the scar tissue to form around the tip of the electrode*
The need to carry pacemaker ID card
Type of pacemaker, brand name, and model number
Programmed pacing rate
To notify physician/pacemaker follow-up office if pulse rate is at least 5 beats slower than programmed rate or of any signs and symptoms of pacemaker malfunction
Pacemaker longevity and the need for pacemaker battery replacement when elective replacement indication (ERI) time has been reached
That the pulse generator replacement (battery) using the same electrode can be done on an outpatient basis
To avoid strong magnetic field (magnetic resonance, electrocautery equipment, laser, diathermy, lithotripsy, direct radiation [should be shielded], current industrial machinery); *these may cause pulse generator circuitry failure, or certain pacemakers will go into backup mode*
That it is safe to use newer model microwave oven, because it has no reported effect on child; if dizziness is felt while near the appliance being used, advise child to step away from it; *pacemaker will assume normal function without permanent effects*
To alert airport personnel, dentist, and others of presence of pacemaker

NURSING DIAGNOSES/ DEFINING CHARACTERISTICS	NURSING INTERVENTIONS / *RATIONALES*	EXPECTED OUTCOMES
Anxiety/Fear **RELATED TO** Insertion/presence of permanent pacemaker at a very young age Strange environment Lack of understanding Altered body image caused by generator appearance and incision line **DEFINING CHARACTERISTICS** Restlessness Crying Irritability Baffled Helplessness Belligerence	**ONGOING ASSESSMENT** ▪ Assess objective signs of emotional distress. ▪ Assess family's care of the child and their acceptance of the illness. ▪ Evaluate effectiveness of a given therapy. **THERAPEUTIC INTERVENTIONS** ▪ Provide emotional support with full tender loving care. ▪ Allow family member to stay with the patient while in the hospital *to provide feelings of security and decrease feelings of fear and anxiety.* ▪ For older child, orient to environment and to pacemaker device *to reduce fear of unknown equipment.* ▪ For older child, allow him or her to verbalize fears. ▪ Assist family in coping and how to adapt to their child's needs at home.	Anxiety level will be reduced.
High Risk for Infection **RELATED TO** Internal invasion by foreign object Altered skin integrity caused by permanent pacemaker insertion **DEFINING CHARACTERISTICS** Fever Redness, tenderness, swelling, drainage from infected site, skin discoloration Elevated WBC Positive blood/fluid culture Pacemaker/lead erosion	**ONGOING ASSESSMENT** ▪ Assess insertion site for signs of infection (see Defining Characteristics). ▪ Evaluate amount and characteristics of drainage. ▪ Assess body temperature. ▪ Follow up on WBC, blood and fluid cultures if infection is absolutely suspected. **THERAPEUTIC INTERVENTIONS** ▪ Ensure sterile technique when changing dressing *to reduce risk of infection at incision site.* ▪ Keep dressing dry and intact *to reduce chance of migration of pathogens.* ▪ Avoid frequent and unnecessary contact with the incision site. ▪ Notify physician if infection is suspected and to report excessive drainage if any. ▪ Administer antibiotics as ordered. ▪ Before discharge, teach child and family: Avoidance of shower or full bath for a week after implant Proper technique on dressing change if needed Signs and symptoms of infection To avoid frequent contact with the incision site To avoid contact sports that could further harm the affected site	Risk of infection will be reduced.

Marilyn Samson-Hinton, RN, BSN

Shock syndrome: cardiogenic

PUMP FAILURE; CONGESTIVE HEART FAILURE

An acute state of decreased cardiac output and tissue perfusion usually associated with cardiac surgery or cardiac tamponade, massive pulmonary embolism, or myocardial infarction. It is a self-perpetuating condition, because coronary blood flow to the myocardium is compromised, causing further ischemia and ventricular dysfunction. This care plan focuses on the care of an unstable child in a shock state.

NURSING DIAGNOSES/ DEFINING CHARACTERISTICS	NURSING INTERVENTIONS / *RATIONALES*	EXPECTED OUTCOMES

Decreased Cardiac Output **RELATED TO** *Mechanical:* Altered preload Altered afterload Inotropic changes in heart *Electrical:* Altered cardiac rate Altered cardiac rhythm Altered conduction *Structural:* Valvular dysfunction Septal defects
 	
 DEFINING CHARACTERISTICS Mental status changes: confusion, restlessness, apathy Variations in hemo-dynamic parameters (BP, heart rate, CVP, pulmonary artery pressures, cardiac output, neck veins) Pale, cool, clammy skin Cyanosis, mottling of extremities Oliguria, anuria Sustained hypotension with narrowing of pulse pressure Pulmonary congestion, rales Respiratory alkalosis or metabolic acidosis
	ONGOING ASSESSMENT
	• Assess age and developmental level.
	• Assess mental status.
	• Assess hemodynamic parameters (BP, heart rate, CVP, pulmonary artery pressures, cardiac output, neck veins).
	• Assess skin color, temperature, moisture.
	• Assess I&O.
	• Assess respiratory rate, rhythm, breath sounds.
	• Assess ABGs.
	
	 THERAPEUTIC INTERVENTIONS
	• Place child in optimal position, usually supine with head of bed slightly elevated *to promote venous return and facilitate ventilation.*
	• Initiate and titrate drug therapy as ordered. *Therapy can be more effective when initiated early.*
	  Dopamine: *Positive inotropic and chronotropic effect on the heart, which improves stroke volume and cardiac output. High dose, however, can cause peripheral vasoconstriction and can be arrhythmiogenic.*
	  Dobutamine: *Positive inotropic effect increases cardiac output. Reduces afterload by decreasing peripheral vasoconstriction, also resulting in higher cardiac output.*
	  Inocor: *Increased contractility and vasodilation.*
	  Nipride: *Increases cardiac output by decreasing afterload. It produces peripheral and systemic vasodilation by direct action on smooth muscles of blood vessels.*
	  Nitroglycerin IV: *May be used to reduce excess preload if contributing to pump failure and to reduce afterload.*
	  Diuretics: *Used when volume overload is contributing to pump failure.*
	• See Decreased cardiac output, p. 10.
		Adequate cardiac output will be maintained.

Impaired Gas Exchange **RELATED TO** Altered blood flow Alveolar capillary membrane changes	**ONGOING ASSESSMENT** • Assess rate, rhythm, depth of respiration. • Assess for abnormal breath sounds. • Assess vital signs. • Assess skin, nailbeds, or mucous membranes for pallor or cyanosis. • Assess ABGs with changes in respiratory status and 15-20 minutes after each adjustment in oxygen therapy *to evaluate effectiveness of oxygen therapy.*	Adequate gas exchange and oxygenation of body tissues will be achieved.

NURSING DIAGNOSES/ DEFINING CHARACTERISTICS	NURSING INTERVENTIONS / *RATIONALES*	EXPECTED OUTCOMES

DEFINING CHARACTERISTICS
Fast, labored breathing
May have Cheyne-Stokes respirations
Rales
Tachycardia
Hypoxia
Restlessness
Confusion
	THERAPEUTIC INTERVENTIONS
	• Place child in optimal position for ventilation. *Slightly elevated head of bed facilitates diaphragmatic movement.*
	• Initiate oxygen therapy as prescribed.
	• Prepare child for mechanical ventilation if noninvasive oxygen therapy is not effective:
	    Explain need for mechanical ventilation to child and family *to allay anxiety and gain compliance.*
	    Assist in intubation procedure.
	• See Mechanical ventilation, p. 155.	

Fear/Anxiety **RELATED TO** Guarded prognosis; mortality is 80% Unfamiliar environment Dyspnea Dependence on CPAP or mechanical ventilation Fear of death **DEFINING CHARACTERISTICS** Sympathetic stimulation Restlessness Increased awareness Increased questioning Uncooperative behavior Avoids looking at equipment or keeps vigilant watch over equipment	**ONGOING ASSESSMENT** • Assess child's level of anxiety. **THERAPEUTIC INTERVENTIONS** • See Anxiety, p. 4. *Controlling anxiety will help decrease physiological reactions that can aggravate condition.* • Assure child and family of close, continuous monitoring that will ensure prompt interventions. • Avoid unnecessary conversations between team members in front of child. *This will reduce misconceptions and fear/anxiety.* • Contact religious representative/counselor *to provide spiritual care and support, if appropriate.* • Keep parent/significant others informed of changes in condition or treatment.	Fear and anxiety will be reduced.

Knowledge Deficit
RELATED TO
Disease process
Prescribed therapy
 	
DEFINING CHARACTERISTICS
Verbalization of lack of knowledge or misconceptions
Questions
Lack of questions
	ONGOING ASSESSMENT
	• Assess child's/family's level of understanding of disease process and prescribed therapy.
	• Assess readiness for learning. *Teaching in the acute stage may be limited to family or significant others. This will minimize their feelings of helplessness and assist them in providing support to child.*
	
	THERAPEUTIC INTERVENTIONS
	• When appropriate, provide information regarding:
	    Disease process and rationale for prescribed therapy *to help allay anxiety*
	    Follow-up care
	• Structure teaching to allow for answering questions.
	• Use teaching aids (pamphlets, visual aids, etc.) *to facilitate learning.*
		Child/significant others will verbalize understanding of disease process and treatment.

Kimberly P. Souder, RN, BSN

Shock syndrome: septic

SEPSIS; SHOCK; BACTEREMIA; WARM SHOCK;
COLD SHOCK; DIC

Septic shock occurs after bacteremia of gram-negative bacilli (most common) or gram-positive cocci that results in a systolic blood pressure <90 mm Hg (or a drop >25%), urine output <1 ml/kg/hr, and metabolic acidosis. The circulatory insufficiency is initiated by endotoxin, which causes an increase in capillary permeability and a decrease in systemic vascular resistance (SVR). Hyperdynamic, warm shock is present in 30% to 50% of children in early septic shock and is characterized by a strong beta-adrenergic stimulation of the heart, with tachycardia and an increased cardiac output if adequate blood volume is available. Hypodynamic, cold septic shock tends to occur relatively late in septic shock as a result of hypovolemia and release of myocardial depressant factors, causing a fall in cardiac output.

NURSING DIAGNOSES/ DEFINING CHARACTERISTICS	NURSING INTERVENTIONS / *RATIONALES*	EXPECTED OUTCOMES
Actual Infection RELATED TO Infectious process of either gram-negative or gram-positive bacteria Most common causative organisms and their related factors are: *Escherichia coli*—commonly occurs in GU tract, biliary tract, IV catheter, colon or intraabdominal abscesses *Klebsiella*—from the lungs, GI tract, intravenous catheter, urinary tract, or surgical wounds *Proteus*—GU tract, respiratory tract, abscesses, or biliary tract *Bacteroides fragilis*—female genital tract, colon, liver abscesses, pressure ulcers *Pseudomonas aeruginosa*—lungs, urinary tract, skin, and IV catheter *Candida albicans*—line-related infection, especially hyperalimentation infusion, pulmonary and urinary abscesses	**ONGOING ASSESSMENT** • Assess age and developmental level. • Assess general status; document and report significant changes: Assess LOC/mentation. Use neurological checklist, using Glasgow Coma Scale; adjust to age/developmental level. Assess skin turgor, color, temperature, and peripheral pulses. Monitor temperature every 4 hours. Assess related factors thoroughly *to identify a source for the sepsis.* **THERAPEUTIC INTERVENTIONS** • Initiate appropriate antibiotics as ordered. Monitor for toxicity, especially with hepatic and/or renal insufficiency/failure: *Aminoglycocides should be followed with urinalysis, and serum creatinine levels at least 3 times/week; chloramphenicol should be restricted from children with liver disease.* • Remove any possible source of infection (e.g., urinary catheter, IV catheter). • Manage the cause of infection and anticipate surgical consultation as necessary: *To drain pus/abscess* *To resolve obstruction* *To repair perforated organ* • Maintain temperature in adequate range *to prevent stress on the cardiovascular system:* Administer antipyretics as ordered. Use cooling mattress. Administer tepid sponge baths. Limit number of blankets/linens used to cover child. • Initiate appropriate isolation measures *to prevent the spread of infection.* • Draw peak and trough antibiotic titers as needed.	Cause of infection will be determined and appropriate treatment initiated.

NURSING DIAGNOSES/ DEFINING CHARACTERISTICS	NURSING INTERVENTIONS / *RATIONALES*	EXPECTED OUTCOMES
DEFINING CHARACTERISTICS Changes in LOC: lethargy, confusion Fever/chills may or may not be present Ruddy appearance with warm, dry skin Leukocytosis		

Fluid Volume Deficit
RELATED TO
 	
Early septic shock (warm shock)
Decrease in systemic vascular resistance (SVR)
Increased capillary permeability
 	
DEFINING CHARACTERISTICS
 	
Hypotension
Tachycardia
Decreased urine output <1 ml/kg/hr
Concentrated urine
	ONGOING ASSESSMENT
	- Assess for presence of hypotension and tachycardia.
	- Closely monitor I&O, assessing urine for concentration.
	- Weigh daily and record weights.
	- When initiating fluid challenges, closely monitor child *to prevent iatrogenic volume overload;* monitor CVP.
	- Assess serum electrolytes, pH, and osmolality.
	
	THERAPEUTIC INTERVENTIONS
	- Notify physician of any signs of fluid volume deficit.
	- Provide aggressive fluid resuscitation as ordered:
	  Administer IV bolus of normal saline or lactated Ringers at 10-20 ml/kg over 30 min to 1 hour.
	  Administer 20-30 ml/kg IV bolus fluids to the child exhibiting signs of circulatory collapse.
	  Monitor response to fluids and notify physician. *For a child in shock, a second or third fluid bolus may be needed to prevent cardiovascular collapse.*
	  Administer plasma volume expanders as ordered (5% albumin).
	  For iatrogenic fluid volume overload, consider administration of diuretics (furosemide [Lasix] or mannitol).
	- Administer vasoactive substances, such as dopamine, phenylephrine HCl (Neo-Synephrine), norepinephrine bitartrate (Levophed) as ordered, if there is poor or no response to fluid resuscitation. *In early septic shock the cardiac output is high or normal. At this point, the vasoactive agents are administered for their alpha effect.*
		Fluid volume deficit will be reduced.

Decreased Cardiac Output
RELATED TO
 	
Late septic shock: Decrease in tissue perfusion leads to increased lactic acid production and systemic acidosis, which causes decrease in myocardial contractility
Gram-negative infections may cause direct myocardial toxic effect
	ONGOING ASSESSMENT
	- Monitor vital signs and hemodynamic parameters every hour and report to physician if out of the following ranges:
	  BP mean <40
	  Pulse <60 or >180
	  Resp <10 or >30
	  Temp <36° or >38.5° C
	  CVP >4-12 mm Hg
	  PCWP >4-12 mm Hg
	  CO >2-5 L/min/m²
	- Monitor for dysrhythmias.
	- Assess skin warmth and peripheral pulses every hour.
	- Assess level of consciousness every hour.
	- Monitor ABG results.
	- Monitor blood lactate levels.
	- Monitor urine output every hour and maintain accurate record.
		Cardiac output will be increased.

Continued.

NURSING DIAGNOSES/ DEFINING CHARACTERISTICS	NURSING INTERVENTIONS / *RATIONALES*	EXPECTED OUTCOMES

DEFINING CHARACTERISTICS
Decreased peripheral pulses
Capillary refill >2 sec
Slightly cyanotic extremities may be present
Cold, clammy skin
Hypotension
Agitation/confusion
Decreased urinary output <1 ml/kg/ hr
Abnormal ABGs:
  Acidosis
  Hypoxemia
	THERAPEUTIC INTERVENTIONS
	• Place child in the physiological position for shock: head of bed flat with the trunk horizontal and lower extremities elevated 20 to 30 degrees with knees straight. Do not use reverse Trendelenburg's (head down) position *because it causes pressure against the diaphragm. A reflex vasoconstrictive action that decreases the blood supply to the brain after the initial increase in blood flow can occur.*
	• Administer inotropic agents (dobutamine HCl [Dobutrex], dopamine, digoxin, or amrinone [Inocor]) *to improve myocardial contractility.* Continuously monitor their effectiveness.
	• Treat acidosis with sodium bicarbonate.	

Altered Breathing Pattern
RELATED TO
Lactic acidosis
 	
DEFINING CHARACTERISTICS
Tachypnea
Change in depth of breathing
Respiratory distress
Use of accessory muscles/retractions
Nasal flaring
	ONGOING ASSESSMENT
	• Assess respiratory rate, rhythm, and depth every hour.
	• Assess for any increase in work of breathing:
	  Shortness of breath
	  Use of accessory muscles
	
	THERAPEUTIC INTERVENTIONS
	• Position child in proper body alignment *for optimal lung expansion.*
	• Provide reassurance and allay anxiety by staying with child during acute episodes of respiratory distress. *Air hunger can produce an extremely anxious state.*
	• Maintain oxygen delivery system *so that the appropriate amount of oxygen is applied continuously and the child's system does not desaturate.*
	• Anticipate the need for intubation and mechanical ventilation. (See Mechanical ventilation, p. 155.)
		Optimal breathing pattern will be maintained.

High Risk for Impaired Gas Exchange **RELATED TO** Respiratory distress syndrome Pneumonia Pulmonary edema **DEFINING CHARACTERISTICS** Hypercapnia Hypoxia Rales Tachypnea Irritability Restlessness	**ONGOING ASSESSMENT** • Assess respirations every hour, noting quality, rate, pattern, depth, and use of accessory muscles. • Assess breath sounds every hour. • Assess for changes in orientation and behavior. • Monitor ABGs and note changes. • Use pulse oximetry, as available, *to monitor oxygen saturation and pulse rate continuously.* **THERAPEUTIC INTERVENTIONS** • Maintain the prescribed oxygen delivery system or ventilator setting *so that child's system does not desaturate.* • Change position every 2 hours *to facilitate movement and drainage of secretions.* Be sure to position child in proper body alignment *for optimal respiratory excursion.* • Suction as needed *to clear secretions.*	Optimal gas exchange will be maintained.

NURSING DIAGNOSES/ DEFINING CHARACTERISTICS	NURSING INTERVENTIONS / *RATIONALES*	EXPECTED OUTCOMES
Altered Level of Consciousness **RELATED TO** Hypotension Hypoxemia Sepsis **DEFINING CHARACTERISTICS** Confusion Lethargy Agitation Impaired judgment Glasgow Coma Scale score <11	**ONGOING ASSESSMENT** • Assess LOC/responsiveness/increased sleepiness every hour. • Assess for confusion/impaired judgment. **THERAPEUTIC INTERVENTIONS** • Reorient child to environment as needed. • Report any change in LOC. • Use protective safety measures: Keep side rails up at all times and bed in low position. If restraints are used, position child on side. Never restrain on back *to lessen the possibility of aspiration.* • See Decreased level of consciousness, p. 173.	Optimal state of consciousness will be maintained.
Urinary Retention **RELATED TO** Hypotension Nephrotoxic drugs (antibiotics) **DEFINING CHARACTERISTICS** Urine output <1 ml/ kg/hr Elevated BUN and creatinine Hematuria, proteinuria Tubular casts in urine Fixed specific gravity	**ONGOING ASSESSMENT** • Monitor and record I&O every hour. • Assess for patency of Foley catheter. • Monitor blood and urine chemistries (BUN, creatinine, electrolytes). • Monitor urine specific gravity and check for blood and protein every 4 hours. **THERAPEUTIC INTERVENTIONS** • Maintain IV fluids and inotropic agents at prescribed rates *to maintain BP, cardiac output, and, ultimately, renal perfusion.* • Notify physician of any abnormalities. • See Renal failure, acute, p. 358.	Optimal urine elimination will be maintained.
High Risk for Injury: Bleeding **RELATED TO** Sepsis: Deficiency in clotting factors DIC **DEFINING CHARACTERISTICS** Oozing of blood from drains, wounds, IV sites Bleeding from mucous membranes PT >25 sec PTT >60-90 sec Thrombocytopenia Elevated fibrin split products Prolonged bleeding time	**ONGOING ASSESSMENT** • Assess for signs of bleeding: Petechiae, purpura, hematomas Blood oozing from IV sites, drains, or wounds Bleeding from mucous membranes: Hemoptysis Blood obtained during suctioning Bleeding from GI/GU tract • Determine blood loss and report to physician. • Monitor PT, PTT, FSP; bleeding time, and hemoglobin/hematocrit. **THERAPEUTIC INTERVENTIONS** • Administer colloids as ordered/obtain blood type and cross match. • If bleeding is present, refer to Disseminated intravascular coagulation, p. 396. • Minimize amount of stimulation and movement *to decrease amount of blood (e.g., cerebral bleeding).* • Avoid taking temperature rectally.	Risk of bleeding will be reduced.

Continued.

Shock syndrome: septic cont'd

NURSING DIAGNOSES/ DEFINING CHARACTERISTICS	NURSING INTERVENTIONS / *RATIONALES*	EXPECTED OUTCOMES
Knowledge Deficit **RELATED TO** New condition	**ONGOING ASSESSMENT** • Assess readiness of child/family to learn. • Evaluate understanding of child's overall condition.	Child/significant others will demonstrate understanding of disease process and treatment methods.
DEFINING CHARACTERISTICS Increased frequency of questions posed by child and significant others Inability to correctly respond to questions asked Family/significant others avoidance of child's condition	**THERAPEUTIC INTERVENTIONS** • Explain all procedures before performing them *to decrease the fear of the unknown.* • Orient child to ICU surroundings, routines, equipment alarms, and noises. *The ICU is a busy and noisy environment that can be very upsetting to child and family.* • Keep child/family informed of the disease process and present status.	

Kimberly P. Souder, RN, BSN

Supraventricular tachycardia (SVT)

One of the most common dysrhythmias in children. It is a regular rapid rate (above 300 beats/min in infants), arising from an atrial or nodal focus. The QRS complex is usually narrow. Children usually can withstand SVT for 24-28 hours before they develop congestive heart failure. Vagal maneuvers can often convert the abnormal rhythm. Medical management is most often with digitalis, propranolol, and/or verapamil. If medical management does not successfully control SVT, then cardioversion, overdrive pacing, or surgical interruption of accessory AV conduction pathways may be required. This care plan covers only the monitoring of a patient with SVT and its medical management. Alternate therapies should be explored in detail if medical management is unsuccessful.

NURSING DIAGNOSES/ DEFINING CHARACTERISTICS	NURSING INTERVENTIONS / *RATIONALES*	EXPECTED OUTCOMES
Decreased Cardiac Output **RELATED TO** Chronic dysrhythmia **DEFINING CHARACTERISTICS** Respiratory difficulty Decreased blood pressure Rapid, weak pulses Prolonged capillary refill Irritability Lethargy Feeding difficulty Pale, cool skin	**ONGOING ASSESSMENT** • Assess age and developmental level. • Assess and record heart rate, BP, and any signs of decreased CO every 2 hours. • Monitor ECG rhythm strip. • Measure I&O and maintain accurate record. **THERAPEUTIC INTERVENTIONS** • Ensure that IV is placed and patent *for administration of emergency medication.* • Place child on continuous cardiac monitor *to monitor changes in rhythm accurately.* • Administer antiarrhythmic medications if ordered and record response and/or side effects. *The most common side effects of digoxin and propranolol are bradycardia, hypotension, and GI upset. Verapamil should not be used in infants and young children because it can cause cardiovascular collapse.* • Assist cardiologist with any procedures or treatments (e.g., vagal stimulation). *Vagal maneuvers often convert SVT by interrupting the recurrent pathway.* • Have emergency equipment and defibrillator available *in case child's system decompensates further.* • Keep child comfortable, warm, and well fed *to maintain adequate cardiac output as much as possible.*	An adequate cardiac output will be maintained.
Patient and Family Anxiety **RELATED TO** Diagnosis of SVT and treatment **DEFINING CHARACTERISTICS** Asking many questions Hesitant to respond or verbalize feelings Excessive worry Feelings of helplessness	**ONGOING ASSESSMENT** • Assess child's and family's level of understanding of diagnosis. • Assess family's desire to learn about treatment and long-term management. **THERAPEUTIC INTERVENTIONS** • Maintain a calm manner while interacting with child/family. • Reassure child/family that child is safe. • Support child and family throughout hospitalization. • Use educational materials to explain supraventricular tachycardia and its treatment *to facilitate learning and retention of information.* • Notify physician of undue anxiety levels *to allay fears and questions by family.*	Child and family express understanding of the diagnosis, verbalize feelings, and ask questions as necessary.

Susan P. Maloney, RN, BSN

Cardiac catheterization

A specialized diagnostic procedure in which the internal structures of the heart and coronary arteries are viewed to determine myocardial function, valvular competency, and presence or absence of suspected congenital heart disease.

NURSING DIAGNOSES/ DEFINING CHARACTERISTICS	NURSING INTERVENTIONS / *RATIONALES*	EXPECTED OUTCOMES
High Risk for Altered Tissue Perfusion **RELATED TO** *Postcatheterization:* Arterial vasospasm Thrombus formation Embolus **DEFINING CHARACTERISTICS** Decrease or absence of peripheral pulses Lessening in temperature of affected extremity Presence of mottling, pallor, rubor, or cyanosis in affected extremity Decrease or absence of motion in affected extremity	**ONGOING ASSESSMENT** ▪ Assess age and developmental level. *Precatheterization:* ▪ Assess and record presence or absence and quality of peripheral pulses. ▪ Mark pedal pulses with an *X*. ▪ Assess and record skin color, temperature, capillary refill of all extremities. ▪ Assess and record baseline range of motion of all extremities. ▪ Assess baseline vital signs, especially temperature. ▪ Assess patency of peripheral IV of prostaglandin (PGE₁) if in use. *Postcatheterization:* ▪ Assess and monitor affected extremity for occlusion every 15 min for 1 hour, then every 30 min for 1 hour, then every hour until stable. ▪ Assess and record presence and quality of pulses distal to catheter insertion site (dorsalis pedis for femoral site). ▪ If dorsalis pedis pulse is being monitored, mark site with *X*. ▪ Assess and record color, temperature, and capillary refill of affected extremity. ▪ Assess motion of affected extremity. Check cannulation site for swelling. *Severe edema can hinder peripheral circulation by constricting the vessels.* ▪ Assess for changes in vital signs. **THERAPEUTIC INTERVENTIONS** *Precatheterization:* ▪ Establish described assessment data *to have necessary baseline information.* ▪ Maintain peripheral IV prostaglandins (PGE₁) as ordered. *Prostaglandin (PGE₁) is a cardiovascular vasodilator used to promote dilation of the ductus arteriosus in infants with ductal-dependent congenital heart disease.* ▪ Assist with umbilical artery catheter (UAC) or umbilical venous catheter (UVC) insertion, to be used during the catheterization procedure *to provide stable lines for PGE₁ administration.* *Postcatheterization:* ▪ Immediately report to physician any decrease in or absence of pulse, change in skin color or temperature, and decrease or absence of motion in affected extremity. *These signs may indicate complications related to the catheterization procedure.* ▪ Avoid heelstick blood-drawing in affected leg *because of possible decreased perfusion.* ▪ Maintain prostaglandin (PGE₁) infusion, if in use, until further orders, *because of ductal-dependent needs for oxygenation/perfusion.* ▪ See Thermoregulation in the low-birth-weight infant, p. 379.	Tissue perfusion of affected extremity will be maintained.
High Risk for Injury: Bleeding **RELATED TO** Disruption of vessel integrity	**ONGOING ASSESSMENT** ▪ Assess insertion site and dressing for evidence of bleeding every 15 min for 1 hour, then every 30 min for 1 hour, then every hour until stable. ▪ Assess for change in vital signs. ▪ Monitor Hct and CBC with platelets following catheterization. ▪ Procure type and cross-match for 1 unit of packed RBCs (send 50 ml to catheterization laboratory with infant; remainder of unit should be placed on hold in blood bank).	Risk of bleeding will be reduced.

NURSING DIAGNOSES/ DEFINING CHARACTERISTICS	NURSING INTERVENTIONS / *RATIONALES*	EXPECTED OUTCOMES

DEFINING CHARACTERISTICS
Significant bleeding noted on dressing
Apprehension and restlessness
Hematoma at site of insertion
Increased heart rate, increased respiratory rate, decreased BP
	THERAPEUTIC INTERVENTIONS
	▪ Maintain bed rest with affected extremity straight for 6 hours *to minimize risk of bleeding.*
	▪ Use an armboard behind the knee *to keep the leg extended. Soft restraints will help to reduce movement.*
	▪ If arterial catheterization has been performed, apply warm packs to affected leg *to reduce swelling.* If venous catheterization has been performed, elevate extremity *to reduce swelling.*
	▪ If femoral site is used, do not elevate head of bed >30 degrees for 6 hours.
	▪ Maintain occlusive pressure dressing to cannulation site *to facilitate clot formation.*
	▪ Avoid sudden movements with affected extremity *to facilitate clot formation and wound closure at insertion site.*
	▪ For bleeding:
	    Circle, date, and time the amount of drainage or size of hematoma.
	    Estimate blood loss.
	    Reinforce dressing; apply pressure to site.
	    Notify physician if bleeding is significant.	

Fluid Volume Deficit **RELATED TO** Dye-induced diuresis Restricted intake before procedure **DEFINING CHARACTERISTICS** Poor skin turgor Dry, sticky mucous membranes Decrease in urine output Decrease in BP; increase in heart rate and respiratory rate Pale, cool, clammy skin	**ONGOING ASSESSMENT** ▪ Assess and monitor hydration status, skin turgor, and hemodynamic status. ▪ Obtain urine specific gravity measurement every 4 hours until normal. *Concentrated urine with high specific gravity may indicate presence of dye in system and/or hypovolemia.* ▪ Monitor BP closely, anticipating drop in BP and need for additional fluids *secondary to hypovolemic state.* **THERAPEUTIC INTERVENTIONS** ▪ Maintain strict I&O record for several hours after catheterization. ▪ Give oral feedings as tolerated. ▪ Institute IV fluids as ordered, monitoring flow rate *to prevent accidental fluid overload.*	Potential for dehydration will be reduced.

Pain/Discomfort
RELATED TO
Interruption of integument
Incision/catheterization performed with mild sedative
 	
DEFINING CHARACTERISTICS
Crying
Irritability
Short periods of sleep or restless sleep
Decreased appetite
Emesis
Flushing of skin
	ONGOING ASSESSMENT
	▪ Assess for discomfort/pain using defining characteristics.
	
	THERAPEUTIC INTERVENTIONS
	▪ Implement comfort measures following catheterization:
	    Offer pacifier.
	    Rock, cuddle, and talk to infant.
	    Administer appropriate analgesia *to relieve pain.*
	▪ Prevent infant from disrupting catheterization site by swaddling or using cloth restraints (as a last resort) *to avoid discomfort and bleeding.*
	▪ Instruct parents on comfort techniques *to promote effective parental care.*
		Discomfort/pain will be reduced or relieved.

Continued.

Cardiac catheterization cont'd

NURSING DIAGNOSES/ DEFINING CHARACTERISTICS	NURSING INTERVENTIONS / *RATIONALES*	EXPECTED OUTCOMES
Parental Anxiety/ Fear **RELATED TO** Unknown outcome of cardiac catheterization on their infant **DEFINING CHARACTERISTICS** Parents exhibit: Increased questioning Increased irritability Restlessness Anger Withdrawal	**ONGOING ASSESSMENT** • Assess parents' level of anxiety. **THERAPEUTIC INTERVENTIONS** • Provide emotional support as needed *to decrease anxiety.* • Be with parents when physician returns *to reinforce and explain information.* • See Parenting in the Special Care Nursery, p. 72.	Parental anxiety/fear will be reduced.
Parental Knowledge Deficit **RELATED TO** Precatheterization: Lack of familiarity with cardiac catheterization and congenital heart disease **DEFINING CHARACTERISTICS** Parents: Express need for information Numerous questions Inability to ask questions (shock) Increased anxiety level	**ONGOING ASSESSMENT** • Assess parental readiness to learn. • Assess parents' knowledge of their infant's cardiac status and heart anatomy. • Assess parents' knowledge of cardiac catheterization procedure. • Assess parents' knowledge of risk/benefits of cardiac catheterization. **THERAPEUTIC INTERVENTIONS** *Before procedure:* • Provide parents with information about: Heart anatomy and physiology Cardiac catheterization: indications; precatheterization preparation; procedure; postcatheterization care: *This provides parents with the necessary information about their infant's requirements.* • Explain rationale and risks/benefits of procedure, *because parents need adequate information to make an informed decision.* • Ascertain that a consent form has been signed by parents. • Encourage parents to ask questions and express concerns. *After procedure:* • Be with parents when catheterization findings are revealed *so clarification and reinforcement of information about infant's future needs can be provided.* • Explain care of site following catheterization. • Discuss comfort measures with parents *to provide them with appropriate comfort techniques to offer to their infant.*	Parents will verbalize basic understanding of procedure and outcome.

Phyllis Lawlor-Klean, RN, MS

Cardiac surgery

CONGENITAL HEART DEFECTS; PEDIATRIC CARDIAC SURGERY

Congenital heart defects (CHD) are fetal malformations of the heart and great vessels present at birth in approximately 8 to 10 of every 1000 newborns. These defects may vary from simple asymptomatic conditions to more complex and life-threatening anomalies. Surgical interventions may be corrective or palliative. Total correction ("open heart") of complex CHD involves the use of extracorporeal circulation, otherwise known as the "heart-lung machine." (For these procedures, see the nursing care plan for Pediatric cardiac surgery.) Palliative procedures—patent ductus arteriosus ligation, pulmonary artery banding, and shunts—are done to maximize oxygenation and minimize cardiopulmonary overload until the child reaches optimal condition for total correction.

NURSING DIAGNOSES/ DEFINING CHARACTERISTICS	NURSING INTERVENTIONS / *RATIONALES*	EXPECTED OUTCOMES

Impaired Gas Exchange
Related To
Pneumothorax
Hemothorax
Atelectasis
 	
Defining Characteristics
Hypercapnea
Hypoxia
Ineffective spontaneous respirations
Increased need for ventilatory support
Decreased or absent breath sounds on affected side
Positive transillumination of chest
Asymmetrical chest movement
Decrease in BP
	Ongoing Assessment
	• Assess age and developmental level.
	• Assess respiratory status every 1-2 hours:
	 Note rate, grunting, flaring retracting, breath sounds, chest movement.
	 Transilluminate chest prn.
	 Assess central and peripheral color.
	 Assess oxygenation:
	  Monitor transcutaneous PO_2 and PCO_2.
	  Measure blood gases every 1-2 hours and prn.
	  Note oximeter reading every 2 hours and prn (oxygen saturation).
	• Monitor chest x-ray films in the immediate postoperative period and follow up prn.
	
	Therapeutic Interventions
	• Do not perform chest physiotherapy unless radiographic evidence of atelectasis exists. If indicated, use electric toothbrush for percussion and vibration *to help move secretions toward the trachea and facilitate removal by suctioning.*
	• Suction endotracheal tube every 2 hours and prn *to prevent airway resistance and promote adequate ventilation.*
	• Change position every 1-2 hours *to evenly ventilate and perfuse the lungs.*
	• Keep temperature of inspired air at 36°-37° C (96.8°-98.6° F) *to provide adequate humidity. This will prevent drying and injury to the respiratory mucosa, impairment of ciliary activity, retention of secretions, atelectasis, and infection.*
	• Maintain ventilatory support *to facilitate normal gas exchange, avoid air leaks and oxygen injury, and maintain oxygen delivery until respiratory compromise or lung injury resolves.*
	• Gently "milk" chest tube every 15-30 min while drainage is bloody and prn *to ensure patency and promote effective drainage. (Neonatal tubes have small lumens and therefore have more tendency to occlude.)*
	• Notify physician if thoracic drainage is excessive: >3 ml/kg/hr for 3 hours or more, or 5 ml/kg/hr in any 1 hour. *(Bleeding totalling 2 ml/kg/hr for 3 hours constitutes a 12%-15% hemorrhage and will compromise systemic perfusion.)*
	• Maintain water seal at 10-15 mm H_2O negative pressure *for effective drainage.*
		Impairment of gas exchange will be absent or minimal.

Continued.

Cardiac surgery cont'd

NURSING DIAGNOSES/ DEFINING CHARACTERISTICS	NURSING INTERVENTIONS / *RATIONALES*	EXPECTED OUTCOMES
Ineffective Breathing Pattern **RELATED TO** Neuromuscular impairment Decreased lung expansion **DEFINING CHARACTERISTICS** Inadequate/ineffective spontaneous respiration Abnormal arterial blood gas Cyanosis	**ONGOING ASSESSMENT** • Assess respiratory status every 1-2 hours: Note rate, grunting, flaring, retractions, breath sounds, chest movement. Transilluminate chest prn. Assess central and peripheral color. Assess oxygenation: Monitor transcutaneous Po_2 and Pco_2. Measure blood gases every 1-2 hours and prn. Note oximeter (oxygen saturation) readings every 2 hours and prn. • Obtain report of type and amount of anesthetic agents used. • Observe child for spontaneous chest movement. **THERAPEUTIC INTERVENTIONS** • Wean child from ventilator when (1) he or she is awake and having spontaneous and effective respirations, (2) blood gases are near normal range, and (3) cardiovascular status is stabilized. • To avoid excessive blood sampling, use transcutaneous Po_2/Pco_2 monitor and pulse oximeter Sao_2 monitor in weaning. • Decrease as needed or indicated: IMV Fio_2 PIP	Respiratory status will be optimized.
Fluid Volume Deficit **RELATED TO** Hemorrhage Inadequate fluid replacement **DEFINING CHARACTERISTICS** Decreased urine output Rising hematocrit or stable hematocrit in spite of blood loss Low blood pressure Capillary refill >3 sec Metabolic acidosis Increased drainage from thoracic drain Inadequate pulses Pallor Prolonged bleeding time Bloody nasogastric drainage Edema Depressed fontanel Low platelet count	**ONGOING ASSESSMENT** • Assess vital signs, with BP and central venous pressure, every 1-2 hours. • Obtain report of blood loss from operating room and type and amount of fluid replacement. • Assess color and perfusion: Temperature of extremities Capillary refill Peripheral pulses • Monitor I&O every 1 hour: Urine specific gravity, pH, and protein Type and amount of thoracic drainage Blood loss for labs and loss from other sites • Monitor laboratory data: Hematocrit on admission and every 2-4 hours until stable Complete blood count on admission and prn Blood urea nitrogen and creatinine on admission and prn • Observe for alternate sites of bleeding/fluid loss (nasogastric, chest tube, or puncture sites). **THERAPEUTIC INTERVENTIONS** • Administer parenteral fluids as needed (usually 50%-75% of maintenance during first 24 hours postoperatively, *because the stress of surgery increases antidiuretic hormone secretion and consequently sodium and water retention*). • Maintain urine output of 0.5 ml to 1 ml/kg/hr (*less may indicate fluid volume depletion or decreased renal perfusion*). • Maintain specific gravity between 1.003 and 1.010. Report specific gravity >1.010 or output <0.5 ml/kg/hr to physician. • Report excessive thoracic drainage (75 ml/kg/hr in 1 hour or >3 ml/ kg/hr for the following 3 hours).	Fluid volume deficit will be reduced.

NURSING DIAGNOSES/ DEFINING CHARACTERISTICS	NURSING INTERVENTIONS / *RATIONALES*	EXPECTED OUTCOMES
High Risk for Ineffective Cardiac Contractility **RELATED TO** Cardiac tamponade **DEFINING CHARACTERISTICS** Increased respiratory rate Tachycardia Decreased blood pressure Narrowing pulse pressure Distant heart sounds Abrupt decrease in thoracic drainage Widening mediastinal shadow Decreased QRS voltage Decreased peripheral perfusion	**ONGOING ASSESSMENT** • Assess respiratory rate, apical pulse, BP, central venous pressure every hour. • Assess for decreased intensity of heart sounds. • Assess peripheral perfusion and pulses. • Assess for cessation or significant decrease in thoracic drainage. • Monitor chest serial x-ray films. • Observe for ECG changes. • Follow hematocrit every shift. • Assess clinical status, using defining characteristics. **THERAPEUTIC INTERVENTIONS** • Notify physician of abrupt decrease in chest tube drainage and/or presence of symptoms listed under defining characteristics. *Cardiac tamponade requires immediate intervention.* • Prepare for and assist physician with emergency pericardiocentesis (needle evacuation of pericardial fluid) *to help restore cardiac contractility and function.* • Maintain ventilatory support *to enhance oxygenation until cardiac function is restored.* • Administer IV fluids and blood products *for intravascular volume expansion and replacement of lost blood.*	Effective cardiac contractility will be maintained.

Altered Electrical Conduction, Rate, or Rhythm **RELATED TO** Low calcium Digoxin toxicity Acidosis High or low potassium Myocardial dysfunction Presence of central venous catheter **DEFINING CHARACTERISTICS** Irregular pulse ECG changes Tachycardia >160 Bradycardia <100 Low blood pressure Pallor Abnormal blood gases Decreased or absent peripheral pulses Abnormal electrolyte and calcium levels	**ONGOING ASSESSMENT**
	• Assess calcium and electrolyte levels on admission and as needed.
	• Assess chest x-ray films on admission and prn for central venous line placement. *Presence of catheter may stimulate myocardial irritability.*
	• Monitor ECG configuration.
	• Monitor digoxin level if toxicity is suspected.
	
	THERAPEUTIC INTERVENTIONS
	• Document dysrhythmias with rhythm strip *to provide baseline information and indicate progression or resolution of abnormality.*
	• Give calcium gluconate as ordered. *Hypocalcemia may increase myocardial spontaneous discharge and prolong myocardial repolarization, causing an increase in QT interval.*
	• Supplement electrolytes as ordered:
	   Hypokalemia *potentiates digoxin effect and causes myocardial irritability.*
	   Hyperkalemia *can slow conduction time and increase potential for heart block.*
		Cardiovascular compromise will be prevented.

Continued.

Cardiovascular Care Plans (Neonatal)

NURSING DIAGNOSES/ DEFINING CHARACTERISTICS	NURSING INTERVENTIONS / *RATIONALES*	EXPECTED OUTCOMES
Altered Cardiac Output Secondary to Ineffective Shunt **RELATED TO** Shunt too large Shunt inadequate because of size and/ or occlusion too small **DEFINING CHARACTERISTICS** *Shunt too large:* Change in quality or radiation of murmur Tachycardia Bounding peripheral pulses Ventricular gallop Hepatomegaly >2 cm below right costal margin Oliguria Peripheral vasoconstriction Tachypnea >60 Rales Retractions Cyanosis *Shunt inadequate secondary to size and/or occlusion:* Clinical deterioration with decreased PO_2, decreased pH, decreased platelet count	**ONGOING ASSESSMENT** • Assess arterial blood gases on admission and every 1-2 hours prn. • Asses vital signs with BP and central venous pressure on admission, every hour, and prn. • Assess color, perfusion, and capillary refill. • See Congestive heart failure, p. 118. **THERAPEUTIC INTERVENTIONS** • Maintain hematocrit level between 45 and 60. • Administer prostaglandin E at 0.05-0.1 µg/kg/min, if it is determined that shunt is nonfunctional, *to produce vasodilation, smooth muscle relaxation, and effective pulmonary or systemic perfusion.* • Titrate prostaglandin E at lowest dose that maintains oxygenation. *(Incidence of complications increases with higher doses.)*	Optimal cardiac output will be maintained.
High Risk for Altered Level of Consciousness **RELATED TO** Impaired cerebral blood flow **DEFINING CHARACTERISTICS** Seizure activity Flaccidity and/or lethargy not attributable to drug therapy Extreme irritability Fluctuations in blood pressure, heart rate, respiration	**ONGOING ASSESSMENT** • See Seizures, p. 214. • Observe for unexplained changes in blood pressure, heart rate, oxygenation, perfusion. • Check pupils for size and reactivity to light. **THERAPEUTIC INTERVENTIONS** • Keep hematocrit level >45 *(lower count diminishes the oxygen-carrying capacity of the blood)* and <60 *(polycythemia characterized by increased hematocrit and blood viscosity produces increased peripheral vascular resistance, decreased oxygen to the body, and ultimately thrombosis or cerebral infarction in particular).* • Do not allow any air to enter arterial circulation *to prevent injury from cerebral air embolus.* • Do not allow air to enter venous circulation (particularly important if infant has right-to-left shunt). *This potentiates danger for pulmonary air embolism and eventually contributes to impaired cerebral blood flow.* • Document type/amount of anesthetic agents and medications given. *Drugs may cause depression of respiratory and cardiovascular functions (decreased BP, increased heart rate, apnea).*	Changes in the cerebral blood flow will be detected early.

NURSING DIAGNOSES/ DEFINING CHARACTERISTICS	NURSING INTERVENTIONS / *RATIONALES*	EXPECTED OUTCOMES
DEFINING CHARACTERISTICS cont'd Change in pupil size and/or reactivity to light not caused by medications, *e.g., atropine administration will produce pupillary dilation* Hemiparesis/hemiplegia		

High Risk for Infection
RELATED TO
Disruption of skin and iatrogenic sources of infection
 	
DEFINING CHARACTERISTICS
Temperature instability
Increased or decreased white blood cell count
Inflammation of and/ or drainage from incision
Foul-smelling or green/yellow drainage from endotracheal tube or thoracic drain
	ONGOING ASSESSMENT
	- Assess vital signs with temperature every 1-2 hours.
	- Assess all skin incisions for signs of inflammation and/or drainage.
	- Note color, type, amount of thoracic drainage.
	- Monitor CBC and culture results.
	- Collect culture specimen of suspicious drainage.
	- Monitor antibiotic levels *to prevent subtherapeutic or toxic levels.*
	
	THERAPEUTIC INTERVENTIONS
	- Administer antibiotics as ordered.
	- Maintain strict handwashing by all individuals handling infant. *(Handwashing is the most effective way of controlling spread of infection.)*
	- Maintain aseptic technique when changing:
	    IV lines/bags/dressings
	    Surgical dressings
	    Preparing/administering medications
		Infectious process will be prevented or reduced.

High Risk for Altered Glucose Metabolism **RELATED TO** *Hyperglycemia:* Stress Epinephrine Iatrogenic factors *Hypoglycemia:* Cold stress Inadequate glucose intake **DEFINING CHARACTERISTICS** *Hyperglycemia:* Osmotic diuresis Chemstrip >120 Glucosuria >1+	**ONGOING ASSESSMENT** - Assess chemstrips and send blood glucose to laboratory on admission. - Monitor chemstrip every 30 min until stable, then every 2 hours. - Obtain report of all medications and fluids administered in operating room. - Assess temperature on admission, every hour until stable, then every 2 hours. **THERAPEUTIC INTERVENTIONS** - See Altered glucose metabolism, p. 372. - Decrease IV glucose as ordered if Chemstrip >240 or glycosuria >1+. - Increase IV glucose as ordered if Chemstrip <40.	Adequate glucose metabolism will be maintained.

Continued.

Cardiac surgery cont'd

NURSING DIAGNOSES/ DEFINING CHARACTERISTICS	NURSING INTERVENTIONS / *RATIONALES*	EXPECTED OUTCOMES
DEFINING CHARACTERISTICS cont'd *Hypoglycemia:* Chemstrip <40 Tremors Temperature instability Pallor Apnea Tachypnea		
High Risk for Altered Calcium Metabolism: Hypocalcemia RELATED TO Stress Administration of citrated blood Metabolic acidosis treated with sodium bicarbonate **DEFINING CHARACTERISTICS** Muscle twitching/ jitters Compromised myocardial function Calcium level <8 mg/dl	**ONGOING ASSESSMENT** • Assess calcium level on admission and as ordered by physician. **THERAPEUTIC INTERVENTIONS** • See Altered calcium metabolism, p. 372.	Calcium level stable at 8-10 mg/dl.
Pain/Discomfort RELATED TO Incision Painful positioning resulting from pressure of drainage tubes, dressings, central lines Painful procedures **DEFINING CHARACTERISTICS** Crying Facial expressions consistent with distress Autonomic responses: HR may increase for severe stimuli HR may decrease for mild pain Agitation Decreased O_2/CO_2 Increased respiratory effort	**ONGOING ASSESSMENT** • Assess presence of pain/discomfort (see defining characteristics). • Assess whether defining characteristics are minimized or resolved on withdrawal of painful stimuli. *Some of these characteristics may also occur secondary to respiratory or cardiac problems.* **THERAPEUTIC INTERVENTIONS** • The following may be attempted before resorting to medications: Offer pacifier. Provide quiet environment *to reduce stimulation and promote rest.* Change position or swaddle if appropriate. *Chest tubes, UAC, and CVP lines need to be closely monitored for proper functioning and detection of complications such as bleeding.* Provide comforting tactile stimulation, e.g., mild rubbing or holding. • Administer pharmacological interventions as indicated and note response.	Pain or discomfort will be reduced or eliminated.

NURSING DIAGNOSES/ DEFINING CHARACTERISTICS	NURSING INTERVENTIONS / *RATIONALES*	EXPECTED OUTCOMES

Altered Parenting and Parent/Infant Bonding
RELATED TO
Hospitalization of infant with life-threatening illness
Possible inability of parents to visit
Infant transported from another hospital
 	
DEFINING CHARACTERISTICS
Verbal/nonverbal expression of fear/anxiety of intensive care environment
Parents blame themselves for infant's condition
Parents express guilt feelings at having a "less than perfect" infant
Parents express feeling of failure or inadequacy in nurturing infant
Single parent or substitute visitation by relatives
Withdrawal
Grief
Sadness
Limited involvement with infant
Does not call or visit regularly
Delays in naming infant
	ONGOING ASSESSMENT
	• Assess level of comprehension.
	• Assess level of anxiety.
	• Assess existing support systems.
	• Assess knowledge of illness/condition.
	• Assess previous experience with hospitalized family members.
	• Assess mother's condition:
	  Ability to come to special care nursery
	  Probable discharge date if in another hospital
	• Assess distance parents live from hospital.
	• Assess availability of transportation.
	• If mother cannot visit, assess her knowledge of infant's condition.
	
	THERAPEUTIC INTERVENTIONS
	• Explain to parents:
	  Infant's current condition
	  Equipment used
	  Immediate treatment
	• Have them describe their understanding of information. Clarify confusing or misinterpreted information.
	• Encourage visitation and phone calls. *Many units have 24-hour open visit/call policy to help alleviate family anxiety.*
	• Encourage parents to touch infant and to bring toys, clothes, etc. for infant. *This will help parents to feel that they are participating in infant's care.*
	• Encourage verbalization of fears/anxieties, but in reassuring them, be careful not to provide false hope.
	• Identify available support systems and make appropriate referral (e.g., social worker, clergy, parent support group). *This will help them feel they are not alone and also improve their coping abilities.*
	• Send picture of infant to mother.
	• Facilitate communication between parents as appropriate.
	• Arrange for overnight accommodations if parents live a long distance from the hospital.
	• Arrange for hospital to call family if long-distance calls present a financial problem.
	• Refer parents to social worker.
	• Encourage attendance at parent support group.
		Parents verbalize an understanding of infant's illness/condition and possible outcome.
		Achievement of optimal parent role.

Laura L. Rybicki, RN, BSN; Racquel Gabriel-Bennewitz, RN, BSN, CCRN

Congestive heart failure

A clinical syndrome in which the myocardium is unable to meet the metabolic requirements of the body. Possible etiological factors may include cardiomyopathy, volume overload, asphyxia, and anemia.

NURSING DIAGNOSES/ DEFINING CHARACTERISTICS	NURSING INTERVENTIONS / *RATIONALES*	EXPECTED OUTCOMES
Altered Breathing Pattern **RELATED TO** Pulmonary venous congestion **DEFINING CHARACTERISTICS** Tachypnea (respiratory rate >60/min) Increased respiratory effort: Retractions Nasal flaring Grunting (indicates significant distress) Rales (rare in infants) Inadequate blood gases Cyanosis	**ONGOING ASSESSMENT** ▪ Assess age and developmental level. ▪ Count respirations for 1 full minute. ▪ Auscultate breath sounds in all lung fields, noting quality of aeration, rales. ▪ Auscultate for heart sounds. ▪ Note any nasal flaring, location, and severity of retractions. ▪ Note general skin and mucous membrane color. ▪ Monitor blood gases to evaluate metabolic/respiratory status. *Early detection/correction will prevent further respiratory compromise.* **THERAPEUTIC INTERVENTIONS** ▪ Maintain infant in semi-Fowler's position or in infant seat *to allow maximal diaphragmatic excursion and lung expansion.* ▪ Place small linen roll under infant's shoulders *to extend airway, which will help infant breathe with less difficulty.* ▪ Suction secretions as needed *to maintain patent airway (endotracheal, nasopharyngeal, oropharyngeal).* ▪ Administer oxygen as needed to maintain PaO₂ at prescribed level *to maximize oxygenation.* ▪ Maintain axillary temperature at 36.4°-36.8° C (97.5°-98.2° F), *because the infant's oxygen requirements increase when temperature is excessively high or low.* ▪ Organize care *to minimize handling and provide for long rest periods.* ▪ Observe for early signs of superimposed infection: Temperature instability/hypothermia Peripheral vasoconstriction Need for increased amount of oxygen and/or increased ventilator pressure	Improved respiratory status will be achieved.
Decreased Cardiac Output **RELATED TO** Decreased contractility Increased/decreased preload Increased afterload Myocardial ischemia Decreased renal perfusion	**ONGOING ASSESSMENT** ▪ Count heart rate for 1 full minute every 2 hours and prn. ▪ Note recent digoxin level and monitor for signs of digoxin toxicity: Dysrhythmias Diarrhea Vomiting ▪ Monitor serum electrolytes, BUN, creatinine and hematocrit. ▪ Monitor weight daily. ▪ Document strict I&O. ▪ Monitor BP every shift. ▪ Assess for edema every shift; document findings. ▪ Palpate liver edge at right costal margin and mark liver edge daily. ▪ Assess heart sounds every 2 hours and prn. ▪ Assess temperature and color of extremities every 2 hours and prn. ▪ Note strength of peripheral pulses every 2 hours and prn. ▪ Obtain urine pH, specific gravity, and protein every 6-8 hours.	Adequate cardiac output will be achieved.

Maintain PaO₂ note: Administer oxygen as needed to maintain PaO_2 at prescribed level.

NURSING DIAGNOSES/ DEFINING CHARACTERISTICS	NURSING INTERVENTIONS / *RATIONALES*	EXPECTED OUTCOMES

DEFINING CHARACTERISTICS
Presence of or change for the worse in quality/radiation of murmur
Presence of ventricular gallop
Tachycardic rhythm
Bounding peripheral pulses (PDA, VSD)
Hepatomegaly >2 cm below right costal margin
Peripheral vasoconstriction and poor systemic perfusion:
  Pale and mottled skin
  Pale mucous membranes and nailbeds
  Cool extremities
  Weak or thready peripheral pulses
  Prolonged capillary refill (>3 sec)
Dependent or periorbital edema
Hypotension
Oliguria (urine output <0.5-1 ml/kg/hr)
Metabolic acidosis with or without hypoxemia
	THERAPEUTIC INTERVENTIONS
	• For infants receiving digoxin:
	  If heart rate is <100/min, or 30 beats below baseline *before* administration, hold dose until physician is notified. *Digoxin can further slow the cardiac electrical conduction.*
	• Notify physician if serum potassium is less than 3.5. *(Hypokalemia potentiates digoxin toxicity.)*
	• Report significant weight changes to the physician (< or >50 g/day).
	• Administer fluids as appropriate:
	  100-150 ml/kg/day, providing there is adequate renal and cardiac functioning. *Hypovolemia decreases cardiac output.*
	  Fluid restrictions between 80-100 ml/kg/day if there is renal or cardiac dysfunction. *Hypervolemia produces systemic and pulmonary congestion and may reactivate a patent ductus arteriosus.*
	• Administer diuretics as ordered *to increase urine output.*
	• Administer sympathomimetic agents such as dopamine, as ordered, *to increase cardiac output.*	

Altered Nutrition: Less Than Body Requirements **RELATED TO** Caloric loss as a result of increased cardiorespiratory demand **DEFINING CHARACTERISTICS** Increased tachypnea, severity of retraction, nasal flaring with feedings Tachycardia during feedings Cyanosis	**ONGOING ASSESSMENT** • Assess respiratory status during feedings. • Monitor for severe/persistent tachycardia. • Plot daily weight on Dancis curve. **THERAPEUTIC INTERVENTIONS** • Organize care *to provide longer rest periods between feedings.* • Feed infant every 3 hours as ordered. • Use nipple sized for premature infants and enlarge the hole. • Keep infant in upright position during feedings. • If infant is distressed, finish feeding by gavage. *Caloric expenditure may exceed intake.* • Consider MCT oil, Polycose, or 24-hour calorie formula for infants with slow or absent weight gain for a more easily absorbed, high-caloric intake. *(These have more calories per ounce.)*	Optimal nutrition will be attained.

Continued.

Congestive heart failure cont'd

NURSING DIAGNOSES/ DEFINING CHARACTERISTICS	NURSING INTERVENTIONS / *RATIONALES*	EXPECTED OUTCOMES
Knowledge Deficit: Parents **RELATED TO** Lack of exposure to condition Special situation affecting infant care **DEFINING CHARACTERISTICS** Increased "questioning" Lack of questions, fear of touching or caring for infant Lack of eye contact with infant Lack of or absence of calls or visits from parents	**ONGOING ASSESSMENT** · Assess parents' level of knowledge related to infant's illness. · Assess parents' available support systems. · Assess parents' coping abilities. **THERAPEUTIC INTERVENTIONS** · Explain to parents the symptoms of heart failure that the infant is exhibiting. · Explain how the physical characteristics affect the special needs of the baby (e.g., feeding, rest, and medication). · Assist parents with infant feeding and care. · Begin documenting information in planning tool soon after admission. · Involve social services in infant's care early in hospitalization.	Parents will verbalize understanding of infant's condition, the mode of treatment, and demonstrate participation in infant's care.

Terri L. Russell, RN; Racquel Gabriel-Bennewitz, RN, BSN, CCRN

Patent ductus arteriosus (PDA)

Persistence of fetal vascular channel between the left pulmonary artery and aorta (left-to-right shunt).

PATENCY OF DUCTUS ARTERIOSUS

NURSING DIAGNOSES/ DEFINING CHARACTERISTICS	NURSING INTERVENTIONS / *RATIONALES*	EXPECTED OUTCOMES
Decreased Cardiac Output **RELATED TO** Prematurity (increased risk with decreased gestational age) Excessive fluid administration Respiratory distress syndrome **DEFINING CHARACTERISTICS** *Physical examination*: Hyperactive precordium Tachycardia Bounding pulses Heart murmur Gallop rhythm Wide pulse pressure Decreased urinary output Hepatomegaly Rales *Chest x-ray evaluation*: Increased pulmonary blood flow Enlarged heart *Electrocardiogram*: Left ventricular hypertrophy	**ONGOING ASSESSMENT** • Assess age and developmental level. • Assess vital signs and blood pressure every 2 hours. • Report tachycardia *because this may be indicative of congestive heart failure (CHF).* • Report wide pulse pressure; *this is suggestive of PDA.* • Palpate precordium and peripheral pulses every 2 hours and document. • Palpate liver edge at right costal margin and mark liver edge daily *to detect presence of hepatomegaly; this is a sign of severe CHF.* • Auscultate breath sounds for presence of rales. • Determine fluid intake in ml/24 hr/kg of body weight. • Monitor urine output in ml/hr/kg of body weight. *Inadequate urine output (<1 ml/kg/hr) may be a sign of congestive heart failure, and is also a contraindication to or a side effect of indomethacin administration.* • Monitor serum electrolytes, creatinine, BUN, and platelet count as ordered. • Assess for GI bleeding by checking stools and aspirated gastric content for blood. • Observe for prolonged bleeding from venipuncture sites. • Monitor for signs of feeding intolerance. • Monitor hematocrit as ordered. *Anemia is associated with PDA.* **THERAPEUTIC INTERVENTIONS** • Maintain appropriate fluid restriction. *Fluid restriction is supportive care for the infant with PDA, to prevent cardiovascular overload.* • Give indomethacin sodium as ordered *to facilitate nonsurgical closure of the PDA in premature infants. Indomethacin administration is contraindicated in the presence of active bleeding, a pathological condition of the GI tract, and/or impaired renal function.* • Transfuse with packed red blood cells as ordered to *facilitate ductal closure by increasing the arterial oxygen content.* • Report abnormal laboratory results, bleeding, and feeding intolerance to physician. • Report any signs of CHF to the physician, *because this may result from volume overload of the left ventricle.* (See CHF, p. 118.) • If infant continues to be symptomatic and medical management is not successful, anticipate possible surgical ligation of the ductus arteriosus.	Adequate cardiac output will be achieved.

Altered Breathing Pattern **RELATED TO** Pulmonary venous congestion
 	
 DEFINING CHARACTERISTICS *Increased respiratory effort*: Tachypnea Nasal flaring Increased $PaCO_2$ Apnea Cyanosis Reduced oxygen saturation
	ONGOING ASSESSMENT
	 • Assess for respiratory distress, using defining characteristics.
	 • Monitor blood gases *to evaluate metabolic/respiratory status; early detection/collection will prevent further compromise.*
	 • Monitor pulse oximeter readings every 2 hours. *This is a noninvasive monitoring device that measures oxygen saturation of arterial blood.*
	
	 THERAPEUTIC INTERVENTIONS
	 • Maintain patent airway:
	   Chest physical therapy/postural drainage
	   Suction
	 • Administer oxygen as needed *to maintain PaO_2 at prescribed levels to maximize oxygenation.*
	 • Minimize handling *to avoid agitation and subsequent hypoxia.*
		Respiratory compromise will be reduced.

Continued.

Cardiovascular Care Plans (Neonatal)

NURSING DIAGNOSES/ DEFINING CHARACTERISTICS	NURSING INTERVENTIONS / *RATIONALES*	EXPECTED OUTCOMES
Altered Nutrition: Less Than Body Requirements **RELATED TO** Caloric loss due to increased respiratory demand **DEFINING CHARACTERISTICS** Increased tachypnea, retractions, and nasal flaring with feedings Tachycardia during feedings Poor tolerance to feedings Documented inadequate weight gain Failure to gain weight according to the growth curve	**ONGOING ASSESSMENT** - Assess respiratory status during feedings, using defining characteristics. - Plot daily weight on Dancis curve *to determine patterns of weight gain or loss.* - Calculate fluid and caloric intake daily. **THERAPEUTIC INTERVENTIONS** - Organize care *to provide longer rest periods between feedings.* - Use a premature-size nipple, *which offers the least resistance to sucking.* - If signs of respiratory distress are present, finish feeding by gavage.	Optimal nutrition will be attained.
Altered Parenting **RELATED TO** Interruption of normal adaptation of new family unit **DEFINING CHARACTERISTICS** Withdrawal Grief Sadness Limited involvement with infant Does not visit or call regularly Delays in naming infant	**ONGOING ASSESSMENT** - Assess parents for: Developmental stage Feelings regarding impact of pregnancy on the family Level of anxiety Existing support systems Cultural backgrounds Knowledge of illness or condition **THERAPEUTIC INTERVENTIONS** - Explain to parents: Reasons for admission Equipment used Immediate treatment *to provide parents with information that will assist in decreasing anxiety* - Familiarize parents with staff of special care nursery *to increase comfort with unit.* - Inform parents of 24-hour calling and visitation policy. - Encourage parents to touch, kiss, and talk to infant. Allow them to hold infant. - Encourage parents to take pictures or give them pictures of infant *to promote parent/infant bonding and to encourage appropriate parenting behaviors.* - Encourage participation in basic caretaking skills: diapering, bathing, and applying lotion *to promote parenting skills and initiate discharge teaching.* - Promote parents' verbalization of feelings and use of support systems. - Show available parent movies. *Movies will reinforce information and provide emotional support.* - See Parenting in the special care nursery, p. 72.	Ability to parent will be maximized.

Terry Griffin, RN, MS; Cynthia R. Wilson, RN, BSN

4

Pulmonary Care Plans

PEDIATRIC PATIENT
Asthma, bronchial
Bronchopulmonary dysplasia (BPD)
Carbon monoxide poisoning/smoke
    inhalation
Epiglottitis
Near-drowning
Near-miss sudden infant death syndrome
    (SIDS)
Pneumonia
Pneumothorax/chest tubes
Respiratory failure
Tracheostomy
Ventilation, high-frequency jet (HFJV)
Ventilation, mechanical

NEONATAL PATIENT
Meconium aspiration syndrome (MAS)
Persistent pulmonary hypertension (PPHN)
Respiratory distress syndrome
Transient tachypnea of the newborn

Asthma, bronchial

STATUS ASTHMATICUS

Paroxysmal dyspnea accompanied by adventitious sounds (wheezing) caused by the swelling and spasm of bronchial tubes. This reversible condition is commonly precipitated by antigen-antibody reactions, respiratory infection, cold weather, physical exertion, emotions, and some drugs.

NURSING DIAGNOSES/ DEFINING CHARACTERISTICS	NURSING INTERVENTIONS / *RATIONALES*	EXPECTED OUTCOMES
Ineffective Airway Clearance **RELATED TO** Swelling and spasm of the bronchial tubes in response to allergies, drugs, stress, infection, inhaled irritants **DEFINING CHARACTERISTICS** Irritability Retractions Grunting Stridor Nasal flaring Wheezing Cough Dyspnea Abnormal breath sounds, rate, and depth Verbalized tightness in chest Decreased air exchange	**ONGOING ASSESSMENT** • Assess age and developmental level. • Assess vital signs every hour when child is in distress. • Note color changes (lips, buccal mucosa, nail beds). • Look for and document signs of respiratory dysfunction: Irritability Retractions Grunting Stridor Nasal flaring Wheezing Cyanosis Decreased air exchange Decreased alertness Abnormal blood gases Restlessness • Evaluate breath sounds. • Monitor laboratory work: Theophylline level ABGs (monitor frequently while child is in distress) CBC Electrolytes • Assess whether medication used for treatment is effectively relieving symptoms leading to distress. • Notify physician immediately of any changes in condition. • Use respiratory scoring system to assess distress. • Follow peak pressures. **THERAPEUTIC INTERVENTIONS** • Keep head of bed elevated *to help with expansion of lungs.* • Keep child as calm as possible. • Check that respiratory treatments are given as ordered; notify the respiratory therapist as needed. • Encourage child to cough, especially after treatments. • Give humidified oxygen as ordered. • Give medications and IV fluids as ordered. • Use appropriate clinical resources. • If child is in severe distress: Assist with intubation and possible administration of paralyzing agents. Admit to PICU as needed. Assist with arterial lines as needed *for quick access.* Maintain patent airway (see Airway clearance, ineffective, p. 3).	Effective airway clearance will be maintained.
High Risk for Fluid Volume Deficit **RELATED TO** Decreased fluid intake Increased respiratory distress Diaphoresis	**ONGOING ASSESSMENT** • Monitor vital signs every hour while in PICU and every 4 hours while on floor. • Measure I&O every hour while in PICU. • Assess urine specific gravity. • Monitor electrolytes. • Assess skin turgor. • Monitor weight.	Hydration will be maximized.

NURSING DIAGNOSES/ DEFINING CHARACTERISTICS	NURSING INTERVENTIONS / *RATIONALES*	EXPECTED OUTCOMES
DEFINING CHARACTERISTICS Decreased urine output <30 ml/hr Complaint of thirst Complaint of dryness to lips and mouth Decreased skin turgor Increased specific gravity Sunken eyes Sunken fontanel in infant Lack of tears in infant	**ONGOING ASSESSMENT cont'd** ▪ Assess sputum for color, tenacity, liquefaction, amount. ▪ Follow ABGs to check for metabolic acidosis. ▪ Observe for signs of dehydration. ▪ Assess parenteral fluid administration. **THERAPEUTIC INTERVENTIONS** ▪ Encourage oral fluid intake by providing water and preferred liquids at bedside. ▪ Maintain IV infusion at proper rate. *Adequate intake will enhance liquefaction of bronchial secretions. Thinner liquid secretions are more easily expectorated.* ▪ Provide assistance with bedpan/commode at frequent intervals. *Some children decrease intake to decrease frequent need for urination.* ▪ Be careful not to overhydrate, causing fluid overload and pulmonary edema *(related to high negative pleural pressures).*	

Anxiety
RELATED TO
Respiratory distress
Change in health status
Change in environment
 	
DEFINING CHARACTERISTICS
Complaints of inability to breathe
Verbalized feelings of impending doom
Restlessness
Apprehensiveness
Insomnia
Increased heart rate
Frequently asking for someone to be in room
Diaphoresis
	ONGOING ASSESSMENT
	▪ Assess anxiety level every hour while in PICU and every 4 hours when on floor, including:
	    Vital signs
	    Respiratory status
	    Irritability
	    Apprehension
	    Orientation
	    Need for sedation
	
	THERAPEUTIC INTERVENTIONS
	▪ Help relieve respiratory distress as soon as possible.
	▪ Explain all procedures before starting.
	▪ Make as comfortable as possible:
	    Be available.
	    Reassure the child and parents as appropriate.
	    Provide quiet diversional activities.
	    Explain importance of remaining as calm as possible. *Maintaining calm will decrease oxygen consumption and the work of breathing.*
	▪ Explain that a nurse will be available if needed.
		Anxiety will be reduced.

Pain
RELATED TO
Excessive exertion of accessory respiratory musculature as a result of acute asthma attack
 	
DEFINING CHARACTERISTICS
Complaints of pain when breathing
Complaints of inability to get comfortable
Restlessness
Position child assumes
	ONGOING ASSESSMENT
	▪ Monitor respiratory function.
	▪ Evaluate ability to relax.
	▪ Assess complaints of pain: degree, location, and effectiveness of interventions.
	▪ Assess for changes in physical tolerance. *Fatigue may indicate increasing distress and can lead to status asthmaticus and respiratory failure.*
	▪ Assess child's need for reassurance.
	▪ Evaluate need for sedation.
	
	THERAPEUTIC INTERVENTIONS
	▪ Make child as comfortable as possible:
	    Raise head of bed.
	    Position with pillows.
	    Hold/rock in upright position.
		Pain will be relieved or reduced.

Continued.

Asthma, bronchial cont'd

NURSING DIAGNOSES/ DEFINING CHARACTERISTICS	NURSING INTERVENTIONS / *RATIONALES*	EXPECTED OUTCOMES
DEFINING CHARACTERISTICS cont'd Insomnia Increased respiratory distress Complaints of inability to breathe; can't catch breath	**THERAPEUTIC INTERVENTIONS cont'd** • Be available to: Answer questions simply. Explain all procedures. Explain all equipment used. • Provide medications as ordered—sedation if needed. • Explain need to remain as calm as possible. • Explain need to inform nurses of any discomfort. *Relief of respiratory distress will relieve the source of pain.* • Allow parents to remain with child if they are able. • Keep parents informed of child's progress *to relieve apprehension. Parental anxiety is readily transmitted to the child.*	
Knowledge Deficit RELATED TO Chronicity of disease Long-term medical management **DEFINING CHARACTERISTICS** Absence of questions Anxious Inability to answer questions properly Ineffective self-care	**ONGOING ASSESSMENT** • Assess knowledge of disease process. • Assess knowledge of medications. • Evaluate self-care activities: Preventive care Home management of acute attack • Assess ability to learn. • Assess knowledge of care when in status asthmaticus. • Assess parents' knowledge of CPR. **THERAPEUTIC INTERVENTIONS** • Explain disease to child/family. • Reinforce need for taking prescribed medications as ordered *to minimize incidence of full-blown attacks.* • Teach warning signs and symptoms of asthma attack and importance of early treatment for impending attack. • Reinforce what is to be done in an asthma attack: Home management When to come to emergency room Prevention • Reinforce need for keeping follow-up appointments. • Refer to social services if needed. • Refer to support groups if needed. • Address long-term management issues: Environmental controls Avoidance of precipitators Good health habits • Keep emergency phone numbers by telephone. • Teach parents/caregivers CPR if needed. • Teach family how to administer respiratory treatments, inhalers.	Child/parent will verbalize knowledge about disease and its management.

Kathleen Jaffrey, RN

Bronchopulmonary dysplasia (BPD)

A chronic and progressive generalized lung disease that is a sequela of respiratory distress syndrome (RDS), following mechanical ventilation in premature and very-low-birth-weight infants. BPD occasionally occurs in term infants following pneumonia, meconium aspiration, persistent pulmonary hypertension, tracheoesophageal fistula, and congenital heart disease. BPD results in thickening and necrosis of the alveolar walls and the basement membranes.

NURSING DIAGNOSES/ DEFINING CHARACTERISTICS	NURSING INTERVENTIONS / *RATIONALES*	EXPECTED OUTCOMES
Impaired Gas Exchange **RELATED TO** Long-term ventilator therapy Barotrauma from mechanical ventilation High oxygen concentration Alveolar rupture or pulmonary interstitial emphysema **DEFINING CHARACTERISTICS** Tachypnea Retractions Nasal flaring Pallor Diminished or unequal breath sounds Deterioration of arterial blood gas values Cyanosis Chest x-ray film ultimately reveals opacification, cystic infiltrates, and increased density	**ONGOING ASSESSMENT** • Assess age and developmental level. • Assess and record: Respiratory rate and breath sounds every 2 hours and prn Signs and symptoms of impaired gas exchange Arterial blood gas values when indicated. Notify physician if results are out of the stated range. • Assess patency of endotracheal tube or tracheostomy by listening to breath sounds frequently. • Check ventilator settings (FiO_2, rate, intermittent mandatory ventilation [IMV], peak inspiratory pressure [PIP], tidal volume [V$_T$], positive end expiratory pressure [PEEP], continuous positive airway pressure [CPAP]), and record every 1-2 hours. • Monitor oxygen saturation per pulse oximeter and end tidal CO_2 as indicated. • Check and record results of chest x-ray examination when indicated. **THERAPEUTIC INTERVENTIONS** • Ensure that O_2 is being delivered in the correct amount and route. • Suction endotracheal tube or trachea using sterile technique every 2-3 hours and prn. Record amount, consistency, and characteristics of secretions. • Ensure that chest physiotherapy and respiratory treatments are being done effectively and gently on schedule.	Infant will maintain adequate gas exchange.
Decreased Cardiac Output **RELATED TO** Increased pulmonary vascular resistance **DEFINING CHARACTERISTICS** Tachycardia >160 Tachypnea >60 Dyspnea Cyanosis Feeding difficulties Fatigue	**ONGOING ASSESSMENT** • Assess and record every two hours and prn: Heart and respiratory rate Breath sounds Femoral, brachial, pedal pulses Any signs and symptoms of decreased cardiac output (such as those listed under defining characteristics) **THERAPEUTIC INTERVENTIONS** • Organize nursing care *to allow rest periods and decrease workload on the heart.* • Elevate head of bed at 30-degree angle. • Inform physician of any signs or symptoms of decreased cardiac output (such as those listed under defining characteristics).	Infant will maintain an adequate cardiac output.

Continued.

Bronchopulmonary dysplasia (BPD) cont'd

NURSING DIAGNOSES/ DEFINING CHARACTERISTICS	NURSING INTERVENTIONS / *RATIONALES*	EXPECTED OUTCOMES
High Risk for Infection **RELATED TO** Increased pulmonary secretions Tissue necrosis **DEFINING CHARACTERISTICS** Temperature instability Tachypnea Apnea Tachycardia Lethargy Elevated WBC count >300,000 mm³ Increased sputum production	**ONGOING ASSESSMENT** ▪ Assess and record every 2 hours and prn: Vital signs Signs and symptoms of infection (such as those listed under defining characteristics) ▪ Assess tracheal secretions for changes in amount, color, consistency, and odor. **THERAPEUTIC INTERVENTIONS** ▪ Maintain a neutral thermal environment. ▪ Ensure that antibiotics are given on schedule. Assess and record any side effects. ▪ Use sterile technique when doing procedures such as suctioning and changing IV tubing. ▪ Maintain good handwashing technique, especially between patients. ▪ Assess parents'/visitors' knowledge of handwashing technique; correct as needed.	Child will be free of infection.
Altered Nutrition: Less Than Body Requirements **RELATED TO** Respiratory distress Inability to tolerate feedings by mouth Increased energy expenditure (alveolar regeneration) **DEFINING CHARACTERISTICS** Failure to gain weight Abdominal distention Increased gastric residual contents Loss of weight with adequate intake	**ONGOING ASSESSMENT** ▪ Assess and record weight every day at same time of day without clothes. Assess abdominal girth (distention) every shift and prn. ▪ Keep accurate record of intake and output, including gastric residual contents before tube feeding. ▪ Monitor placement of NGT before feeding. ▪ Check for bowel sounds before feeding and NGT residual. Record characteristics of any drainage. **THERAPEUTIC INTERVENTIONS** ▪ Obtain dietary consult. *High-calorie, high-protein formula is needed to maintain positive nitrogen balance.* ▪ Establish appropriate feeding route (may require tube feeding) tolerant of hyperosmolar fluids. ▪ Administer vitamins, minerals, and calorie supplements (e.g., MCT oil, Polycose). ▪ Provide pacifier *to strengthen suck and satiate suck reflex.*	Infant will be free of signs and symptoms of nutritional deficit.
Ineffective Family Coping **RELATED TO** Long-term hospitalization of infant Unknown cause of illness Chronic illness **DEFINING CHARACTERISTICS** Inability to leave infant Inappropriate anger toward staff members Inability to express fears and concerns Failure to understand repeated explanations regarding the illness, treatments, and procedures	**ONGOING ASSESSMENT** ▪ Identify and record any past or usually successful coping strategies used by the family. **THERAPEUTIC INTERVENTIONS** ▪ Explain the course of the illness, treatments, and procedures to the family. Include reasons for treatments and procedures. ▪ Encourage family to express their feelings, fears, and concerns. ▪ Communicate with family concerning their infant's condition at least once per shift and prn as the infant's condition demands. Be open, honest, and straightforward *to establish trusting relationship with family.* ▪ Involve social services to assist in obtaining economic relief and home care equipment when needed. ▪ Involve family in child's care. ▪ See Ineffective family coping, p. 14.	Family's ability to cope successfully will be enhanced.

Bronchopulmonary dysplasia (BPD) cont'd

NURSING DIAGNOSES/ DEFINING CHARACTERISTICS	NURSING INTERVENTIONS / *RATIONALES*	EXPECTED OUTCOMES
Knowledge Deficit: Family **RELATED TO** Chronic illness Unfamiliar diagnosis New skills required **DEFINING CHARACTERISTICS** Questions Hesitant caretaking Absence	**ONGOING ASSESSMENT** • Assess family's knowledge and skill level. • Determine skills needed for home care. • Determine family's readiness for learning. **THERAPEUTIC INTERVENTIONS** • Teach family how to: Feed Suction Administer medications and oxygen Apply apnea monitor • Obtain home assistance if needed. • Instruct family on signs of respiratory distress and when to contact physician or obtain medical assistance.	Family will understand hospital and home care needs.

Joan Marie Fogata, RN, BSN

Carbon monoxide poisoning/smoke inhalation

Carbon monoxide (CO) poisoning resulting from smoke inhalation or gas leak (as in a furnace malfunction) causes normal hemoglobin to bind with CO, forming Hbco (carboxyhemoglobin). Oxygen is displaced to the extracellular fluid. Mild CO saturation produces headache, slight dyspnea, decreased visual acuity, and confusion. Moderate CO saturation produces irritability, fatigue, poor visual acuity, and nausea. Severe CO saturation produces severe neurological changes, including ataxia, confusion, hallucinations, and coma. Fires produce other gases and toxic chemicals that can be irritating to the airway such as wood smoke or burning plastics (polyvinyl chloride gas). Inhalation of chlorine or cyanide gas by-products can be fatal if prolonged, and thermal/burn injury to the airway should always be suspected in a victim of smoke inhalation.

NURSING DIAGNOSES/ DEFINING CHARACTERISTICS	NURSING INTERVENTIONS / *RATIONALES*	EXPECTED OUTCOMES
Impaired Gas Exchange **RELATED TO** Potentially fatal inhalation of gases **DEFINING CHARACTERISTICS** *Mild:* Slight confusion Mild dyspnea Visual changes Headache *Moderate:* Fatigue Irritability Poor vision Nausea	**ONGOING ASSESSMENT** • Assess age and developmental level. • Assess respirations for rate, pattern, depth, dyspnea, retractions, nasal flaring. • Inspect oral and nasal airway. *Smoke inhalation resulting from fires increases risk of thermal injury to airway.* • Assess breath sounds. • Assess orientation and behavior (see Defining Characteristics). **THERAPEUTIC INTERVENTIONS** • Apply cardiopulmonary monitor. • Maintain humidified 100% oxygen delivery. *Hemoglobin has a greater affinity for carbon monoxide versus oxygen and easily displaces oxygen, creating Hbco (carboxyhemoglobin), which will not sustain life; 100% oxygen is required to decrease the half-life of the circulating Hbco molecules from 4 hours to 1 hour.* • Prepare for intubation and mechanical ventilation. • See Mechanical ventilation, p. 155, and Decreased level of consciousness, p. 173.	Optimal gas exchange will be maintained.

Continued.

Carbon monoxide poisoning/smoke inhalation cont'd

NURSING DIAGNOSES/ DEFINING CHARACTERISTICS	NURSING INTERVENTIONS / *RATIONALES*	EXPECTED OUTCOMES
DEFINING CHARACTERISTICS cont'd *Severe:* Confusion Ataxia Hallucinations Decreased LOC Coma		
Ineffective Breathing Patterns **RELATED TO** Smoke inhalation Poisonous gases Tissue damage **DEFINING CHARACTERISTICS** Dyspnea Retractions Tachypnea Pain Nasal flaring Diminished lung sounds Rales Rhonchi Copious secretions	**ONGOING ASSESSMENT** • Assess respiration rate/rhythm. • Assess lung sounds, all quadrants every hour. • Assess oral/nasal airway for thermal injury and edema. **THERAPETIC INTERVENTIONS** • Apply 100% humidified oxygen. • Notify physician of changes in lung sounds, breathing patterns. • Suction as needed *to maintain airway.* • Provide chest PT, obtain respiratory therapy consultation. • Encourage use of incentive spirometer or other technique *to establish breathing pattern.*	Optimal breathing pattern will be maintained.
Fluid Volume Deficit **RELATED TO** Edema (fluid shifts) Insensible water loss Bronchial secretions **DEFINING CHARACTERISTICS** Intake < output Concentrated urine Hemoconcentration Increased hemo- globin Increased hematocrit Increased serum Na Thirst Hypotension Increased heart rate Poor skin turgor Sunken eyeballs Sunken fontanels	**ONGOING ASSESSMENT** • Monitor respiratory rate. *Tachypnea increases insensible water loss.* • Assess for increasing bronchial secretions *contributing to fluid loss.* • Assess CBC, electrolytes. • Monitor I&O and urine specific gravity. • Monitor for signs of dehydration. **THERAPEUTIC INTERVENTIONS** • Administer humidified oxygen *to decrease insensible water loss of respiration.* • Maintain IV fluids as ordered. • Encourage oral fluids if able. *(Burn injury or neurological deficit may preclude oral intake.)* • Administer volume expanders and/or other medications as ordered.	Adequate fluid volume will be maintained.

Carbon monoxide poisoning/smoke inhalation cont'd

NURSING DIAGNOSES/ DEFINING CHARACTERISTICS	NURSING INTERVENTIONS / *RATIONALES*	EXPECTED OUTCOMES
High Risk for Infection **RELATED TO** Tissue damage/necrosis Copious secretions **DEFINING CHARACTERISTICS** Increased WBCs Malodorous secretions Fever Radiological evidence	**ONGOING ASSESSMENT** • Assess breath sounds in all lung fields. • Monitor CBC with differential count. • Monitor secretions for change in amount, color, odor. Send sample for culture and sensitivity. • Monitor chest x-ray films. • Assess temperature every 4 hours. **THERAPEUTIC INTERVENTIONS** • Provide chest PT if possible. • Suction as needed *to remove offending secretions and prevent aspiration.* • Administer antibiotics as ordered. • Encourage use of incentive spirometer or other lung expansion techniques.	Risk for infection will be reduced.
Knowledge Deficit: Family **RELATED TO** New problem/injury New situation **DEFINING CHARACTERISTICS** Asks questions Verbalized lack of knowledge Fearful Hesitant involvement in care	**ONGOING ASSESSMENT** • Assess child and family for current understanding and readiness to learn. • Assess for circumstances of injury. *Parents may need to work through guilt and/or grief before they can learn about current needs.* **THERAPEUTIC INTERVENTIONS** • Provide information on an ongoing basis. • Involve child in self-care or parents in child's care if they are able. • Discuss home care needs; arrange home care assistance if necessary. *Needs depend entirely on extent of damage and residual effects, including respiratory and neurological support.* • Obtain social service consult.	Family will understand current situation and learn home care requirements.

Michele Knoll Puzas, RNC, MHPE

Epiglottitis

RESPIRATORY DISTRESS; OBSTRUCTED AIRWAY; CROUP

Severe, life-threatening, rapidly progressive bacterial infection of the epiglottis and surrounding structures usually caused by Haemophilus influenzae type B in children 3 to 7 years of age.

NURSING DIAGNOSES/ DEFINING CHARACTERISTICS	NURSING INTERVENTIONS / *RATIONALES*	EXPECTED OUTCOMES

High Risk for Injury: Airway Obstruction
RELATED TO
Inflammation
Edema of epiglottis
 	
DEFINING CHARACTERISTICS
Dysphagia
Drooling
Dyspnea
	ONGOING ASSESSMENT
	• Assess age and developmental level.
	• Assess respiratory rate every hour or more often as condition worsens.
	• Auscultate breath sounds every hour or more often as condition worsens.
	• Assess for respiratory distress:
	    Retractions
	    Stridor
	    Anxiety
	    Cyanosis
	    Nasal flaring
	    Use of accessory muscles
		A patent airway and adequate oxygenation will be maintained.

Continued.

Pulmonary Care Plans (Pediatric)

NURSING DIAGNOSES/ DEFINING CHARACTERISTICS	NURSING INTERVENTIONS / *RATIONALES*	EXPECTED OUTCOMES
DEFINING CHARACTERISTICS **cont'd** Restlessness Fever Increased WBCs Cough (unusual) Positive throat culture for *Haemophilus influenzae* type B Abrupt onset (6-24 hours) Stridor Sore throat Anxious appearance Tachycardia	**ONGOING ASSESSMENT cont'd** ▪ Monitor WBCs. ▪ Assess results of throat and blood cultures. ▪ Check x-ray film results. ▪ Monitor ABG results. **THERAPEUTIC INTERVENTIONS** *Preintubation:* ▪ Withhold all therapeutic interventions (such as initiating IV fluids or taking a temperature) until the patient is intubated. *A slight agitation of the patient may cause an airway obstruction by further traumatizing an already swollen epiglottis.* *Postintubation:* ▪ Administer oxygen and/or humidity via endotracheal tube. ▪ Institute suctioning of airway *to ensure tube patency.* ▪ Place elbow restraints on child *to prevent accidental extubation.* ▪ Administer antipyretics for temperature greater than *38.5° C (101.3° F).* ▪ Sponge patient with tepid water for temperature greater than *39° C (102.2° F).* ▪ Administer antibiotics as ordered.	
High Risk for Fluid Volume Deficit **RELATED TO** Respiratory distress Inability to maintain oral intake **DEFINING CHARACTERISTICS** Thirst Drooling Inability to swallow Increased insensible fluid loss	**ONGOING ASSESSMENT** ▪ Monitor vital signs every hour or more often as condition worsens. ▪ Monitor daily weight for a large increase or decrease *that may relate to overhydration or underhydration.* ▪ Monitor I&O every 2 hours. ▪ Monitor laboratory values. **THERAPEUTIC INTERVENTIONS** ▪ Administer IV fluids. ▪ Control insensible water losses: Keep child dry and warm. Keep respiratory rate within normal range. Sedate child if needed *to decrease metabolic demand/rate.*	Adequate fluid and electrolyte balance will be maintained.
Knowledge Deficit About Disease Process and Treatment **RELATED TO** Lack of knowledge about the illness **DEFINING CHARACTERISTICS** Request for information Statements of misconceptions	**ONGOING ASSESSMENT** ▪ Assess level of understanding about the illness and hospitalization. ▪ Assess previous **exp**erience with coping with illness and hospitalization. **THERAPEUTIC INTERVENTIONS** ▪ Orient family to unit and staff. ▪ Provide accurate information about disease process and the possibility of recurrence. ▪ Provide information about the disease and the treatment to other family members, friends, schoolmates, etc. ▪ Maintain consistent caregivers *to establish rapport with child and family.*	Child and family will verbalize an increased awareness about the disease and treatment.
Anxiety/Fear **RELATED TO** Acute illness and the need for immediate hospitalization	**ONGOING ASSESSMENT** ▪ Assess degree of stress and the ability to cope. ▪ Assess the quantity and quality of support available to the family.	Family's anxiety will be decreased.

Epiglottitis cont'd

NURSING DIAGNOSES/ DEFINING CHARACTERISTICS	NURSING INTERVENTIONS / *RATIONALES*	EXPECTED OUTCOMES
DEFINING CHARACTERISTICS Insomnia Crying Clinging Withdrawal Restlessness Poor eye contact Tachycardia Pupil dilation	**THERAPEUTIC INTERVENTIONS** • Encourage ventilation of feelings and concerns. • Assist family to mobilize support systems. • Allow family to remain with child *to promote involvement in the child's care.* • Offer factual information *to dispel misconceptions.* • Decrease amount of stimuli. • Inform family of child's progress.	

Nedra Skale, RN, MS, CNA

Near-drowning

Survival after prolonged submersion in a fluid medium. Aspiration of saltwater causes plasma to be drawn into the lungs, resulting in hypoxemia and hypovolemia. Freshwater aspiration causes hypervolemia as a result of absorption of water through alveoli into the vascular system. These fluids are further absorbed into the interstitial space. Hypoxemia results from the decreased lung surfactant washed away by the absorbed water. Severe hypoxia also results from the asphyxia related to submersion without aspiration of fluid. Survival is influenced by the length of time submerged, water temperature, performance of CPR by rescuers, and the child's age. Infants and young children will experience the diving reflex, limiting aspiration. Cold water decreases metabolic demands for oxygen.

NURSING DIAGNOSES/ DEFINING CHARACTERISTICS	NURSING INTERVENTIONS / *RATIONALES*	EXPECTED OUTCOMES
Impaired Gas Exchange **RELATED TO** Surfactant elimination Bronchospasm Aspiration Pulmonary edema **DEFINING CHARACTERISTICS** Cyanosis Retractions Tachypnea Stridor Hypoxemia Frothy, pink-tinged expectorant (saltwater-induced pulmonary edema)	**ONGOING ASSESSMENT** • Assess age and developmental level. • Assess breath sounds every 2 hours. • Assess for signs of respiratory distress: Retractions Stridor Nasal flaring Use of accessory muscles • Assess for signs of hypoxemia: Altered level of consciousness Tachycardia Deteriorating serial ABGs Tachypnea Cyanosis Increasing respiratory distress • Assess serial chest x-ray examination reports. • Monitor for evidence of increasing pulmonary edema, *which may indicate the need for mechanical ventilation.* **THERAPEUTIC INTERVENTIONS** • Place child in high Fowler's position, *which would allow for maximum chest expansion.* • Notify physician of changes in respiratory status. • Administer humidified oxygen as ordered. • Provide chest PT and frequent suctioning. • Maintain CPAP as ordered; prepare for mechanical ventilation if needed.	Adequate gas exchange will be maintained.

Continued.

NURSING DIAGNOSES/ DEFINING CHARACTERISTICS	NURSING INTERVENTIONS / *RATIONALES*	EXPECTED OUTCOMES
Altered Cerebral Tissue Perfusion **RELATED TO** Impaired gas exchange Increased intracranial pressure resulting from fluid shifts Hypoxia Prolonged hypoxemia **DEFINING CHARACTERISTICS** Deficit in cranial nerve responses Altered level of consciousness Inappropriate behavior Altered pupillary response	**ONGOING ASSESSMENT** ▪ Assess LOC, using Glasgow Coma Scale. *Use measures appropriate to age/level of development.* ▪ Determine cranial nerve response, especially vagus (breathing, gag, cough). *Absence indicates need for artificial airway maintenance.* ▪ Monitor for increasing intracranial pressure: Increased ICP monitor readings Narrowed pulse pressure and decreased heart and respiratory rates Alteration of pupil response LOC altered (from admission level) ▪ Assess for seizure activity. ▪ Assess environment for degree of stimulation. **THERAPEUTIC INTERVENTIONS** ▪ Prepare for intubation. *The comatose child will be unable to maintain airway/breathing.* ▪ Hyperventilate as ordered. *Increased PaO$_2$ should decrease cerebral blood flow, limiting cerebral edema.* ▪ Elevate head of bed 30 degrees and maintain midline head and body alignment. ▪ Notify physician of any signs of increasing ICP. ▪ Administer corticosteroids as ordered *to treat increased ICP.* ▪ Administer anticonvulsants as ordered *to prevent seizure activity.* ▪ Maintain seizure precautions *to prevent patient from injuring self in the event of seizure.* ▪ Minimize frequency of suctioning. *Hypoxia and Valsalva maneuver can be associated with suctioning and may elevate ICP.* ▪ Minimize exposure to unnecessary stimuli. ▪ Sedate child before beginning procedures as ordered (e.g., blood drawing, invasive procedures) *to prevent elevating ICP.* ▪ Administer medications as ordered to maintain child in barbiturate coma, *that protects the brain from the athetoid movements, grunting, and straining that may increase ICP.* ▪ Maintain body temperature between *31° and 32° C (87.8° and 89.6° F), to reduce the total oxygen requirements.*	Cerebral perfusion will be maximized.
Fluid Volume, Excess **RELATED TO** Aspiration of fresh water Fluid shift from interstitial to intravascular space **Fluid Volume, Deficit** **RELATED TO** Aspiration of salt water Fluid shift from intravascular to interstitial space **DEFINING CHARACTERISTICS** Abnormal vital signs Poor peripheral vascular tone leading to edema Dysrhythmias	**ONGOING ASSESSMENT** ▪ Assess heart rate/rhythm. ▪ Assess serial electrolytes. ▪ Assess pH results for acidosis/alkalosis. ▪ Assess Hct *to determine level of hemodilution/concentration.* ▪ Assess urine output every hour; maintain accurate I&O record. ▪ Assess specific gravity. ▪ Assess urine electrolytes, BUN, and creatinine. ▪ Assess weight on admission, then every day once neurological signs are stable. ▪ Monitor CVP. *Severe hypovolemia will cause decreasing CVP and indicates the need for volume expanders.* **THERAPEUTIC INTERVENTIONS** ▪ Notify physician of laboratory results and changes in output or cardiac function. ▪ Administer IV fluids as ordered *to correct fluid imbalance.* ▪ Place on cardiopulmonary monitor. ▪ Administer sodium bicarbonate as ordered *to correct metabolic acidosis.* ▪ Prepare for central line placement. ▪ Administer fluid volume expanders as ordered. ▪ See Fluid volume excess, p. 19, and Deficit, p. 21.	Fluid volume imbalances will be reduced.

NURSING DIAGNOSES/ DEFINING CHARACTERISTICS	NURSING INTERVENTIONS / *RATIONALES*	EXPECTED OUTCOMES
High Risk for Impaired Skin Integrity **RELATED TO** Imposed hypothermia Immobility Prolonged exposure **DEFINING CHARACTERISTICS** Reddened areas of skin Rashes Edema Blisters	**ONGOING ASSESSMENT** ▪ Assess rectal temperature every 2 to 4 hours. ▪ Assess skin every 2 hours for pressure areas, redness, blisters, edema, rashes. **THERAPEUTIC INTERVENTIONS** ▪ Do not allow child's temperature to go below prescribed limit. ▪ Reposition child every 2 hours *to reduce risk of skin breakdown from pressure areas.* ▪ Protect bony prominences with padding. ▪ Apply lotion to pressure areas. ▪ See Impaired skin integrity, p. 39.	Skin will remain intact.
High Risk for Infection **RELATED TO** Aspiration of contaminated water **DEFINING CHARACTERISTICS** Temperature Rales, rhonchi Positive results to culture tests	**ONGOING ASSESSMENT** ▪ Monitor temperature every 2-4 hours. ▪ Monitor results of culture tests and serial white counts, *which may indicate infection.* ▪ Assess for increased respiratory distress. ▪ Obtain chest x-ray films; *aspiration of contaminated water puts child at risk for developing pneumonia.* ▪ Record color, odor, and amount of sputum. **THERAPEUTIC INTERVENTIONS** ▪ Suction secretions as needed; send secretion sample for culture and sensitivity. ▪ Notify physician of fever, positive culture results, x-ray films, or clinical findings. ▪ Administer antibiotics as ordered. ▪ Position child *for ease in lung expansion.* ▪ Reposition *to promote drainage* (postural drainage) and perform chest PT as needed. ▪ Encourage the use of an incentive spirometer when child is neurologically stable.	Risk of infection will be reduced.
Knowledge Deficit: Family **RELATED TO** Near-drowning Child's critical status Admission to PICU **DEFINING CHARACTERISTICS** Continual questions Excessive talking Constant demands Inability to come into unit Pacing Withdrawal Inability to leave child's bedside	**ONGOING ASSESSMENT** ▪ Assess degree of stress. ▪ Assess support systems available. ▪ Assess level of understanding about child's illness and treatment. ▪ Assess degree of involvement in child's care. **THERAPEUTIC INTERVENTIONS** ▪ Establish a good rapport with parents. ▪ Encourage expression of feelings about condition and treatment. ▪ Reassure and support family. ▪ Allow for questions and answer as honestly as possible. ▪ Include family in child's care. ▪ Include clergy and social worker in meetings with family *so they may better answer questions and help family remember details of care.* ▪ Assist family in anticipating mourning if applicable. ▪ Provide information for follow-up care and home care as necessary.	Family will understand treatments, prognosis, and follow-up care.

Michele Knoll Puzas, RNC, MHPE

Near-miss sudden infant death syndrome (SIDS)

CRIB DEATH

Sudden infant death syndrome (SIDS) is the sudden, unexpected death of an infant, usually under 6 months of age, from no known cause determined through history and postmortem examination. "Near-miss" can be defined as an interrupted SIDS, when the infant is found not breathing and is resuscitated.

NURSING DIAGNOSES/ DEFINING CHARACTERISTICS	NURSING INTERVENTIONS / *RATIONALES*	EXPECTED OUTCOMES

Ineffective Breathing Pattern
RELATED TO
True cause is unknown but may be related to prematurity, family history, sleep or neurological disorder, or viral infection
 	
DEFINING CHARACTERISTICS
Apnea
Limpness
Cyanosis
Pallor
Skin warm and dry to cool and dry
	ONGOING ASSESSMENT
	• Assess age and developmental level.
	• Assess vital signs, especially respiratory rate.
	• Note color changes (lips, buccal mucosa, nailbeds).
	• Observe for and document signs of respiratory dysfunction:
	    Apnea
	    Slow, shallow breathing
	    Retractions
	    Nasal flaring
	• Determine type of apnea when present and stimulation required to resume normal breathing:
	    Central or diaphragmatic: Chest movement ceases, absence of air flow
	    Obstructive: Chest and diaphragm move but there is no air exchange
	    Mixed: Cessation of air flow and chest movement followed by respiratory effect without air flow
	• Monitor laboratory work:
	    Theophylline level
	    ABGs
	    CBC
	    Electrolytes
	• Obtain chest x-ray evaluation *to rule out aspiration.*
	
	THERAPEUTIC INTERVENTIONS
	• Keep head of bed elevated *to help with expansion of lungs.*
	• Prepare for resuscitation.
	• Keep infant as calm as possible.
	• Administer medications and IV fluids as ordered.
	• Keep infant NPO until stabilized.
	• Apply cardiopulmonary (CP) monitor.
	• Assist with tests (pneumogram, trend).
	• Plan for possible admission to PICU with intubation.
	• Obtain clinical consultations/resources as needed.
		Adequate breathing pattern will be maintained.

Ineffective Family Coping **RELATED TO** Unfamiliar environment Loss of role as primary caretaker Change in infant's health status Knowledge deficit Guilt Overwhelming situation	**ONGOING ASSESSMENT** • Assess for defining characteristics. • Assess level of anxiety and normal family coping strategies. **THERAPEUTIC INTERVENTIONS** • Approach in a calm, reassuring, nonjudgmental manner. • Provide ongoing information in simple, honest terms. • Provide flexible visiting hours and encourage participation in the infant's care *to maintain parental role/bonds and self-esteem.* • See Ineffective family coping, p. 14.	Coping abilities will be acknowledged and demonstrated.

NURSING DIAGNOSES/ DEFINING CHARACTERISTICS	NURSING INTERVENTIONS / *RATIONALES*	EXPECTED OUTCOMES
DEFINING CHARACTERISTICS Distortion of reality Restlessness Verbalization of problem or guilt Limited interaction with infant/other family members Statement of misconception Agitation Depression Abandonment		
Fear: Parental **RELATED TO** Change in infant's health status Change in environment (from PICU to general unit or general unit to home) **DEFINING CHARACTERISTICS** Verbalized fears Verbalized lack of confidence Hesitance to care for infant Demanding behaviors Avoidance Increased respiratory/heart rates Diaphoresis Tremors Crying Denial	**ONGOING ASSESSMENT** ▪ Assess parents' fears and coping ability. *Parents will need to work through their fears in order to provide adequate care for their child and themselves.* ▪ Identify coping mechanisms and support systems useful to the parents. **THERAPEUTIC INTERVENTIONS** ▪ Provide comfort measures for infant and parents. ▪ Assign infant to room near the desk/nurses' station if transferring from PICU. *Parents may be fearful that with fewer nurses in attendance their child may be at risk.* ▪ Reassure parents that a nurse will be available; establish primary care relationship if possible. ▪ Demonstrate confidence while caring for infant and in the use of monitors/other equipment. ▪ Encourage parents' participation in their child's care as they are able. ▪ See Fear, p. 18.	Fears will be acknowledged and managed or reduced.

Knowledge Deficit: Parental
RELATED TO
New situation/diagnosis
Home care requirements
 	
DEFINING CHARACTERISTICS
Stated lack of understanding
Requests for information
Lack of questions
Incorrect responses
Ineffective care
	ONGOING ASSESSMENT
	▪ Assess knowledge of disorder and potential for recurrence.
	▪ Assess cognitive abilities and readiness to learn.
	▪ Evaluate self-care activities:
	    Preventive care/equipment
	    Home management of acute scenario
	
	THERAPEUTIC INTERVENTIONS
	▪ Explain disorder and that parents are not to blame themselves.
	▪ Teach parents to document apneic events and intervention, including:
	    If infant was awake or asleep
	    Respiratory status—no respirations, normal, shallow, infant's color, muscle tone
	    Monitor display—apneic episodes, bradycardic episodes
	    Interventions—none required, gentle stimulation, vigorous stimulation, resuscitation required
		Parents/significant others will demonstrate adequate home care management skills.

Continued.

Near-miss sudden infant death syndrome (SIDS) cont'd

NURSING DIAGNOSES/ DEFINING CHARACTERISTICS	NURSING INTERVENTIONS / *RATIONALES*	EXPECTED OUTCOMES
	THERAPEUTIC INTERVENTIONS cont'd	
	• Demonstrate and require return demonstration of: Home monitoring equipment CPR EMS system	
	• Encourage parents to maintain infant's normal activities whenever possible *to enhance growth and development.*	
	• Provide information concerning available resources: National Sudden Infant Death Syndrome Foundation (local chapters available) The International Guild for Infant Survival	

Kathleen Jaffrey, RN

Pneumonia

PNEUMONITIS; LOBAR PNEUMONIA; BRONCHOPNEUMONIA; PNEUMOCOCCAL PNEUMONIA; STAPHYLOCOCCAL PNEUMONIA; KLEBSIELLA PNEUMONIA; RSV PNEUMONIA

Pneumonia is caused by a bacterial or viral infection that results in an inflammatory process in the lungs. It is an infectious process spread by droplets or by contact. Some predisposing factors to the development of pneumonia include upper respiratory infection, CNS depression, cardiac failure, any debilitating illness, prolonged bed rest, and a depressed immune system. Newborns are particularly susceptible to respiratory syncytial virus (RSV), which frequently causes severe lower respiratory tract infections/ pneumonia.

NURSING DIAGNOSES/ DEFINING CHARACTERISTICS	NURSING INTERVENTIONS / *RATIONALES*	EXPECTED OUTCOMES
Ineffective Airway Clearance **RELATED TO** Increased production of sputum in response to respiratory infection Decreased energy and increased fatigue resulting from prolonged immobilization, cardiac failure, postoperative effect of general anesthesia, chronic illness, depression of CNS Aspiration **DEFINING CHARACTERISTICS** Abnormal breath sounds, e.g., rhonchi, bronchial breath sounds Retractions, nasal flaring	**ONGOING ASSESSMENT** • Assess age and developmental level. • Assess breath sounds. • Assess respiratory movements and use of accessory muscles. • Monitor chest x-ray reports. • Monitor sputum: Gram's stain and culture and sensitivity reports. **THERAPEUTIC INTERVENTIONS** • Assist child with coughing and deep breathing, splinting as necessary *to improve coughing.* • Encourage child to cough unless cough is frequent and nonproductive. *Frequent nonproductive coughing can result in hypoxemia.* • Use positioning *to facilitate clearing secretions.* Avoid use of infant seats for the newborn; *these have been found to decrease lung expansion and further hypoxia.* • Use respiratory therapist for chest physiotherapy and nebulizer treatments, as appropriate. • Use humidified oxygen *to loosen secretions.* • Maintain adequate hydration. *Fluids are lost from diaphoresis, fever, and tachypnea.* Encourage oral fluids. Administer IV fluids as ordered. • Administer medication (e.g., antibiotics, expectorants) as ordered, noting effectiveness. • Institute suctioning of airway as needed *to remove sputum and mucus plugs.* • Use nasopharyngeal/oropharyngeal airway as needed. • Anticipate possible need for intubation *if child's condition deteriorates.*	Airway will be freed of secretions.

Pneumonia cont'd

NURSING DIAGNOSES/ DEFINING CHARACTERISTICS	NURSING INTERVENTIONS / *RATIONALES*	EXPECTED OUTCOMES
DEFINING CHARACTERISTICS cont'd Decreased breath sounds over affected areas Cough Dyspnea Cyanosis Change in respiratory status Infiltrates on chest x-ray film		

Impaired Gas Exchange
RELATED TO
Collection of mucus in airways
 	
DEFINING CHARACTERISTICS
Dyspnea
Decreased PaO$_2$
Increased PaCO$_2$
Cyanosis
Tachypnea
Air hunger
Tachycardia
Pallor
Decreased activity tolerance
Restlessness
Disorientation/confusion
	ONGOING ASSESSMENT
	- Assess respiratory status:
	   Rate
	   Depth
	   Breath sounds
	   Pattern of respiration
	- Assess skin color and capillary refill.
	- Assess for changes in orientation, and note increasing restlessness. *These can be early signs of hypoxia and/or hypercarbia.*
	- Assess for changes in activity.
	- Monitor changes in vital signs.
	- Monitor ABGs, and note differences.
	
	THERAPEUTIC INTERVENTIONS
	- Notify physician if child's condition worsens.
	- Pace activities to child's tolerance. *Activities will increase oxygen consumption and should be planned so that the child does not become hypoxic.*
	- Maintain oxygen administration device as ordered. *Mist tent with oxygen and Ribavirin will be ordered for infants with RSV infection.*
	- Anticipate the need for intubation and possible mechanical ventilation if condition worsens. (See Mechanical ventilation, p. 155.)
		Gas exchange will be enhanced.

Infection
RELATED TO
Invading bacterial/ viral organisms
 	
DEFINING CHARACTERISTICS
Elevated temperature
Elevated WBC
Tachycardia
Chills
Positive sputum culture report
Changing character of sputum
	ONGOING ASSESSMENT
	- Elicit parent's/child's description of illness including:
	   Onset
	   Chills
	   Chest pain
	   Medications *(Patients receiving high dosages of corticosteroids have a reduced resistance to infections.)*
	   Recent exposure to illness
	   Chronic illness
	- Assess vital signs.
	- Monitor Gram stain, sputum, and culture and sensitivity reports.
	- Monitor WBCs.
	- Monitor temperature. *Continued fever may be caused by drug allergy, drug-resistant bacteria, superinfection, or inadequate lung drainage.*
	
	THERAPEUTIC INTERVENTIONS
	- Use appropriate therapy for elevated temperature—antipyretics, cold therapy.
	- Obtain fresh sputum for Gram stain/culture and sensitivity, as ordered. Instruct child to expectorate into sterile container. Be sure the specimen is coughed up and is not saliva.
		Infection will be reduced.

Continued.

Pneumonia cont'd

NURSING DIAGNOSES/ DEFINING CHARACTERISTICS	NURSING INTERVENTIONS / *RATIONALES*	EXPECTED OUTCOMES
	THERAPEUTIC INTERVENTIONS cont'd If child/infant is unable to effectively cough up a specimen, use sterile nasotracheal suctioning with a Lukens' tube. Call respiratory therapist for assistance. ▪ Administer prescribed antimicrobial agent(s) at scheduled times *so that a blood level is maintained.* ▪ Isolate child as necessary following review of culture and sensitivity results.	

Pain/Discomfort
RELATED TO
Respiratory distress
Coughing
 	
DEFINING CHARACTERISTICS
Complaints of discomfort
Guarding
Withdrawal
Moaning
Facial grimace
Irritability
Anxiety
Tachycardia
Increased BP
Increased temperature
	ONGOING ASSESSMENT
	▪ Assess complaints of discomfort.
	▪ Determine quality, severity, location, onset, duration, and precipitating factors for child's discomfort.
	▪ Assess infant for irritability, tolerance to touch, feeding.
	
	THERAPEUTIC INTERVENTIONS
	▪ Ask child/parent to verbalize any complaints of discomfort.
	▪ Examine for objective signs of discomfort.
	▪ Administer appropriate medications to treat the cough:
	  Do not suppress a productive cough, but do use moderate amounts of analgesics to relieve pleuritic pain.
	  Use cough suppressants and humidity for a dry, hacking cough. *An unproductive hacking cough irritates the airways and should be suppressed.*
	▪ Administer analgesics as ordered and as needed. Encourage child to take analgesics before discomfort becomes severe *to prevent peak periods of pain.*
	▪ Evaluate effectiveness of medications. Use additional measures to relieve discomfort, including positioning and relaxation.
		Discomfort will be relieved.

High Risk for Altered Levels of Consciousness **RELATED TO** Cerebral hypoxia Meningitis **DEFINING CHARACTERISTICS** Decreasing PaO_2 Change in alertness, orientation, verbal response Agitation Restlessness Irritability	**ONGOING ASSESSMENT** ▪ Assess for presence of defining characteristics; if they are present, notify physician. **THERAPEUTIC INTERVENTIONS** ▪ For a decrease in PaO_2, see Gas exchange, impaired, p. 23. ▪ See Decreased level of consciousness, altered level of, p. 173. ▪ If appropriate, see Meningitis, p. 193.	Risk of altered level of consciousness will be reduced.

High Risk for Altered Nutrition: Less Than Body Requirements
RELATED TO
Pneumonia, resulting in:
  Increased metabolic needs
  Lack of appetite
  Decreased intake
	ONGOING ASSESSMENT
	▪ Document child's actual weight.
	▪ Obtain nutritional history.
	▪ Obtain baseline laboratory values:
	  Serum total protein
	  Serum albumin
	  Serum osmolarity
	  Vitamin assays (as appropriate)
	  Mineral and trace element levels (as appropriate)
		Optimal nutritional status will be maintained.

NURSING DIAGNOSES/ DEFINING CHARACTERISTICS	NURSING INTERVENTIONS / *RATIONALES*	EXPECTED OUTCOMES
DEFINING CHARACTERISTICS Anorexia Loss of weight Decreased caloric intake Feeding difficulties Feeding intolerance	**THERAPEUTIC INTERVENTIONS** ▪ Minimize activity *to decrease metabolic needs.* ▪ Increase activity gradually as tolerated. ▪ Provide high-protein/high-carbohydrate diet. Provide high-calorie formula for infants, if tolerated. ▪ Provide small, frequent feedings. *Infants may have difficulty sucking and may require tube feeding.* ▪ Maintain oxygen delivery system while the child eats (e.g., nasal cannula if appropriate). *This will help keep the child from desaturating and becoming short of breath, with a resultant loss of appetite.* ▪ Administer vitamin supplements as ordered. ▪ Administer enteral supplements and parenteral nutrition as ordered. ▪ See Altered nutrition: less than body requirements, p. 33.	
Diversional Activity Deficit **RELATED TO** Isolation Bed rest **DEFINING CHARACTERISTICS** Child complains of: Boredom Isolation Irritability	**ONGOING ASSESSMENT** ▪ Assess for signs of diversional activity deficit (see Defining Characteristics). **THERAPEUTIC INTERVENTIONS** ▪ Consult child life therapist. ▪ Provide activities at bedside. ▪ Encourage family participation.	Diversional activities will be available.

Knowledge Deficit
RELATED TO
New condition and procedures
Unfamiliarity with disease process and transmission of disease
 	
DEFINING CHARACTERISTICS
Questions
Confusion about treatment
Inability to comply with treatment regimen, including any appropriate isolation procedures
Lack of questions
	ONGOING ASSESSMENT
	▪ Determine understanding by child/family of disease process, complications, and treatment regimen.
	
	THERAPEUTIC INTERVENTIONS
	▪ Provide information to child/family in teaching sessions regarding the need to:
	  Maintain natural resistance to infection through adequate nutrition, rest, exercise.
	  Avoid contact with people with upper respiratory infections.
	  Obtain immunizations on schedule.
	▪ Encourage questions.
	▪ Evaluate understanding of information following teaching sessions *to determine knowledge level.* Repeat teaching as needed *to reinforce the information* and use handouts *for the child/parent to refer to at a later time.*
	▪ Observe for compliance with treatment regimen.
	▪ Instruct the child/family on isolation procedure being used, *so that they understand the importance of protecting the child and themselves as appropriate.*
		Child/family will demonstrate understanding of disease process and compliance with treatment regimen and any isolation procedures.

Susan Galanes, RN, MS, CCRN; Michele Knoll Puzas, RNC, MHPE

Pneumothorax/chest tubes

COLLAPSED LUNG

Air in the pleural space resulting from injury or disease. The child's clinical status depends on the size of the wound and on the rate of air leakage.

NURSING DIAGNOSES/ DEFINING CHARACTERISTICS	NURSING INTERVENTIONS / *RATIONALES*	EXPECTED OUTCOMES
Ineffective Breathing Pattern **RELATED TO** Chest trauma Pneumonia Emphysema Bronchitis Airway obstruction Needle aspiration Central line placement Positive pressure ventilation **DEFINING CHARACTERISTICS** Chest pain on affected side Dyspnea Asymmetrical chest expansion Severe hypoxemia Drastic reduction in cardiac output Bradycardia Nasal flaring and intercostal retractions Venous engorgement Decreased breath sounds on side of injured lung Confusion, anxiety, restlessness, irritability Fatigue, lethargy Changes in chest x-ray films Cyanosis	**ONGOING ASSESSMENT** • Assess age and developmental level. • Obtain a thorough patient history to assist in a definitive diagnosis. • Auscultate breath sounds carefully. *Chest wall of infant and young child is thin, and breath sounds are easily referred from other areas of lungs. Decreased breath sounds may not necessarily be heard over involved area of lung; instead may note a difference in quality or pitch of breath sounds over area of pneumothorax.* • Assess intactness of chest. *Spontaneous or closed pneumothorax can result from ruptured pulmonary blebs.* • Assess for signs and symptoms of respiratory distress: Altered breathing pattern Presence/absence of breath sounds Use of accessory muscles Changes in orientation, restlessness Skin color changes Change in ABGs • Assess vital signs frequently. • After needle aspiration, monitor vital signs at a minimum of every 15 minutes for the first hour. • Assess need to increase FiO_2. • Evaluate serial monitoring of oxygen saturation by pulse oximetry. • Monitor chest x-ray films *to confirm signs of pneumothorax or correct placement of chest tubes.* • After needle aspiration, assess for dizziness, tightness in chest, increased respirations, tachycardia, and signs and symptoms of hypoxemia, *all of which could indicate recurrence of pneumothorax.* **THERAPEUTIC INTERVENTIONS** • Elevate head of bed. • Provide oxygen or increase FiO_2 (whichever is indicated). • Insert large-bore venous catheter *to ensure venous access.* • Assist with needle aspiration for small pneumothorax: Inform child and/or family about the procedure. Obtain a signed consent from parents. Administer sedatives as ordered. Gather equipment and chest x-ray films. *Equipment will include sterile drape and gloves, disinfectant, gauze, 1%-2% Lidocaine, 14- to 18-gauge needle attached to stopcock on 20-50 ml syringe. Through this setup air can be aspirated from chest; stopcock port to chest can be turned off, and air can be flushed from syringe out to stopcock.* Instruct child to refrain from coughing during the procedure. Help with positioning. Provide emotional support. Provide pacifier (age appropriate). Record amount of air and/or fluid removed. Document color and viscosity of fluid. Provide adequate explanation and support before, during, and after procedure. Once air and/or fluid is removed, apply pressure and dressing to the site. Facilitate bed rest for child.	Effective breathing pattern and gas exchange will be restored.

NURSING DIAGNOSES/ DEFINING CHARACTERISTICS	NURSING INTERVENTIONS / *RATIONALES*	EXPECTED OUTCOMES

THERAPEUTIC INTERVENTIONS cont'd

- Assist with insertion of chest tube to underwater seal and suction. *This is necessary if pneumothorax is greater than 10% or if accompanied by significant respiratory distress. The chest tube will be used to drain any air, blood, or fluid that accumulates in the lungs.*
    - Assemble all appropriate equipment at bedside and have it prepared for immediate use. *Equipment will include chest bottle or disposable pleural drainage system with both water seal and suction chambers, appropriate fluid levels, adequate lighting, sterile gloves and gown, masks, tape, suture material, appropriate-sized chest tube, and thoracotomy tray.*
    - Explain procedure to child and family and obtain consent from parent.
    - Assist with the procedure.
    - If water seal drainage is used, be sure that water fluctuates in the water seal unit on respiration. *Bubbling in the water seal unit may indicate an air leak.*
    - Examine drainage unit for any blood or air. Mark fluid level on the outside of the drainage bottle to show fluid loss.
    - Have follow-up chest x-ray done *to confirm tube placement and to see if the lung has reexpanded.*
    - Inspect the tube insertion site for bleeding, redness, and air or fluid leakage.
    - Keep the tubing patent.
    - Suction airway as needed *to keep it patent.*
    - Perform chest physiotherapy *to promote lung expansion.*
    - Administer pain medication as ordered.
    - Replace any pleural blood evacuated *to prevent hypovolemic shock.*
    - Secure chest tube with tape on chest, on bed, or crib. Tape pleurovac to floor. Use restraints as needed.
    - Keep an extra chest tube clamp at bedside.
- Prepare child for removal of chest tube once lung has reexpanded. Apply an airtight bandage with petroleum-impregnated gauze on incision site:
    - Encourage child to turn, cough, deep breath frequently *to prevent further complications.*
    - Provide activities that will enhance deep breathing or coughing such as blowing up a balloon or bubbles.

PATIENT/PARENT EDUCATION

- Inform child and parents of the importance of follow-up examination; *the physician will need to test for resolution of pneumothorax.*
- Instruct family on symptoms to observe and to call the physician if they recur or if new ones develop.

Jacqueline Santiago-Tan, RN, BSN

Respiratory failure

RDS; SHOCK LUNG; NONCARDIOGENIC PULMONARY EDEMA; ADULT HYALINE MEMBRANE DISEASE; OXYGEN PNEUMONITIS; POSTTRAUMATIC PULMONARY INSUFFICIENCY

Respiratory distress syndrome (RDS) is a form of respiratory failure that was not recognized as a syndrome until the 1960s, when advances in medical care allowed for prolonged survival of trauma victims who previously would have died. Many causal factors have been related to RDS, but the exact causative event is unknown. The most common pediatric disorders associated with RDS include near-drowning; trauma; viral, bacterial, or fungal pneumonias; and sepsis. Nursing care must focus on maintenance of pulmonary function as well as treatment of the causal factor; even then mortality remains at 50% to 60%.

NURSING DIAGNOSES/ DEFINING CHARACTERISTICS	NURSING INTERVENTIONS / *RATIONALES*	EXPECTED OUTCOMES
Ineffective Breathing Patterns **RELATED TO** Decreased lung compliance: Low amounts of surfactant Fluid transudation Fatigue and decreased energy: Increased work of breathing Primary medical problem **DEFINING CHARACTERISTICS** Dyspnea Shortness of breath Tachypnea Abnormal ABGs Cyanosis Cough Use of accessory muscles	**ONGOING ASSESSMENT** • Assess age and developmental level. • Assess respiratory rate and depth every hour. • Assess for dyspnea, shortness of breath, cough, and use of accessory muscles. *Initially, respiratory rate increases with the decreasing lung compliance. Work of breathing increases greatly as compliance decreases.* • Assess for cyanosis and monitor ABGs. *As the child becomes fatigued from the increased work of breathing, he or she may no longer be capable of adequately maintaining his or her own ventilation: CO_2 begins to elevate on ABGs.* **THERAPEUTIC INTERVENTIONS** • Maintain the oxygen delivery system applied to the child *so that his or her system does not desaturate.* • Provide reassurance and allay anxiety: Have an agreed-upon method for the child to call for assistance (e.g., call light or bell). Stay with the child during episodes of respiratory distress. • Keep physician informed of respiratory status. • Anticipate the need for intubation and mechanical ventilation. *Being prepared for intubation will prevent full decompensation of the child to cardiopulmonary arrest. Early intubation and mechanical ventilation are recommended.* (See Mechanical ventilation, p. 155, as appropriate.)	Optimal breathing pattern will be maintained.
Impaired Gas Exchange **RELATED TO** Diffusion defect: Hyaline membrane formation Increased shunting: Collapsed alveoli Fluid-filled alveoli Increased dead space: Microembolization in the pulmonary vasculature	**ONGOING ASSESSMENT** • Assess respirations every hour, noting quality, rate, pattern, depth, and breathing effort. • Assess breath sounds and note changes. • Monitor chest x-ray reports. *Keep in mind that radiographic studies of lung water lag behind the clinical presentation by 24 hours.* • Assess for changes in orientation and behavior. • Closely monitor ABGs and note changes. • Use pulse oximetry to monitor oxygen saturation and pulse rate continuously. Keep alarms on at all times. *Pulse oximetry has been found to be a useful tool in the clinical setting to detect changes in oxygenation.* **THERAPEUTIC INTERVENTIONS** • Use a team approach in planning care with the physician and respiratory therapist. *Timely and accurate communication of assessments is a must to adequately keep pace with the needed ventilator setting changes: FiO_2 and CPAP.* • Administer sedation as ordered *to decrease the child's energy expenditure during mechanical ventilation and to deliver adequate CPAP.*	Impaired gas exchange will be reduced.

NURSING DIAGNOSES/ DEFINING CHARACTERISTICS	NURSING INTERVENTIONS / *RATIONALES*	EXPECTED OUTCOMES
DEFINING CHARACTERISTICS Confusion Somnolence Restlessness Irritability Inability to move secretions Hypercapnia Hypoxia	**THERAPEUTIC INTERVENTIONS cont'd** • Combine nursing actions (e.g., bath, bed, and dressing changes), and intersperse with rest periods *to minimize energy expended by child and to prevent a decrease in oxygen saturation.* Temporarily discontinue activity if saturation drops, *to decrease oxygen consumption,* and make any necessary FiO_2, CPAP, or sedation changes *to improve saturation.* • Change position every 2 hours *to facilitate movement and drainage of secretions.* • Suction as needed *to clear secretions.*	
High Risk for Decreased Cardiac Output RELATED TO Positive pressure ventilation **DEFINING CHARACTERISTICS** Variations in hemodynamic parameters (BP, heart rate, CVP, pulmonary artery pressures, cardiac output) Dysrhythmias Weight gain, edema Decreased peripheral pulses, cold clammy skin	**ONGOING ASSESSMENT** • Assess vital signs and hemodynamic pressures (CVP, pulmonary artery pressures) every hour; with changes in positive pressure ventilation; and with any changes in inotrope administration. • Obtain cardiac output measurement as ordered, after positive pressure ventilation changes, and with inotrope administration change. • Closely monitor ABGs. **THERAPEUTIC INTERVENTIONS** • Notify physician of changes in child's status. • Administer inotropic agent as ordered, noting response and observing for side effects. • Administer IV fluids as ordered *to maintain optimal fluid balance.* • Anticipate need to decrease level of CPAP to a range that allows for an improved cardiac output if fluid administration and inotropes are not successful. • See Decreased cardiac output, p. 10, as appropriate.	Optimal cardiac output will be maintained.
High Risk for Injury: Barotrauma RELATED TO Positive pressure ventilation Decreased pulmonary compliance **DEFINING CHARACTERISTICS** Crepitus Subcutaneous emphysema Altered chest excursion: asymmetrical chest Abnormal ABGs Shift in trachea Restlessness Evidence of pneumothorax on chest x-ray evaluation	**ONGOING ASSESSMENT** • Assess for signs of barotrauma every hour. *Frequent assessments are needed, since barotrauma can occur at any time and the child will not show signs of dyspnea, shortness of breath, or tachypnea if heavily sedated to maintain ventilation.* • Monitor chest x-ray reports daily and obtain a stat portable chest x-ray examination if barotrauma is suspected. **THERAPEUTIC INTERVENTIONS** • Notify physician of signs of barotrauma immediately. • Anticipate need for chest tube placement and prepare as needed. *If barotrauma is suspected, intervention must follow immediately to prevent tension pneumothorax.*	Potential for injury from barotrauma will be reduced.

Continued.

NURSING DIAGNOSES/ DEFINING CHARACTERISTICS	NURSING INTERVENTIONS / *RATIONALES*	EXPECTED OUTCOMES
High Risk for Altered Nutrition: Less Than Body Requirements **RELATED TO** Intubation **DEFINING CHARACTERISTICS** Loss of weight >10% to 20% under ideal body weight Documented inadequate caloric intake Caloric intake inadequate to keep pace with abnormal disease/metabolic state	**ONGOING ASSESSMENT** • Obtain and document child's weight. • Obtain nutritional history. • Assess for bowel sounds. • Check for abdominal distension and tenderness. **THERAPEUTIC INTERVENTIONS** • Give enteral or parenteral feedings as ordered. • See Altered nutrition: less than body requirement, p. 33; Enteral tube feeding, p. 225.	Nutritional deficit will be reduced or prevented.

Impaired Physical Mobility **RELATED TO** Acute respiratory failure Monitoring devices Mechanical ventilation **DEFINING CHARACTERISTICS** Imposed restriction of movement Decreased muscle strength Limited ROM	**ONGOING ASSESSMENT**
	 • Assess for any imposed restriction of movement.
	 • Assess muscle strength.
	 • Assess range of motion of extremities.
	
	 THERAPEUTIC INTERVENTIONS
	 • Turn and reposition child every 2 hours.
	 • Maintain limbs in functional alignment (with pillows).
	     Support feet in dorsiflexed position *to prevent footdrop.*
	     Perform/assist with passive ROM exercises to extremities *to prevent contractures.*
	 • Initiate activity increases (dangling, sitting in chair, ambulation) as condition and age allows.
		Optimal physical mobility will be maintained.

High Risk for Impaired Skin Integrity **RELATED TO** Prolonged bed rest Immobility Sensory deficit Altered vasomotor tone Altered nutritional state Prolonged intubation	**ONGOING ASSESSMENT**
	 • Assess bony prominences for signs of threatened or actual breakdown of skin.
	 • Assess around endotracheal (ET) tube for crusting of secretions, redness, or irritation.
	 • Assess for signs of skin breakdown beneath ET tube securing tape.
	
	 THERAPEUTIC INTERVENTIONS
	 • Turn and reposition child every 2 hours.
	 • Institute prophylactic use of pressure-relieving devices.
	 • Maintain skin integrity:
	     If child is nasally intubated, notify physician if skin is red or irritated or breakdown is noted.
	     If child is orally intubated, the tube should be repositioned from side to side every 24-48 hours *(will help to prevent pressure necrosis on the lower lip).*
	 • Provide mouth care every 2 hours.
	 • Keep ET tube free of crusting secretions.
	 • See Impaired skin integrity, p. 39, as appropriate.
		Skin integrity will be maintained.

NURSING DIAGNOSES/ DEFINING CHARACTERISTICS	NURSING INTERVENTIONS / *RATIONALES*	EXPECTED OUTCOMES

DEFINING CHARACTERISTICS
Actual skin break-
down:
  Stage I—redness,
    skin intact
  Stage II—blisters
  Stage III—necrosis
  Stage IV—necrosis
    involving bones
    and joints		

Anxiety/Fear
RELATED TO
Threat of death
Change in health
  status
Change in environ-
  ment
Change in interaction
  patterns
Unmet needs
 	
DEFINING CHARACTERISTICS
Restlessness
Diaporesis
Pointing to his/her
  throat (possibly un-
  able to speak)
Uncooperative be-
  havior
Withdrawal
Watches equipment
  vigilantly
	ONGOING ASSESSMENT
	• Assess child for any signs that could indicate increased fear or increased anxiety.
	
	THERAPEUTIC INTERVENTIONS
	• If child is unable to speak because of respiratory status:
	  Provide pencil and pad to write, or use picture board or alphabet board as age appropriate.
	  Establish some form of nonverbal communication if child is too sick to write. *Maintaining an avenue for communication is important to alleviate anxiety/fear.*
	• Assist the child/parents by:
	  Explaining mechanical ventilation
	  Explaining alarm systems on monitors and ventilators
	  Reassuring child/parents of your presence
	• Display a confident, calm manner and tolerant, understanding attitude.
	• Allow parents/family to visit and involve them in the care.
	• Use other supportive measures as indicated (e.g., medications, psychiatric liaison, clergy, social services).
		Absence or decrease in fear and anxiety will be evidenced.

Knowledge Deficit
RELATED TO
New equipment
New environment
New condition
 	
DEFINING CHARACTERISTICS
Increased frequency
  of questions posed
  by child and signifi-
  cant others
Inability to correctly
  respond to ques-
  tions asked
	ONGOING ASSESSMENT
	• Evaluate child's/parents' understanding of child's overall condition.
	• Assess child's/parents' readiness for learning.
	
	THERAPEUTIC INTERVENTIONS
	• Explain all procedures to child before performing them. *This will help to decrease the child's anxiety. Fear of the unknown can make the child extremely anxious, uncooperative.*
	• Orient child and parents to PICU surroundings, routines, equipment alarms, and noises. *The PICU is a busy and noisy environment which can be very upsetting to child and significant others.*
	• Keep the child/parents informed of current status. *RDS is a very serious syndrome with high mortality. Parents must be informed of changes as they occur.*
		Child/parent will demonstrate understanding of serious nature of disease and treatments.

Susan Galanes, RN, MS, CCRN

Tracheostomy

ARTIFICIAL AIRWAY

A surgical opening into the trachea that is created to relieve airway obstruction, to protect, and/or to serve as an access for suctioning and for mechanical ventilation.

NURSING DIAGNOSES/ DEFINING CHARACTERISTICS	NURSING INTERVENTIONS / *RATIONALES*	EXPECTED OUTCOMES
Ineffective Airway Clearance **RELATED TO** Copious secretions Thick secretions Fatigue; weakness Uncooperative child Confused child Tracheostomy Inability to cough **DEFINING CHARACTERISTICS** Increasing restlessness and irritability Change in mental status Pallor, cyanosis Diaphoresis Tachypnea Increased work of breathing: use of accessory muscles, intercostal retractions, nasal flaring Tachycardia Inconsolability	**ONGOING ASSESSMENT** ▪ Assess age and developmental level. ▪ Assess for evidence of respiratory distress (tachypnea, nasal flaring, and increased use of accessory muscles of respiration). ▪ Assess vital signs every 4 hours and prn. Notify physician if out of prescribed range. ▪ Auscultate chest *for normal and adventitious sounds.* ▪ Assess for changes in mental status (increasing lethargy, confusion, restlessness, and irritability). ▪ Record amount, color, and consistency of secretions. **THERAPEUTIC INTERVENTIONS** ▪ Keep suction and Ambu equipment at bedside. ▪ Provide humidified air *to prevent drying and crusting of secretions.* Use proper-sized tracheostomy collar while child is in bed or asleep. Apply an artificial nose (HME [heat moisture exchanger]) while awake and/or ambulating. ▪ Administer oxygen as needed. ▪ Encourage the child to cough out secretions. ▪ Institute suctioning of airway as needed *to clear secretions.* Instill sterile saline if secretions are thick. *This will help to loosen secretions and induce coughing.* Administer oxygen between suctioning *to prevent hypoxemia.* ▪ Administer stoma care: Clean area around and under phlanges of tube and stoma with a swab and half-strength hydrogen peroxide. If applicable, clean inner cannula with half-strength hydrogen peroxide. Rinse with sterile water or saline. Dry area thoroughly using a sterile gauze or swab. Secure tracheostomy tube with twill tape *to prevent inhalation of loose threads into the tracheostomy opening.* Use a square knot to one side of the child's neck. ▪ Keep small objects out of child's reach *to prevent possible aspiration.* ▪ Keep tracheal obturator taped at head of bed *for emergency use.* ▪ Change trach tube weekly after initial trach change has been performed and sutures have been removed. ▪ Obtain a spare tracheostomy tube of same size and brand to keep at bedside. ▪ Transport child with portable oxygen, suction, Ambu bag, suction catheters, and an extra trach tube.	Patent airway will be maintained.
Ineffective Breathing Pattern **RELATED TO** Superimposed infection Copious tracheal secretions Tracheostomy leak **DEFINING CHARACTERISTICS** Hyperventilation Decreased breath sounds	**ONGOING ASSESSMENT** ▪ Monitor respirations, pulse, and temperature every 4 hours and assess changes. ▪ Assess changes in orientation and behavior pattern. ▪ Auscultate breath sounds every 4 hours. ▪ Monitor blood oxygen concentration: Pulse oximeter Arterial blood gases **THERAPEUTIC INTERVENTIONS** ▪ Maintain adequate airway. ▪ Position child with proper body alignment *for optimal breathing pattern.* ▪ If abnormal breath sounds are present, use tracheal suction as needed *to clear secretions.* ▪ Decrease anxiety by staying with, stroking, or holding child during episodes of respiratory distress.	Optimal breathing pattern will be maintained.

NURSING DIAGNOSES/ DEFINING CHARACTERISTICS	NURSING INTERVENTIONS / *RATIONALES*	EXPECTED OUTCOMES
DEFINING CHARACTERISTICS cont'd Adventitious breath sounds Intercostal retractions Fever Tachycardia Tachypnea Audible tracheostomy leak Behavior changes		
High Risk for Impaired Gas Exchange **RELATED TO** Pneumothorax **DEFINING CHARACTERISTICS** Recent tracheostomy Shortness of breath Tachypnea Increased work of breathing Anxiety Diaphoresis, pallor, vertigo Absence of breath sounds on affected side	**ONGOING ASSESSMENT** ▪ Assess child for evidence of respiratory distress. ▪ Assess vital signs every 4 hours. **THERAPEUTIC INTERVENTIONS** ▪ Stay with child and notify physician if signs of respiratory distress are present. ▪ Place child in semi- to high-Fowler's position *to promote full lung expansion.* ▪ Administer humidified oxygen as needed *to maintain oxygenation and to prevent drying of mucosal membranes.* ▪ Assist in proper positioning when portable chest x-ray film is needed *so that the entire lung field will be x-rayed and optimal lung expansion will occur.* ▪ Set up chest tube placement as needed *to evacuate air from the pleural cavity and reexpand a collapsed lung.*	Optimal gas exchange will be maintained.
High Risk for Altered Nutrition: Less Than Body Requirements **RELATED TO** Possible dysphagia secondary to tracheostomy Depression Anorexia Fatigue **DEFINING CHARACTERISTICS** Loss of weight with or without adequate caloric intake >10%-20% under ideal body weight Caloric intake inadequate to keep pace with abnormal disease/metabolic state	**ONGOING ASSESSMENT** ▪ Compare admission weight with present weight. ▪ Obtain nutritional history. ▪ Assess child's present nutritional intake: oral feeding, enteral, parenteral. ▪ Assess infant's ability to suck and swallow. **THERAPEUTIC INTERVENTIONS** ▪ If signs of altered nutrition are present, see Altered nutrition, less than body requirements, p. 33. ▪ See Enteral tube feedings, p. 225. ▪ Refer to speech therapist for sucking and swallowing evaluation. ▪ Obtain dietary consultation as needed.	Optimal nutrition will be maintained.

Continued.

NURSING DIAGNOSES/ DEFINING CHARACTERISTICS	NURSING INTERVENTIONS / *RATIONALES*	EXPECTED OUTCOMES
High Risk for Infection **RELATED TO** Surgical incision of tracheostomy Skin excoriation from tracheal ties **DEFINING CHARACTERISTICS** Inability of wound to heal Abnormal appearance of wound drainage Purulent drainage from wound Fever and chills Elevated WBC count Stoma red, warm, and tender to touch Redness or breakdown of skin under tracheal ties	**ONGOING ASSESSMENT** <ul><li>Observe stoma for erythema, exudates, odor, and crusting lesions. If present, culture stoma and notify physician.</li><li>Assess vital signs every 4 hours and notify physician of abnormalities.</li><li>Assess laboratory values of WBCs and differential.</li><li>Assess for fever and chills and monitor blood cultures.</li><li>Assess skin integrity under tracheal ties every 8 hours.</li></ul> **THERAPEUTIC INTERVENTIONS** <ul><li>Provide routine tracheostomy care every 8 hours and prn *to prevent airway obstruction and infection.*</li><li>Do not allow secretions to pool around stoma. Suction area or wipe area with aseptic technique *to keep stoma clean and dry.*</li><li>Keep skin under tracheostomy ties clean and dry *to prevent skin irritation.*</li><li>Use Reston foam or Duoderm under trach ties *to prevent breakdown if redness is present.*</li><li>If signs of infection are present, apply topical antifungal or antibacterial agent as ordered.</li></ul>	Potential for infection will be reduced.
Impaired Communication: Verbal **RELATED TO** Tracheostomy **DEFINING CHARACTERISTICS** Difficulty in making himself or herself understood Withdrawal Restlessness Frustration	**ONGOING ASSESSMENT** <ul><li>Assess child's ability to understand spoken word.</li><li>Assess child's ability to express ideas.</li></ul> **THERAPEUTIC INTERVENTIONS** <ul><li>Provide call light within easy reach at all times.</li><li>Obtain a room close to the nurse's station *to provide easy observation of child by nursing staff.*</li><li>Provide child with pad and pencil. Use picture or alphabet board if child does not understand.</li><li>Provide child with reassurance and be patient in interactions *to allay frustration.*</li><li>Consult speech therapist for possible artificial larynx.</li></ul>	Alternative methods of communication will be facilitated.
Knowledge Deficit of Tracheostomy **RELATED TO** New procedure/ intervention	**ONGOING ASSESSMENT** <ul><li>Assess knowledge of significant other(s) concerning tracheostomy.</li><li>Assess ability of significant other(s) to provide adequate home health care of child.</li><li>Assess interest and readiness to learn.</li><li>Assess ability to respond to emergency situations.</li></ul>	Patient/significant others will demonstrate skills appropriate for tracheostomy.

Tracheostomy cont'd

NURSING DIAGNOSES/ DEFINING CHARACTERISTICS	NURSING INTERVENTIONS / *RATIONALES*	EXPECTED OUTCOMES
DEFINING CHARACTERISTICS Anxiety Lack of questioning Increased questioning Expressed need for more information	**THERAPEUTIC INTERVENTIONS** • Discuss the need for the child to have a tracheostomy and its particular purpose. • Begin teaching skills one at a time and reinforce them daily. *The child/ parent can then begin to acquire the skills at a pace that is not overwhelming.* • Provide instruction on sterile tracheostomy care and suctioning; include step-by-step care guidelines. • Reinforce knowledge of emergency techniques. • Provide list of resource persons to contact, including who they are and why/when they should be contacted. • Explain importance of follow-up appointments. • Use social services as appropriate *to attain equipment and arrange for visiting nurses.* • Encourage a 24-hour in-hospital trial of total care before discharge.	

Ruth E. Schumacher, RNC, MSN

Ventilation: high-frequency jet (HFJV)

JET VENTILATION; HIGH-FREQUENCY VENTILATION; VENTILATION MODES; HFJV

A type of mechanical ventilation that uses high-frequency rates (40 to 900 cycles/min) with very low tidal volumes (3 to 5 ml/ kg) to achieve ventilation. It is useful for children with bronchopleural fistulas or large pulmonary air leaks and is indicated for children who have failed on conventional ventilation.

NURSING DIAGNOSES/ DEFINING CHARACTERISTICS	NURSING INTERVENTIONS / *RATIONALES*	EXPECTED OUTCOMES
Impaired Gas Exchange Requiring HFJV **RELATED TO** Respiratory distress syndrome Barotrauma Aspiration pneumonitis Bronchopleural fistula Interstitial air leak syndromes **DEFINING CHARACTERISTICS** Hypercapnia Hypoxia Abnormal ABGs Low pulmonary compliance exhibited by high peak pressures (≤ 55 cm H_2O) Presence of increased intrathoracic pressures	**ONGOING ASSESSMENT** • Assess age and developmental level. • Assess respiratory rate, rhythm, and character every hour. • Auscultate lungs every hour to check for aeration both before and after jet ventilation is begun. • Observe for abnormal breathing patterns (Cheyne-Stokes, Kussmaul, sternal retractions). • Assess LOC and level of anxiety. • Assess skin color (presence/absence of cyanosis), temperature, capillary refill, and peripheral perfusion. • Monitor vital signs every hour, watching for increased central venous pressure, increased pulmonary capillary wedge pressure (PCWP), decreased BP, and decreased cardiac output; notify physician if these occur. • Monitor for complaints of pain, *which may increase respirations, making it more difficult to ventilate child's lungs.* Assess location and duration. • Monitor ABGs frequently or as indicated (e.g., after changes in FiO_2 rate, drive pressure, or continuous positive airway pressure). • Monitor cardiac output as indicated or ordered, especially after ventilator changes or changes in child's condition. **THERAPEUTIC INTERVENTIONS** • Administer oxygen as ordered and indicated. • Obtain informed consent for jet therapy if possible.	Optimal gas exchange will be maintained.

Continued.

151

Pulmonary Care Plans (Pediatric)

NURSING DIAGNOSES/ DEFINING CHARACTERISTICS	NURSING INTERVENTIONS / *RATIONALES*	EXPECTED OUTCOMES
	THERAPEUTIC INTERVENTIONS cont'd	
	▪ If not already intubated, prepare child for intubation. *The endotracheal tube is prepared with two additional ports; one for the jet-drive line, and one for continuous monitoring of intratracheal pressures.* Administer sedation or neuromuscular blocking agent as ordered, e.g., diazepam (Valium), pancuronium (Pavulon), or succinylcholine. Provide comfort measures/reassurance (verbal and nonverbal contact). Obtain baseline status before institution of therapy (PCWP, cardiac output, and ABGs) as ordered.	
	▪ Maintain adequate blood volume, treating any sources of hemorrhage or changes in vascular compartments with appropriate fluids as ordered (i.e., blood, crystalloid, colloid).	
	▪ Combine nursing actions (e.g., bath, bed, and dressing changes) *to minimize energy expended by child and allow frequent periods of rest.*	
	▪ Provide frequent attendance, *since there are few alarms on present jet system to detect patient disconnect or low volumes.* Be prepared to use Ambu bag *in case of emergency failure of machinery or an acute change in the child's condition. Ambu bag ventilation may be difficult because of decreased compliance and elasticity.*	
	▪ Administer antibiotics and medications as ordered.	
	▪ Administer pain relievers as ordered, and provide other comfort measures as needed.	
	▪ Be aware that sedation to maintain ventilation control will decrease with jet ventilation. *Most children placed on HFJV have a cessation of their own ventilatory effort at the supraphysiological ventilatory rates. However, when weaning back to conventional ventilation, the need for sedation may return.*	
Ineffective Airway Clearance **RELATED TO** Presence/irritation by ET tube Secretions Drying of mucosa Decreased energy and fatigue	**ONGOING ASSESSMENT** ▪ Assess for alteration in airway clearance. ▪ Assess ET tube placement and, on older children, the adequacy of cuff to prevent air leakage: *Underinflation may cause aspiration of oral secretions.* *Overinflation of cuff may obliterate perfusion to left or right bronchus, resulting in deterioration of ABGs.* Notify respiratory therapist to check cuff pressure. Notify physician if there are any problems with ET tube maintenance (e.g., placement, suctioning, cuff).	Airway will be free of secretions.
DEFINING CHARACTERISTICS Abnormal breath sounds Change in rates, depth, and character of respirations Tachypnea Cough Cyanosis Dyspnea or shortness of breath	**THERAPEUTIC INTERVENTIONS** ▪ Institute aseptic suctioning of airway as needed *to prevent airway obstruction. Potential for mucus plug is present because of drying of mucosa from high-frequency ventilation* (respiratory therapist will maintain humidification). ▪ Turn off jet ventilator or disconnect during suctioning; *otherwise increased airway resistance may increase potential for pneumothorax.* ▪ Be aware that the respiratory therapist will use Ambu bag or "sigh" every hour, with the jet off, *to prevent atelectasis or atrophy of respiratory muscles as a result of low tidal volumes.*	
High Risk for Injury: Barotrauma **RELATED TO** Pressure cycled ventilation High peak airway pressures	**ONGOING ASSESSMENT** ▪ Assess for signs of barotrauma. *Frequent assessments are needed, since barotrauma can occur at any time, and the child may not show signs of dyspnea, shortness of breath, or tachypnea while on HFJV.* ▪ Monitor chest x-ray reports daily, and obtain a stat portable chest x-ray evaluation if barotrauma is suspected.	Potential for injury from barotrauma will be reduced.

NURSING DIAGNOSES/ DEFINING CHARACTERISTICS	NURSING INTERVENTIONS / *RATIONALES*	EXPECTED OUTCOMES
DEFINING CHARACTERISTICS Crepitus Subcutaneous emphysema Altered chest excursion: asymmetrical chest Abnormal ABGs Shift in trachea Restlessness Chest x-ray report shows evidence of pneumothorax	**THERAPEUTIC INTERVENTIONS** • Notify physician immediately of any signs of barotrauma. • Anticipate the need for chest tube placement, and prepare as needed. *If barotrauma is suspected, intervention must be immediate to prevent a tension pneumothorax.*	
High Risk for Impaired Skin Integrity **RELATED TO** Prolonged bed rest Immobility Sensory deficit Altered vasomotor tone and/or altered nutritional state Prolonged intubation **DEFINING CHARACTERISTICS** Actual skin breakdown: 　Stage I—redness, skin intact 　Stage II—blisters 　Stage III—necrosis 　Stage IV—necrosis involving bones and joints	**ONGOING ASSESSMENT** • Assess bony prominences for signs of threatened or actual breakdown of skin. • Assess around ET tube for crusting of secretions, redness, or irritation. • Assess for signs of skin breakdown beneath ET tube-securing tape. **THERAPEUTIC INTERVENTIONS** • Institute changes in position carefully *because of limitations in length of ventilator tubing (which is designed to minimize compressible volume, increasing efficiency). Changes in position may change ability to ventilate but should be made every 2 hours.* • Institute prophylactic usage of pressure-relieving devices. (See Impaired skin integrity, p. 39, as appropriate.) • Change tape securing ET tube when loosened or soiled, taking care to maintain tube position. 　If child is nasally intubated, notify physician if skin is red, irritated, or breakdown is noted. 　If child is orally intubated, the tube should be repositioned from side to side every 24 to 48 hours. *This will help to prevent pressure necrosis from occurring on the lower lip.* • Provide mouth care every 2 hours *to decrease oral bacteria.* • Keep ET tube free from crusting of secretions.	Skin integrity will be maintained.
High Risk for Altered Nutrition: Less Than Body Requirements **RELATED TO** Intubation **DEFINING CHARACTERISTICS** Loss of weight ≥10% to 20% under ideal body weight Documented inadequate caloric intake Caloric intake inadequate to keep pace with abnormal disease/metabolic state	**ONGOING ASSESSMENT** • Obtain daily weight and document. • Obtain nutritional history. • Assess for bowel sounds. • Check for abdominal distension and tenderness. **THERAPEUTIC INTERVENTIONS** • Give enteral or parenteral feedings as ordered. • See Altered nutrition: less than body requirement, p. 33.	Nutritional deficit will be reduced or prevented.

Continued.

Pulmonary Care Plans (Pediatric)

NURSING DIAGNOSES/ DEFINING CHARACTERISTICS	NURSING INTERVENTIONS / *RATIONALES*	EXPECTED OUTCOMES
Knowledge Deficit **RELATED TO** New equipment New environment **DEFINING** **CHARACTERISTICS** Increased frequency of questions posed by child and/or parents Inability to correctly respond to questions asked by medical personnel	**ONGOING ASSESSMENT** • Evaluate understanding by child/parents of child's overall condition and the need for jet ventilation. • Evaluate readiness for learning by child/parents. **THERAPEUTIC INTERVENTIONS** • Explain all procedures to child/parents before performing them, especially during period of intubation and initial start of jet ventilation. *This will help to decrease their anxiety. Fear of the unknown could otherwise result in an extremely anxious, uncooperative child and family.* • Provide reassurance of safety of jet ventilatory system. • Orient and reorient child to PICU surroundings, routines, equipment alarms, and noises. *The PICU is a busy and noisy environment that can be very upsetting to the child if he or she does not know what the noises and alarms mean.* • Include parents in explanations of the jet therapy. • Allow child to ventilate feelings through alternative methods of communication, as age appropriate (picture board, written messages, alphabet board). • Explain methods/procedures of "weaning off" HFJV. Be aware that sedation, which may have been used before the jet therapy, may need to be reinstituted during weaning process. Reassure that sedation is not meant as a means of punishment but may provide an easier transition to conventional ventilation and eventual extubation.	Child/parents will demonstrate understanding of rationale for jet ventilation.

Susan Galanes, RN, MS, CCRN

Ventilation: mechanical

VENTILATORS; RESPIRATORY FAILURE; INTUBATION

The child requiring mechanical ventilation must have an artificial airway (endotracheal [ET tube] or tracheostomy) in place. A mechanical ventilator will facilitate the movement of gases into and out of the pulmonary system (ventilation), but it cannot ensure gas exchange at the pulmonary and tissue level (respiration). It provides either partial or total ventilatory support for patients with respiratory failure. Management of the child includes preventing further lung injury, pulmonary hypertension, cor pulmonale, and fluid overload and maintaining adequate nutrition.

NURSING DIAGNOSES/ DEFINING CHARACTERISTICS	NURSING INTERVENTIONS / *RATIONALES*	EXPECTED OUTCOMES

Impaired Gas Exchange/ Ineffective Breathing Pattern Requiring Mechanical Ventilation **RELATED TO** Acute respiratory failure Pneumonia: viral or bacterial RDS Aspiration Various CNS disorders: Guillian Barré Myasthenia gravis Muscular dystrophies Trauma Status asthmaticus Drug overdose Near-drowning Smoke inhalation Bronchopulmonary dysplasia and chronic lung disease Postoperative effects of cardiac surgery Pulmonary edema Airway obstruction Diabetic coma Uremia **DEFINING CHARACTERISTICS** pH <7.35 P_{O_2} <50-60 P_{CO_2} ≥50-60 Decrease in available Hgb, resulting in a decreased oxygen content Changes in mental status Increased or decreased respiratory rate	**ONGOING ASSESSMENT**
	• Assess age and developmental level.
	• Assess vital signs every hour and prn. *In the presence of hypoxia and/ or hypocarbia, hypotension, tachycardia, and tachypnea may result.*
	• Assess lung sounds every 1-2 hours. *This enables early detection of any deterioration or improvement.*
	• Listen closely for rhonchi, rales, wheezing, and diminished breath sounds in each lobe assessing right to left *to compare lung sounds. Reassess lung sounds following coughing/suctioning to determine whether they have improved/cleared.*
	• Assess breathing rate, pattern, depth; note position assumed for breathing.
	• Observe ABGs for any abrupt changes or deteriorations. Normal ranges:
	  pH 7.35-7.45
	  P_{O_2} 80-90 mm Hg
	  P_{CO_2} 35-45 mm Hg
	  O_2 sat 85%-98%
	  O_2 content 16-23 vol%
	  H_{CO_3} 23-29 mEq/L
	  Base excess O ± 2 mEq/L
	  Oxygenation must be closely monitored to prevent hypoxia or hyperoxia, both of which could cause more lung injury.
	• Assess for changes in mental status and LOC. *Signs of hypoxia include anxiety, restlessness, disorientation, somnolence, lethargy, and/or coma.*
	• Assess skin color, checking nailbeds and lips for cyanosis.
	• Use pulse oximetry or transcutaneous oxygen monitoring, as available, *to continuously monitor oxygenation to have information immediately available to prevent acute or chronic hypoxia. Chronic hypoxia can cause pulmonary hypertension and cor pulmonale.*
	• Observe laboratory data, especially noting changes in Hgb, electrolytes, and blood glucose.
	• If child has hemodynamic monitoring, assess pressures every hour and notify physician if out of prescribed ranges.
	Postintubation:
	• Assess good ET tube position following intubation:
	  For the older child in which a cuffed ET tube is used, inflate cuff until no audible leaks are heard. The cuff pressure should not exceed 30 mm Hg. *Overinflation of the cuff increases incidence of tracheal erosions.*
	• Auscultate for bilateral breath sounds while the child's lungs are being manually ventilated by Ambu bag *to ensure good ET tube position. If diminished breath sounds are present over the left lung field, the ET tube is most likely below the carina in the right mainstem bronchus and needs to be pulled back.*
		Altered gas exchange will be reduced.

Continued.

NURSING DIAGNOSES/ DEFINING CHARACTERISTICS	NURSING INTERVENTIONS / *RATIONALES*	EXPECTED OUTCOMES

DEFINING CHARACTERISTICS cont'd

Apnea

Inability to maintain airway, i.e., depressed gag, depressed cough, emesis

Forced vital capacity <10 cc/kg

Rales, rhonchi, wheezing

Diminished breath sounds

ONGOING ASSESSMENT cont'd

- Observe for abdominal distention, *which may be indicative of gastric intubation and can also occur following CPR when air is inadvertently blown/bagged into the esophagus as well as the trachea.*
- Ensure that chest x-ray evaluation is obtained *for determination of ET tube placement. A right mainstem intubation frequently occurs in young children, and breath sounds may seem equal because of transmission of sound. ET tube placement needs to be determined by x-ray evaluation.*

THERAPEUTIC INTERVENTIONS

Before intubation:
- Maintain airway:
    Encourage child to cough and deep breathe.
    If coughing and deep breathing are not effective, use nasotracheal suction as needed *to clear airway.* Do not suction deeply when inspiratory stridor and barky cough are present. *Suction could result in laryngospasm, leading to partial or complete airway obstruction.*
    Use oral or nasal airway as needed *to prevent tongue from occluding the oropharynx.*
    See Ineffective airway clearance, p. 3.
    Provide oxygen therapy as ordered and indicated. *Increasing the oxygen tension in the alveoli may result in more oxygen being diffused into the capillaries.*
    Coordinate respiratory therapy treatments.
- Place child in a high-Fowler's position, if tolerated, *to promote lung expansion.* Check the positioning frequently, *so that child does not slide down, causing the abdomen to compress the diaphragm, which would cause respiratory embarrassment.*
- Notify physician:
    If vital signs are out of prescribed range or trending from baseline
    Immediately for signs of impending respiratory failure
- Prepare for endotracheal intubation:
    Notify respiratory therapist to bring a mechanical ventilator.
    If possible, before intubation explain to child and parent:
        Need for intubation
        Steps involved
        Temporary inability to speak
    Place equipment:
        ET tubes of various sizes; note size used
        Benzoin and waterproof tape or other methods *for securing ET tube*
        A syringe for inflating balloon after ET tube is in position (for the older child in which a cuffed ET tube is used). *In a child under 8 years, a cuffed ET tube is not generally used because of the anatomical differences in the airway (under 8 years of age, the cricoid diameter is narrower and provides a natural seal).*
        Local anesthetic agent, e.g., Cetacaine spray, cocaine, lidocaine (Xylocaine) spray or jelly, and cotton-tipped applicators *for comfort and to suppress the gag reflex*
        Sedation as prescribed by physician *to decrease combative resistance to intubation*
        Stylet *to make ET tube firmer and to give additional support to direction*
        Laryngoscope and blades
        Ambu bag and mask connected to oxygen *to provide assisted ventilation with 100% oxygen*
        Suction equipment *to maintain airway*
        Oral airway if child is being orally intubated *to prevent occlusion or biting of ET tube*
        Bilateral soft wrist restraints *to prevent self-extubation of ET tube*

NURSING DIAGNOSES/ DEFINING CHARACTERISTICS	NURSING INTERVENTIONS / *RATIONALES*	EXPECTED OUTCOMES
	THERAPEUTIC INTERVENTIONS cont'd *Postintubation:* ▪ Continue with manual ventilation until ET tube is stabilized. ▪ *To prevent child from biting down on ET tube,* insert oral airway for child who is orally intubated. ▪ Assist in securing ET tube (if in proper placement per examination). *Securing an ET tube in a child is critical. Care must be taken to maintain the tube position.* Document ET tube position and level *for continuity of care.* ▪ Institute aseptic suctioning of airway. ▪ Institute mechanical ventilation, with setting as ordered. ▪ Apply bilateral soft wrist restraints as needed, explaining to child/parent reason for use. ▪ Anticipate need for NG drainage *to prevent abdominal distention.*	
High Risk for Injury **RELATED TO** Improper ventilator settings Improper alarm settings Disconnection of ventilator **DEFINING CHARACTERISTICS** Reduction of PO_2 Increase in PCO_2 Acidosis Tachypnea Apnea Changes in mental state Tachycardia	**ONGOING ASSESSMENT** ▪ Check ventilator settings *to see that child is receiving the correct:* Mode Rate of mechanical breaths (frequency) Tidal volume Inspiratory time and I:E ratio FIO_2 Continuous positive airway pressure *(2-4 cm H_2O pressure is considered physiologic in children)* Pressure support **THERAPEUTIC INTERVENTIONS** ▪ Notify respiratory therapist immediately of any discrepancy in ventilator settings. ▪ Listen for alarms, know the range in which the ventilator will alarm, and respond to alarms as they occur: High peak−pressure alarm: If child is agitated, give sedation as ordered. Auscultate breath sounds and institute suctioning as needed. Notify respiratory therapist and physician if high-pressure alarm persists. *This could indicate a decrease in lung compliance, which could result in barotrauma or could be a partial airway obstruction.* Low-pressure alarm: *indicates possible disconnection or mechanical ventilatory malfunction:* If disconnected, reconnect to mechanical ventilator. If malfunctioning, remove from mechanical ventilator, and use Ambu bag. Notify respiratory therapist to correct malfunction. Low exhale volume: *indicates that the patient is not returning delivered tidal volume, i.e., a leak or disconnection:* NOTE: *A small air leak should be present in children without cuffed ET tubes. Submucosal ischemia can occur quickly with tight tubes.* Reconnect to the ventilator if disconnected, or reconnect the exhale tubing to the ventilator. If the problem is not resolved, notify the physician and the respiratory therapist. On older children with cuffed ET tubes, check cuff volume by assessing whether the child is able to talk or make sounds around the tube or if exhaled volumes are significantly less than volumes delivered. To correct, slowly reinflate cuff with air until no leak is detected. Notify respiratory therapist to check cuff pressure; *cuff pressure should be maintained at <30 mm Hg. Maintenance of low-pressure cuffs prevents many tracheal complications that in the past have been associated with ET tubes.* Notify physician if leak persists. *The ET tube cuff may be defective, requiring the physician to change the tube.*	Injury will be prevented.

Continued.

NURSING DIAGNOSES/ DEFINING CHARACTERISTICS	NURSING INTERVENTIONS / *RATIONALES*	EXPECTED OUTCOMES

	THERAPEUTIC INTERVENTIONS cont'd
	Apnea alarm: *is indicative of disconnection or absence of sponta-neous respirations:*
	  If disconnected, reconnect to ventilator.
	  If apnea persists, use Ambu ventilation and notify physician.	

Ineffective Airway Clearance
RELATED TO
Endotracheal intuba-tion
 	
DEFINING CHARACTERISTICS
Copious secretions
Abnormal breath sounds
Dyspnea
	ONGOING ASSESSMENT
	▪ Assess breath sounds every hour and as needed.
	▪ Note quantity, color, consistency, and odor of sputum.
	
	THERAPEUTIC INTERVENTIONS
	▪ Institute suctioning of airway as needed:
	  Hyperoxygenate before and after each suctioning attempt.
	    For neonatal patients, use approximately 0.10 greater FiO_2 than receiving from ventilator.
	    For >6 months old, use 100% oxygen.
	  Use appropriate suction pressures *to prevent further trauma or collapse of the airways:*
	    Neonatal: −60 to −80 mm Hg
	    Pediatrics: −80 to −100 mm Hg
	▪ Turn every 2 hours *to mobilize secretions.*
	▪ Use sterile saline instillations during suctioning as needed *to help facili-tate the removal of tenacious sputum:*
	  Neonatal: A few drops to 0.33 ml
	  Older children: 1 to 3 ml may be appropriate, depending on size.
		Airway will remain patent.

Impaired Communication: Verbal
RELATED TO
Endotracheal intu-bation
 	
DEFINING CHARACTERISTICS
Child is unable to communicate ver-bally because of in-tubation
Difficulty in being un-derstood with non-verbal methods
Increasing frustration and/or anxiety
	ONGOING ASSESSMENT
	▪ Assess child's ability to use nonverbal communication.
	
	THERAPEUTIC INTERVENTIONS
	▪ Provide nonverbal means of communication as is age appropriate:
	  Picture board/cards
	  Writing equipment
	  Communication board
	  Artificial larynx
	  Generalized list of questions/answers
	▪ Reassure child and parent that the inability to speak *is a temporary ef-fect of the ET tube passing the vocal cords.*
	▪ Enlist parents' assistance in understanding child's needs/communica-tion.
	▪ See Impaired communication, p. 11.
		Nonverbal means to express needs and concerns will be at-tained.

High Risk for Anxiety/Fear **RELATED TO** Inability to ade-quately breathe without support Unable to maintain adequate gas ex-change Fear of the unknown outcome	**ONGOING ASSESSMENT** ▪ Assess for signs of fear/anxiety. **THERAPEUTIC INTERVENTIONS** ▪ Display a confident, calm manner and an understanding attitude. ▪ Inform child/parent of alarms in the ventilatory system and reassure them of the close proximity of health care personnel *to respond to those alarms.* ▪ Reduce distracting stimuli *to provide a quiet environment.* ▪ Encourage visiting by family/friends. ▪ See Anxiety, p. 4, and Fear, p. 18.	Anxiety will be re-duced.

Ventilation: mechanical cont'd

NURSING DIAGNOSES/ DEFINING CHARACTERISTICS	NURSING INTERVENTIONS / *RATIONALES*	EXPECTED OUTCOMES
DEFINING CHARACTERISTICS Restlessness Afraid to sleep at night Uncooperative behavior Withdrawal Indifference Watches equipment vigilantly		

High Risk for Decrease in Cardiac Output
RELATED TO
Mechanical ventilation
Positive pressure ventilation
 	
DEFINING CHARACTERISTICS
Hypotension
Tachycardia
Dysrhythmias, ECG changes
Anxiety, restlessness
Decrease in peripheral pulses
Weight gain
Edema
	ONGOING ASSESSMENT
	• Assess vital signs and hemodynamic parameters (CVP, pulmonary artery pressures, cardiac output). *Mechanical ventilation can cause a decrease in venous return to the heart, resulting in a decreased cardiac output. This can occur abruptly with ventilator changes (rate, tidal volume, or positive pressure ventilation). Close monitoring during ventilator changes is imperative.*
	• Assess skin color, temperature, and note quality of peripheral pulses.
	• Assess fluid balance through:
	  Daily weights
	  I&O *(After the initial decrease in venous return to the heart, the volume receptors in the right atrium signal a decrease in volume that triggers an increase in the release of antidiuretic hormone from the posterior pituitary and a retention of water by the kidneys.)*
	• Assess mentation.
	
	THERAPEUTIC INTERVENTIONS
	• Maintain optimal fluid balance. *Fluid challenges may initially be used to add volume. However, if the pulmonary artery pressures rise and the cardiac output remains low, fluid restriction may be necessary.*
	• Notify physician immediately of signs of a decrease in cardiac output and anticipate possible ventilator setting changes.
	• Administer medications as ordered (diuretics, inotropic agents, bronchodilator).
	• See Cardiac output, decreased, p. 10.
		Cardiac output will be maintained.

High Risk for Impairment of Skin Integrity **RELATED TO** Prolonged intubation **DEFINING CHARACTERISTICS** "Crusting" of secretions around ET tube Redness or irritation around ET tube and/or beneath securing tape Skin breakdown under or around ET tube and/or tape	**ONGOING ASSESSMENT** • Observe skin for buildup of secretions, redness, or breakdown. **THERAPEUTIC INTERVENTIONS** • If child is nasally intubated, notify physician if skin is red or irritated, or if breakdown is noted. • If child is orally intubated, the tube should be repositioned from side to side every 24-48 hours, using care to maintain tube at correct level. • Support ventilator tubing *to prevent pressure on nose or lips.* • Change tape as needed when loosened or soiled *to ensure adequate stabilization of ET tube.* • Provide mouth care every 2 hours. *This will help to decrease oral bacteria as well as to prevent crusting of secretions.*	Skin integrity will be maintained.

Continued.

Pulmonary Care Plans (Pediatric)

NURSING DIAGNOSES/ DEFINING CHARACTERISTICS	NURSING INTERVENTIONS / *RATIONALES*	EXPECTED OUTCOMES
High Risk for Altered Nutrition: Less Than Body Requirements **RELATED TO** Endotracheal intubation	**ONGOING ASSESSMENT** • Document weight on admission and every day. • Obtain nutritional history. • Assess for bowel sounds. • Check for abdominal distention and tenderness and, if present, notify physician. *This could be indicative of a paralytic ileus, bowel obstruction, or acute abdomen.*	Nutritional deficit will be reduced or prevented.
DEFINING CHARACTERISTICS Loss of weight with or without caloric intake ≥10%-20% under ideal body weight Documented inadequate caloric intake Caloric intake inadequate to keep pace with abnormal disease/metabolic state	**THERAPEUTIC INTERVENTIONS** • Give enteral or parenteral feedings as ordered. *Be aware that children with elevated CO_2 will need a low-carbohydrate diet to reduce CO_2 production. Use specially formulated enteral feeding formula that provides low carbohydrate, high polyunsaturated fats, moderate protein, and high calories.* • See Altered nutrition: less than body requirements, p. 33; Enteral tube feeding, p. 225.	
High Risk for Infection **RELATED TO** ET intubation Suctioning of airway	**ONGOING ASSESSMENT** • Monitor temperature every 4 hours and notify physician if temperature is above 38.5° C (101.3° F). • Monitor WBC and notify physician of elevation. • Monitor sputum culture and sensitivity reports.	Risk of infection will be reduced.
DEFINING CHARACTERISTICS Increased temperature Increased WBC Changes in tracheal secretions, color, consistency, and amount Tachycardia Infiltrates on chest x-ray examination	**THERAPEUTIC INTERVENTIONS** • Maintain aseptic suctioning techniques *to lessen the probability of child's acquiring an infection.* • Administer antibiotics as ordered.	
Knowledge Deficit **RELATED TO** New treatment New environment	**ONGOING ASSESSMENT** • Assess child's/significant others' perception and understanding of mechanical ventilation.	Child/parent will state a basic understanding of mechanical ventilation and the care involved.
DEFINING CHARACTERISTICS Multiple questions Lack of concern Anxiety		

Ventilation: mechanical cont'd

NURSING DIAGNOSES/ DEFINING CHARACTERISTICS	NURSING INTERVENTIONS / *RATIONALES*	EXPECTED OUTCOMES
	THERAPEUTIC INTERVENTIONS	

- Allow child/parents to express feelings and ask questions.
- Explain that child will not be able to eat or drink while intubated, but assure him or her that alternative measures will be taken to provide nourishment, i.e., gastric feedings or hyperalimentation. *The risk of aspiration is high if the child eats or drinks while intubated.*
- Explain to child/parents the necessity for procedures, e.g., obtaining ABGs.
- Explain to child/parents the inability to talk while intubated: *the ET tube passes through the vocal cords, and attempting to talk could cause more trauma to the cords.*
- Explain that the alarms may periodically sound, which may be normal, and the staff will be in close proximity.
- Explain the need for frequent assessments, e.g., vital signs, auscultating breath sounds.
- Explain the probable need for restraints *to gain cooperation to prevent an accidental extubation.*
- Explain to child the need for suctioning as needed.
- Explain the weaning process to child and parents and that extubation will be attempted after the child has demonstrated good respiratory function and a decrease in pulmonary secretions.

Susan Galanes, RN, MS, CCRN; Michelle McGhee, RN, BSN

Meconium aspiration syndrome (MAS)

This condition occurs more often in term or postterm infants. Pulmonary disease may result from meconium being aspirated into the airway, either from gasping efforts of the asphyxiated fetus or with the first breaths after birth.

NURSING DIAGNOSES/ DEFINING CHARACTERISTICS	NURSING INTERVENTIONS / *RATIONALES*	EXPECTED OUTCOMES

Ineffective Breathing Pattern **RELATED TO** Meconium aspiration **DEFINING CHARACTERISTICS** Tachypnea Grunting Nasal flaring Retractions Mild to profound cyanosis Rales Chest hyperexpanded and barrel-shaped	**ONGOING ASSESSMENT**
	 • Assess vital signs and BP.
	 • Assess for grunting. Document if audible with or without stethoscope.
	 • Assess for presence of nasal flaring.
	 • Assess depth and location of retractions:
	     Mild, moderate, or severe
	     Substernal or subcostal
	 • Assess for cyanosis (room air, oxygen).
	 • Assess breath sounds and air entry:
	     Equality
	     Rales (fine, coarse)
	 • Monitor arterial or capillary blood gases every 4 hours and prn.
	 • Monitor transcutaneous PO_2 during suctioning or during periods of agitation.
		Respiratory compromise will be reduced.

Continued.

Meconium aspiration syndrome (MAS) cont'd

NURSING DIAGNOSES/ DEFINING CHARACTERISTICS	NURSING INTERVENTIONS / *RATIONALES*	EXPECTED OUTCOMES
	THERAPEUTIC INTERVENTIONS • Maintain patent airway: 　Chest physical therapy/postural drainage 　Suction • Maintain oxygen therapy, continuous positive airway pressure, or ventilatory settings as ordered. • Minimize handling *to avoid agitation and subsequent hypoxia.* • Maintain ABGs: 　pH 7.40 to 7.45 　P_{CO_2} 35-45 mm Hg 　P_{O_2} 70-80 mm Hg 　*to prevent pulmonary vasoconstriction.* • For persistent hypoxia administer pancuronium (Pavulon) per order. 　NOTE: *Infants receiving Pavulon must be maintained on mechanical ventilation as ordered. Since these infants are usually term or postterm, they may fight assisted ventilation and require paralyzation to ventilate and oxygenate the lungs adequately.*	
High Risk for Injury: Systemic Complications **RELATED TO** Meconium aspiration **DEFINING CHARACTERISTICS** *Metabolic complications:* Metabolic acidosis Hypocalcemia Hypoglycemia/hyperglycemia Electrolyte imbalance *Neurologic complications:* Postasphyxia cerebral edema Syndrome of inappropriate antidiuretic hormone Seizures *Circulatory complications:* Profound hypoxia Hypovolemia Fluid shifts Anemia Disseminated intravascular coagulation Hematuria Oliguria Anuria Necrotizing enterocolitis	**ONGOING ASSESSMENT** • Assess the following: 　Serum calcium 　Chemstrip bG or serum glucose 　Peripheral perfusion, total serum solute, and presence of edema 　Hematocrit 　Urine specific gravity and Labstix 　Abdominal circumference 　Stools and/or gastric drainage *for bleeding* • Monitor electrolytes. • Document type and duration of seizure activity. **THERAPEUTIC INTERVENTIONS** • Provide or administer electrolytes, fluids, and medications as ordered *to prevent pulmonary vasoconstriction.* • See Seizures, p. 214.	Risk for injury will be reduced.

NURSING DIAGNOSES/ DEFINING CHARACTERISTICS	NURSING INTERVENTIONS / *RATIONALES*	EXPECTED OUTCOMES
High Risk for Fluid Volume Deficit **RELATED TO** Increased water loss via respiratory tract in tachypneic infant Use of radiant warmer **DEFINING CHARACTERISTICS** Poor tissue turgor Decreased urine output Increased specific gravity Weight loss Sunken fontanels	**ONGOING ASSESSMENT** ▪ Assess hydration status: Skin turgor Mucous membranes Quality of mouth secretions Fontanels Specific gravity. ▪ Assess I&O every 1-2 hours. Document urine output <1 ml/kg/hr. ▪ Monitor daily weight. Document excessive weight gain or loss. **THERAPEUTIC INTERVENTIONS** ▪ Maintain parenteral therapy as ordered, taking into consideration baby's weight, intake and output, and electrolytes. *Fluids may be restricted in cases of cerebral edema or syndrome of inappropriate antidiuretic hormone.* ▪ Notify physician of urine output <1 ml/kg/hr.	Appropriate fluid volume will be maintained.
Knowledge Deficit: Meconium Aspiration **RELATED TO** New condition New illness **DEFINING CHARACTERISTICS** Asking same questions of different members of health team Apparent confusion over events Lack of questions Expressed need for more information	**ONGOING ASSESSMENT** ▪ Assess parents' experience with well and ill infants. ▪ Determine parents' knowledge of infant's illness and condition. ▪ Assess parents' knowledge of procedures and equipment. **THERAPEUTIC INTERVENTIONS** ▪ Orient parents to unit, staff, procedures, and equipment. ▪ Provide parents with unit booklet. ▪ Provide parents with information about: Meconium aspiration as it relates to their infant's illness Rationale behind procedures How procedures are performed Expected outcome of infant's condition ▪ Provide explanations appropriate for parents' level of understanding. ▪ Encourage parents to ask questions. ▪ Reinforce information given by other members of health care team *to help parents understand expected outcome regarding infant's condition.*	Knowledge deficit will be reduced.
Altered Parenting **RELATED TO** Interruption of normal adaptation of new family unit **DEFINING CHARACTERISTICS** Withdrawal Grief Indifference Sadness Limited involvement with infant Delay in choosing a name for infant	**ONGOING ASSESSMENT** ▪ Assess maturity level of parents. ▪ Note degree of parental self-esteem. ▪ Evaluate parental support system: Other family members Friends/peers Religious beliefs ▪ Assess infant's growth and development. ▪ Document parents' involvement with infant. ▪ Assess parents' need for referrals to other services: social services, Dysfunctioning Child Center. **THERAPEUTIC INTERVENTIONS** ▪ Encourage parents to express feelings. ▪ Facilitate open lines of communication between parents and health care team. ▪ Demonstrate nonjudgmental, supportive attitude. ▪ Encourage parents to visit and telephone. ▪ Encourage attendance and participation in parents' support group. ▪ Encourage parents to interact with infant as physical condition permits *to promote parent/infant bonding.* ▪ Emphasize positive aspects of infant. ▪ Encourage parents to choose name.	Positive parent/infant bonding behaviors will be attempted.

Deborah Rickard, RN, BSN

Persistent pulmonary hypertension (PPHN)

PULMONARY HYPERTENSION

Increased pulmonary pressure results in fetal circulation where blood is shunted from the right to the left side of the heart through the patent ductus arteriosus and/or foramen ovale. This leads to an inadequate pulmonary blood flow, causing hypoxemia and acidemia.

NURSING DIAGNOSES/ DEFINING CHARACTERISTICS	NURSING INTERVENTIONS / *RATIONALES*	EXPECTED OUTCOMES
Impaired Gas Exchange **RELATED TO** High pulmonary vascular resistance Inadequate pulmonary blood flow Asphyxia **DEFINING CHARACTERISTICS** Tachypnea Cyanosis Acidosis Respiratory distress Possible murmur	**ONGOING ASSESSMENT** • Review perinatal history and Apgar scores. • Monitor vital signs and blood pressure every 1 to 2 hours. • Assess cardiac status: 　Rate 　Variability 　Absence or presence of murmur 　Point of maximum impulse 　Perfusion • Assess respiratory status: 　Spontaneous respiration 　Respiratory effort 　Breath sounds 　Chest expansion 　Grunting, flaring, retracting • Assess need for chest physiotherapy; adapt procedure based on infant's tolerance level and need. • Assess tolerance of activity and degree of duskiness or cyanosis with increased handling or activity. • Monitor I&O. • Collect laboratory data as needed: 　Hematocrit 　Blood gas (preductal and postductal) 　Electrolytes 　Chemstrip 　Chest x-ray evaluation **THERAPEUTIC INTERVENTIONS** • Maintain clear airway: 　Reposition infant every 2 hours. 　Suction secretions prn. 　Perform gentle chest physiotherapy as necessary. • Minimize handling *to limit bouts of crying, which increases pulmonary pressure and consequently a right-to-left shunt of blood.* • Ensure that blood pressure is appropriate for size and gestational age and capillary refill is less than 3 seconds. *Hypotension and hypovolemia can contribute to increased pulmonary vascular resistance.* • Report any changes in cardiac status to physician. *Infant with PPHN may have congestive heart failure because of pressure overload of the right ventricle.* • Maintain body temperature at 36.5° to 37° C (97.7° F to 98.6° F). *Body temperature <36.5° C may cause pulmonary vasoconstriction, whereas temperatures >37.5° C lead to increased metabolic rate and oxygen consumption.* • Report to physician a specific gravity >1.008 or urine output <1-2 ml/kg/hr *to recognize early signs of renal failure resulting from hypoperfusion and acidosis.*	Improved respiratory status will be achieved.

Persistent pulmonary hypertension (PPHN) cont'd

NURSING DIAGNOSES/ DEFINING CHARACTERISTICS	NURSING INTERVENTIONS / *RATIONALES*	EXPECTED OUTCOMES
High Risk for Injury **RELATED TO** Side effects of tolazoline HCl (Priscoline) therapy **DEFINING CHARACTERISTICS** Side effects: GI bleeding Decrease in cardiac output Skin rash or flushed skin Renal failure, hematuria Thrombocytopenia Pulmonary hemorrhage Hypotension and shock Diarrhea Tachycardia	**ONGOING ASSESSMENT** • Assess for side effects and/or complications of tolazoline HCl using defining characteristics. **THERAPEUTIC INTERVENTIONS** • Calculate appropriate dose: 0.5 to 1 mg/kg/hr. • Correlate BP with tolazoline HCl infusion rate. *This medication is both a potent systemic and pulmonary vasodilator.* • Infuse medication into upper extremities or scalp veins *to avoid generalized vasodilation.* • If infant becomes hypotensive, the drug should be discontinued, and physician notified immediately.	Risk for injury will be reduced.
Knowledge Deficit: Parental **RELATED TO** Unfamiliarity with persistent pulmonary hypertension **DEFINING CHARACTERISTICS** Parents ask frequent questions Lack of questions Repetitive questions	**ONGOING ASSESSMENT** • Assess parents' understanding of infant's condition. **THERAPEUTIC INTERVENTIONS** • Explain infant's condition and plan of care to parents. • Refer parents to physician for questions as necessary. • Explain equipment and nursery routine *to decrease parental anxiety.* • See Parenting in the special care nursery, p. 72.	Parents will be able to verbalize understanding of infant's condition.
Anxiety: Parental **RELATED TO** New condition Change in health status **DEFINING CHARACTERISTICS** Fear of touching infant Infrequent calling Expression of guilt feelings Criticism of care given to infant Silence	**ONGOING ASSESSMENT** • Assess coping mechanism of family. • Assess family/infant interactions. **THERAPEUTIC INTERVENTIONS** • Encourage parents to: Touch infant Talk to infant Call and visit whenever they can Bring toys Participate in care (e.g., breastfeeding, blood donor program) *to help facilitate bonding.* • Encourage parents to verbalize concerns. • Refer to special care nursery parents' support group.	Parental anxiety will be reduced.

Vanida Komutanon, RN

Respiratory distress syndrome

HYALINE MEMBRANE DISEASE (HMD); RDS

A neonatal pulmonary disease caused by decreased surfactant synthesis, storage and/or release from type II alveolar cells. Surfactant deficiency leads to increased alveolar tension, predisposing to diffuse atelectasis and ventilation/perfusion imbalance with hypoventilation. The most important cause of RDS is prematurity. Other predisposing factors may include intrapartum stress, maternal diabetes, a history of RDS in a sibling, severe hypothermia in immediate newborn period, and male gender.

NURSING DIAGNOSES/ DEFINING CHARACTERISTICS	NURSING INTERVENTIONS / *RATIONALES*	EXPECTED OUTCOMES
Impaired Gas Exchange **RELATED TO** Alveolar atelectasis **DEFINING CHARACTERISTICS** Tachypnea Subcostal and intra-costal retractions Nasal flaring Cyanosis Pallor Expiratory grunt Apnea PaO_2 <50 mm Hg $PaCO_2$ >50 mm Hg	**ONGOING ASSESSMENT** • Monitor temperature, heart rate, respiration, and BP. • Assess breath sounds for quality of air exchange, equality, and presence of grunting. • Apply continuous noninvasive monitoring of oxygenation. • Serially monitor work of breathing. • Obtain blood gases. • Follow hematocrit. • Review chest x-ray films for reticulogranular pattern with air bronchograms. • Assess for other cause of respiratory disturbances, e.g., infection, congenital heart disease. **THERAPEUTIC INTERVENTIONS** • Maintain neutral thermal environment (NTE). *Metabolic rate and oxygen consumption are decreased when an infant is cared for in an optimal thermal environment.* • Administer oxygen to maintain SaO_2-88%-92% *to ensure adequate cellular oxygenation and support aerobic metabolism.* • Use assisted ventilation (CPAP or ventilator) *to promote alveolar expansion and CO_2 elimination.* • Use minimal ventilatory support to maintain pH >7.30, PO_2 >50, PCO_2 <50. *Excessive support can produce oxygen toxicity and barotrauma in the lungs and contribute to the development of retinopathy of prematurity (ROP).* • Administer exogenous surfactant as ordered *to correct deficiency state and promote alveolar expansion.* • Correct metabolic acidosis. *Acidosis may result in pulmonary vasoconstriction, right-to-left shunting, hypoperfusion, and further impairment of surfactant availability.* • Maintain mean arterial BP <30 mm Hg for infants less than 1000 g, >35 mm Hg for infants above 1000 g. *Normovolemia enhances pulmonary and tissue perfusion.* • Maintain Hct >40%. *Decreased red cell mass limits oxygen delivery to cells.* • Minimize handling. *Increased activity can lead to increased oxygen demands.* • Maintain patent airway. Suction intubated infants prn. • Administer sedatives and/or analgesic to infants cautiously. *Fighting the ventilator may be an indicator of inadequate support or a problem in the system.* • Obtain cultures before giving first dose of broad-spectrum antibiotics. *Sepsis and/or pneumonia may initially present like RDS.*	Improved respiratory status will be achieved.
High Risk for Fluid Volume Deficit **RELATED TO** Renal inability to concentrate urine Large insensible fluid losses via skin Inadequate fluid intake	**ONGOING ASSESSMENT** • Weigh every 12 to 24 hours. • Maintain I&O. Record all volumes of intake from any source; weigh diapers to measure output. • Monitor urine specific gravity every 4 hours. • Calculate intake in ml/kg/24 hours. • Test urine for glucose. • Monitor serum electrolytes. • Monitor vital signs for tachycardia and hypotension.	Fluid volume deficit will be reduced.

Respiratory distress syndrome cont'd

NURSING DIAGNOSES/ DEFINING CHARACTERISTICS	NURSING INTERVENTIONS / *RATIONALES*	EXPECTED OUTCOMES
DEFINING CHARACTERISTICS Excessive weight loss Hypernatremia Urine output less than 1 ml/kg/hr Increase urine specific gravity in infants older than 32 weeks Tachycardia (HR >150) Hypotension (birth weight ≤1000 g, mean arterial pressure ≤30; birth weight ≥1000 g, mean arterial pressure ≥35)	**THERAPEUTIC INTERVENTIONS** • Use in-bed scale *to minimize handling while following weight closely.* • Initiate stable venous access and provide IV fluids at rate of 60-100 ml/kg/day with glucose intake of 4-6 mg/kg/min. *This intake will meet basic metabolic needs and provide adequate glucose. Excess glucose can lead to an osmotic diuresis and dehydration.* • Cover infant on radiant warmer with heat shield, hat, and/or plastic wrap; place in warmed and humidified isolette as soon as possible. *These measures will decrease insensible fluid losses.* • Notify physician of signs of hypovolemia and anticipate orders for volume expansion.	
High Risk for Fluid Volume Excess **RELATED TO** Renal inability to excrete any volume overload Iatrogenic fluid volume excess **DEFINING CHARACTERISTICS** Failure to lose weight during first days of life Weight gain in excess of 10-15 g/kg/day Hyponatremia Edema Hyperglycemia	**ONGOING ASSESSMENT** • Weigh every 12 to 24 hours. • Monitor I&O. • Monitor urine specific gravity every 4 hours. • Calculate intake in ml/kg/24 hours. • Test urine for glucose. • Monitor serum electrolytes. • Monitor for hyperglycemia. • Assess for patent ductus arteriosus, presence of murmur, bounding pulses, widened pulse pressure (>30 mm Hg), and signs of congestive heart failure. **THERAPEUTIC INTERVENTIONS** • During acute phase of RDS, maintain fluid intake at minimum volume required to prevent hypotension and hypoglycemia. *Fluid volume excess has been associated with the development of patent ductus arteriosus, bronchopulmonary dysplasia, intraventricular hemorrhage, and necrotizing enterocolitis.* • Limit fluid intake as ordered if signs of fluid excess are noted.	Potential for fluid volume excess will be reduced.
Altered Nutrition: Less Than Body Requirements **RELATED TO** Immature GI system Compromised perfusion of gut during acute phase of RDS resulting in feeding intolerance Immature suck/swallow reflexes **DEFINING CHARACTERISTICS** Weight loss greater than 10%-15% of birth weight in first week Abdominal distention	**ONGOING ASSESSMENT** • Weigh daily. • Obtain Chemstrip on admission and every 30 minutes until infant is stable. • Assess bowel sounds. • Measure abdominal girth every 3-4 hours when feedings are started. • Administer guaiac and Clinitest to stools. • Check gastric residual before each feeding. • Record accurate I&O. • Inspect IV site every hour. **THERAPEUTIC INTERVENTIONS** • Initially, keep infant NPO. *GI perfusion may be inadequate, especially if infant is or has been hypoxic.* • Initiate and maintain IV glucose infusion. *Chemstrip results should be 45-100. IV glucose will prevent hypoglycemia.* • Provide long-term stable venous access (e.g., PCVC) if prolonged period of NPO is expected. *Secure intravenous line will ensure uninterrupted delivery of nutrients and decrease the stress of repeated peripheral IV attempts.*	Maintenance of adequate calorie requirement will be achieved.

Continued.

Respiratory distress syndrome cont'd

NURSING DIAGNOSES/ DEFINING CHARACTERISTICS	NURSING INTERVENTIONS / *RATIONALES*	EXPECTED OUTCOMES
DEFINING CHARACTERISTICS cont'd Vomiting Guaiac-positive stools Clinitest positive stools Large gastric residuals Hypoglycemia	**THERAPEUTIC INTERVENTIONS cont'd** • Insert nasal gastric tube (size 5 Fr) for feedings. *Nasogastric feeding will be given until infant is capable of coordinating suck, swallow, and breathing.* • Advance feedings slowly over several days. *Gradual increases allow for GI adaptation to enteral nutrition.* • Provide parenteral nutrition until full enteral feedings are established. • Notify physician of signs of feeding intolerance. *NPO status will be ordered for infant if feedings are not tolerated.*	
High Risk for Injury RELATED TO Fragile, immature capillary network in germinal matrix; rupture leads to intraventricular hemorrhage (IVH)	**ONGOING ASSESSMENT** • Monitor serial Hct determinations. • Record blood drawn for laboratory testing. • Palpate fontanel every shift. • Monitor serial measurements of head circumferences. • Obtain head ultrasound evaluation. • Monitor blood pressure. • Monitor blood gases.	Potential for injury will be reduced.
DEFINING CHARACTERISTICS Unexplained fall in Hct Failure to see improvement in Hct following transfusion Full/bulging fontanel Split sutures Change in LOC Metabolic acidosis Hypotension Seizures	**THERAPEUTIC INTERVENTIONS** • Maintain blood gas values within normal limits. *Hypoxia can damage endothelial cells of capillaries in germinal matrix. Hypercarbia can cause dilation of cerebral blood vessels predisposing to rupture of vessels.* • Avoid rapid infusion of volume expander. *Rapid volume expansion can cause increased intravascular pressure and lead to IVH. Risk may be increased if a history of hypoxia and hypotension exists.* • Position with head in midline and head of bed slightly elevated during first four days when risk of IVH is highest. *Intracranial pressure is lowest with head in midline and head of bed elevated 30 degrees. Turning the head sharply to the side causes an obstruction of the ipsilateral jugular vein and can increase ICP.* • Avoid interventions that cause crying. Use analgesia for painful procedures. *Crying can impede venous return, increase cerebral blood volume, and compromise cerebral oxygenation in sick infants.* • When $NaHCO_3$ is necessary to correct a documented metabolic acidosis, slowly give 4.2% solution. *Rapid infusions may cause elevations in CO_2, which can dilate cerebral vessels and contribute to a pressure-passive cerebral circulation.* • Notify physician of changes in BP. Avoid interventions that cause fluctuations in BP. *A fluctuating pattern has been associated with development of IVH.* • Suction only as needed. *Suctioning can increase cerebral blood flow velocity, increase BP, increase ICP, and decrease oxygenation.*	
High Risk for Injury: Air Leaks RELATED TO Surfactant deficiency results in uneven compliance, predisposing to air leaks	**ONGOING ASSESSMENT** • Maintain continuous HR, RR, BP, and SaO_2 or $TcPO_2$ monitoring. • Provide serial assessment of PMI. • Provide serial assessment of breath sounds. • Monitor blood gases daily and prn.	Potential for air leak will be reduced.

NURSING DIAGNOSES/ DEFINING CHARACTERISTICS	NURSING INTERVENTIONS / *RATIONALES*	EXPECTED OUTCOMES

DEFINING CHARACTERISTICS
Decreased PO_2
Increased PCO_2
Decreased breath sounds
Shift in point of maximum impulse (PMI)
Sudden deterioration
Change in vital signs:
  Early—increased diastolic BP, tachycardia, increased signs of respiratory distress
  Late—hypotension, bradycardia
Positive transillumination
X-ray findings consistent with pulmonary air leak
	THERAPEUTIC INTERVENTIONS
	• Prevent barotrauma by using lowest possible ventilator rates and pressures. *Alveolar injury and rupture will be avoided.*
	• Use pressure manometer with bag and do not exceed preset inspiratory pressure. *Prevents use of excessive pressure during manual bag ventilation.*
	• Do not advance suction catheter past end of endotracheal tube. *Correct suctioning technique prevents injury to bronchial lining.*
	• Prepare equipment for needle aspiration of pneumothorax and place at bedside.
	• Ensure proper placement of endotracheal tube. *ET tube malposition in right mainstem bronchus will permit delivery of excessive pressure to one lung and lead to atelectasis in the nonventilated lung.*
	• Investigate causes for early changes in vital signs. *Early recognition of air leaks can prevent acute deterioration.*	

High Risk for Altered Parent/ Infant Attachment **RELATED TO** Premature birth Fear of infant's death Separation **DEFINING CHARACTERISTICS** Express verbal/nonverbal fear/anxiety with intensive care environment Exhibit reluctance to look at infant Blame themselves for infant's condition Verbalize infant may be in pain or staff is hurting infant Absence of parental attachment behaviors Do not visit or call regularly	**ONGOING ASSESSMENT** • Assess for presence of defining characteristics. **THERAPEUTIC INTERVENTIONS** • See Parenting in the special care nursery, p. 72.	Parent/infant bonding will be achieved.

Patricia Kling, RNC, MSN, NNP

Transient tachypnea of the newborn

TYPE II RESPIRATORY DISTRESS SYNDROME;
WET LUNG

A clinical condition of term or near-term infants in which there is a delayed reabsorption of normal lung fluid, which will cause neonate to manifest symptoms of respiratory distress.

NURSING DIAGNOSES/ DEFINING CHARACTERISTICS	NURSING INTERVENTIONS / *RATIONALES*	EXPECTED OUTCOMES
High Risk for Ineffective Breathing Pattern **RELATED TO** Delivered by cesarean section Precipitous delivery **DEFINING CHARACTERISTICS** Tachypnea Retractions Grunting Nasal flaring Varying degrees of cyanosis Barrel chest Chest x-ray film reveals: Increased lung fluid Hyperexpansion with streaky infiltrates Mild to moderately enlarged heart	**ONGOING ASSESSMENT** ▪ Assess respiratory and cardiac status every 1-2 hours: Note rate, grunting, retractions, and nasal flaring. Assess central and peripheral color. Auscultate breath sounds. Monitor oxygenation: Transcutaneous Po_2 and Pco_2 Blood gases every shift and prn Pulse oximetry ▪ Obtain complete blood count and differential *to help rule out any other infectious process.* ▪ Obtain urine Wellcogen test *to assist in ruling out group B streptococcal pneumonia.* **THERAPEUTIC INTERVENTIONS** ▪ Administer oxygen as needed to maintain Pao_2 in the range of 80, *as hypoxemia will constrict the pulmonary vasculature.* ▪ Report changes in infant's respiratory and cardiovascular status, *because transient tachypnea is difficult to distinguish from other lung diseases that increase in severity. This is usually a benign disease and lasts 3 to 5 days.* ▪ Suction as needed *to maintain patent airway.* ▪ Maintain infant in semi-Fowler's position *to allow maximal diaphragmatic excursion and lung expansion.*	Optimal breathing pattern will be maintained.
Altered Nutrition: Less Than Body Requirements **RELATED TO** Possible caloric loss as a result of increased cardiorespiratory demand **DEFINING CHARACTERISTICS** Failure to gain weight according to the growth curve Documented inadequate caloric intake Inability to eat orally	**ONGOING ASSESSMENT** ▪ Monitor respiratory rate and signs of distress (increased tachypnea [respirations greater than 80/min], nasal flaring, retractions). ▪ Weigh infant daily. **THERAPEUTIC INTERVENTIONS** ▪ If the respiratory rate is over 60/min, do not feed infant by mouth *because of the risk for aspiration.* Institute NGT feedings as indicated. ▪ If the respiratory rate is over 80/min, initiate intravenous nutrition as indicated *to provide appropriate volume and calories.*	Adequate nutritional intake will be maintained.

NURSING DIAGNOSES/ DEFINING CHARACTERISTICS	NURSING INTERVENTIONS / *RATIONALES*	EXPECTED OUTCOMES
Altered Parenting RELATED TO Separation/hospital- ization of infant **DEFINING CHARACTERISTICS** Expresses verbal/ nonverbal fear/anx- iety with intensive care environment Exhibits reluctance to look at infant Verbalizes concern that infant may be in pain Asks inappropriate questions Holds unrealistic view of infant's condition/illness Blames self for in- fant's condition Does not demon- strate parental at- tachment behaviors Verbalizes resent- ment toward infant Verbalizes guilt feel- ings for having a "less than perfect" infant Does not visit or call regularly Delays in naming in- fant	**ONGOING ASSESSMENT** • Assess parents': Developmental stage Feelings regarding impact of pregnancy on the family Level of anxiety Existing support system Cultural background Knowledge of illness or condition **THERAPEUTIC INTERVENTIONS** • Explain to parents: Reasons for admission Equipment used Immediate treatment *to provide parents with information that will as- sist in decreasing anxiety* • Familiarize parents with staff in NICU *to increase comfort with unit and begin to develop relationships.* • Encourage reading of parent booklet *to clarify answers to their ques- tions, to increase comfort with medical terminology used, and to alle- viate anxiety.* • Inform parents of calling and visitation policy. Encourage frequent visit- ing and/or calling *to promote parent/infant bonding.* • Explain the infant's prognosis *to encourage communication and de- crease anxiety of the unknown.* • Offer additional support systems such as: Social service Developmental support services Parent support group Parent CPR classes • Encourage verbalization of perceptions regarding infant *to clarify con- cerns and provide support systems as indicated.* • Encourage parents to touch, kiss, and talk to infant. Allow them to hold infant if possible. • Encourage parents to take pictures or give them pictures of infant *to promote parent/infant bonding and to encourage appropriate parenting behaviors.* • Encourage participation in basic caretaking skills, e.g., diapering, bath- ing, and applying lotion, *to promote parenting skills and initiate dis- charge teaching.* • Promote parents' verbalization of feelings and use of support systems. • Show parents educational movies. *Movies will reinforce information and provide emotional support.*	Ability to parent will be maximized.

Sophia A. Spencer, RN, BSN

5

Neurological Care Plans

PEDIATRIC PATIENT
Consciousness, decreased level of
Craniotomy: postoperative
Guillain Barré syndrome
Head trauma
Hydrocephalus
Increased intracranial pressure
Lead poisoning
Meningitis
Reye's syndrome
Seizure activity
Status epilepticus
Toxic ingestion

NEONATAL PATIENT
Bacterial meningitis, acute
Hydrocephalus
Seizures
Substance abuse withdrawal

Consciousness: decreased level of

COMA; IMPAIRED MENTAL STATUS;
RESPONSIVENESS; REDUCED AWARENESS

Normal consciousness can be defined as the condition of the normal person when awake. In this state, the child is fully responsive to stimuli and indicates by his behavior and, in the older child, speech, that he has an accurate awareness of himself and his environment. There are two components of consciousness: (1) arousal or wakefulness, which reflects the integrity of the reticular activating system (RAS) located in the upper brainstem and diencephalon, and (2) cognition or awareness, which reflects the integrity of the cortical cerebral hemispheres.

NURSING DIAGNOSES/ DEFINING CHARACTERISTICS	NURSING INTERVENTIONS / *RATIONALES*	EXPECTED OUTCOMES
Decreased Level of Consciousness **RELATED TO** *Structural:* Head trauma Tumor Cerebral edema Increased ICP Infection: meningitis, encephalitis, Reye's syndrome, abscess *Metabolic:* Anoxia Profound hypoglycemia Profound hyponatremia or hypernatremia Hypercalcemia Toxic agent (e.g., lead intoxication) **DEFINING CHARACTERISTICS** Change in alertness, orientation, verbal response, eye opening in response to command, motor response Impaired memory Impaired judgment Agitation Inappropriate affect Impaired thought processes Glasgow Coma score <11 *Infant:* Reduced awareness Decreased interaction with environment Decreased response to stimulation Irritability, crying, which may be inconsolable and inappropriate Listlessness	**ONGOING ASSESSMENT** • Assess age and developmental level. • Assess LOC/responsiveness as indicated. • To evaluate the coma scale in a child younger than 4 years of age: (1) eye and motor evaluation are the same parameters as in an older child (eye opening and motor response); (2) verbal response differs: use smiles, oriented to sound, follows objects, interacts = 5-6 points; crying (consolable vs. inappropriate) = 4 points; moaning = 3 points; restless with reduced interaction = 2 points; no response to stimulation = 1 point. • Determine contributing factors to any change (e.g., anesthesia, medications, awakening from sound sleep, not understanding questions). • Assess understanding by child/significant others of events surrounding change in LOC. • Assess potential for physical injury. • Assess vital signs, especially respiratory status. **THERAPEUTIC INTERVENTIONS** • Record serial assessments. • Report/record any change or deterioration. • Keep side rails up at all times, bed in low position, and functioning call light within reach. • If restraints are needed, child must be positioned on side, never on back. *Restraints should be used judiciously, since their use may increase agitation/anxiety and contribute to increased ICP.* • Reorient to environment as needed *to decrease apprehension and anxiety. Short-term memory may be affected by pathological conditions.* • Explain all nursing activities before initiating in age-appropriate manner. *Use of anatomically specific dolls or books with simple pictures will be helpful for the younger child who is not yet capable of abstract thinking.* • Protect child from possible injury (seizure activity, decreased corneal reflex, decreased blink, decreased gag reflex, airway obstruction/aspiration). • Avoid contributing to confusion/disorientation by agreeing with misinterpretations. *Reality orientation decreases false sensory perception and enhances child's sense of personal dignity and self-esteem.* • Use calendars, television, radio, clocks, lights *to help with reorientation.* • Call neurological resource personnel if instructions are needed. • Involve child/significant others in goal setting and care planning. • Encourage significant others to bring in things familiar to patient (e.g., pictures, favorite dolls, teddy bears, pajamas). • Consult rehabilitation medicine, social service, play therapist as needed. • Encourage and support verbalization by child and significant others.	Optimal state of consciousness will be maintained.

Linda Arsenault, RN, MSN, CNRN

Craniotomy: postoperative

CRANIECTOMY; BURR HOLE; TREPHINATION

Surgical opening of a part of the cranium made by the neurosurgeon to gain access to disease or injury affecting the brain, the ventricles, or intracranial blood vessels. Craniectomy is removal of part of the cranium, which may be indicated for fractures or infection.

NURSING DIAGNOSES/ DEFINING CHARACTERISTICS	NURSING INTERVENTIONS / *RATIONALES*	EXPECTED OUTCOMES
Altered Tissue Perfusion: Cerebral **RELATED TO** Cerebral edema Intracranial bleeding Cerebral ischemia/infarction Increased intracranial pressure Metabolic abnormalities Hydrocephalus **DEFINING CHARACTERISTICS** Changed LOC/responsiveness Changed pupil size, reaction to light, gaze preference/deviation Focal or generalized motor weakness Presence of pathological reflexes (Babinski) Seizures Increased BP and bradycardia Changed respiratory pattern	**ONGOING ASSESSMENT** ▪ Assess age and developmental level. ▪ Assess and document baseline LOC: pupil size, position, reaction to light; motor movement and strength of limbs; and vital signs. *Early detection of changes is necessary to prevent fixed neurological dysfunction.* ▪ Compare current assessment with previous assessment. Report any deviations. ▪ Evaluate contributing factors to change in responsiveness, and reevaluate in 5-10 min *to see if change persists as a result of such factors as anesthesia, medications, awakening from sound sleep, not understanding question.* ▪ Check head dressing for presence of drains. *Intraventricular drains, self-contained bulb suction, and drainage system (e.g., Jackson-Pratt) are most commonly used. All drains and catheters should be secured to the patient/bed to prevent falls to the floor, negative gravity suctioning, and increased risk of bleeding or dislodging of drain.* ▪ Evaluate function of catheter placed to monitor intracranial pressure. *Normal ICP is below 15 mm Hg.* ▪ Evaluate for lash reflex. ▪ Monitor CBC, electrolytes, and ABGs. Report ABGs: PaO_2 <80 mm Hg; $PaCO_2$ >45 mm Hg; CBC: Hct <30; electrolytes: Na <130 >150 mEq/L; glucose: <180 or >200 mg/dl; osmolalities: <185 >310 mOsm/L. ▪ Assess current medications and compare with preoperative medications, with specific attention to thyroid replacement medications, anticonvulsants, and steroids. **THERAPEUTIC INTERVENTIONS** ▪ Report temperature >39° C (102.2° F). Report and maintain normothermia with tepid sponge/antipyretics or hypothermia blanket as ordered. Turn blanket off at patient temperature of 38° C (100° F) rectally. ▪ Maintain head of bed at 30 degrees unless contraindicated (e.g., *patient is hemodynamically unstable*). If child has altered LOC and is receiving tube feeding, maintain head elevation during feedings *to prevent aspiration.* Clamp tube during transport. ▪ Turn and reposition child on side, with head supported in neutral alignment, every 2 hours *to prevent venous outflow obstruction and increased intracranial pressure.* ▪ Reorient child to environment as needed. ▪ If soft restraints are needed, position child on side, *never on back, to minimize danger of aspiration if child should vomit.* ▪ Avoid nursing activities that may trigger increased intracranial pressure excursions (*ICP >15 mm Hg*) by straining, strenuous coughing, positioning with neck in flexion, head flat. ▪ If child has difficulty closing eye (cranial nerve VII palsy), administer artificial tears (methylcellulose drops) every 2 hours. Glad-Wrap or Saran-Wrap (or facsimile) can be applied over the eye *to protect the exposed cornea and prevent dryness,* or the eyelids can be taped shut. ▪ See Decreased levels of consciousness, p. 173.	Optimal cerebral perfusion will be maintained.

NURSING DIAGNOSES/ DEFINING CHARACTERISTICS	NURSING INTERVENTIONS / *RATIONALES*	EXPECTED OUTCOMES

High Risk for Fluid Volume Deficit

RELATED TO

Neurogenic diabetes insipidus

Dehydration secondary to hyperosmotic diuretics, emesis

DEFINING CHARACTERISTICS

Polyuria

Polydipsia

Urine specific gravity <1.005

Dehydration

Thirst

Increased serum Na >145 mEq/L

Increased serum osmolarity >300

Dry mucous membranes

Poor skin turgor

Weight loss

Tachycardia, hypotension

Sunken fontanel

Weak peripheral pulses

Delayed capillary refill >2-3 sec

ONGOING ASSESSMENT

- Monitor I&O every hour, with specific attention to fluid volume infused over output. Report urine output >200 ml/hr for 2 consecutive hours.
- Check urine specific gravity every 2-4 hours. *Specific gravity is decreased with diabetes insipidus to <1.005.*
- Monitor serum and urine electrolytes and osmolarity.
- Monitor for signs of dehydration (decreased skin turgor, weight loss, increased heart rate, decreased blood pressure, depressed fontanel, etc.).
- Monitor heart rate and BP every 2 hours and prn.
- Weigh daily and record.

THERAPEUTIC INTERVENTIONS

- Replace fluid output as directed.
- Administer vasopressin (Pitressin) as ordered. *This is an exogenous synthetic antidiuretic hormone that will cause a decrease in urinary output.*
- Record effectiveness of vasopressin in decreasing urinary output and any side effects, e.g., change in heart rate or abdominal cramping.
- See Fluid volume deficit, p. 19.

Optimal fluid volume will be maintained.

Fluid Volume Excess

RELATED TO

Syndrome of inappropriate antidiuretic hormone secretion (SIADH)

Free H$_2$O excess

DEFINING CHARACTERISTICS

Changed sensorium

Decreased serum Na <130 mEq/L

Decreased serum osmolarity <285

Increased urine Na

Seizures

Lethargy

Nausea and vomiting

Muscle twitching

ONGOING ASSESSMENT

- Assess child for fluid volume excess. *This is usually determined by hyponatremia/hyposmolarity. Edema is usually not present in SIADH.*
- Monitor serum and urine electrolytes and osmolarity at least daily.
- Monitor I&O.
- Assess vital signs and neurological changes every 2 hours and prn.

THERAPEUTIC INTERVENTIONS

- Restrict oral/IV fluids as ordered. *Fluid restriction usually corrects the hyponatremia associated with SIADH.*
- Weigh patient daily.
- If fluid restriction fails, 3% saline with concomitant administration of potassium and IV furosemide (Lasix) may be administered. In this instance serial sodium, potassium, and serum osmolarity should be monitored every 6-8 hours.

Optimal fluid balance will be maintained.

Continued.

Neurological Care Plans (Pediatric)

NURSING DIAGNOSES/ DEFINING CHARACTERISTICS	NURSING INTERVENTIONS / *RATIONALES*	EXPECTED OUTCOMES
High Risk for Impaired Physical Mobility **RELATED TO** Decreased LOC Weakness/paralysis of extremities Imposed restrictions **DEFINING CHARACTERISTICS** Inability to move purposefully within the physical environment Decreased muscle strength Impaired coordination; verbalization of inability to perform Limited ROM	**ONGOING ASSESSMENT** • Assess for alteration in mobility. **THERAPEUTIC INTERVENTIONS** • Do not position child in prone or semiprone position. *This increases intrathoracic pressure and may increase intracranial pressure.* • Encourage active range of motion of affected joints *to maintain muscle strength and prevent contractures.* • Establish a turning schedule *to prevent skin breakdown, respiratory complications, bone demineralization, and muscle wasting.*	Mobility will be maximized.
Ineffective Airway Clearance **RELATED TO** Decreased LOC Postoperative atelectasis, pneumonia Predisposition for lung infection, especially in premature infant: Immature development of intercostal and abdominal muscles Small length and diameter of airway **DEFINING CHARACTERISTICS** Abnormal breath sounds (rhonchi, wheezing) Change in rate and depth of respirations, tachypnea, apnea Cough, cyanosis, dyspnea Nasal flaring Grunting Intercostal/abdominal retractions Cyanosis Tachycardia Feeding difficulties Abdominal distention Increased secretions	**ONGOING ASSESSMENT** • Assess for signs of ineffective airway clearance (see Defining Characteristics). • Assess breath sounds, respirations, heart rate every 2 hours and prn. • Monitor amount and characteristics of secretions. **THERAPEUTIC INTERVENTIONS** • Suction secretions prn. *Nasotracheal suctioning is contraindicated for child having surgery proximal to frontal sinuses (e.g., pituitary tumor, basal frontal meningioma, basal skull fracture). This could result in the introduction of catheter tips into the brain or allow for bacterial communication.* • See Ineffective airway clearance, p. 3, Ineffective breathing pattern, p. 8.	Airway will be free of secretions.

NURSING DIAGNOSES/ DEFINING CHARACTERISTICS	NURSING INTERVENTIONS / *RATIONALES*	EXPECTED OUTCOMES
High Risk for Injury: Seizures **RELATED TO** Intracranial bleeding Infarction Tumor Trauma **DEFINING CHARACTERISTICS** Focal and/or generalized seizures with/ without loss of consciousness Cyanosis Grunting Apnea Increased oral secretions Eye rolling Staring Hyperventilation	**ONGOING ASSESSMENT** • Observe for seizure activity. Record and report observations: Note time and signs of attack. Observe parts of body involved: order of involvement and character of movement. Check deviation of eyes; note change in pupil size. Assess airway and respiratory pattern. Note tonic-clonic stages. Assess postictal state (e.g., loss of consciousness, alertness, airway). Note incontinence. Note length of seizure. Assess for postictal paralysis. • Observe for any signs of respiratory distress. **THERAPEUTIC INTERVENTIONS** • Maintain child's safety, e.g., pad side rails, protect head from injury, padded helmet if indicated. *If a craniectomy is performed in a young child, a padded helmet should be ordered.* • Maintain airway during postictal state. Turn child on side, suction as needed. • Maintain minimal environmental stimuli: Noise reduction Curtains closed Private room (when available/advisable) Dim lights • Administer anticonvulsants as indicated. *Phenytoin (Dilantin) can only be administered orally or intravenously. When given IV it should be administered in NS. It will precipitate in any dextrose solution. Administer no faster than 50 mg/min to prevent hypotension. IV diazepam (Valium) or midazolam (Versed) is often used to control recurrent seizures and should not be administered any faster than 10 mg/min to avoid respiratory compromise.* • If seizure occurs, remain with child, protect head from injury. Do not attempt to introduce anything into the child's mouth during the seizure—*carries increased risk of aspiration, broken teeth, soft tissue injury.* • Suction secretions and administer oxygen if needed after seizure.	Risk of seizures will be reduced.
Knowledge Deficit **RELATED TO** New procedures/ treatments **DEFINING CHARACTERISTICS** Child/significant others verbalizing questions and concerns	**ONGOING ASSESSMENT** • Assess child/significant others for knowledge base and readiness for teaching. **THERAPEUTIC INTERVENTIONS** • Discuss change in body image related to head dressing and loss of hair, potential for and duration of facial edema. • Discuss need for monitoring equipment and frequent assessments. • Explain unit visiting hours and reasons for restrictions. • Instruct in deep breathing and leg exercises. • Explain use of medications such as dexamethasone (Decadron), anticonvulsants, antibiotics. • Discuss need for frequent assessment, reorientation, etc. • Encourage significant others to participate in reorientation, rehabilitation, etc. • Reinforce discussion of neurological definitions/progress given by physician to significant others.	Child/significant others will verbalize understanding of postoperative expectations and experiences.

Linda Arsenault, RN, MSN, CNRN

Guillain Barré syndrome

POLYNEURITIS; GBS

A rapidly evolving reversible paralytic illness of unknown origin. The disease is thought to be autoimmune in origin and has been reported to be related to the occurrence of varicella, the Epstein Barr virus, swine flu vaccines, or following respiratory or gastro-intestinal illnesses, mumps, or mycoplasma pneumonia. The disease occurs as a result of destruction of peripheral nerve myelin sheaths. The onset of neurological symptoms is abrupt, with a tendency for the paralysis to ascend the body symmetrically. Paralysis may last 4 weeks or longer. Recovery tends to be slow.

NURSING DIAGNOSES/ DEFINING CHARACTERISTICS	NURSING INTERVENTIONS / *RATIONALES*	EXPECTED OUTCOMES
Ineffective Breathing Pattern **RELATED TO** Increasing weakness of respiratory muscles Progression to total motor paralysis resulting in respiratory failure **DEFINING CHARACTERISTICS** Shortness of breath Decreasing tidal volume Decreasing vital capacity Dyspnea Tachypnea Hypercapnia Hypoxia Change in mental status	**ONGOING ASSESSMENT** ▪ Assess age and developmental level. ▪ Assess respiratory rate, pattern, and depth. ▪ Monitor tidal volume and vital capacity daily and prn. *A significant amount of respiratory muscle insufficiency may exist without being apparent clinically.* ▪ Monitor ABGs and watch closely for the development of hypercapnia and hypoxia. ▪ Observe for mental status changes *that may be indicative of a change in the adequacy of ventilation.* **THERAPEUTIC INTERVENTIONS** ▪ Elevate head of bed *for optimal ventilatory excursion to occur.* ▪ Anticipate the need for intubation and mechanical ventilation if respirations become shallow with a decreasing tidal volume and vital capacity. *Intercostal and diaphragmatic paralysis produce progressive alveolar hypoventilation, which can occur within 36 hours. The patient may not be disturbed by the weakness because of the gradual onset and slow progression.* ▪ See Mechanical ventilation, p. 155, as appropriate.	Optimal breathing pattern will be maintained.
High Risk for Aspiration **RELATED TO** Ascending muscle paralysis **DEFINING CHARACTERISTICS** Depressed gag and cough reflex Dysphagia	**ONGOING ASSESSMENT** ▪ Assess for presence of gag and cough reflex every shift. ▪ Assess for any difficulty in swallowing every shift and before any oral intake. *Paralysis of cranial nerves IX and X may occur.* ▪ Assess for increased nerve paralysis involving respiratory muscles and facial nerves. **THERAPEUTIC INTERVENTIONS** ▪ Notify physician immediately of noted decreases in cough and gag reflexes or for any difficulty in swallowing. *Early intervention will protect the airway and prevent aspiration.* ▪ Assist child with any oral intake *to detect abnormalities early.* ▪ Anticipate need for plasmapheresis *to minimize the immune response of cells to the offending virus. It is believed that the immune response causes the demyelination of peripheral nerves.*	Aspiration will be prevented.
Ineffective Airway Clearance **RELATED TO** Increasing weakness of respiratory muscles Loss of gag or cough reflex	**ONGOING ASSESSMENT** ▪ Auscultate lungs for breath sounds every shift. ▪ Assess respiratory rate and depth. ▪ Assess for presence of cough: Effectiveness Productivity	Airway clearance will be maintained.

Guillain Barré syndrome cont'd

NURSING DIAGNOSES/ DEFINING CHARACTERISTICS	NURSING INTERVENTIONS / *RATIONALES*	EXPECTED OUTCOMES
DEFINING CHARACTERISTICS Abnormal breath sounds (rales, rhonchi, wheezes) Changes in respiratory rate or depth Cough Cyanosis Dyspnea	**THERAPEUTIC INTERVENTIONS** • Elevate head of bed *to promote effective coughing.* • If cough is ineffective, use oropharyngeal or tracheal suction as needed *to clear secretions.* • Anticipate need for intubation and mechanical ventilation *to maintain the airway.* • See Mechanical ventilation, p. 155.	
High Risk for Decrease in Cardiac Output **RELATED TO** Vasomotor instability Autonomic dysfunction, which reflects involvement of the myelinated preganglionic fibers and the ganglia **DEFINING CHARACTERISTICS** Instability of BP (increased or decreased) Dysrhythmias Decreased peripheral pulses Confusion, agitation, restlessness Anxiety Fatigue, lethargy	**ONGOING ASSESSMENT** • Monitor BP and heart rate continuously. • Continuously monitor ECG rhythm for development of dysrhythmias. • Assess peripheral pulses. • Observe for profuse diaphoresis or loss of sweating. • Observe for mental status changes and signs of fatigue/lethargy. • Monitor pulmonary artery wedge pressure and cardiac output, as available. **THERAPEUTIC INTERVENTIONS** • Be prepared for labile heart rate and BP *as a result of autonomic dysfunction.* • Administer inotropic medications as ordered *to maintain hemodynamic parameters* (heart rate, BP, cardiac output, CVP, pulmonary artery pressures). • Place the older child/adolescent on sequential or Venodyne pump to legs *to increase venous return, decrease peripheral pooling of blood, and decrease the risk of thrombosis.* • Maintain adequate ventilation; provide oxygen as needed.	Cardiac output will be maximized.

Impaired Physical Mobility **RELATED TO** Muscle weakness or total paralysis as a result of the disease process **DEFINING CHARACTERISTICS** Symmetrical weakness Hyporeflexia Ascending paralysis Verbalization of generalized weakness	**ONGOING ASSESSMENT**
	• Assess motor strength and reflexes, checking for:
	  Level of progression
	  Symmetry
	  Ascending paralysis
	  Paresthesia
	• Assess baseline ROM and note deterioration or improvement.
	
	THERAPEUTIC INTERVENTIONS
	• Turn and reposition child every 2 hours.
	• Maintain limbs in functional alignment and begin passive range of motion *to prevent contractures.*
	• Use physical therapy *to assist in maintaining muscle tone.*
	• Use occupational therapy *to assist in maintaining position of upper extremities, e.g., hand rolls/splints rotating every hour.*
	• Administer medications as ordered. *A trial course of prednisone may be ordered to minimize effects of disease.*
		Optimal physical mobility will be maintained.

Continued.

Neurological Care Plans (Pediatric)

NURSING DIAGNOSES/ DEFINING CHARACTERISTICS	NURSING INTERVENTIONS / *RATIONALES*	EXPECTED OUTCOMES
High Risk for Impaired Skin Integrity **RELATED TO** Complete bed rest Impaired physical mobility Paresthesia **DEFINING CHARACTERISTICS** Stage I: redness, skin intact Stage II: blisters Stage III: necrosis Stage IV: necrosis involving muscle, bone, joint, or body cavity	**ONGOING ASSESSMENT** • Assess skin integrity every shift, noting color, moisture, texture, and temperature. **THERAPEUTIC INTERVENTIONS** • Maintain good skin care, keeping skin clean and dry. • Turn every 2 hours according to an established turning schedule. • Provide prophylactic use of pressure-relieving devices *to assist in preventing skin breakdown.*	Skin integrity will be maintained.
Altered Nutrition: Less Than Body Requirements **RELATED TO** Dysphagia Paralysis **DEFINING CHARACTERISTICS** Loss of weight with/ without adequate caloric intake Documented inadequate caloric intake Caloric intake inadequate to keep pace with abnormal disease/metabolic state	**ONGOING ASSESSMENT** • Obtain nutritional history. • Weigh daily and record. • Assess nutritional needs, consulting dietitian when appropriate. **THERAPEUTIC INTERVENTIONS** • See Altered nutrition, less than body requirements, p. 33.	Optimal caloric intake will be maintained.
High Risk for Constipation **RELATED TO** Increasing muscle weakness/paralysis **DEFINING CHARACTERISTICS** Decrease in soft formed stools Abdominal pain Fecal impaction Abdominal distention Nausea/vomiting	**ONGOING ASSESSMENT** • Assess bowel sounds every shift. • Assess frequency of bowel movements, checking color, consistency, and amount. • Observe for nausea/vomiting, abdominal pain, or distention. • Assess for presence of fecal impaction, as needed. **THERAPEUTIC INTERVENTIONS** • Provide adequate fluid intake as ordered *to prevent dehydration.* • Administer prescribed medications as needed. • See Constipation, p. 12.	Constipation will be prevented.

Guillain Barré syndrome cont'd

NURSING DIAGNOSES/ DEFINING CHARACTERISTICS	NURSING INTERVENTIONS / *RATIONALES*	EXPECTED OUTCOMES
Anxiety/Fear **RELATED TO** Change in health status Fear of unknown **DEFINING CHARACTERISTICS** Restlessness Fear Crying Trembling Withdrawal Facial tension	**ONGOING ASSESSMENT** • Assess level of fear/anxiety. • Assess normal coping patterns (by interview with child/family). **THERAPEUTIC INTERVENTIONS** • Display a confident, calm manner *to reassure child.* • Allow child/family to express feelings through talking, writing, or using an alphabet board. • Keep child informed of his or her condition and treatment regimen *to help decrease anxiety.* • Reduce distracting stimuli *to provide a quiet environment.* • Provide diversional activities as appropriate (e.g., television, dolls, toys, books, radio, magazines). • Allow parents or significant others to be involved with the child throughout the hospitalization.	Anxiety/fear will be reduced.
Knowledge Deficit **RELATED TO** Disease of sudden onset **DEFINING CHARACTERISTICS** Request for information Multiple questions Lack of questions	**ONGOING ASSESSMENT** • Assess child for current status of disease/stability of condition (in early stages may be deteriorating). • Assess child's/parents' readiness to learn. • Assess current knowledge of illness. • Assess level of understanding of therapeutic regimen. **THERAPEUTIC INTERVENTIONS** • Ensure physical comfort and maintain quiet atmosphere *to provide an environment conducive to learning.* • Establish rapport with child/parents. • Explain the disease process as simply as possible. • Inform child/parents of the treatment regimen. *The child/parents need to be aware that prognosis for recovery is good, but that recovery tends to be slow.*	The child/family will state a basic understanding of the disease and its treatment.

Caramen E. Billheimer, RN, BSN

Head trauma

Head injuries are the leading cause of death in the United States for persons aged 1 to 42. Most head injuries are blunt (closed) trauma to the brain. Damage to the scalp, skull, meninges, and brain run the gamut of skull fracture, concussion, and/or extra-cerebral or intracerebral pathological conditions.

NURSING DIAGNOSES/ DEFINING CHARACTERISTICS	NURSING INTERVENTIONS / *RATIONALES*	EXPECTED OUTCOMES

Altered Tissue Perfusion: Cerebral
✓ **RELATED TO**
Increased intracranial pressure (ICP)
Cerebral edema
Decreased cerebral perfusion pressure (CPP)
	ONGOING ASSESSMENT
	▪ Assess neurological status as follows:
	  ✓ Level of consciousness (Glasgow Coma Scale)
	  Orientation to person, place, and time
	  Motor signs: drift, decreased movement, abnormal or absent movement, increased reflexes
	  ✓ Pupil size, symmetry, and reaction to light
	  Extraocular movement
	  Speech, thought processes, and memory changes
	  ✓ Bulging fontanel/sutures
		Optimal cerebral tissue perfusion will be maintained.

Continued.

Neurological Care Plans (Pediatric)

NURSING DIAGNOSES/ DEFINING CHARACTERISTICS	NURSING INTERVENTIONS / *RATIONALES*	EXPECTED OUTCOMES

DEFINING CHARACTERISTICS

Decreased level of consciousness (confusion, disorientation, somnolence, lethargy, coma)
Headache
Papilledema
Bulging fontanel
Vomiting
Pupillary asymmetry
Changes in pupillary reaction
ICP >15 mm Hg
CPP <60 mm Hg

ONGOING ASSESSMENT cont'd

- Monitor ICP.
- Calculate the cerebral perfusion pressure (CPP) (CPP = mean systemic arterial pressure − ICP). CPP should be 80-100 mm Hg.
- Evaluate presence/absence of protective reflexes: corneal, gag, blink, cough, startle, grab, Babinski. *Babinski reflex is normal in an infant <18 months and abnormal in any child who is walking.*
- Monitor oxygen and CO_2 levels via an arterial blood gas assessment. *Normal levels are Pao_2 >80 mm Hg and $Paco_2$ <35 mm Hg in a child with a normal ICP. Goal of hyperventilation is $Paco_2$ between 25-30.*
- Monitor I&O every 1-2 hours or more frequently when needed. Assess urine specific gravity and urine glucose.
- Assess the child for pain, fever, and shivering.
- Monitor serum electrolytes, BUN, creatinine, osmolarity, glucose, and hemoglobin and hematocrit.
- Monitor the child closely with induction of treatment and when titrating treatment.

THERAPEUTIC INTERVENTIONS

- Document information derived from assessment every 1-4 hours or as needed.
- Report ICP >15 mm Hg sustained for >5 min. Elevate head of bed 30 degrees and keep head in midline position *to prevent a decrease in venous drainage from the head, unless the child is hemodynamically unstable.* Recheck equipment if ICP remains elevated.
- Notify physician for urine specific gravity >1.025 or urine output <½ ml/kg/hr or for large increase in urine output.
- Administer pain relief agents and neuromuscular blocking agents as ordered. Maintain normothermia. *Fever, pain, and the mechanical effect of shivering elevate ICP. Infants tend to lose more heat to their environment because of their large surface area. Keep covered or under warming lights.*
- Administer mannitol as indicated by physician. *Mannitol is a hyperosmotic agent and must be given carefully. Monitor serum osmolality and electrolyte levels carefully. Accurate and close assessment of urine output is mandatory. A Foley catheter should be in place. Mannitol should also be infused through a filter.*
- Avoid maneuvers that would increase intrathoracic pressure and thereby increase ICP.
- Maintain calm, peaceful environment. Allow parents to be at bedside.

Decreased Level of Consciousness
RELATED TO
Head trauma
Cerebral edema
Increased ICP

DEFINING CHARACTERISTICS
Change in alertness, orientation, verbal response, eye opening, motor response
Agitation
Inappropriate affect
Reduced awareness

ONGOING ASSESSMENT

- Assess LOC and perform neurological assessment every 1-2 hours.
- Assess for contributing factors that may affect LOC (e.g., anesthesia, medications).
- Assess vital signs.
- Assess for communication barriers.
- Assess for rhinorrhea, otorrhea, battle sign (*ecchymosis over the mastoid process is often seen with basal skull fracture*).

THERAPEUTIC INTERVENTIONS

- Record all assessment changes and/or deteriorations. *The Glasgow Coma Scale uses the same parameters for eye opening and motor movement. Verbal response must be evaluated by smiles, orientation to sound, appropriate interactions.*
- Protect child from injury by:
  Maintaining side rails in high position
  Bed in low position
  Protecting for decreased corneal and gag reflex and seizure activity

Optimal state of consciousness will be achieved.

NURSING DIAGNOSES/ DEFINING CHARACTERISTICS	NURSING INTERVENTIONS / *RATIONALES*	EXPECTED OUTCOMES
DEFINING CHARACTERISTICS cont'd Irritability, crying that may be inappropriate and inconsolable Decreased response to stimulation Lethargy	**THERAPEUTIC INTERVENTIONS cont'd** • If restraints are needed, child must be positioned on side. *Restraints should be used judiciously, since they may increase agitation and anxiety, thereby increasing ICP.* • Reorient child to environment as needed *to decrease anxiety.* Provide familiar objects in the child's environment (toys, pictures). • Explain all nursing activities in an age appropriate manner. Use anatomically specific dolls and books. Do not try to explain the whole procedure at once. Take one step at a time before proceeding to the next step. • Encourage and support interaction and verbalization by child, family, and significant others.	
High Risk for Fluid Volume Deficit **RELATED TO** Diabetes insipidus **DEFINING CHARACTERISTICS** Polyuria Polydypsia Dehydration Increased serum Na+ Increased serum osmolarity Sunken fontanel Tachycardia, hypotension	**ONGOING ASSESSMENT** • Monitor I&O every hour. • Assess urine specific gravity every 2-4 hours. • Monitor serum and urine electrolytes and osmolarity. • Monitor for signs of dehydration (decreased skin turgor, weight loss, increased heart rate, decreased BP, decreased fontanel). • Monitor vital signs every hour. • Assess urine for glucose. • Monitor daily weights. **THERAPEUTIC INTERVENTIONS** • Notify physician of urine output >200 ml/hr for 2 consecutive hours. Maintain an indwelling Foley catheter *to provide accurate assessment of urine output.* • Replace fluid output as directed. • Notify physician of urine specific gravity <1.005. *Diabetes insipidus will result in a decrease in urine specific gravity.* • Notify physician of positive urine glucose. *Glucosuria may lead to dehydration and increased urine output, mimicking diabetes insipidus.* • Administer vasopressin as ordered. *Vasopressin is a synthetic antidiuretic hormone that will induce concentration and decrease urine output. Careful monitoring of the urine output and serum Na and osmolarity is mandatory when vasopressin is administered.* • Keep accurate records of all fluid losses (blood draws, vomiting, diarrhea).	Optimal fluid volume will be obtained.
High Risk for Fluid Volume Excess **RELATED TO** Free water excess Syndrome of inappropriate secretion of antidiuretic hormone (SIADH) **DEFINING CHARACTERISTICS** Change in LOC or sensorium Decreased serum sodium <130 mEq/L Increased urine sodium Seizures Lethargy Nausea/vomiting	**ONGOING ASSESSMENT** • Assess intake and output. • Assess electrolytes and osmolality at least daily. • Monitor vital signs and neurological status every 1-2 hours. • Assess for edema. • Monitor weight daily. **THERAPEUTIC INTERVENTIONS** • Restrict fluid intake as directed by physician. • Limit free water intake. 0.9% NS fluids over D_5W as ordered. • Anticipate 3% saline with potassium and furosemide (Lasix) if fluid restriction fails.	Optimal fluid balance will be maintained.

Continued.

Neurological Care Plans (Pediatric)

NURSING DIAGNOSES/ DEFINING CHARACTERISTICS	NURSING INTERVENTIONS / *RATIONALES*	EXPECTED OUTCOMES
Ineffective Airway Clearance **RELATED TO** Decreased LOC Possible mechanical obstruction resulting from facial trauma Facial edema Use of paralytic agents **DEFINING CHARACTERISTICS** Abnormal or ineffective breathing pattern Decreased PaO$_2$ or increased PaCO$_2$ Change in rate of respiration (tachypnea or apnea) Change in heart rate (tachycardia or bradycardia) Cyanosis Use of accessory muscles of respiration Nasal flaring, grunting Intercostal retractions Feeding difficulties	**ONGOING ASSESSMENT** ▪ Assess rate and quality of respirations every 1-2 hours. ▪ Monitor breath sounds every 2 hours and prn. ▪ Monitor neurological status every 2-4 hours. ▪ Monitor ABGs as needed. ▪ Assess child's ability to cough and for gag reflex. **THERAPEUTIC INTERVENTIONS** ▪ Administer oxygen as directed. ▪ Suction secretions prn. *Nasotracheal suctioning is contraindicated in child with head trauma resulting from possible basilar skull fracture. This could result in the introduction of the catheter tip into the brain.*	Airway will be free of secretions.

High Risk for Injury: Seizures
RELATED TO
Cortical laceration
Temporal lobe contusion
Intracranial bleeding
Fluid/electrolyte imbalance
Hypoxia
Multiple contusions
Penetrating injuries to brain
 	
DEFINING CHARACTERISTICS
Focal and/or generalized seizures with/ without loss of consciousness
Eye deviation
Hyperventilation
Staring
Increased oral secretions
Decreased LOC
Apnea
	ONGOING ASSESSMENT
	▪ Observe child for seizure activity. Record and report observations:
	  Length of seizure
	  Body part involved, pattern and order of movement
	  Preictal activity
	  Direction of eye deviation and change in pupil size
	  Airway and respiratory pattern
	  Length of postictal state and characteristics
	  Incontinence
	
	THERAPEUTIC INTERVENTIONS
	▪ Protect child's head from injury. Give a padded helmet when appropriate (e.g., after craniectomy for compound depressed skull fracture). Pad side rails.
	▪ Maintain patent airway during the postictal state. Turn the child's head to the side and suction secretions as necessary.
	▪ Administer anticonvulsants as directed. *Phenytoin (Dilantin) can only be mixed in NS. Precipitation will be noted when mixed with D$_5$W. Observe for hypotension during the administration and administer <50 mg/min.*
	▪ If seizure occurs, protect the child's head and body from injury. Do not attempt to stick anything into the mouth.
	▪ Suction the child as indicated.
		Potential for additional injuries to head from seizures will be reduced.

NURSING DIAGNOSES/ DEFINING CHARACTERISTICS	NURSING INTERVENTIONS / *RATIONALES*	EXPECTED OUTCOMES
High Risk for Altered Nutrition: Less Than Body Requirements **RELATED TO** Facial trauma Restriction of intake Physical immobility Impaired LOC Multisystem trauma **DEFINING CHARACTERISTICS** Decreased daily weight Increased protein loss in urine Decreased muscle mass Poor skin turgor	**ONGOING ASSESSMENT** • Monitor child's albumin, urine, urea nitrogen level, glucose, electrolytes. • Assess skin color, turgor, and muscle mass. • Assess rate and quality of wound healing. • Observe for signs of infection and local infection at catheter insertion site. *Wound healing and immunocompetence depend on good nutrition.* • Monitor daily weights. • Verify placement of oral gastric (OG) or gastric (G) tube before initiation of tube feedings. Avoid insertion of feeding tube through the nose on a child with head injury unless the possibility of a basal skull fracture has been excluded. **THERAPEUTIC INTERVENTIONS** • Administer tube feedings or total parenteral nutrition (TPN) as directed. *Children have increased energy requirements and less nutritional reserves.* • Maintain head of bed at 30 degrees *to prevent risk of aspiration.*	Optimal nutritional support will be maintained.
Knowledge Deficit **RELATED TO** Lack of prior experience **DEFINING CHARACTERISTICS** Questioning members of health care team or other family members Verbalization of incorrect information Withdrawal from environment Frustration with health care and other family members	**ONGOING ASSESSMENT** • Assess current knowledge of equipment and health care status by asking the individual to describe what has been explained to him or her in the past. • Identify misconceptions. • Assess readiness for learning about head trauma, treatment, and equipment. • Assess intellectual and emotional ability to learn. • Identify priority of learning needs. **THERAPEUTIC INTERVENTIONS** • Inform family of the equipment and monitors used in the environment. • Provide an open, unthreatening atmosphere and encourage questions. • Provide physical comfort and quiet environment. • Provide an accessible time for questions. • Explain about their child's condition in simple, concise terms that are understandable by child or family. • Repeat the information as needed and request feedback. • Discuss need for quiet, calm environment *to conserve child's energy and minimize discomfort.* • Discuss diagnosis as appropriate. • Refer family to social service, financial counselor as appropriate.	Child/family will be able to discuss the illness, treatment, and expected outcome.

Jan Colip, RN, MSN, CCRN; Linda Arsenault, RN, MSN, CNRN

Hydrocephalus

A condition in which cerebrospinal fluid (CSF) production exceeds absorption. Noncommunicating hydrocephalus refers to an obstruction in the ventricular system between the lateral ventricles, third ventricle, fourth ventricle, or the outflow ports of the fourth ventricle. Communicating hydrocephalus usually connotes a problem with flow and absorption within the subarachnoid pathway and superior sagittal sinus.

NURSING DIAGNOSES/ DEFINING CHARACTERISTICS	NURSING INTERVENTIONS / *RATIONALES*	EXPECTED OUTCOMES

Altered Tissue Perfusion: Cerebral
 	
 RELATED TO
 	
 Increased intracranial pressure (ICP)
 Decreased cerebral perfusion pressure (CPP)
 Untreated hydrocephalus
 Obstructed shunt
 Subdural hematoma after shunt complication
 	
 DEFINING CHARACTERISTICS
 	
 Decreased level of consciousness (lethargy, decreased Glasgow Coma score, coma)
 Headache
 Vomiting
 Bulging fontanel in infant <18 months
 Parinaud's sign (sunsetting, failure of upward gaze)
 Impaired thought processes
 Increased blood pressure with bradycardia
 Motor weakness
	ONGOING ASSESSMENT
	 ▪ Assess age and developmental level.
	 ▪ Assess the child for signs/symptoms of increased ICP by evaluation of the following:
	     LOC (Glasgow Coma score)
	     Extraocular movements
	     Speech, thought processes
	     Fontanel/head circumference in child <18 months
	     Vital sign changes: increased BP and bradycardia
	     Motor strength
	     Headache/emesis
	 ▪ If child has a ventricular shunt in place, locate reservoir pump and press down in pumping fashion—should depress and refill within seconds. *If unable to depress or fails to refill, shunt may be obstructed.*
	
	 THERAPEUTIC INTERVENTIONS
	 ▪ Document serial assessment every 1-4 hours as indicated.
	 ▪ Report deterioration in child's assessment (e.g., increased lethargy, sunsetting, vital sign changes, respiratory distress).
	 ▪ Administer medications as ordered, e.g., furosemide (Lasix), mannitol *used to decrease ICP.*
	 ▪ Place child on cardiopulmonary monitor.
	 ▪ See Increased intracranial pressure, p. 189.
		Optimal cerebral tissue perfusion will be maintained.

High Risk for Fluid Volume Deficit **RELATED TO** Externalization of ventricular shunt for CSF drainage Use of diuretics/hyperosmotic agents to control ICP	**ONGOING ASSESSMENT** ▪ Monitor I&O hourly. *Urine output should normally be >0.5 ml/kg/hr. CSF drainage will vary, depending on external drainage bag position. Normal CSF production ~ 20 ml/hr (500 ml/day).* ▪ Monitor serum Na, osmolality, and urine specific gravity as indicated. ▪ Monitor for signs of dehydration (see Defining Characteristics). **THERAPEUTIC INTERVENTIONS** ▪ Administer IV fluids as ordered. *If ventricular shunt has been externalized, it is usually recommended that child receive IV normal saline replacement, milliliter per milliliter of CSF output. CSF is high in sodium.*	Optimal fluid volume will be maintained.

NURSING DIAGNOSES/ DEFINING CHARACTERISTICS	NURSING INTERVENTIONS / *RATIONALES*	EXPECTED OUTCOMES
DEFINING CHARACTERISTICS Thirst Polyuria Polydypsia Poor skin turgor Weight loss Tachycardia, hypotension Sunken fontanel <18 months Weak peripheral pulses Decreased urine output <0.5 ml/kg/hr Urine specific gravity >1.025 Serum Na >155 mEq/L Serum Osm >310 mOsm/L		

High Risk for Injury
RELATED TO
Rapid increase in cerebrospinal fluid volume and pressure by shunting
Revision of shunt or externalization of shunt
 	
DEFINING CHARACTERISTICS
Headache
Dizziness
Vomiting
Restlessness
Lethargy
	ONGOING ASSESSMENT
	• Assess child for signs of disequilibrium related to sudden drop in CSF pressure:
	    Headache that worsens when child sits up
	    Dizziness
	    Emesis with or without nausea
	    Restlessness
	
	THERAPEUTIC INTERVENTIONS
	• Administer IV fluids as ordered.
	• Administer antiemetics as ordered.
	• If child complains of headache when sitting up, keep head of bed flat with gradual elevation as child tolerates over several days.
	• Accompany child for follow-up CT scan as indicated. *A CT scan may be ordered to evaluate ventricular size and rule out subdural hematoma following shunting or revision of shunt.*
		Potential for injury will be reduced.

Actual and High Risk for Impaired Skin Integrity **RELATED TO** *Actual:* Surgical incisions for insertion of shunt—usually head and abdomen, occasionally also neck *High Risk:* Shunt tubing tunnelled subcutaneously under the skin from the scalp, down the neck and chest, into the peritoneum (or the atrium of the heart)	**ONGOING ASSESSMENT** • Monitor suture lines for healing, redness, swelling, leakage. *Leakage of CSF from the suture line should be promptly reported to the physician.* • Monitor skin surface over pathway of shunt tubing and reservoir for any signs of focal erythema or erosion. • Monitor temperature every 1-4 hours. **THERAPEUTIC INTERVENTIONS** • Administer IV antibiotics as ordered. *Postoperative antibiotics are commonly given for 24-48 hours after shunting or revision of shunt.* • If child is young infant, keep infant from lying on site of reservoir/ pump *because of danger of focal pressure and breakdown related to thinness of scalp.* • In young child, try to keep dressings dry, *e.g., may need frequent diapering or external urinary collection device.* • Turn child frequently, as appropriate.	Skin integrity will remain intact or healing without signs of infection.

Continued.

Hydrocephalus cont'd

NURSING DIAGNOSES/ DEFINING CHARACTERISTICS	NURSING INTERVENTIONS / *RATIONALES*	EXPECTED OUTCOMES
DEFINING CHARACTERISTICS Mechanical pressure from the shunt reservoir (pump) and length of tubing with *mild* erythema, tenderness, swelling Recent incisions		

Knowledge Deficit RELATED TO Lack of prior experience New shunt **DEFINING CHARACTERISTICS** Questioning health care members Verbalization of incorrect information Expressions of frustration Expressions of apprehension, anxiety, fear	**ONGOING ASSESSMENT** • Assess readiness for learning about hydrocephalus causes and its treatment (ventriculoperitoneal or atrial shunting). • Assess child's/family's current knowledge base. • Assess intellectual and emotional resources and ability to learn. • Identify priority of learning needs. • Assess willingness of child/family to learn. • Assess misconceptions about child's illness. • Evaluate knowledge of caregiver regarding signs and symptoms of shunt obstruction and follow-up before discharge. **THERAPEUTIC INTERVENTIONS** • Provide quiet, comfortable environment. • Encourage questions. • Keep explanations about child's illness and treatment simple, concise, and at level of understanding appropriate to individuals. • Provide frequent communication about child's status to family. • Allow adequate time for assimilation of new information. • Provide frequent feedback. • Use pictures and written materials as available. • Provide written information regarding shunt malfunction for the family: *Infant:* Bulging fontanel—soft spot on head Enlarging head Irritability Excessive sleepiness High-pitched cry Vomiting Decreased appetite Fever, puffiness, redness, swelling at incision or along shunt tubing *Older child/adolescent:* Vomiting Decreased appetite Unusual irritability or restlessness Persistent headache Difficulty walking Blurred/double vision Inability to retain urine (if toilet trained) Fever, puffiness, redness, swelling at incisions or along shunt tubing Unusual sleepiness • Provide child and family with follow-up appointments and information for emergency access to health care system. • Involve social worker as indicated.	Child/family will be able to discuss hydrocephalus, shunting treatment, and possible signs of shunt malfunction before discharge.

Linda Arsenault, RN, MSN, CNRN

Increased intracranial pressure

Intracranial pressure (ICP) reflects the pressure exerted by the intracranial components of blood, brain, cerebrospinal fluid (CSF), and any other fluid/mass (subdural, tumor, abscess, etc.). Increases in ICP occur when compensation mechanisms fail (mostly blood and CSF buffering). The normal range of ICP is up to 15 mm Hg; excursions above that level occur normally, but readily return to baseline parameters. In the event of disease, trauma, or a pathological condition, a disturbance in autoregulation occurs and ICP is increased and sustained.

NURSING DIAGNOSES/ DEFINING CHARACTERISTICS	NURSING INTERVENTIONS / *RATIONALES*	EXPECTED OUTCOMES

Altered Tissue Perfusion: Cerebral **RELATED TO** Increased ICP Increased cerebral blood flow (CBF) Cerebral edema Decreased CBF and cerebral perfusion pressure (CPP) **DEFINING CHARACTERISTICS** Decreased LOC (confusion, disorientation, somnolence, lethargy, coma) Headache Vomiting Papilledema Pupil asymmetry Decreased pupil reactivity Impaired memory, judgment, thought processes Glasgow Coma Scale <11 Bulging fontanel Split sutures Unilateral or bilateral VI nerve palsy	**ONGOING ASSESSMENT**
	• Assess age and developmental level.
	• Assess neurological status as follows:
	  LOC per Glasgow Coma Scale
	  Pupil size, symmetry, reaction to light
	  Extraocular movement (EOM)
	  Gaze preference
	  Speech, thought processes, memory
	  Fontanel/sutures
	  Motor-sensory signs—drift, increased tone, increased reflexes, Babinski
	  Head circumference increased in child <18 months.
	• Monitor ICP if ICP monitor in place.
	• Evaluate presence/absence of protective reflexes: swallow, gag, blink, cough, etc.
	• Monitor ABGs. *Recommended parameters of PaO_2 of >80 mm Hg and $PaCO_2$ of <35 mm Hg in a child with normal ICP. If patient's lungs are being hyperventilated to decrease ICP, $PaCO_2$ should be between 25 and 30 mm Hg. A $PaCO_2$ of <20 mm Hg may decrease CBF because of profound vasoconstriction → hypoxia. $PaCO_2$ >45 mm Hg induces vasodilation with increase in CBF, which may trigger increase in ICP.*
	• Monitor I&O every 1-2 hours with urine specific gravity. Report urine specific gravity >1.025 or urine output <½ ml/kg/hr.
	• Calculate CPP. *Should be ~90-100 mm Hg and not <50 mm Hg to ensure blood flow to brain. Calculate CPP by subtracting ICP from the mean systemic arterial pressure (MSAP): CPP = MSAP − ICP. To calculate MSAP, use the following formula:* $$\left(\frac{\text{Diastolic BP} - \text{Systolic BP}}{3}\right) + \text{Diastolic BP}$$
	• Monitor serum electrolytes, BUN, creatinine, glucose, osmolality, Hgb, and Hct as indicated.
	• Monitor the child closely when treatment of increased ICP begins to be tapered, i.e., once ICP is stabilized at normal pressure for 48 hours.
	
	THERAPEUTIC INTERVENTIONS
	• Document serial assessment of LOC, Glasgow Coma Scale, pupil evaluation, EOM, speech, motor, sensory status every 1-4 hours as indicated.
	• Report ICP >15 mm Hg for 5 minutes.
	• Elevate head of bed 30 degrees and keep head in neutral alignment *to prevent decrease in venous outflow with increase in ICP.*
	• Avoid Valsalva maneuvers, *which increase intrathoracic pressure and increase CBF, thereby increasing ICP.*
	• If ICP increases and fails to respond to repositioning of head in neutral alignment and head elevation, recheck equipment. If ICP is increased, one or more of the following may be ordered by the physician:
	  Hyperventilate the child's lungs *to decrease $PaCO_2$ to between 25 and 30 mm Hg; this induces vasoconstriction and decrease in CBF.*
		Optimal cerebral tissue perfusion will be maintained.

Continued.

Increased intracranial pressure cont'd

NURSING DIAGNOSES/ DEFINING CHARACTERISTICS	NURSING INTERVENTIONS / *RATIONALES*	EXPECTED OUTCOMES
	THERAPEUTIC INTERVENTIONS cont'd	

Administer mannitol 0.25 g/kg-1 g/kg given over 30-60 min. *This is a hyperosmotic agent and needs to be given with caution; it is contraindicated with hypovolemic symptoms: hypotension, tachycardia, CHF, renal failure, hypernatremia. A diuretic response can be anticipated within 30-60 min. A Foley catheter should be in place. An IV filter should be used when mannitol is infused. Electrolytes, osmolality, and serum glucose must be monitored every 4-6 hours during mannitol infusion.*

- Administer barbiturates, additional diuretics such as furosemide as ordered by physician if ICP is refractory to hyperventilation/mannitol regimen.
- If patient is intubated, administer neuromuscular blocking agent as ordered every 1-4 hours *to reduce shivering, coughing, bucking, Valsalva maneuver. Remember, however, that neuromuscular blocking agents have no effect on cerebration; therefore, patient should receive short-acting sedation before noxious stimulation.*
- Administer a short-acting pain reliever, e.g., morphine, midazolam (Versed), before painful stimulation or stress-related care such as suctioning, IV line changes.
- If ICP elevated 12-15 mm Hg, reduce nursing and medical procedures to those absolutely necessary. *Counteract noxious stimulation with preoxygenation, hyperventilation, analgesia.*

Knowledge Deficit RELATED TO

Lack of prior experience

DEFINING CHARACTERISTICS

Questioning members of health care team
Verbalization of incorrect information
Anger/hostility
Depression
Withdrawal from environment
Expressions of frustration

ONGOING ASSESSMENT

- Assess readiness for learning about increased ICP, causes, treatment, and outcome.
- Assess current knowledge base of child/family/significant others.
- Assess intellectual and emotional ability to learn.
- Identify priority of learning needs.
- Assess willingness of child/family to learn.
- Identify misconceptions about child's illness.

THERAPEUTIC INTERVENTIONS

- Provide physical comfort, quiet environment.
- Encourage questions.
- Keep explanations about child's condition simple, concise, and at a level of understanding of child/significant other.
- Provide frequent communication about child's status to family.
- Allow adequate time for assimilation of new information.
- Request feedback regarding information given.
- Discuss need for calm, quiet environment and restriction of visitors *to conserve child's energy and minimize discomfort.*
- Discuss prognosis as appropriate.

Child/family will be able to discuss illness, treatment, and expected outcome if known.

Linda Arsenault, RN, MSN, CNRN

Lead poisoning

PLUMBISM

Often a result of chronic ingestion or inhalation of lead-bearing products. Lead poisoning is a chronic process that is most commonly seen in children exhibiting pica behaviors. Accidental ingestion can occur from serving acidic liquids from lead-containing pottery or antique pewter. Lead salts are absorbed by the blood, interfere with hemoglobin production, and destroy kidney and brain tissue. About 30% of children treated for lead poisoning will suffer irreversible damage to the nervous system, including mental retardation, hyperactivity, cerebral palsy, seizures, and optic atrophy.

NURSING DIAGNOSES/ DEFINING CHARACTERISTICS	NURSING INTERVENTIONS / *RATIONALES*	EXPECTED OUTCOMES
Altered Hematological Status **RELATED TO** Ingestion of substances containing lead **DEFINING CHARACTERISTICS** Decreased Hct Decreased Hgb Increased lead level >15-50 µg/dl History of pica	**ONGOING ASSESSMENT** • Check vital signs with BP every 4 hours. • Monitor daily laboratory values, i.e., CBC, lead levels <50 µg/dl after 5 days of chelation therapy. • Observe skin for pallor/anemia. • Monitor for side effects/complications of these agents. **THERAPEUTIC INTERVENTIONS** • Administer chelating agents (IM injections) such as dimercaprol (BAL in oil) or edetate calcium disodium (CaEDTA), or an oral chelator, such as succimer (Chemet). *These form a highly soluble compound that causes free lead to be readily excreted in the urine.* • Assist with exchange transfusion if appropriate. *This will decrease lead level in the bloodstream and keep lead from being readily absorbed by the soft tissue. Anything over 25 µg/dl will cause nerve damage, with cognitive changes seen at levels less than 25 µg/dl.*	Blood lead level will be decreased.
High Risk for Altered Urinary Elimination **RELATED TO** Toxic levels of dimercaprol (BAL) and/or edetate calcium disodium (CaEDTA) **DEFINING CHARACTERISTICS** Decreased urine output Proteinuria Hematuria	**ONGOING ASSESSMENT** • Monitor vital signs every 4 hours (especially for increased heart rate and change in BP). • Monitor I&O every 8 hours. • Check urine specific gravity and dipstick for protein/blood every void. • Monitor laboratory results: urinalysis, electrolytes, BUN, and creatinine, *since the chelating agents are toxic to kidneys.* **THERAPEUTIC INTERVENTIONS** • Review potential renal side effects of all drugs before administration. • Do not administer chelators to dehydrated child. *Decreased kidney function severely limits the effectiveness of chelation therapy.* • Ensure adequate oral/IV intake. *Fluids ensure excretion of the lead via urine.* • Report significant change in I&O or a urine output <30 ml/hr. *Chelating agents are nephrotoxic.*	Adequate urinary elimination will be maintained.
Pain/Discomfort **RELATED TO** Multiple injections Side effects of drug therapy	**ONGOING ASSESSMENT** • Observe injection areas for swelling, redness, inflammation, abscess formation. • Check for skin rash in children receiving succimer (Chemet).	Discomfort and complications will be reduced.

Continued.

Lead poisoning cont'd

NURSING DIAGNOSES/ DEFINING CHARACTERISTICS	NURSING INTERVENTIONS / *RATIONALES*	EXPECTED OUTCOMES
DEFINING CHARACTERISTICS Irritability Crying Swelling, inflammation, and redness at the injection sites Skin rash	**THERAPEUTIC INTERVENTIONS** • Palpate muscle area before preparing site *to locate and avoid fibrous tissue from previous injections.* • Rotate all injection sites and use large muscle groups. • Obtain order for use of local anesthetic with injection (draw this up last in syringe and do not mix). *This would help lessen the pain during administration.* • Administer BAL and CaEDTA by deep IM injection as ordered *for adequate absorption.* CaEDTA can also be given IV. • Apply warm soaks to injection sites as needed *to relieve discomfort.* • Avoid activity *to prevent strain or exertion on painful muscle areas.* • Notify physician of side effects of therapy, especially rash. *Therapy may need to be changed.* • Apply topical ointments as ordered.	

High Risk for Altered Levels of Consciousness RELATED TO
Chronic lead ingestion
 	
DEFINING CHARACTERISTICS
Falling, clumsiness, loss of coordination
Irritability
Seizures
Drowsiness/lethargy
Coma
Peripheral nerve palsy/paralysis
Nonspecific:
Headache, vomiting
	ONGOING ASSESSMENT
	• Interview parent regarding child's level of development before ingestion. *This will help in determining current neurologic deficit.*
	• Assess LOC every 4 hours or more frequently if any deterioration, increased toxicity, or encephalopathy noted.
	• Assess vital signs, especially respiratory status, every 2-4 hours.
	• Compare present neurological assessment with previous level from history. Document serial assessments.
	
	THERAPEUTIC INTERVENTIONS
	• Use seizure precautions and safety measures, e.g., side rails up and padded, *since seizure activity, loss of coordination, drowsiness may occur.*
	• If actual altered level of consciousness is noted:
	    Obtain emergency equipment; place Ambu bag at bedside.
	    Report to physician.
	    Consult neurology clinical specialist.
	• See Consciousness, decreased level of, p. 173.
		Maximum neurological functioning will be maintained.

Knowledge Deficit RELATED TO
Unfamiliarity with diagnosis, source of exposure
 	
DEFINING CHARACTERISTICS
Verbalized lack of understanding of diagnosis and cause
Multiple questions or comments
Repeated episodes of ingestion
	ONGOING ASSESSMENT
	• Assess knowledge of lead poisoning and source of ingestion.
	• Assess for pica behavior and general nutrition.
	• Elicit information for possible lead sources.
	• Screen all siblings for increased lead levels.
	• Observe family interaction/relationships.
	
	THERAPEUTIC INTERVENTIONS
	• Explain the cause of lead poisoning, e.g., pica, improperly glazed pottery, toxic fumes (paint), lead pipes.
	• Emphasize the need for a good diet *to decrease pica behaviors and minimize lead uptake in body tissues.*
	• Explain the environmental factors that contribute to lead poisoning, such as:
	    Poorly maintained older dwellings
	    Fumes from toxic waste
	• Review and emphasize the hazards of lead, signs of lead intoxication, and long-term complications.
	• Inform parent of the importance of proper medication administration at home.
	• Initiate referrals with social worker, public health nurse, Board of Health, and other agencies that can assist in overall management.
	• Emphasize the need for continued follow-up to monitor lead levels; usually once/week during therapy.
	• Provide telephone number for local emergency room and poison control.
		An understanding of lead poisoning, environmental hazard, long-term complications, medications, and resources available for follow-up will be achieved.

Gina Stevens, RN, BSN

Meningitis

**INTRACRANIAL INFECTION,
MENINGOENCEPHALITIS, MENINGOCEREBRITIS
ENCEPHALITIS**

Inflammation/infection of the membranes of the brain or spinal cord (meninges) caused by bacteria, viruses, or other organisms. Encephalitis is an inflammation/infection of the brain and meninges. The bacterial organisms most commonly involved in meningitis in children are Haemophilus influenzae type B, Streptococcus pneumoniae, and Neisseria meningitidis.

NURSING DIAGNOSES/ DEFINING CHARACTERISTICS	NURSING INTERVENTIONS / *RATIONALES*	EXPECTED OUTCOMES

Altered Tissue Perfusion: Cerebral
RELATED TO
Central nervous system infection
Cerebral edema
Hydrocephalus
Increased ICP
 	
DEFINING CHARACTERISTICS
Fever
Elevated WBC
Rash
Chills
Emesis
Seizures
Nuchal rigidity
Headache
Photophobia
Impaired mentation
	ONGOING ASSESSMENT
	▪ Assess age and developmental level.
	▪ Assess for signs of infection:
	  Fever
	  Increased WBC
	  Chills
	  Emesis
	▪ Assess for meningeal signs:
	  Nuchal rigidity
	  Headache
	  Pain with flexion of neck
	  Kernig's sign
	  Brudzinski's sign
	  Photophobia
	  Hyperirritability
	  High-pitched cry
	▪ Assess for any neurological deficits:
	  Change in LOC, Glasgow Coma Scale
	  Cranial nerve paresis
	  Seizure activity
	▪ Assess for signs of increased ICP:
	  Bulging fontanel in infants <18 months
	  Vomiting
	  Bradycardia with increased blood pressure
	  Decreased LOC
	  Increasing head circumference in infants (<18 months)
	  Pupil asymmetry
	
	THERAPEUTIC INTERVENTIONS
	▪ Report temperature >39° C (102.2° F).
	▪ Maintain normothermia with tepid sponge bath and antipyretics or hypothermia blanket as ordered. *Fever increases cerebral metabolic demand.*
	▪ Document baseline and serial neurological assessment every 1-4 hours. Report alteration in mentation, seizures, bradycardia, increasing BP, *since one or more of these events may indicate increasing intracranial pressure with a decrease in cerebral perfusion pressure.*
	▪ Administer antibiotics and antiemetics as ordered.
	▪ Isolate child if appropriate for 24-48 hours after start of antibiotic therapy.
	▪ Record urine specific gravity every shift. *Child may become dehydrated because of fever, emesis, impaired mental status.*
		Optimal cerebral perfusion will be maintained.

Pain/Discomfort
RELATED TO
Meningeal irritation
Increased ICP
	ONGOING ASSESSMENT
	▪ Assess for:
	  Headache
	  Photophobia
	  Restlessness
	  Irritability
	  Crying
	  Vital sign changes
	  Diaphoresis
	▪ Evaluate response to analgesics.
		Comfort will be maintained.

Continued.

Meningitis cont'd

NURSING DIAGNOSES/ DEFINING CHARACTERISTICS	NURSING INTERVENTIONS / *RATIONALES*	EXPECTED OUTCOMES
DEFINING CHARACTERISTICS Headache Photophobia Nuchal rigidity Irritability Crying unrelieved by usual comfort measures Vital sign changes (e.g., increased HR, respiration, BP, pupil dilation) Diaphoresis	**THERAPEUTIC INTERVENTIONS** • Restrict visitors as deemed appropriate. • Reduce noise in the environment. • Keep child's room darkened/ask family to bring in sunglasses *to minimize effects of photophobia, if age appropriate.* • Administer analgesics as ordered and document response. • Discourage Valsalva maneuvers, e.g., instruct older child to exhale when moving up in bed; provide with stool softeners *to prevent increase in cerebral blood flow and increase in ICP.* • Encourage family to stay with and comfort child when appropriate. • See Pain, p. 35.	
High Risk for Fluid Volume Deficit **RELATED TO** Reduced LOC Lack of oral intake, poor feeding Fever Vomiting Diarrhea **DEFINING CHARACTERISTICS** Poor skin turgor Increased urine specific gravity Decreased urine output Change in mental status Tachycardia Hypotension Increased BUN Hypernatremia Increased serum osmolality Increased urine specific gravity Weight loss Sunken anterior fontanel	**ONGOING ASSESSMENT** • Assess skin turgor. *Loss of interstitial fluid causes loss of skin elasticity.* • Assess for presence of one or more defining characteristics. • Monitor I&O. • Monitor weight. *Changes in weight may reflect fluid volume changes.* • Monitor serum electrolytes, urine specific gravity, and blood urea nitrogen (BUN). • Record urine specific gravity every shift and check laboratory results that may reflect dehydration, e.g., urine specific gravity of >1.025, serum Na >150 mEq/L, serum osmolality >310 mOsm/L, BUN >18 mg/dl, creatinine >0.4 mg/dl. **THERAPEUTIC INTERVENTIONS** • Encourage fluid intake as appropriate. May require intravenous or nasogastric feedings *to ensure hydration. The average daily fluid loss is 1500 ml urine, 200 ml stool, and 1300 ml perspiration/respiration/insensible water loss.* • Provide oral care, lubrication to lips. • Document and report any changes in BP, heart rate. *Reduction in circulating blood volume can cause changes in vital signs.*	Optimal fluid volume will be maintained.
High Risk for Altered Nutrition: Less Than Body Requirements **RELATED TO** Reduced oral intake Vomiting Loss of appetite Fever with increased metabolic demand	**ONGOING ASSESSMENT** • Assess child's ability to swallow. • Inquire about food and fluid preferences. • Assess child's admission weight and compare with normal range for age and height. • Weigh daily. • Monitor I&O. • Compare normal caloric requirements for body weight with present weight.	Weight loss will be reduced and nutritional requirements maintained.

Meningitis cont'd

NURSING DIAGNOSES/ DEFINING CHARACTERISTICS	NURSING INTERVENTIONS / *RATIONALES*	EXPECTED OUTCOMES
DEFINING CHARACTERISTICS Weight loss Documented reduction in intake Diarrhea Vomiting Ileus, abdominal distention Bradycardia Failure to gain weight	**THERAPEUTIC INTERVENTIONS** • Encourage food intake. Provide small frequent meals and supplements as tolerated. *Child may experience a sense of fullness related to decreased digestive secretions or altered glucose metabolism. Smaller meals may facilitate gastric emptying and improve appetite.* • Administer IV fluids as ordered. • Assist child with eating as appropriate. • Provide adaptive or assistive devices as needed. • Consult dietitian when appropriate. • See Altered nutrition: less than body requirements, p. 33.	
Knowledge Deficit RELATED TO Lack of prior similar experience **DEFINING CHARACTERISTICS** Probing questions Request for information Expression of misconceptions	**ONGOING ASSESSMENT** • Assess current knowledge base of child/significant others. • Assess readiness for learning. **THERAPEUTIC INTERVENTIONS** • Discuss need for calm, quiet environment and restriction of visitors *to conserve child's energy and minimize discomfort.* • Discuss course prognosis as appropriate. • Identify exposed contact individuals and refer for prophylactic treatment if appropriate. • Instruct parents/caretakers in medication to be taken, dose, frequency, time, route, and side effects. • Ask for feedback from parents regarding information given.	Child/family will understand disease process.

Linda Arsenault, RN, MSN, CNRN

Reye's syndrome

A fulminant biphasic illness, usually characterized by an antecedent viral infection followed by hepatic, metabolic, and neurological dysfunction. The cause is unknown; it is thought to be pleurifactorial. Reye's syndrome can occur in infants to adults; it is most often seen in 6- to 12-year-old children. Mild symptoms of malaise, nausea, vomiting, and irritability may rapidly progress to personality changes, impaired level of consciousness, and coma. Biochemical abnormalities include elevated ammonia levels, SGOT, SGPT, and prolonged prothrombin time. Clinical staging has been developed to evaluate the child's presentation, progression, and outcome and to evaluate response to treatment.

NURSING DIAGNOSES/ DEFINING CHARACTERISTICS	NURSING INTERVENTIONS / *RATIONALES*	EXPECTED OUTCOMES
Altered Level of Consciousness RELATED TO Encephalopathy Increased ICP Cerebral edema	**ONGOING ASSESSMENT** • Assess age and developmental level. • Assess LOC/responsiveness every 1-4 hours. • Assess vital signs every 1-4 hours with temperature. • Assess pupil size, symmetry, reaction to light, extraocular movement every 1-4 hours. • Evaluate speech, motor movement, and strength every 1-4 hours. • Monitor child for characteristics listed from stages I through V every 1-4 hours.	Optimal level of consciousness will be maintained.

Continued.

NURSING DIAGNOSES/ DEFINING CHARACTERISTICS	NURSING INTERVENTIONS / *RATIONALES*	EXPECTED OUTCOMES

DEFINING CHARACTERISTICS
Stage I:
  Vomiting
  Lethargy
  Sleepiness
  Obeys commands
  Increased liver en-
  zymes
Stage II:
  Disorientation, agi-
  tation, delirium
  Combativeness
  Tachypnea
  Hyperreflexia
  Purposeful re-
  sponse to pain
  Increased ammo-
  nia and liver en-
  zymes
Stage III:
  Obtunded
  Comatose
  Decorticate posturing
  Hyperventilation
  Reactive pupils
  Intact oculovestib-
  ular responses
Stage IV:
  Deepening coma
  Decerebrate rigidity
  Loss of oculoce-
  phalic reflexes
  Dilated, fixed
  pupils
Stage V:
  Seizures
  Flaccidity (are-
  flexia)
  Dilated, fixed
  pupils
  Apnea
  No withdrawal to
  pain
	THERAPEUTIC INTERVENTIONS
	• Document serial assessment parameters.
	• Notify physician if child's condition deteriorates/changes.
	• If child needs to be restrained, avoid doing so with child flat on back *(danger of aspiration).*
	• Reorient to environment as needed *to minimize apprehension and anxiety. Use of TV, radio, clocks may help with reorientation.*
	• Protect child from possible injury (seizure activity; diminished protective reflexes such as blink, gag, swallowing, aspiration).
	• Encourage significant others to bring in things familiar to child, e.g., favorite dolls, teddy bear, pajamas.
	• Encourage and support verbalization by child/family.
	• Consult rehabilitation therapists, social service, play therapists, etc. as indicated.	

Altered Tissue Perfusion: Cerebral
RELATED TO
Increased intracranial pressure (ICP)
Increased/decreased cerebral blood flow (CBF)
Cerebral edema
Decreased cerebral perfusion pressure (CPP)
	ONGOING ASSESSMENT
	• Assess child for signs/symptoms of increased ICP by monitoring the following:
	  LOC (Glasgow Coma score)
	  Pupil size, symmetry, reaction to light
	  Extraocular movement (EOM)
	  Speech, thought processes, memory
	  Fontanel/head circumference (in child <18 months)
	  Motor/sensory integrity *The hallmark of a structural pathological condition is focal signs of dysfunction (e.g., asymmetric pupils, gaze preference, facial weakness, Babinski's sign).*
	  Evaluate presence/absence of protective reflexes (e.g., swallow, gag, blink, cough).
	• If an intracranial pressure (ICP) monitor is in situ, assess ICP serially. *Normal ICP should be <15 mm Hg.*
	• Calculate cerebral perfusion pressure (CPP = MSAP − ICP) every hour and prn. *CPP should be >60 mm Hg. Normal CPP: 90-100 mm Hg.*
		Optimal cerebral tissue perfusion will be maintained.

NURSING DIAGNOSES/ DEFINING CHARACTERISTICS	NURSING INTERVENTIONS / *RATIONALES*	EXPECTED OUTCOMES
DEFINING CHARACTERISTICS Decreased level of consciousness (confusion, disorientation, lethargy, coma, Glasgow Coma score) Headache Vomiting Impaired memory, judgment, thought processes, speech Bulging fontanel/split sutures in child <18 months Unilateral or bilateral VI nerve palsy Gaze preference Motor weakness Increased deep tendon reflexes Babinski's sign	**ONGOING ASSESSMENT cont'd** • Monitor ABG's as indicated. *Pao_2 of >80 mm Hg and $Paco_2$ of <40 mm Hg is recommended in a child with potential risk for increased ICP. If the child is receiving hyperventilation therapy to decrease ICP, the $Paco_2$ should be between 25-30 mm Hg. A $Paco_2$ of <20 mm Hg may result in vasoconstriction, ↓ in CBF, and ischemia. A $Paco_2$ of >45 mm Hg may cause vasodilation, increase in CBF, and an increase in ICP.* • Monitor I&O every 1-4 hours. • Monitor serum electrolytes, glucose, BUN, creatinine, osmolality, ammonia level, PT, PTT, liver function studies, and anticonvulsant levels as indicated. • Monitor the child closely when treatment of increased ICP begins to be tapered (e.g., once ICP stabilized at normal pressure for approximately 48 hours). **THERAPEUTIC INTERVENTIONS** • Document serial assessment every 1-4 hours as indicated. • Report changes in child's assessment. • Elevate head of bed 30 degrees and support the child's head in neutral position *to prevent a decrease in venous outflow with an increase in ICP.* • Avoid Valsalva maneuvers, *which increase intrathoracic pressure and increase CBF, leading to an increase in ICP.* • Hyperventilate the patient's lungs as ordered to decrease $Paco_2$ to between 25 and 30 mm Hg. • Administer hyperosmotic agent such as mannitol as ordered. Needs to be given cautiously. *Contraindicated with hypovolemic signs (such as hypotension, tachycardia), CHF, renal failure, hypernatremia. A diuretic response can be anticipated within 30-60 minutes. A Foley catheter should be in place. An IV filter should be utilized when mannitol is administered.* • Administer additional diuretics such as furosemide (Lasix) as ordered, if ICP is refractory to hyperventilation/mannitol regimen. • Administer a short-acting pain reliever (e.g., morphine sulfate or midazolam [Versed]) before painful stimulation or stress-related care (e.g., suctioning secretions). • If child is intubated, administer neuromuscular blocking agent every 1-4 hours as ordered *to reduce shivering, coughing, bucking. Remember that neuromuscular blocking agents have no effect on cerebration; therefore, child should receive short-acting sedation before noxious stimulation.* • If ICP is elevated 12-15 mm Hg or more, reduce nursing/medical procedures to those absolutely necessary.	
Impaired Gas Exchange **RELATED TO** Central hyperventilation or hypoventilation associated with increased ICP, medullary-pontine ischemia/pressure Apnea related to increased ICP Status epilepticus Use of neuromuscular paralytic agents Aspiration	**ONGOING ASSESSMENT** • Monitor respiratory rate, rhythm. • Auscultate for breath sounds every 1-4 hours as indicated. • Assess presence/absence of protective reflexes such as swallowing/gag. • Observe child for restlessness, confusion, nasal flaring, grunting, intercostal and/or abdominal contraction. • Monitor ABG results as ordered. **THERAPEUTIC INTERVENTIONS** • Suction as needed. *Preoxygenation and hyperventilation/sedation will help to counteract increases in ICP related to noxious stimulation and help to minimize decreases in Pao_2.* • Elevate head of bed 30 degrees *to facilitate breathing as well as to promote cerebral venous drainage.* • Encourage slow deep-breathing exercises, as appropriate.	Adequate gas exchange will be maintained.

Continued.

Neurological Care Plans (Pediatric)

NURSING DIAGNOSES/ DEFINING CHARACTERISTICS	NURSING INTERVENTIONS / *RATIONALES*	EXPECTED OUTCOMES
DEFINING CHARACTERISTICS Tachypnea Abnormal respiratory rate/rhythm Restlessness Confusion Rhonchi, wheezes, congestion Impaired protective reflexes such as cough, gag Hypoxia/hypercarbia Acid-base imbalances		
Altered Nutrition: Less Than Body Requirements **RELATED TO** NPO status Emesis Altered level of consciousness **DEFINING CHARACTERISTICS** Weight loss (10%-20% of ideal body weight) Decreased serum albumin Decreased serum transferrin or TIBC Decreased total protein Electrolyte imbalance Poor appetite/intake	**ONGOING ASSESSMENT** • Monitor caloric intake and food intake each meal. • Monitor appropriate laboratory parameters (e.g., serum albumin, total protein, iron, and electrolytes). • Monitor I&O every shift. • Weigh child on admission. If scale is incorporated into the bed, obtain daily weights. Otherwise, do two times/week, or weekly depending upon the status of the child's ICP. *Should avoid lowering the head of the bed if ICP is elevated.* **THERAPEUTIC INTERVENTIONS** • Encourage food appropriate for age. • Elevate head of bed for meals and for 1 hour after. *This helps prevent epigastric discomfort/feeling of fullness and minimizes the potential for aspiration.* • Consult dietitian as appropriate. • Offer high-protein supplements between meals as appropriate.	Optimal nutrition will be maintained.
High Risk for Fluid Volume Deficit **RELATED TO** Use of hyperosmotic agents such as mannitol or diuretics to control ICP NPO status	**ONGOING ASSESSMENT** • Monitor I&O hourly. *Urine output should not fall below 0.5-1 ml/kg/hr. Check urine specific gravity every 8 hours; normal = 1.015-1.025.* • Monitor for clinical signs of dehydration (see defining characteristics). • Weigh child daily if ICP has normalized or scale is incorporated into the bed. Otherwise, defer weights until ICP is within normal limits. • Monitor central venous pressure (CVP) every 1-2 hours. • Monitor serum glucose, electrolytes, osmolarity as ordered. **THERAPEUTIC INTERVENTIONS** • Administer IV fluids as ordered. *Children with Reye's are at risk for hypoglycemia. Hypertonic solutions with 10%-15% glucose may be ordered to maintain serum glucose levels at 150-200 mg/dl.*	Optimal fluid volume will be maintained.

NURSING DIAGNOSES/ DEFINING CHARACTERISTICS	NURSING INTERVENTIONS / *RATIONALES*	EXPECTED OUTCOMES

DEFINING CHARACTERISTICS
Thirst
Polyuria
Polydipsia
Poor skin turgor
Weight loss
Tachycardia, hypo-
  tension
Sunken fontanel
  (<18 months)
Weak peripheral
  pulses		

Ineffective Family Coping
RELATED TO
Sudden severe illness
  of child
Uncertain prognosis
Guilt
 	
DEFINING CHARACTERISTICS
Facial tension
Increased alertness/
  vigilance
Expressions of
  worry/fear
Restlessness
Insomnia
Extraneous motion
  (e.g., repetitive
  hand/leg motion)
Tearfulness
Loss of appetite
	ONGOING ASSESSMENT
	• Assess family/significant others for defining characteristics.
	• Monitor family response to information given by staff.
	• Monitor family response to child.
	• Assess child's/family's ability to openly express feelings about this illness.
	
	THERAPEUTIC INTERVENTIONS
	• Encourage questions.
	• Orient to hospital environment and to PICU equipment, etc.
	• Elicit feedback, questions regarding information transmitted.
	• Discuss ways parents can be involved in daily care (e.g., bathing, skin care, feeding).
	• Answer all questions patiently and repeat explanations as needed.
	• Communicate with family on a regular basis even if nothing has changed.
	• Refer to social service for help and support.
	• Refer to local chapter of Reye's Syndrome Foundation for information/ support.
		Family will be able to discuss methods of coping with this po-tentially life-threat-ening illness.

Knowledge Deficit: Illness, Hospitalization Procedures, Prognosis **RELATED TO** Lack of prior experi-ence **DEFINING CHARACTERISTICS** Questioning Expression of incor-rect/inaccurate in-formation	**ONGOING ASSESSMENT** • Assess the child's/family's knowledge base, readiness for learning, pre-vious experience. **THERAPEUTIC INTERVENTIONS** • Provide explanation of disease process, hospitalization, treatments as often as necessary. • Allow time for feedback and further questioning. • Refer family to local chapter of the Reye's Syndrome Foundation/Na-tional Reye's Syndrome Foundation *for additional literature and poten-tial source of guidance and comfort for parents.*	Child/family will be able to verbalize understanding of disease process, treatment, and re-covery experiences.

Linda Arsenault, RN, MSN, CNRN

Seizure activity

CONVULSION; EPILEPSY; SEIZURE DISORDER

A seizure is an occasional, excessive disorderly discharge of neuronal activity. Recurrent seizures (epilepsy) may be classified as partial, generalized, or partial complex.

NURSING DIAGNOSES/ DEFINING CHARACTERISTICS	NURSING INTERVENTIONS / *RATIONALES*	EXPECTED OUTCOMES
High Risk for Injury **RELATED TO** Seizure activity Postictal state Altered level of consciousness Impaired judgment **DEFINING CHARACTERISTICS** Increased rhythmic motor activity— jerking of arms and legs Repetitive psychomotor activity Tonic-clonic movements Change in alertness, orientation, verbal response, eye opening, motor response Aspiration of oral secretions	**ONGOING ASSESSMENT** • Assess age and developmental level. • Assess frequency, duration, and type of seizure activity. • Note the following: Change in LOC Child's preceding seizure activity Where seizure started Epileptic cry Automatism Length of seizure Head and eye turning Pupillary reaction Associated falls Foam from mouth Urinary or fecal incontinence Cyanosis Postictal state Any postseizure focal abnormality (e.g., Todd's paralysis) **THERAPEUTIC INTERVENTIONS** • Document observations and frequency of seizures; notify physician as indicated. • Roll child to side following cessation of muscle twitching. • If child is in bed: Pad side rails. Remove sharp objects from bed. Keep bed in low position. • If child is on floor, remove furniture or other potentially harmful objects from area. • Do not restrain. *Physical restraint applied during seizure activity can cause pathogenic trauma.* • Allow child to have seizure. Do not place tongue blade or other objects in mouth. • If airway is occluded, open airway, then insert oral airway.	Potential for physical injury will be reduced.
Health Maintenance **RELATED TO** Perceptual and/or cognitive impairment Lack of fine motor ability Lack of material resources Physiologic derangement	**ONGOING ASSESSMENT** • Assess perceptual and cognitive abilities. • Note alterations in fine motor ability. • Inquire as to material resources that would influence ability to obtain medications—money or transportation. • Assess for presence/history of prolonged vomiting. • Monitor blood levels of anticonvulsant. **THERAPEUTIC INTERVENTIONS** • Administer anticonvulsant as ordered during hospitalization. • Suggest alternate routes if child is vomiting. • Involve parent, significant others/friends/social support in solving home care needs, where appropriate. • Consult social service as appropriate. *May be helpful in securing transportation or in application for financial assistance necessary for compliance.*	Therapeutic level of anticonvulsant will be maintained.

NURSING DIAGNOSES/ DEFINING CHARACTERISTICS	NURSING INTERVENTIONS / *RATIONALES*	EXPECTED OUTCOMES
DEFINING CHARACTERISTICS Inadequate serum anticonvulsant levels (below therapeutic range) Oral intake altered to the degree of affecting medication intake Vomiting Demonstrated inability to take or obtain medications		
High Risk for Disturbance in Self-Esteem **RELATED TO** Seizure activity Dependence on medications **DEFINING CHARACTERISTICS** Nonparticipation in therapy Lack of responsibility for self-care Self-destructive behavior Lack of eye contact	**ONGOING ASSESSMENT** ▪ Assess child's feelings about self and disorder. ▪ Assess perceived implications of disorder and need for long-term therapy. **THERAPEUTIC INTERVENTIONS** ▪ Encourage ventilation of feelings. ▪ Incorporate family and significant others in care plan. *May be helpful in assisting/giving support.* ▪ Assist child and others in understanding nature of disorder. ▪ Dispel common myths and fears about convulsive disorders.	Effect of consulvant disorder on self-esteem will be reduced.

Knowledge Deficit
RELATED TO
 	
Lack of exposure
Information misinterpretation
Unfamiliarity with information resources
 	
DEFINING CHARACTERISTICS
 	
Verbalization of problem
Inappropriate or exaggerated behavior
Request for information
Statement of misconception
	ONGOING ASSESSMENT
	▪ Assess child's/family's knowledge concerning disorder and treatment.
	▪ Assess readiness for learning, *so that information is presented at a time when comprehension will be optimal for child and parent.*
	
	THERAPEUTIC INTERVENTIONS
	▪ Discuss disease process.
	▪ Review with child and parent need for medication and schedule:
	    Right medication at right time and dosage
	    Drug levels
	    Danger of seizure activity with abrupt withdrawal
	    Possible side effects and interactions of medication
	▪ Educate about safety measures:
	    Diving
	    Swimming with companion
	    Driving (as adolescent reaches appropriate age)
	    Medic-Alert tag
	    Home safety
	▪ Refer to Epilepsy Foundation of America, Landover, MD 20785.
		Child and/or parent will understand and be able to verbalize the disorder process, treatment, and safety measures.

Caramen E. Billheimer, RN, BSN

Status epilepticus

Recurrent seizures that fail to allow recovery from previous seizure and in which the level of consciousness is not regained, or a series of seizures that last longer than 30 minutes. Status epilepticus is a medical emergency, with mortality ranging from 6% to 30% and high morbidity, both of which are duration dependent; therefore, prompt intervention is imperative. Factors that contribute to high morbidity are hypoxia, fractures, aspiration, cardiac dysrhythmias, and acidosis.

NURSING DIAGNOSES/ DEFINING CHARACTERISTICS	NURSING INTERVENTIONS / *RATIONALES*	EXPECTED OUTCOMES

Impaired Gas Exchange **Related To** Aspiration related to prolonged seizure activity Hypoxia during seizure activity Hypoventilation secondary to prolonged muscle contraction **Defining Characteristics** Increased secretions Grunting Tachypnea Irregular respirations Choking Dyspnea Cyanosis	**Ongoing Assessment**
	• Assess age and developmental level.
	• Assess respirations during and after seizure activity.
	• Monitor child for presence of any of the defining characteristics during and after seizure activity.
	• Monitor arterial blood gases as indicated.
	• Monitor breath sounds hourly as indicated.
	• Monitor closely during administration of medications to halt seizures. *Most common side effects are depressed respirations, apnea, hypotension. The combination of prolonged seizure activity and the administration of medications intravenously to stop them may precipitate sudden respiratory failure and necessitate rapid intubation.*
	• Monitor ECG as needed.
	
	Therapeutic Interventions
	• During seizure:
	  Stay with the child.
	  Loosen clothing.
	  Try to roll child onto a side-lying position *to facilitate drainage of secretions.*
	  Administer oxygen if necessary.
	  Suction as indicated.
	  Assist with intubation.
	  Apply pulse oximeter if possible.
	• Administer medications to stop seizures as ordered. The following medications are generally used:
	  Lorazepam (Ativan) 0.05 mg/kg IV over 2 min; may be repeated every 2-3 min × 3 doses total.
	  Diazepam (Valium) 0.2-0.5 mg/kg/dose/min with maximum of 5 mg if <5 years old; maximum 10 mg if >5 years old.
	  Simultaneous administration of phenytoin (Dilantin): 18 mg/kg at no faster than 50 mg/min in saline solution. *Dilantin will precipitate in any dextrose solution.*
	  Alternate medication to phenytoin is phenobarbital 5-10 mg/kg every 20-30 min to maximum dose of 30-40 mg/kg.
	  If seizures persist, anticipate need for a general inhalation anesthetic agent.
	  Additional medications that may be used:
	    Lidocaine, valproic acid, and carbamazepine (Tegretol)
	    For neonates: glucose, pyridoxine, calcium gluconate, magnesium sulfate
		Adequate ventilation and oxygenation will be maintained.

NURSING DIAGNOSES/ DEFINING CHARACTERISTICS	NURSING INTERVENTIONS / *RATIONALES*	EXPECTED OUTCOMES

High Risk for Injury from Fall: Lacerations, Abrasions, Fractures **RELATED TO** Seizures with impaired level of consciousness Prolonged involuntary muscle contractions **DEFINING CHARACTERISTICS** Fall Bruises on body Swelling skin areas Abrasions Lacerations	**ONGOING ASSESSMENT**
	 • Assess child for presence of any of the defining characteristics.
	 • Observe child for details of seizure:
	   Duration
	   Types of movement
	   Respiratory distress
	   Incontinence
	   Sleep between seizures
	   Length of time between seizures
	   Frequency
	 • Monitor respirations and vital signs closely.
	 • Evaluate child's ability to move all extremities without evidence of abnormal movement/pain, which may be related to a fracture.
	
	 THERAPEUTIC INTERVENTIONS
	 • Remain with child.
	 • Do not attempt to restrain child or use force.
	 • Protect child's head from injury, e.g., place on folded blanket, your lap, flat pillow.
	 • Keep side rails up and padded if child is in bed.
	 • Move any sharp objects or furniture away from child.
	 • Do not place anything into child's mouth.
		Absence of injury to child during seizures will be attained.

Altered Tissue Perfusion: Cerebral **RELATED TO** Cerebral hypoxia secondary to prolonged seizure activity Cerebral edema **DEFINING CHARACTERISTICS** Impaired LOC Confusion, disorientation Impaired memory, judgment, speech Glasgow Coma Scale <11 Motor-sensory impairment Incontinence Pupillary asymmetry, dilation, decreased light activity Gaze preference	**ONGOING ASSESSMENT**
	 • Assess child once seizure activity has ceased for:
	   Level of orientation
	   Memory, judgment
	   Speech appropriateness
	   Motor-sensory integrity
	   Incontinence
	   Glasgow Coma score
	   Pupillary size, reaction to light
	 • Monitor child throughout for signs of cyanosis, emesis, respiratory difficulties.
	 • Monitor arterial blood gases.
	
	 THERAPEUTIC INTERVENTIONS
	 • Remain with child.
	 • Turn onto side with head down *to promote drainage of secretions and maintain open airway*.
	 • Remove restrictive clothing.
	 • Support head.
	 • Suction as needed.
	 • Provide oxygen as indicated.
		Optimal cerebral perfusion will be maintained.

Linda Arsenault, RN, MSN, CNRN

Toxic ingestion

POISONING; DRUG OVERDOSE

Toxic ingestion refers to the accidental or purposeful consumption of potentially life-threatening substances. Older infants test their environment by putting things in their mouths. Toddlers mistake medications for food or candy, and while accidents occur with older children and adolescents, these age groups are capable of purposeful self-harm.

NURSING DIAGNOSES/ DEFINING CHARACTERISTICS	NURSING INTERVENTIONS / *RATIONALES*	EXPECTED OUTCOMES

High Risk for Injury: Self

RELATED TO

Accidental or intentional ingestion of potentially life-threatening substance

DEFINING CHARACTERISTICS

Decreased LOC
Cardiac disturbance
Tachypnea
Dyspnea
Respiratory failure
Abdominal pain
Decreased urinary output
Hypotension or hypertension

ONGOING ASSESSMENT

- Assess age and developmental level.
- Monitor vital signs.
- Elicit circumstances of ingestion from child or family.
- Elicit initial symptoms of ingestion.
- Assess time of onset, estimated time of ingestion.
- Assess prior attempts at treatment.
- Assess type and amount of drug ingested:
    Send blood and urine for toxicology screening immediately.
    Ask for empty bottles left nearby; question whether any drugs are missing from home.
    Ask if child is taking any prescription drugs and, if so, what type.
    Evaluate the possibility of street drug use.
- Monitor I&O.
- Obtain child's age and weight.
- Repeat screening of urine/blood toxicology levels as needed.
- Monitor ABGs.

THERAPEUTIC INTERVENTIONS

- Place child on cardiopulmonary monitor.
- Prepare for emergent intubation.
- Induce emesis as ordered:
    Do not attempt if child is convulsing or if neurological status is significantly depressed.
    Do not induce vomiting if ingested substance is caustic.
    Provide ipecac, as ordered, for emesis induction.
    Provide abundant clear liquids if ipecac is given.
- Provide gastric lavage as ordered (*effective in child with significantly depressed level of consciousness; is method of choice if ingested substance is caustic*):
    Attempt nasogastric insertion after checking gag reflex; if sluggish, child should be intubated first.
    Provide appropriate-sized nasogastric tube; check for placement before beginning lavage.
- Administer absorption-inhibiting medications, as ordered and as appropriate for type of ingestion, at safe dosage for child's age and weight:
    Administer activated charcoal within 1 hour of aspirin ingestion.
    Administer acetylcysteine (Mucomyst) every 4 hours for 24 hours if patient has ingested acetaminophen.
- Promote catharsis as ordered (unless neurologically contraindicated) *to decrease amount of substance absorbed in the gut*:
    Provide medications as ordered: *drug of choice is magnesium sulfate solution.*
    Tell child and parent to expect abdominal cramping, diarrhea-like syndromes.
    Provide privacy, bedpan, cleaning materials.
    Assist as needed.
- Promote diuresis as ordered *to enhance renal excretion of toxic substance:*
    Push oral fluids if child is alert.
    Maintain IV fluids if LOC is depressed (usually 1-1½ times maintenance fluid required for weight).
    Assist with bedpan/urinal.
    Catheterize if necessary.

Risk of further injury will be reduced.

NURSING DIAGNOSES/ DEFINING CHARACTERISTICS	NURSING INTERVENTIONS / *RATIONALES*	EXPECTED OUTCOMES
	THERAPEUTIC INTERVENTIONS cont'd ▪ If substance ingested is renal-toxic, another method of elimination should be considered, such as peritoneal lavage or hemodialysis. *Hypertension and decreasing urine output may indicate kidney failure.*	

High Risk for Altered Tissue Perfusion: Cardiopulmonary
RELATED TO
Drug ingestion:
  Street drugs
  Over-the-counter medications
  Psychotropic medications
  Seizure-controlling medications
  Other poisonous substances
 	
DEFINING CHARACTERISTICS
Change in LOC
Hyperventilation or hypoventilation
Tachycardia and hypertension
Bradycardia and hypotension
	ONGOING ASSESSMENT
	▪ Assess respiratory function: rate and pattern, airway, lung sounds.
	▪ Assess cardiac function: rate, rhythm, and BP. *Most drug overdoses cause cardiac and respiratory depression. The ingestion of a corrosive material may cause an acute obstruction, necessitating emergency tracheostomy and intubation.*
	
	THERAPEUTIC INTERVENTIONS
	▪ Place child on cardiopulmonary monitor.
	▪ Prepare for intubation and mechanical ventilation.
	▪ Place patient in semi-Fowler's position *to assist in lung expansion and avoid aspiration if vomiting occurs.*
	▪ Administer oxygen as necessary. Keep Ambu bag at bedside.
	▪ Maintain quiet environment.
	▪ Notify physician of changes in vital signs.
		Respiratory function will be maintained.

Altered Levels of Consciousness
RELATED TO
Toxic levels of ingested drugs
 	
DEFINING CHARACTERISTICS
Restlessness
Delirium
Convulsions
Marked constriction or dilation of pupils
Lethargy, confusion, disorientation
Coma (likely with ingestion of salicylate, sedatives, narcotics, narcotic-like drugs, and anticholinergic and cholinergic agents)
	ONGOING ASSESSMENT
	▪ Assess neurological status every 2 hours, including:
	  LOC
	  Pupil size and reactivity
	  Visual acuity
	  Muscle strength
	  Behavioral changes, irritability
	  Headache
	  Response to stimuli
	  Orientation
	  Tinnitus
	
	THERAPEUTIC INTERVENTIONS
	▪ Avoid excessive stimulation by:
	  Dimming lights
	  Limiting visitors
	  Maintaining quiet environment
	▪ Provide seizure precautions:
	  Keep side rails up at all times; pad if necessary.
	  Keep bed in lowest position.
	  Keep head of bed slightly elevated.
	▪ Record responses to questions. *These may be useful later during psychiatric evaluation.*
	▪ Reorient child to environment as needed.
	▪ Provide antidote or perform procedures (lavage, dialysis) *that will decrease amount of drug available to circulation.*
		Consciousness will be maintained.

Continued.

205

Toxic ingestion cont'd

NURSING DIAGNOSES/ DEFINING CHARACTERISTICS	NURSING INTERVENTIONS / *RATIONALES*	EXPECTED OUTCOMES
High Risk for Fluid Volume Deficit **RELATED TO** Side effects of ingested toxins or of treatment modalities Decreased fluid intake **DEFINING CHARACTERISTICS** Tachycardia Hypotension Decreased urine output Increased urine specific gravity Elevated serum Na Dry mucous membranes Weakness	**ONGOING ASSESSMENT** • Assess level of hydration every 2 hours: Urine specific gravity Urine pH Skin turgor Mucous membranes I&O • Assess vital signs every 2 hours. • Monitor for nausea and vomiting. • Measure and record type of emesis. • Check laboratory values: CBC Electrolytes Toxicology levels **THERAPEUTIC INTERVENTIONS** • Maintain fluid intake (oral if possible) or IV fluids as ordered *to prevent circulatory collapse. Plasma or blood may be required if patient is severely dehydrated and/or losing blood in emesis/stool.*	Risk of fluid volume deficit will be reduced.
Ineffective Family Coping **RELATED TO** Temporary family separation/disorganization Situational crisis Attempted suicide of family member New awareness of drug use/addictions of family member **DEFINING CHARACTERISTICS** Verbalizes inadequate understanding of situation Displays inappropriate or overly protective behaviors Appears withdrawn Appears preoccupied with personal guilt, fears, and grief	**ONGOING ASSESSMENT** • Assess family's immediate understanding of child's situation/physical status. • Assess available coping mechanisms and supports. **THERAPEUTIC INTERVENTIONS** • Provide family with support personnel, clergy, ombudsman, volunteer, psychiatric nurse liaison, physician. • Keep family informed of child's status and of care being provided *to decrease fear and anxiety and increase understanding of situation.* • Allow visitation as soon as possible. • Provide privacy during discussion of further treatment, hospitalization. • Support family's use of adaptive coping mechanisms.	Anxiety/fear will be reduced.

NURSING DIAGNOSES/ DEFINING CHARACTERISTICS	NURSING INTERVENTIONS / *RATIONALES*	EXPECTED OUTCOMES
Ineffective Individual Coping **RELATED TO** Circumstances of intentional ingestion: Suicide attempt Suicide gesture **DEFINING CHARACTERISTICS** Suicidal ideation Depression Behavior changes	**ONGOING ASSESSMENT** ▪ Assess type and amount of chemical ingested; *this may indicate an intentional vs. accidental ingestion.* ▪ Assess previous behaviors and relationships. ▪ Assess current coping mechanisms if possible. ▪ Assess developmental level. **THERAPEUTIC INTERVENTIONS** ▪ Provide a safe, structured environment, especially after initial physical crisis is resolved. ▪ Provide a sitter if suicide is suspected, or transfer to psychiatric unit if possible. ▪ Allow expression of feelings and concerns. ▪ Obtain psychiatric consultation. *Intentional ingestion is suggestive of psychiatric illness, and counseling should be initiated before discharge.*	Anxiety/fear will be reduced.
Knowledge Deficit **RELATED TO** Circumstances of accidental poisoning: Medications unlabeled; misunderstanding of label or directions Unable to read instructions Harmful substance within reach of child Lack of knowledge of: Prevention Emergency treatment Follow-up treatment **DEFINING CHARACTERISTICS** Verbalized lack of knowledge or ability by child or family Demonstrated threat to self	**ONGOING ASSESSMENT** ▪ Assess current level of understanding. ▪ Assess cognitive abilities. **THERAPEUTIC INTERVENTIONS** ▪ Provide information at a level and in the manner that comprehension will best be achieved. ▪ Initiate home/discharge teaching after crisis is resolved. ▪ Provide information on prevention/safety. ▪ Provide consults and follow-up as appropriate. ▪ If abuse or neglect is suspected, contact proper authorities. Consult social services before discharge. ▪ See Child abuse, p. 48.	Patient will verbalize understanding.

Janet L. McCants, RN, BSN; Michele Knoll Puzas, RNC, MHPE

Bacterial meningitis, acute

SPINAL INFECTION

Inflammation of the membranes of the spinal cord and/or brain, caused by a bacterial infection. It is a potentially fatal disease that demands early diagnosis and prompt intervention to avoid severe neurological sequelae. Onset can be early (less than 7 days after birth) or late (more than 7 days after birth). Contributory factors of early-onset disease include complications during labor and delivery, chorioamnionitis, maternal peripartal infection, and prolonged rupture of membranes (more than 24 hours). Causative organisms are most frequently group B Streptococcus, Escherichia coli, and Listeria monocytogenes. Late-onset disease is commonly a result of contact with humans and equipment. Causative organisms include Staphylococcus aureus, S. epidermidis, and Proteus spp. Other contributing factors to both early- and late-onset disease include an immunocompromised infant and sepsis.

NURSING DIAGNOSES/ DEFINING CHARACTERISTICS	NURSING INTERVENTIONS / *RATIONALES*	EXPECTED OUTCOMES
High Risk for Decreased Level of Consciousness **RELATED TO** Inflammation of the meninges secondary to bacterial infection **DEFINING CHARACTERISTICS** Lethargy Irritability Seizures Nuchal rigidity Bulging anterior fontanel High-pitched cry Temperature instability Poor feeding Increasing blood pressure Pupillary changes	**ONGOING ASSESSMENT** • Perform and document neurological check every 2 hours: Monitor activity level. Monitor neuromuscular tone. Monitor seizure activity. Check whether pupils are equal, round, and respond to light and accommodation. Evaluate pitch of cry. • Obtain laboratory work as needed *to document diagnosis of bacterial meningitis:* CBC with platelets Blood cultures and sensitivities Blood glucose—draw blood glucose just prior to lumbar puncture *because CSF glucose is normally ½ to ⅔ of the serum glucose* Lumbar puncture (cerebrospinal fluid for protein, glucose, cell count, and culture and sensitivity) • Measure and record daily weights, head circumference, and size of anterior fontanel. *Hydrocephalus can be a complication of meningitis.* • Observe for symptoms of increased intracranial pressure: Bulging anterior fontanel Split cranial sutures Vomiting Irritability **THERAPEUTIC INTERVENTIONS** • Report significant change from baseline data, *since neurological status and intracranial pressure can change quickly in patients with meningitis.* • See Seizures, p. 214. • Practice careful handwashing *to prevent spread of infection.* • Assist with lumbar puncture. • Administer prescribed antibiotics immediately after cultures are obtained. *Prompt administration of antibiotics will lessen the incidence of complications by eliminating the causative organism:* Verify that antibiotic dosage is appropriate for the baby's weight and age. Maintain parenteral fluids at a restricted volume as ordered *to minimize the development of cerebral edema.*	Altered level of consciousness will be reduced.

NURSING DIAGNOSES/ DEFINING CHARACTERISTICS	NURSING INTERVENTIONS / *RATIONALES*	EXPECTED OUTCOMES
High Risk for Fluid Volume Excess **RELATED TO** Syndrome of inappropriate antidiuretic hormone secretion (SIADH) **DEFINING CHARACTERISTICS** Oliguria Increased specific gravity Hypoosmolarity Hyponatremia Weight gain Edema Low hematocrit Low total serum solute	**ONGOING ASSESSMENT** • Obtain laboratory work as needed to document the presence of SIADH. *SIADH results in concentrated urine, and electrolyte and fluid imbalance:* Monitor urine specific gravity and I&O. Monitor serum and urine electrolytes and osmolarity. Check hematocrit level and total serum solutes. • Weigh infant daily. • Note presence of edema. **THERAPEUTIC INTERVENTIONS** • Notify physician if specific gravity is <1.012 or urine output is <2 ml/ kg/hr. *Meningitis is associated with SIADH; therefore fluid may be retained.* • Notify physician of a hematocrit level below 40% and total serum solutes below 4. • Maintain fluids at restricted volume as ordered *to decrease overall circulating volume.* • If edema is present, change child's position frequently and institute antipressure devices.	Risk for fluid volume excess will be reduced.
Ineffective Breathing Pattern **RELATED TO** Infection **DEFINING CHARACTERISTICS** Periodic breathing Apnea Cyanosis Tachycardia Bradycardia	**ONGOING ASSESSMENT** • Assess respiratory status. Observe and document episodes of apnea, bradycardia, and cyanosis. *Increasing episodes of apnea and bradycardia suggest a possibility of severe infection or CNS complication.* **THERAPEUTIC INTERVENTIONS** • Institute cardiorespiratory monitoring. • Maintain ventilation as ordered. • Suction as necessary *to maintain patent airway.* • Provide appropriate resuscitation if necessary *to prevent further respiratory failure.* • See Ineffective breathing pattern, p. 8.	Optimal breathing pattern will be achieved.
Altered Nutrition: Less Than Body Requirements **RELATED TO** Feeding intolerance secondary to illness Poor suck Vomiting Abdominal distention **DEFINING CHARACTERISTICS** Lack of interest in feeding Loss of weight with or without adequate caloric intake Documented inadequate caloric intake	**ONGOING ASSESSMENT** • Assess ability to tolerate feedings. • Monitor I&O. Calculate volume and calories received (kilograms per day). • Report increased abdominal girth, vomiting, or gastric residual. *These may be signs of feeding intolerance.* • Weigh daily and record *to document adequate caloric intake needed to facilitate growth.* **THERAPEUTIC INTERVENTIONS** • Administer parenteral fluids as prescribed *to provide infant with appropriate volume and calories per day to supplement or replace feedings. Fluids may be restricted to minimize the risks of cerebral edema and manage SIADH.* • Advance feedings as tolerated. *Absorption is altered in infants with an infection.*	Adequate caloric intake will be achieved.

Continued.

Bacterial meningitis, acute cont'd

NURSING DIAGNOSES/ DEFINING CHARACTERISTICS	NURSING INTERVENTIONS / *RATIONALES*	EXPECTED OUTCOMES
Altered Parenting **RELATED TO** Separation/hospitalization of neonate Fear and anxiety about abruptness and severity of illness Knowledge deficit regarding parental role **DEFINING CHARACTERISTICS** Verbal/nonverbal expressions of fear and anxiety with intensive care environment Self-blame for infant's condition Feelings of guilt for having a "less than perfect" child are verbalized Disbelief Lack of or inappropriate response to infant	**ONGOING ASSESSMENT** • Assess for presence of defining characteristics. **THERAPEUTIC INTERVENTIONS** • See Parenting in special care nursery, p. 72.	Parent/infant bonding will be initiated.

Herminia Inawat, RN

Hydrocephalus

A pathological enlargement of the cranium, caused by an obstruction of the cerebrospinal fluid (CSF) pathway. Obstructions occurring in the subarachnoid space are called communicating; obstructions found in the aqueduct of Sylvius are called noncommunicating.

NURSING DIAGNOSES/ DEFINING CHARACTERISTICS	NURSING INTERVENTIONS / *RATIONALES*	EXPECTED OUTCOMES
High Risk for Neurological Impairment **RELATED TO** Increased intracranial pressure Intracranial bleeding	**ONGOING ASSESSMENT** • Assess for clinical status using defining characteristics. • Assess respiratory and cardiac status every 1-2 hours. • Measure head circumference daily. • Monitor infant during CT scan procedures. *This is a very reliable diagnostic test for detection of ventricular enlargement.* • Assist aseptically with serial lumbar punctures, *which are done to drain cerebrospinal fluid in communicating hydrocephalus.*	Impairment of neurological function will be reduced.

NURSING DIAGNOSES/ DEFINING CHARACTERISTICS	NURSING INTERVENTIONS / *RATIONALES*	EXPECTED OUTCOMES

DEFINING CHARACTERISTICS

Rapidly increasing head circumference
Fontanels become tense and bulging
Transillumination of skull
Dilated scalp veins
Irritability
Lethargy
Sunset eyes
Vomiting
Bradycardia

THERAPEUTIC INTERVENTIONS

- Use the growth chart for plotting the daily head circumference *to determine whether excessive growth is occurring.*
- Notify physician if signs and symptoms of increased intracranial pressure are observed. *This is caused by the blockage or increased volume of CSF in the head.*
- Support head and neck when moving or lifting infant.
- Position infant on side or prone, *so that head does not fall forward, obstructing airway.*
- Give acetazolamide (Diamox) as ordered *to decrease CSF production.*

High Risk for Impaired Skin Integrity

RELATED TO

Increased size and weight of head
Decreased movement of head
Increased movement of extremities resulting from irritability

DEFINING CHARACTERISTICS

Skin breakdown
Reddened areas over bony prominences
Friction burns of exposed extremities

ONGOING ASSESSMENT

- Assess skin integrity using defining characteristics.
- Assess environment for any potential source of pressure or trauma.

THERAPEUTIC INTERVENTIONS

- Use sheepskin or Eggcrate mattress under infant *to help prevent pressure points and skin breakdown.*
- Massage with lotion over bony prominences every 2 to 4 hours *to improve circulation.*
- Reposition gently every 2-4 hours *to redistribute pressure.*
- See Skin integrity, impaired, high risk for, p. 41.

Skin breakdown will be prevented.

High Risk for Fluid Volume Deficit

RELATED TO

Feeding intolerance resulting from increasing intracranial pressure

DEFINING CHARACTERISTICS

Anorexia
Vomiting with feedings
Electrolyte imbalance
Poor skin turgor
Weight loss or minimal weight gain
Lethargy
Poor perfusion
Hypotension
Increased heart rate

ONGOING ASSESSMENT

- Assess weight pattern. Weigh daily. *Excessive weight loss is a symptom of dehydration.*
- Observe skin turgor.
- Assess I&O status. *Urine output should be 1 to 2 ml/kg/hr.*
- Assess nature and amount of secretions.
- Monitor vital signs, including BP, every 2-4 hours.
- Check urine specific gravity every 4-8 hours. *This should range between 1.006 and 1.008.*
- Monitor serum electrolytes every 24-48 hours or prn.
- Determine appropriate feeding route based on:
  Gestational age
  Sensitivity of gag reflex
  Level of irritability
  Respiratory rate
  Level of activity/alertness
- Assess infant's ability to tolerate feedings:
  Observe for vomiting.
  Observe amount of residual contents per nasogastric tube before feedings.
  Measure abdominal circumference *to assess for distention.*

Nutritional/fluid deficit will be reduced.

Continued.

Neurological Care Plans (Neonatal)

NURSING DIAGNOSES/ DEFINING CHARACTERISTICS	NURSING INTERVENTIONS / *RATIONALES*	EXPECTED OUTCOMES

DEFINING CHARACTERISTICS cont'd
Decreased urine output
Increased specific gravity
	THERAPEUTIC INTERVENTIONS
	• Encourage oral feedings when appropriate, using the following criteria:
	    Gestational age of 32 weeks or more
	    Respiratory rate of 40-60/min
	    Tolerance of 5-10 ml at first feeding
	    Progressive weight gain of 10-20 g daily
	• Offer pacifier with nasogastric feedings *to satisfy sucking reflex.*
	• Hold feedings and notify physician if residual content is 3-4 ml or more, *because large amounts are a symptom of feeding intolerance.*
	• Keep infant's head slightly elevated after feedings *to facilitate digestion and minimize regurgitation.*
	• Adjust IV or feedings to provide 80-100 ml/kg/day on the first day of life; 100-120 ml/kg/day thereafter. An additional 10% to 20% may need to be added based on the degree of insensible water loss or dehydration. *(Desired caloric intake for growth is 100-120 cal/kg/day.)*	

Body Temperature: High Risk for Hypothermia **RELATED TO** Increased body surface area Reduced glycogen and brown fat stores Compromised neurological function secondary to increasing intracranial pressure **DEFINING CHARACTERISTICS** Body temperature less than 36.5° C (97.7° F) Pallor or duskiness Lethargy Apnea Bradycardia CO_2 retention Weight loss Low glucose levels	**ONGOING ASSESSMENT** • Assess infant using defining characteristics. • Assess environment for potential causes for hypothermia. • Review laboratory data to identify possible systemic sources of hypothermia. • Monitor blood gases prn. • Monitor glucose levels. **THERAPEUTIC INTERVENTIONS** • Cover head if possible *to minimize heat loss.* • Use isolette or radiant heater if necessary *to control environmental temperature.* • Notify physician of abnormal blood gas results. *The consequences of hypothermia include acidotic states and increased oxygen needs.* • Notify physician of glucose levels less than 40, *because hypoglycemia can result from increased use of carbohydrate stores in an effort to maintain temperature between 36.5° C and 37.5° C (97.7° F and 99.5° F).* • See Thermoregulation in the low-birth-weight infant, p. 379.	Risk for hypothermia will be reduced.
High Risk for Infection **RELATED TO** Surgical procedure to insert ventriculoperitoneal shunt **DEFINING CHARACTERISTICS** Inflammation of and/ or drainage at shunt site	**ONGOING ASSESSMENT** • Assess head, abdominal, and chest dressings for moisture or drainage. • Administer culture tests to suspicious drainage. • Assess vital signs with temperature every 1-2 hours. • Monitor CBC. **THERAPEUTIC INTERVENTIONS** • Notify physician of leakage of CSF. • Administer antibiotics as ordered and follow antibiotic level results *to prevent subtherapeutic or toxic levels.* • Use strict aseptic technique when changing surgical dressing *to help prevent infections.*	Risk for infection will be reduced.

NURSING DIAGNOSES/ DEFINING CHARACTERISTICS	NURSING INTERVENTIONS / *RATIONALES*	EXPECTED OUTCOMES
DEFINING CHARACTERISTICS cont'd Leakage of cerebro-spinal fluid Increased or decreased WBC count Temperature instability Pallor		
High Risk for Injury **RELATED TO** Malfunctioning of ventriculoperitoneal shunt **DEFINING CHARACTERISTICS** Increasing head circumference High-pitched cry Full and/or tense fontanels Irritability Vomiting Poor feeder Sutures more separated	**ONGOING ASSESSMENT** ▪ Assess neurological functioning using defining characteristics. ▪ Measure head circumference daily. ▪ Observe and record characteristics of fontanels. ▪ Weigh daily, *since shunts in infants are revised as their growth proceeds.* **THERAPEUTIC INTERVENTIONS** ▪ Notify physician if signs of defining characteristics are present, *since this could indicate shunt failure.*	Potential for injury will be reduced.

High Risk for Altered Parenting
RELATED TO
 	
Fear of infant's response to parents' handling
Depression over prognosis
Anxiety about how others will view parents and their infant
 	
DEFINING CHARACTERISTICS
 	
Inconsistency or disinterest in visiting or calling
Disinterest or uneasiness in handling infant
Nonverbal/verbal expression of concern for infant's condition
Guilt, hostility, or suspicion
	ONGOING ASSESSMENT
	▪ Observe frequency of visits or calls.
	▪ Observe parents' interaction with infant.
	▪ Assess developmental stages of parents.
	▪ Assess support system of parents:
	    Family members
	    Friends
	    Religious beliefs
	▪ Assess emotional response of parents to the reason for the infant's hospitalization.
	
	THERAPEUTIC INTERVENTIONS
	▪ Initiate calls to parents if necessary and encourage them to visit. *Contact with the infant is important in establishing bonding.*
	▪ Encourage parents to hold the infant and do as much of the care as possible.
	▪ Encourage parents to express their feelings regarding the infant's condition.
	▪ Stress the positive aspects of the infant's condition.
	▪ See Parenting in special care nursery, p. 72.
		Initiation and development of parent-infant bonding will be achieved.

Continued.

Hydrocephalus cont'd

NURSING DIAGNOSES/ DEFINING CHARACTERISTICS	NURSING INTERVENTIONS / *RATIONALES*	EXPECTED OUTCOMES
High Risk for Parental Knowledge Deficit Related to Infant's Condition **RELATED TO** Denial Unfamiliarity with terms Inability to comprehend explanations **DEFINING CHARACTERISTICS** Inappropriate or negative questions Hostility or suspicion toward staff Anxiety Disbelief or denial	**ONGOING ASSESSMENT** • Observe attitude of parents as expressed by comments and behavior. • Assess the level of parents' knowledge as expressed by the appropriateness of their questions. • Observe parents' reactions to changes in infant's condition or treatment. **THERAPEUTIC INTERVENTIONS** • Encourage parents to discuss their feelings and concerns regarding infant and his or her condition. • Offer information and ask for feedback regarding: Baby's condition Unit policies Roles/responsibilities of unit personnel; *asking parents to verbalize this information and to give feedback allows the nurse to assess how well they have understood*	Knowledge deficit will be reduced.

Christine Todd, RN, BS, BGS

Seizures

CONVULSIONS; TONIC-CLONIC SEIZURES; FOCAL CLONIC SEIZURES

Involuntary muscle motion, usually in the form of contractions, but may be loss of tone. Most often seizures in the newborn period are the result of a very significant brain insult. Common causes for neonatal seizures include perinatal asphyxia, intracranial hemorrhage, congenital infections, inherited metabolic conditions, drug withdrawal or drug overdosage problems, kernicterus, specific nongenetic syndromes, and congenital malformations.

NURSING DIAGNOSES/ DEFINING CHARACTERISTICS	NURSING INTERVENTIONS / *RATIONALES*	EXPECTED OUTCOMES
Altered Levels of Consciousness **RELATED TO** Seizure **DEFINING CHARACTERISTICS** Apnea or transient alteration in respiration Sudden eye opening or eye blinking Vasomotor movements like chewing and sucking Tonic-clonic movement Limpness Facial twitching	**ONGOING ASSESSMENT** • Verify seizure activity, using defining characteristics—note location, activity involved, duration, and effect on infant. • Monitor vital signs and neurological status every 2 hours. • Monitor calcium level every 12 hours. • Monitor Chemstrip every 2-4 hours. • Monitor hematocrit every 12 hours. • Assess abnormal respiratory patterns and periods of apnea. • Assess for bradycardia episodes. • Obtain blood culture results. *Antibiotic therapy is needed if infection is bacterial.* • Assist in completing diagnostic workup as ordered: Blood culture *needed to rule out infection as cause of seizure* Lumbar puncture *to rule out infection and hemorrhage as cause of seizure* CBC *to rule out infection and hemorrhage* Electroencephalogram *will help establish diagnosis, evaluate focality, determine cause and prognosis* Skull films	Episodes of seizures will be reduced.

NURSING DIAGNOSES/ DEFINING CHARACTERISTICS	NURSING INTERVENTIONS / *RATIONALES*	EXPECTED OUTCOMES

DEFINING CHARACTERISTICS cont'd
 	
Abnormal cry
Drooling
Bicycle-like movements
Agitation
Changes in alertness
Rhythmic fluctuations in vital signs and degree of oxygenation
	ONGOING ASSESSMENT cont'd
	  Transillumination
	  TORCH titers from mother and infant (toxoplasmosis, rubella, cytomegalovirus, and herpes simplex)
	  Ultrasound and CT scan
	  Serum measurement of magnesium bicarbonate, BUN, creatinine, bilirubin, and NH_3 levels
	
	THERAPEUTIC INTERVENTIONS
	• Minimize stimulation; keep handling and noise to a minimum. *Seizures may be the result of a hyperirritable central nervous system.*
	• Administer anticonvulsants as ordered. (See next nursing diagnosis, High Risk for Injury, for administration of phenobarbital and dilantin.)
	• Notify physician if calcium is <7 and correct imbalance as ordered. *Hypocalcemia can cause seizures.*
	• Notify physician if Chemstrip is <40. *Hypoglycemia can cause seizures.*
	• Notify physician if there is a significant drop from previously recorded hematocrit. *This may signify an intraventricular hemorrhage.*
	• Maintain patent airway:
	  Position infant on side or abdomen, with neck slightly hyperextended.
	  Suction secretions.
	  Assist with ventilation as needed.
	• Remove toxins if indicated by:
	  Peritoneal dialysis
	  Exchange transfusions	

High Risk for Injury RELATED TO Side effects of phenobarbital **DEFINING CHARACTERISTICS** Drowsiness Diarrhea and other GI symptoms Aggravated psychomotor seizure Hypotension Apnea	**ONGOING ASSESSMENT** • Assess for side effects and/or complications of phenobarbital administration. • Monitor serum phenobarbital level after emergency dose. Notify physician if nontherapeutic or toxic. *If toxic, hold phenobarbital dose. Therapeutic range is 15 to 30 µg/ml.* **THERAPEUTIC INTERVENTIONS** • Administer phenobarbital loading dose: 15-20 mg/kg, slow IV per physician's order. If seizures continue, give additional 5 mg/kg loading dose. • If seizures subside, maintain phenobarbital 3-5 mg/kg/24 hr IV or IM in 2 divided doses every 12 hours.	Risk of injury from side effects will be reduced.
High Risk for Injury RELATED TO Side effects of phenytoin (Dilantin) **DEFINING CHARACTERISTICS** Drowsiness Nausea and vomiting Hypotension Hypotonia Gastritis Liver damage Cardiovascular collapse	**ONGOING ASSESSMENT** • Assess for side effects and/or complications of phenytoin therapy. • Monitor phenytoin level after emergency dose and notify physician of nontherapeutic or toxic level. *Therapeutic level is 10 to 20 µg/ml peak.* **THERAPEUTIC INTERVENTIONS** • Administer loading dose of 15 to 20 mg/kg in normal saline (over 30 minutes) per physician's orders, and give maintenance dose of 5 to 8 mg/kg/24 hr as ordered.	Risk of injury from side effects will be reduced.

Continued.

Neurological Care Plans (Neonatal)

NURSING DIAGNOSES/ DEFINING CHARACTERISTICS	NURSING INTERVENTIONS / *RATIONALES*	EXPECTED OUTCOMES
Altered Nutrition: Less Than Body Requirements **RELATED TO** Inability to nipple food (poor suck and swallow reflex, inability to keep tongue down) **DEFINING CHARACTERISTICS** Loss of weight Documented inadequate caloric intake	**ONGOING ASSESSMENT** ▪ Assess nutritional needs. ▪ Determine need for nipple or nasogastric feeding. ▪ Monitor weight every 24 hours. ▪ Monitor I&O. ▪ Establish degree of wakefulness. *Infant may need readjustment in medication, i.e., phenobarbital/phenytoin.* ▪ Observe for abdominal distention and vomiting. Report any of these occurrences to physician. ▪ Observe respiratory and neurological status during feeding. **THERAPEUTIC INTERVENTIONS** ▪ Administer parenteral fluids as prescribed *to provide appropriate volume and calories.* ▪ Insert nasogastric tube as needed and provide gavage feeding until able to feed by mouth. ▪ Advance feedings as tolerated. ▪ Make adjustment in nipple feeding as needed: Feed in upright position. Put extra hole in nipple. Use nipple designed for premature infants. ▪ Instruct parents on how to feed infant by nipple or nasogastric route.	Adequate caloric requirements will be attained.
High Risk for Impaired Physical Mobility **RELATED TO** Sedation Decreased muscle tone and strength Impaired coordination High phenobarbital or phenytoin level **DEFINING CHARACTERISTICS** Limited ROM Decreased muscle control	**ONGOING ASSESSMENT** ▪ Assess ability to move extremities. ▪ Assess respiratory rate, rhythm, and amplitude. *Immobility can result in pulmonary embolus.* ▪ Assess skin integrity. **THERAPEUTIC INTERVENTIONS** ▪ Turn and position every 2 hours. ▪ Provide range of motion exercises. ▪ Perform chest physiotherapy and suctioning every 2 to 4 hours. ▪ Use antipressure devices *to optimize skin integrity.* ▪ Clean, dry, and moisturize skin every 4 to 8 hours. ▪ If skin integrity becomes a problem, see Skin integrity, impaired, p. 41. ▪ Maintain adequate nutrition *to optimize energy levels.*	Optimal mobility will be maintained.
High Risk for Altered Parent/ Infant Bonding **RELATED TO** Separation Fear of the unknown **DEFINING CHARACTERISTICS** Change in visiting and calling patterns Unrealistic expectations of baby and self Lack of physical contact with baby (touching and holding)	**ONGOING ASSESSMENT** ▪ Assess parental developmental stage. ▪ Assess parents' degree of involvement with infant. **THERAPEUTIC INTERVENTIONS** ▪ Encourage visiting and calling as much as possible, and give an accurate description of baby's appearance and condition. ▪ Encourage touching and holding when possible, especially during feedings. ▪ Recognize any support system; encourage parents to verbalize feelings of anxiety and guilt. ▪ Explain to parents and significant others the disease process: Signs and symptoms Possible complications Treatment and procedures ▪ Encourage participation in the care of baby by letting parents perform simple tasks they can succeed in doing. *This will increase confidence in caretaking abilities.* ▪ Assist parents to make decisions for long-term care as needed.	Parent/infant bonding will be initiated.

NURSING DIAGNOSES/ DEFINING CHARACTERISTICS	NURSING INTERVENTIONS / *RATIONALES*	EXPECTED OUTCOMES
DEFINING CHARACTERISTICS cont'd Feelings of detachment because of fear of death, permanent brain damage, or mental retardation are verbalized Lack of or inappropriate response to infant Resentment toward baby is verbalized Lack of knowledge about disease entity is verbalized		
Knowledge Deficit RELATED TO Short-term and long-term management and care of infant No previous experience Expected outcome/ prognosis **DEFINING CHARACTERISTICS** Questioning Keeping quiet Appear uninvolved	**ONGOING ASSESSMENT** ▪ Assess parents' level of understanding of disease process, management, and care involved. ▪ Assess level of comfort in caring for infant. **THERAPEUTIC INTERVENTIONS** ▪ Explain disease process, management, and care. ▪ Encourage questioning and discussion. ▪ Encourage parental participation in care and decision-making. ▪ Reinforce teaching before discharge and arrange for discharge follow-up.	Parents' understanding of disease process, management, and care will be enhanced.

Ruby Rotor-Cajindos, RN, BSN

Substance abuse withdrawal

DRUG ADDICTION WITHDRAWAL

Occurs in an infant who is born to a mother with acquired dependence on narcotics or other drugs that stimulate/depress mental or physiological function. These substances can cause deleterious affects on the newborn.

NURSING DIAGNOSES/ DEFINING CHARACTERISTICS	NURSING INTERVENTIONS / *RATIONALES*	EXPECTED OUTCOMES
Ineffective Breathing Patterns **RELATED TO** Inhibitory effects of maternal drug ingestion **DEFINING CHARACTERISTICS** Respiratory rate >60/min Respiratory alkalosis Increased secretions Rales Retractions Cyanosis	**ONGOING ASSESSMENT** • Review maternal drug history. • Count respirations for 1 full minute. • Auscultate all lung lobes and compare breath sounds. • Observe location and severity of retraction. • Observe color of trunk, face, extremities, nailbed, and mucous membranes. • Monitor ABGs. • Observe amount and nature of secretions. **THERAPEUTIC INTERVENTIONS** • Perform chest physiotherapy and suction secretions as needed *to keep airway patent.* • Reposition infant frequently, keeping neck slightly hyperextended *to facilitate full expansion of lungs.* • Place bed in semi-Fowler's position, or use infant seat *to prevent mucus from pooling in throat.*	Optimal respiratory status will be achieved.
High Risk for Fluid Volume Deficit **RELATED TO** Effects of drug withdrawal: vomiting, diarrhea, and profuse sweating **DEFINING CHARACTERISTICS** Excessive weight loss Poor skin turgor Decreased urine output Increase urine specific gravity Decrease or concentration of mouth secretions Lethargy Electrolyte imbalance Diarrhea Sweating Vomiting Sunken fontanels Poor perfusion Hypotension Increased heart rate	**ONGOING ASSESSMENT** • Observe skin turgor. • Assess I&O. • Assess fontanels: Are fontanels sunken? Do sutures overlap? • Assess the tenacity and amount of secretions. • Observe activity level. • Weigh every 24 hours. • Check urine specific gravity every 4 hours. *A rise from 1.000 to 1.008 may indicate dehydration.* • Monitor serum electrolytes every 24 to 48 hours, *because excessive fluid loss may cause electrolyte imbalance.* • Monitor vital signs. **THERAPEUTIC INTERVENTIONS** • Adjust IV or feedings to provide 80-100 ml/kg/day on first day of life, 100-120 ml/kg/day on second day of life, and 150 ml/kg/day thereafter. Also add 10%-20% based on severity of dehydration. • Maintain strict I&O.	Optimal fluid balance will be achieved.

NURSING DIAGNOSES/ DEFINING CHARACTERISTICS	NURSING INTERVENTIONS / *RATIONALES*	EXPECTED OUTCOMES
High Risk for Altered Nutrition **RELATED TO** Inability to feed, secondary to: Irritability Lethargy Vomiting Uncoordinated suck/swallow Respiratory distress Increased secretions Hypersensitive gag reflex Abdominal cramps **DEFINING CHARACTERISTICS** Weight loss of 20-30 g/day for more than 2 consecutive days	**ONGOING ASSESSMENT** • Assess ability to handle secretions secondary to inability to swallow, e.g., pooling of secretions. • Determine appropriate feeding route based on: Gestational age Sensitivity of gag reflex Ability to coordinate suck and swallow Respiratory rate • Assess infant's ability to tolerate feedings: Observe for vomiting. Observe amount of residual gastric content before meals if nasogastric feedings are used. Measure abdominal circumference every 4-6 hours. *Distention is an early symptom of feeding intolerance.* **THERAPEUTIC INTERVENTIONS** • Encourage oral formula feedings when appropriate, using assessment data and the following criteria: Gestational age ≥32 weeks Respiratory rate 30 to 60/min Infant's tolerance of 5-10 ml × 1 • Offer pacifier with nasogastric feedings *to satisfy sucking reflex.* • Hold feedings and notify physician if residual gastric content is ≥2-3 ml.	Optimal nutritional status will be achieved.
Pain/Discomfort **RELATED TO** Withdrawal of the drug **DEFINING CHARACTERISTICS** Irritability or hyperactivity Disorganized, vigorous sucking Tremors or hypotonicity Hyperphagia Exaggerated reflexes Fever Sneezing Hiccups Yawning Short, restless sleep Drooling Sensitive gag reflex Abdominal cramps Stuffy nose Flushing	**ONGOING ASSESSMENT** • Assess level of activity. • Assess reactions to stimuli. **THERAPEUTIC INTERVENTIONS** • Use calming techniques: Swaddle infant. Place in prone position. Hold and cuddle as often as possible. • Satisfy sucking desire, using pacifier or infant's hands. • Reduce environmental stimuli: Dim lights near bed if possible. Limit activity and noise near bedside whenever possible. Organize care to limit amount of invasive procedures.	Comfort will be maximized.

Continued.

Substance abuse withdrawal cont'd

NURSING DIAGNOSES/ DEFINING CHARACTERISTICS	NURSING INTERVENTIONS / *RATIONALES*	EXPECTED OUTCOMES
Parental Knowledge Deficit **RELATED TO** Unfamiliarity with infant's condition **DEFINING CHARACTERISTICS** Inappropriate or repetitive questions Hostility or suspicion toward staff Anxiety Disbelief	**ONGOING ASSESSMENT** • Observe attitude of parents as expressed by comments and behavior. • Assess the level of parents' knowledge as expressed by the appropriateness of their questions. • Observe parental reactions to changes in infant's condition or treatment. **THERAPEUTIC INTERVENTIONS** • Encourage parents to discuss their feelings and concerns regarding infant and his or her condition. *This will often highlight problems or concerns that were not obvious from nonverbal behavior of parents.* • Offer information and ask for feedback regarding: Baby's condition Unit policies Role/responsibilities of unit personnel • Contact social service personnel, if indicated.	Knowledge deficit will be reduced.
High Risk for Altered Parenting **RELATED TO** Interruption of normal adaptation of new family member **DEFINING CHARACTERISTICS** Inconsistency or disinterest in visiting or calling Disinterest or uneasiness in handling infant Nonverbal expression of concern about infant's condition Guilt, hostility, or suspicion	**ONGOING ASSESSMENT** • Observe frequency of visits or calls. • Observe interaction of parents with infant. • Assess developmental stage of parents. • Assess support system of parents: Other family members Friends Religious beliefs • Assess emotional response of parents regarding infant's reason for hospitalization. **THERAPEUTIC INTERVENTIONS** • Initiate calls to parents if necessary and encourage them to visit. *Frequent contact with infant is important in bonding.* • Encourage parents to hold infant and do as much of care as possible. • Encourage parents to express their feelings regarding their drug addiction. • Stress the positive aspects of infant's condition. • Make referrals as indicated: Social services Parent support group Drug rehabilitation program	Initiation of parent/ infant bonding will occur.

Christine Todd, RN, BS, BGS

6

Gastrointestinal Care Plans

PEDIATRIC PATIENT
Acute abdomen
Enteral tube feedings
Fecal ostomy
Gastroesophageal reflux
Gastrointestinal bleeding
Inflammatory bowel disease
Pyloric stenosis

NEONATAL PATIENT
Abdominal wall defect: preoperative
Breastfeeding the infant requiring special
   care
Choanal atresia
Cleft lip and palate
Hyperbilirubinemia
Low birth weight and total parenteral
   nutrition
Necrotizing enterocolitis
Percutaneous central venous catheter
Small-for-gestational-age neonate
Tracheoesophageal fistula with esophageal
   atresia: preoperative care

Acute abdomen

PERITONITIS; APPENDICITIS; PANCREATITIS;
ENTERITIS; OBSTRUCTED BOWEL

A condition characterized by abdominal pain, vomiting, anorexia, constipation or diarrhea, changes in bowel sounds, and fever. Accurate diagnosis depends on thorough physical assessment, appropriate testing and observation, and treatment of etiology.

NURSING DIAGNOSES/ DEFINING CHARACTERISTICS	NURSING INTERVENTIONS / *RATIONALES*	EXPECTED OUTCOMES

Pain
RELATED TO
Pancreatitis
Thrombosis
Strangulating/infarcted bowel
Renal/biliary colic
Ruptured aneurysm
Appendicitis
Diverticulitis
Obstruction
Gastroenteritis
 	
DEFINING CHARACTERISTICS
Complaints of abdominal pain
Restlessness
Insomnia
Guarding behavior
Self-focusing
Moaning/crying
Autonomic responses not seen in chronic pain (e.g., diaphoresis, changes in vital signs, pupillary dilation)
	ONGOING ASSESSMENT
	• Assess age and developmental level.
	• Assess pain: degree, location, sudden or gradual onset.
	• Assess for precipitating and relief factors.
	• Monitor for changes in type, degree, location of pain.
	• Evaluate effectiveness of interventions.
	• Assess need for pain medication if allowed.
	• Assess need for nasogastric tube.
	• Assess need for comfort of intubated child.
	• Assess vital signs—note changes from normal.
	• Assess blood gases.
	
	THERAPEUTIC INTERVENTIONS
	• Make child as comfortable as possible:
	  Respond immediately to complaints of pain.
	  Place child in semi-Fowler's position.
	  Support with pillows.
	  Provide analgesics as ordered.
	  Explain the need to remain as calm as possible.
	  Use techniques child identifies as helpful.
	• Be available to answer questions, explain procedures, and prepare for tests.
	• Explain need to inform nurse of any change in discomfort. *Changes may indicate complications (e.g., ruptured appendix).*
	• Notify physician of ineffective pain measures, changes in type, level, location of pain. *Pain is a diagnostic indicator.*
	• Provide mouth care after intubation.
	• Apply lubricant to external nares of intubated child.
		Pain will be reduced.

Anxiety **RELATED TO** Change in health status Change in environment Suddeness of illness **DEFINING CHARACTERISTICS** Restlessness Apprehensiveness Facial tension Increased questioning/awareness Difficulty sleeping Fear of unknown Change in vital signs	**ONGOING ASSESSMENT** • Monitor anxiety level. • Assess vital signs frequently. • Assess behavior for listed defining characteristics. • Document signs and symptoms, including nonverbal communication. • Assess usual coping patterns and support system. • Assess child for signs of respiratory distress. **THERAPEUTIC INTERVENTIONS** • Establish rapport through continuity of care. • Encourage ventilation of feelings, concerns. Acknowledge anxiety and normalcy of this and other feelings. • Explain importance of remaining as calm as possible. *Relaxation of abdominal muscles may help decrease severity of pain.* • Explain that a nurse will be available if needed. • Explain all procedures before starting. • Provide comfort measures including reassurance, quiet environment, and medications. • Prepare for surgery if needed.	Anxiety will be reduced.
High Risk for Fluid Volume Deficit **RELATED TO** NPO status Diaphoresis Vomiting	**ONGOING ASSESSMENT** • Monitor vital signs, skin turgor, mucous membranes. • Assess I&O, specific gravity. • Monitor weight and record daily. • Monitor lab values and electrolytes. • Observe for complications and notify physician.	Risk of dehydration will be reduced.

NURSING DIAGNOSES/ DEFINING CHARACTERISTICS	NURSING INTERVENTIONS / *RATIONALES*	EXPECTED OUTCOMES
High Risk for Fluid Volume Deficit cont'd Diarrhea Increased metabolic needs **DEFINING CHARACTERISTICS** Decreased urine output Increased specific gravity Thirst Tachycardia Weakness Dry mucous membranes Poor skin turgor, tenting Hemoconcentration	**ONGOING ASSESSMENT cont'd** • Assess blood gases for signs of metabolic acidosis if in distress. • Assess for signs of dehydration. • Assess level of consciousness with severe dehydration. • Assess for signs of ileus. **THERAPEUTIC INTERVENTIONS** • Maintain fluid infusion *to prevent dehydration.* • Maintain hydration so as not to overhydrate or hydrate too quickly. • Insert nasogastric tube and attach to low suction *to ease persistent vomiting.* • Measure gastric output and provide ml for ml IV replacement fluids, usually 0.45 NS or 0.9 NS.	

Diarrhea/ Constipation
RELATED TO
Acute abdominal condition
 	
DEFINING CHARACTERISTICS
Vomiting
Pain
Abdominal distention
Change in bowel sounds
Numerous watery stools
No stools
	ONGOING ASSESSMENT
	• Assess vital signs, abdominal circumference, and bowel sounds at least every 4 hours.
	• Maintain accurate I&O, including emesis, gastric output.
	• Assess emesis for odor, frequency, color, consistency, blood.
	• Assess stools for color, frequency, amount, consistency, blood.
	• Monitor lab work:
	    CBC
	    Electrolytes
	    Amylase
	    BUN, creatinine
	    Sedimentation rate
	• Assess for changes in pain characteristics.
	• Assess nasogastric tube placement.
	• Maintain NPO status until bowel sounds present.
	
	THERAPEUTIC INTERVENTIONS
	• Maintain IV fluids.
	• Insert and monitor nasogastric tube if ordered.
	• Maintain NPO status unless otherwise stated.
	• Explain all procedures.
	• Prepare for and assist with diagnostic tests, x-ray, peritoneal tap.
	• Provide comfort measures.
	• Notify physician immediately for changes in condition; *may indicate emergency situation requiring surgical intervention.*
	• Prepare for surgery if needed.
		Gastrointestinal function elimination will be maximized.

High Risk for Ineffective Airway Clearance **RELATED TO** Pain Abdominal distention	**ONGOING ASSESSMENT** • Assess vital signs—note changes. • Assess respiratory function: rate, quality, pattern, depth, use of accessory muscles. • Auscultate lung fields at least every 4 hours to assess airway clearance. • Assess for abdominal distention. • Assess need for oxygen therapy as a result of increased respiratory distress. • Assess blood gases when in distress. • Intubate as needed for severe distress.	Optimal airway clearance will be maintained.

Continued.

Gastrointestinal Care Plans (Pediatric)

NURSING DIAGNOSES/ DEFINING CHARACTERISTICS	NURSING INTERVENTIONS / *RATIONALES*	EXPECTED OUTCOMES
DEFINING CHARACTERISTICS Guarded breathing due to pain Dyspnea Tachypnea	**THERAPEUTIC INTERVENTIONS** • Position *to facilitate lung expansion.* • Encourage child to change position *to facilitate drainage and air exchange.* • Encourage coughing and deep breathing or use of incentive spirometer *to enhance airway clearance and pulmonary toilet.* • Notify physician of abdominal distention and respiratory difficulty. *Sedation may be used to keep child calm.* • Provide oxygen therapy with humidity *to ease the work of breathing and maintain adequate saturation while child exhibits guarding actions.* • Provide necessary suctioning *to prevent obstruction.*	
High Risk for Infection **RELATED TO** Surgical incision Decreased resistance **DEFINING CHARACTERISTICS** Increased heart rate Fever Wound drainage Increased WBC Odor from incision Increased abdominal pain	**ONGOING ASSESSMENT** • Assess incisional wound every 4 hours for signs of redness. • Assess drainage—for color, amount, odor, defining characteristics. • Assess vital signs, especially temperature. • Assess for increase in pain. • Measure abdominal circumference every 4 hours. • Assess suture line for signs of adhesions. • Assess for signs of shock when severe infection is present. • Assess bowel sounds every 4 hours. **THERAPEUTIC INTERVENTIONS** • Keep incision clean and dry. • Use sterile technique when changing dressings. • Note any changes in incision and report to physician. • Teach child/parent signs of infection of incisional line. • Maintain IV line. • Administer antibiotics as ordered.	Risk for infection will be reduced.

Knowledge Deficit
RELATED TO
Acuity of illness
New diagnosis
 	
DEFINING CHARACTERISTICS
Anxious
Questioning
Anger/hostility
Withdrawal/depression
Noncompliance
	ONGOING ASSESSMENT
	• Assess child's/parent's knowledge of:
	  Illness
	  Medications
	  Management of disorder
	• Assess previous experience and health teaching.
	• Assess ability to perform tasks.
	• Assess ability to learn; explore attitude and feelings about condition.
	
	THERAPEUTIC INTERVENTIONS
	• Provide physical comfort and a quiet environment *to enhance ability to concentrate on teaching.*
	• Establish mutual objectives/goals.
	• Allow time for integration of material.
	• Provide home care information:
	  Home management
	  Prevention
	  Follow-up
	  Signs/symptoms necessitating emergency room visit
	• Provide consultation referrals as needed, including appropriate support/ self-help groups.
	• Explain need for surgical intervention if medical intervention ineffective.
		Child/parent will understand current illness and its treatment.

Kathleen Jaffrey, RN

Enteral tube feedings

ENTERAL HYPERALIMENTATION; G-TUBE;
JEJUNOSTOMY; DUODENOSTOMY

A method of providing nutrition using a nasogastric tube, a gastrostomy tube, or a tube placed in the duodenum or jejenum. Feedings may be continuous or intermittent (bolus).

NURSING DIAGNOSES/ DEFINING CHARACTERISTICS	NURSING INTERVENTIONS / *RATIONALES*	EXPECTED OUTCOMES
High Risk for Ineffective Airway Clearance **RELATED TO** Aspiration as a result of: Lack of gag reflex Poor positioning Overfeeding **DEFINING CHARACTERISTICS** Abnormal breath sounds Shortness of breath Coughing Diaphoresis Anxiety Restlessness Poor skin color	**ONGOING ASSESSMENT** • Assess age and developmental level. • Assess correct position of tube before initiation of feeding. • Assess presence of gag reflex before each feeding. • Assess level of consciousness before administration of feeding. • Document child's baseline respiratory status. Monitor child's respiratory status throughout feeding. • Placement of tube: Check tube placement before feeding by injecting air and listening over stomach. *A gurgling sound indicates correct placement.* • Check for residual feeding before each feeding. • Document incorrect tube placement and amount of residual feeding obtained. • See Ineffective airway clearance, p. 3. **THERAPEUTIC INTERVENTIONS** • Hold infant or elevate head of bed to 30 degrees for 30 minutes after feeding (unless contraindicated) *to facilitate gravity flow to stomach.* • In case of aspiration: Stop tube feeding. Monitor vital signs. Assess respiratory status. Notify physician. Keep head of bed elevated. Suction as necessary. Document time feeding was stopped, child's appearance, and changes in respiratory status. *High-risk patients are those who are comatose, who have decreased gag reflex, or who are unable to tolerate elevated head of bed. Nasoduodenal or gastroduodenal feedings are preferred for high-risk patients.*	Potential for aspiration will be reduced.
Altered Nutrition: Less Than Body Requirements **RELATED TO** Mechanical problems during administration of feedings, such as: Clogging of tube Inaccurate flow rate Incorrect tube administration set for pump Defective tube administration set Long-term feeding (i.e., G-tube/ J-tube) **DEFINING CHARACTERISTICS** Continued weight loss or failure to gain Persistent anergy	**ONGOING ASSESSMENT** • Monitor equipment for proper functioning. • Assess tubing for passage of feeding. • Assess nitrogen balance as ordered. • See Altered nutrition: less than body requirements, p. 33. **THERAPEUTIC INTERVENTIONS** • Care of tube: Flush tubing with water after feedings *to reduce risk of clotting.* Crush medications and dilute with water; use elixir form when possible. Flush tube after administration of medications. Check tubing connections. • Care of pump: Keep alarms on. Attach to outlet unless child is walking.	Nutritional support will be maximized.

Continued.

Enteral tube feedings cont'd

NURSING DIAGNOSES/ DEFINING CHARACTERISTICS	NURSING INTERVENTIONS / *RATIONALES*	EXPECTED OUTCOMES

High Risk for Diarrhea
RELATED TO
Intolerance to tube feeding because of:
Hyperosmolarity
Temperature of feeding
Rate of delivery
Anxiety
Bacterial contamination of feeding
 	
DEFINING CHARACTERISTICS
Abdominal cramps
Abdominal pain
Frequency of stools
Loose, liquid stools
Urgency
Hyperactive bowel sounds
	ONGOING ASSESSMENT
	• Assess bowel sounds every 4 hours.
	• Assess number and character of stools.
	• Monitor I&O.
	• Record frequency and consistency of all stools.
	• See Diarrhea, p. 15.
	
	THERAPEUTIC INTERVENTIONS
	• Delivery of formula:
	  Begin feedings slowly; consider a dilute solution.
	  Increase rate and strength to prescribed amount but not at the same time. *High-rate feeding combined with high osmolarity may precipitate diarrhea.*
	  Administer feedings at room temperature. *Cold stimulates peristalsis.*
	  Do not allow formula bag to hang longer than 8 hours at room temperature *to minimize risk of bacterial contamination.*
	  Change setup daily.
	  Administer feedings in a calm, relaxed atmosphere.
	  Notify physician of any intolerance.
	• Patient activity:
	  Encourage light activity after feeding.
	  Document activity tolerance.
		Intolerance to feeding will be reduced.

High Risk for Fluid Volume Deficit **RELATED TO** Osmolarity of feeding formula **DEFINING CHARACTERISTICS** Dry mucous membranes Poor skin turgor Elevated temperature Changes in mental status Azotemia	**ONGOING ASSESSMENT** • Monitor for signs of fluid deficit. • Assess child for change in mental status every shift. • Document baseline mental status. *This is a sensitive indicator of hyperosmolar states.* **THERAPEUTIC INTERVENTIONS** • Provide water through feeding tube between regular feedings. Offer water orally if physiologically/medically acceptable. • Document changes in mental status; notify physician. • See Fluid volume deficit, p. 19.	Fluid volume will be maintained.

Altered Glucose and Fat Metabolism
RELATED TO
Continuous feeding, rather than a physiologic intermittent bolus schedule
 	
DEFINING CHARACTERISTICS
Glucose level >120 mg/dl, flushed skin, headache, nausea, vomiting, fatigue, fruity breath
Glucose <70 mg/dl, hunger, sweating, pallor, cold skin, tremor, blurry vision, fatigue, dizziness
	ONGOING ASSESSMENT
	• Review laboratory values:
	  Monitor blood glucose level as ordered.
	  Monitor urine sugar/acetone four times a day, and notify physician of changes.
	• Assess child for mental status changes and other defining characteristics.
	• Assess stool for odor and greasiness:
	  Monitor bowel sounds every 8 hours.
	  Monitor number and characteristics of stools.
	
	THERAPEUTIC INTERVENTIONS
	• Administer hyperglycemic/antihyperglycemic agents as ordered.
	• Notify physician if feeding is stopped for any reason.
	• Notify physician of any change in stools.
		High risk for altered glucose and fat metabolism will be reduced.

NURSING DIAGNOSES/ DEFINING CHARACTERISTICS	NURSING INTERVENTIONS / *RATIONALES*	EXPECTED OUTCOMES
DEFINING CHARACTERISTICS cont'd Foul-smelling, greasy stools		
Pain **RELATED TO** Dry mucous membranes and tape irritation **DEFINING CHARACTERISTICS** Dry, cracked lips Soiled tape Reddened area where tube is positioned Difficulty swallowing Verbalized discomfort	**ONGOING ASSESSMENT** • Assess mucous membranes/stoma site. • Assess tube insertion site for reddened areas. • See Pain, p. 35. **THERAPEUTIC INTERVENTIONS** • Provide skin/mucous membrane care. Change position of tube at nares, and retape every 12 hours. • Provide mouth care every 4 hours. • Clean skin around G-tube daily with soap and water. • Allow hard candy or gum if permissible, *which stimulates salivary secretion.*	Pain will be reduced or relieved.
Social Isolation **RELATED TO** Change in body image **DEFINING CHARACTERISTICS** Child stays in room and resists environmental changes Child/parent limits visitors or avoids play area	**ONGOING ASSESSMENT** • Assess parent's/child's behavior pattern during contact with significant others or staff. **THERAPEUTIC INTERVENTIONS** • Allow time for verbalization. *Reactions to changed body are normal.* • Arrange privacy for visitation. • Encourage parent and child to participate in daily care. • Encourage activity outside of room if allowable.	Withdrawn behavior will be reduced.
Disturbance in Self-Concept/Self-Image **RELATED TO** Change in body image: feeding tube extending from nose, or G-tube visually present **DEFINING CHARACTERISTICS** Parent/child verbalizes feelings of not being able to eat normally Parent/child will not look at tube Parent/child will not participate in daily hygiene	**ONGOING ASSESSMENT** • Assess parents'/child's use of defense mechanisms in past crises. • Assess parents'/child's response to tube feedings. **THERAPEUTIC INTERVENTIONS** • Explain reason for tube feeding. • Allow parent and child time to express feelings and ask questions. • Allow parent and child to help with feedings. • Allow self-care to the extent possible *to increase/reinforce parent's/ child's capabilities.*	Disturbances in self-concept/self-image will be reduced.

Frankie Harper, RN; Audrey Klopp, RN, PhD, CS, ET

Fecal ostomy

COLOSTOMY; ILEOSTOMY; FECAL DIVERSION;
STOMA; OSTOMY

A surgical procedure that results in an opening into small or large intestine for the purpose of diverting the fecal stream past an area of obstruction or disease, or to protect a distal surgical anastomosis, or to provide an outlet for stool in the absence of a functioning intact rectum. Common reasons that infants and children require colostomy or ileostomy include: necrotizing enterocolitis, Hirschsprung's disease, volvulus, and intussusception. Ostomy may also be indicated for intestinal tumors and abdominal trauma. Infants born with imperforate anus will also require a stoma. Depending on the purpose of the surgery and the integrity and function of anatomical structures, stomas may be temporary or permanent.

NURSING DIAGNOSES/ DEFINING CHARACTERISTICS	NURSING INTERVENTIONS / *RATIONALES*	EXPECTED OUTCOMES
Knowledge Deficit (Preoperative) **RELATED TO** Lack of previous similar experience Need for additional information **DEFINING CHARACTERISTICS** Parent's/child's: Verbalized need for information Verbalized misinformation/ misconceptions	**ONGOING ASSESSMENT** ▪ Assess age and developmental level. ▪ Assess previous surgical experience. ▪ Inquire regarding information given by surgeon regarding formation of ostomy (i.e., purpose, site). ▪ Ascertain (from chart, physician) whether stoma will be permanent or temporary. **THERAPEUTIC INTERVENTIONS** ▪ Reinforce and reexplain proposed procedure. ▪ Answer questions directly and honestly. ▪ Use diagrams, pictures, and audiovisual equipment to explain: Anatomy, physiology of GI tract Pathophysiology necessitating ostomy Proposed location of stoma ▪ Explain need for pouch in terms of loss of sphincter. ▪ Show parent/child actual pouch or one similar to what child will have postoperatively. ▪ Allow child to wear pouch preoperatively. *Stoma site selection is facilitated by observing adhesive faceplate in situ.* ▪ Use doll with "stoma" to allow child *to express concerns and explore feelings.*	Parent and child will understand alteration in normal GI anatomy or physiology requiring the surgical creation of the ostomy, and understand that loss of sphincter will likely necessitate wearing a pouch.
Anxiety/Fear **RELATED TO** Proposed creation of ostomy Previous contact with or knowledge of poorly rehabilitated ostomate **DEFINING CHARACTERISTICS** Parent/child verbally expresses concern/ anxiety Tense facial expression Restlessness Multiple questions Lack of questions Crying	**ONGOING ASSESSMENT** ▪ Assess parent's/child's level of anxiety/fear; note nonverbal signs. ▪ Elicit from parent/child (or other source) normal coping strategies. **THERAPEUTIC INTERVENTIONS** ▪ Ask parent/child to describe in detail the cause of fear/anxiety. ▪ Correct misconceptions, fill in knowledge gaps. ▪ Offer a visit from rehabilitated ostomate/parent of child with an ostomy. *Contact with another individual who has "been there" often is more beneficial in decreasing fear/anxiety than factual information.* ▪ Encourage equipment handling and play with doll with stoma. ▪ See Anxiety, p. 4/Fear, p. 18.	Level of anxiety/fear will be decreased or manageable.

NURSING DIAGNOSES/ DEFINING CHARACTERISTICS	NURSING INTERVENTIONS / *RATIONALES*	EXPECTED OUTCOMES
Anticipatory Grieving **RELATED TO** Proposed loss of fecal continence Anticipated loss of function, love, body image **DEFINING CHARACTERISTICS** Crying Rage Questioning Bargaining with self, God, health care professionals Withdrawal from usual relationships	**ONGOING ASSESSMENT** ▪ Recognize the signs of anticipatory grieving (see Defining Characteristics). ▪ Assess perceived loss of: 　Life 　Function 　Social status 　Love 　Control 　Other **THERAPEUTIC INTERVENTIONS** ▪ Encourage parent/child to verbalize feelings. ▪ Assure parent/child that such grieving is real, expected, and appropriate. *Anticipatory grieving facilitates postoperative grieving, and often follows patterns similar to actual grieving.*	Anticipatory grieving will be recognized and facilitated.
Altered Bowel Elimination **RELATED TO** Preoperative preparation for surgery **DEFINING CHARACTERISTICS** Orders for dietary restriction, cathartics, cleansing enemas	**ONGOING ASSESSMENT** ▪ Assess preparedness of bowel for surgery: clear/near-clear returns on enemas. *Postoperative complications are decreased when the surgical area has been properly emptied and cleansed.* ▪ Observe for weakness, bradycardia, perianal discomfort. **THERAPEUTIC INTERVENTIONS** ▪ Perform necessary bowel preparation. ▪ Explain necessity of bowel preparation. ▪ Provide privacy during evacuation. ▪ Allow for rest periods between enemas. ▪ Treat any perianal discomfort resulting from frequent stooling.	Bowel will be sufficiently prepared for surgical procedure.
High Risk for Self-Care Deficit: Toileting **RELATED TO** Presence of stoma Presence of pouch **DEFINING CHARACTERISTICS** Presence of old abdominal scars Presence of bony prominences on anterior abdominal surface Presence of skin folds over abdomen Extreme obesity Physical deformities that may interfere with self-care Chronologically/developmentally too young to provide self-care	**ONGOING ASSESSMENT** ▪ Assess abdominal surface for presence of: 　Old scars 　Bony prominences 　Skin folds 　Contour 　Visibility to child ▪ Assess child's developmental stage/ability to learn self-ostomy care. ▪ Assess parent's readiness and ability to learn ostomy care. **THERAPEUTIC INTERVENTIONS** ▪ Indelibly mark proposed stoma site where: 　Child can easily see. 　Child can easily reach. 　Scars, bony prominences, and skin folds are avoided. 　Hip flexion does not change contour. 　*Stoma location is a key factor in self-care. A poorly located stoma can delay/preclude self-care abilities.* ▪ Note usual sites for stoma: 　Ileostomy: lower right quadrant 　Ascending colostomy: right upper or lower quadrant 　Transverse colostomy: mid-waist or just below mid-waist 　Descending and sigmoid colostomies: lower left quadrant ▪ If possible, have child wear pouch over proposed site; evaluate effectiveness 12 to 24 hours after applying pouch.	High risk for self-care deficit will be reduced.

Continued.

Fecal ostomy cont'd

NURSING DIAGNOSES/ DEFINING CHARACTERISTICS	NURSING INTERVENTIONS / *RATIONALES*	EXPECTED OUTCOMES

Altered Postoperative Bowel Elimination
RELATED TO
Surgical diversion of fecal stream
 	
DEFINING CHARACTERISTICS
Structural or functional absence of anal sphincter
Presence of stoma
	ONGOING ASSESSMENT
	• Assess stoma every 4 hours postoperatively for:
	    Color
	    Shape
	    Size
	    Presence of supportive device (rod, catheter)
	    Function (flatus, stool)
	    Drainage that is not stool
	
	THERAPEUTIC INTERVENTIONS
	• Apply pouch to stoma as soon as possible postoperatively *to protect other surgical sites from fecal contamination and to protect peristomal skin.*
	• Notify physician if stoma appears dusky or blue. *The stoma (a piece of intestine) should be pink and moist, indicating good perfusion and adequate venous drainage.*
		Bowel function via the stoma will return within 8 hours (ileostomy) or 1 to 4 days (colostomy).

Disturbance in Self-Concept/Body Image **RELATED TO** Presence of stoma: loss of fecal continence **DEFINING CHARACTERISTICS** Verbalized feelings about stoma and altered bowel elimination Parent's refusal to discuss, acknowledge, touch, or care for stoma/pouch	**ONGOING ASSESSMENT** • Assess parent's/child's perception of change in body structure and function. • Assess perceived impact of change. *Assigned importance of body part or importance is a major factor in impact.* • Note verbal references to stoma, altered bowel elimination. **THERAPEUTIC INTERVENTIONS** • Acknowledge appropriateness of emotional response to perceived change in body structure and function. *Because control of elimination is a skill/task of early childhood and a socially private function, loss of control in a previously continent child precipitates a change in body image, and a possible change in self-concept.* • Assist parent/child in looking at, touching, and caring for stoma when ready. • Reoffer a visit from a rehabilitated ostomate/parent. • See Disturbance in body image, p. 7. • Refer family to local ostomy support group. *The United Ostomy Association runs summer camps for children with stomas.*	Feelings about altered bowel function, stoma, and changes in self-concept will be acknowledged.

Knowledge Deficit Regarding Ostomy Self-Care
RELATED TO
Presence of new stoma
Lack of similar experience
	ONGOING ASSESSMENT
	• Assess parent's/child's:
	    Ability to empty and change pouch
	    Ability to care for peristomal skin and identify problems, potential problems
	    Appropriateness in seeking assistance
	    Knowledge regarding:
	        Diet
	        Activity
	        Hygiene
	        Clothing
	        Interpersonal relationships
	        Equipment purchase
	        Financial reimbursement for ostomy equipment
		Parent/child will be capable of ostomy self-care on discharge.

NURSING DIAGNOSES/ DEFINING CHARACTERISTICS	NURSING INTERVENTIONS / *RATIONALES*	EXPECTED OUTCOMES

DEFINING CHARACTERISTICS
Parent's/child's demonstrated inability to empty and change pouch
Verbalized need for information regarding diet, odor, activity, hygiene, clothing, interpersonal relationships, equipment purchase, financial concerns
	THERAPEUTIC INTERVENTIONS
	• Build on information given preoperatively.
	• Plan and share teaching plan with parent/child.
	• Begin psychomotor teaching during first and subsequent applications of pouch.
	• Gradually transfer responsibility for pouch emptying and changing to parent or to child if capable.
	• Allow at least one opportunity for supervised return demonstration of pouch change before discharge. *Ostomy care requires both cognitive and psychomotor skills. Postoperatively, learning ability may be decreased, requiring repetition and opportunity for return demonstrations.*
	• Instruct parent/child on the following:
	  Diet:
	   For ileostomy:
	    Balanced diet—special care in chewing high-fiber foods (popcorn, peanuts, coconut, vegetables, string beans, olives), increased fluid intake during hot weather, vigorous exercise
	   For colostomy:
	    Balanced diet—no foods are specifically contraindicated, although certain foods (eggs, fish, green leafy vegetables, carbonated beverages), may increase flatus and fecal color.
	  Odor control:
	   Best achieved by eliminating odor causing-foods from diet.
	   Oral agents and deodorant are available.
	   Activity should not be restricted because of stoma or pouch; direct forceful blows to the stoma should be avoided.
	   One-piece clothing is often useful in keeping pouch intact for infants and toddlers.	

Pain **RELATED TO** Surgical incision(s) **DEFINING CHARACTERISTICS** Facial mask of pain Verbal complaints of pain Inability to move, cough, deep breathe, get out of bed Decreased concentration Crying Poor feeding	**ONGOING ASSESSMENT** • Assess level of comfort. • Elicit from parent/child possible sources of discomfort/recommendations for relief. **THERAPEUTIC INTERVENTIONS** • Institute pain relief measures, incorporating parent's/child's suggestions when possible. • See Pain, p. 35.	Pain will be reduced or relieved.

Audrey Klopp, RN, PhD, CS, ET

231

Gastroesophageal reflux

CHALASIA

Gastroesophageal reflux (GER) is the pathologic entry of gastric acid into the esophagus that occurs at any time and is not necessarily related to feeding or a full stomach. It is the result of an incompetent lower esophageal sphincter or a relaxed sphincter. This is primarily a disorder in infancy that often resolves without surgical intervention by the time the child is 6 months to 7 years old.

NURSING DIAGNOSES/ DEFINING CHARACTERISTICS	NURSING INTERVENTIONS / *RATIONALES*	EXPECTED OUTCOMES
Altered Nutrition: Less Than Body Requirements **RELATED TO** Reflux with reduced nutrient intake Vomiting Heartburn (crying, irritability, disturbed sleep) Choking/coughing while eating Failure to thrive Rumination **DEFINING CHARACTERISTICS** Loss of weight ≥10%-20% less than ideal body weight Documented inadequate caloric intake Dehydration	**ONGOING ASSESSMENT** ▪ Assess age and developmental level. ▪ Assess feeding patterns and methods. ▪ Assess for congenital defects. ▪ Assess weight, length, head circumference. ▪ Keep accurate I&O. ▪ Assess feeding environment at home. ▪ Assess bedtime/eating routines. ▪ Assess for signs of dehydration. ▪ Assess the abdomen for pain, tenderness, bowel sounds, and masses. ▪ Record amount, characteristics of vomitus, and time since last feeding. ▪ Assess ongoing test results. *Tests commonly ordered:* Upper GI: *Evaluates swallowing mechanism, pharyngeal coordination, and esophageal motility. It also rules out pyloric stenosis, ulcers, hiatal hernia. Does not detect frequency of GER, acidity of refluxed material, or length of time of material in esophagus.* Radionuclide scan: *Evaluates gastric emptying, esophageal clearance, and correlates reflux and aspiration episodes.* pH monitor: *Evaluates the acidity of the material in the esophagus continuously. Normal pH 5.5-7.0; reflux pH <4.0; reliable for determining reflux 90% of the time.* ▪ Note skin turgor, urine specific gravity, presence or absence of tears, and moisture of mucous membranes *to evaluate the hydration of the infant.* ▪ If there is a gastrostomy or nasogastric tube, check for residuals before the administration of the next feeding *to determine the gastric emptying time.* ▪ Monitor stool for blood *because esophageal bleeding secondary to esophagitis is a complication of GER.* **THERAPEUTIC INTERVENTIONS** ▪ Thicken formula with cereal (1 tsp/oz). ▪ Feed slowly in small amounts. ▪ Handle infant gently and burp after every 1-2 oz. ▪ Use prone position with the head of bed elevated 30 degrees *to decrease the reflux by gravity and aid in the clearance of gastric contents.* ▪ Avoid bedtime snacks *because they stimulate gastric secretions and thus increase symptoms.*	The child will maintain normal nutrient intake.
Ineffective Airway Clearance **RELATED TO** Coughing Fever Apnea (SIDS) Pneumonia (chronic or recurrent) Upper respiratory infections— recurrent Asthma/bronchitis	**ONGOING ASSESSMENT** ▪ Assess respiratory symptoms/complaints (coughing, pneumonia, bronchitis). ▪ Assess respiratory status: respiratory rate, depth, oxygen saturation before, during, and after feeding. ▪ Assess breath sounds every 1-4 hours depending on the infant's condition.	Effective airway clearance will be maintained.

NURSING DIAGNOSES/ DEFINING CHARACTERISTICS	NURSING INTERVENTIONS / *RATIONALES*	EXPECTED OUTCOMES
DEFINING CHARACTERISTICS Abnormal breath sounds (rales, rhonchi) Change in rate or depth of respiration Tachypnea Cough Cyanosis Dyspnea	**THERAPEUTIC INTERVENTIONS** ▪ Use apnea monitor *since SIDS may be associated with GER.* ▪ Encourage deep breathing in the infant through imitation and play (blowing bubbles). ▪ Suction prn.	
Impaired Physical Mobility **RELATED TO** Prone position Torticollis Sandifer syndrome Clubbed fingers **DEFINING CHARACTERISTICS** Inability to purpose-fully move Imposed restriction of movement Limited ROM Decreased muscle strength Impaired coordi-nation	**ONGOING ASSESSMENT** ▪ Assess the family's acceptance of the treatment modalities. ▪ Assess the infant for clubbing of fingers, *as a result of the protein-losing enteropathy of GER.* ▪ Assess the infant for torticollis or contortions of the head and neck (neural tics or opisthotonos) known as Sandifer syndrome *associated with the child's attempt to empty the esophagus of refluxed gastric contents.* **THERAPEUTIC INTERVENTIONS** ▪ Schedule active play before meals. ▪ Make child's environment stimulating (mobiles, toys within reach, music). ▪ Talk to child frequently. ▪ Put child in room with others; face crib in different directions *for stimulation and to encourage the child to turn the head, preventing contractures.*	Risks related to im-paired mobility will be reduced.
Anxiety **RELATED TO** Hospitalization Altered feeding pattern **DEFINING CHARACTERISTICS** Apprehension Restlessness Facial tension Difficulty in cognitive functioning Extraneous move-ment	**ONGOING ASSESSMENT** ▪ Assess the implication of the diagnosis for the family. Identify the fami-ly's areas of concern and the availability of support. ▪ Assess parental anxiety. **THERAPEUTIC INTERVENTIONS** ▪ Allow parent to discuss fears and identify coping strategies. ▪ Provide adequate teaching for feeding regimen. ▪ Explain rationale and prepare parent for all procedures, tests, and sur-gery.	The family will have their fears and anx-ieties lessened.
Altered Parenting **RELATED TO** Hospitalization Grieving the loss of a perfect child Child's weight loss Delayed growth and development	**ONGOING ASSESSMENT** ▪ Assess parent/infant interactions. ▪ Assess parent's desire and skills in caring for child. **THERAPEUTIC INTERVENTIONS** ▪ Explain that GER is not uncommon and frequently resolves when the infant eats thicker foods. ▪ Involve parent in feeding and physical care. ▪ Help parent to focus on the infant's positive behaviors. ▪ Encourage parent to ventilate feelings.	The parent will feel adequate in parent-ing skills.

Continued.

Gastroesophageal reflux cont'd

NURSING DIAGNOSES/ DEFINING CHARACTERISTICS	NURSING INTERVENTIONS / *RATIONALES*	EXPECTED OUTCOMES

DEFINING CHARACTERISTICS

Disruption in care-taking routines

Parent expresses concern of feeling inadequate to provide for the child's physical and emotional needs

Concern over loss of control over his or her own child

Knowledge Deficit RELATED TO

New disease/procedures:
  Positioning
  Feeding
  Medications

DEFINING CHARACTERISTICS

Parent states deficiency in knowledge

Parent states inadequate understanding of information

Nonverbal cues indicating lack of understanding

Inadequate recall of information

Inaccurate return performance

ONGOING ASSESSMENT

- Assess the family's readiness and willingness to learn.

THERAPEUTIC INTERVENTIONS

- Explain the anatomy of the stomach and the esophagus.
- Explain the causes of GER.
- Teach proper positioning/feeding.
- Teach infant stimulation exercises to parent and explain developmental milestones.
- If medication is prescribed, teach the parent the correct method and time of administration and the expected results.
- Medications commonly used:
  Reglan *(metoclopramide HCl)*
    Action: Increases gastric emptying.
    Dose: 0.1 mg/kg/dose 15 minutes before each feeding.
    Side effects: Rigidity.
  Zantac *(ranitidine HCl)*
    Action: Inhibits gastric acid secretion.
    Dose: 2.0 mg/kg/dose every 8 hours.
    Side effects: Headaches, abdominal pain, constipation or diarrhea, leukopenia, thrombocytopenia, rash.
  Tagamet *(cimetidine)*
    Action: Inhibits gastric acid secretion.
    Dose: 20-40 mg/kg/dose every 6 hours.
    Side effects: Diarrhea, rash, myalgia, neutropenia, gynecomastia.
  Urecholine *(bethanechol chloride)*
    Action: Increases acid clearance of distal esophagus, little effect on gastric emptying.
    Dose: 0.1 mg/kg/dose before meals and at bedtime.
    Side effects: Tremors, irritability, diarrhea, bronchospasm.

The parent will understand and demonstrate proper techniques in caring for infant.

Nedra Skale, RN, MS, CNA

Gastrointestinal bleeding

LOWER GI BLEEDING; UPPER GI BLEEDING;
GI HEMORRHAGE; ESOPHAGEAL VARICES;
ULCER DISEASE

Loss of blood from the GI tract that is most often the result of erosion or ulceration of the mucosa, but that may be the result of arteriovenous (AV) malformation, malignancies, increased pressures in the portal venous bed, or direct trauma to the gastrointestinal tract.

NURSING DIAGNOSES/ DEFINING CHARACTERISTICS	NURSING INTERVENTIONS / *RATIONALES*	EXPECTED OUTCOMES
Actual Fluid Volume Deficit **RELATED TO** Upper GI bleeding (mouth, esophagus, stomach, duodenum) caused by: Gastric ulcer Duodenal ulcer Gastritis Esophageal varices Blunt or penetrating trauma Cancer Upper GI bleeding (small or large intestine, rectum, anus) caused by: Tumors Inflammatory bowel disease (diverticular disease, Crohn's disease, ulcerative colitis) AV malformations Blunt or penetrating trauma Generalized GI bleeding: Systemic coagulopathies Radiation therapy Chemotherapy Family history of GI bleeding **DEFINING CHARACTERISTICS** Hematemesis, observed or reported Melena Hematochezia (bright red blood per rectum) Abdominal pain History of aspirin, steroid, nonsteroidal, or ibuprofen use/abuse Tachycardia Hypotension	**ONGOING ASSESSMENT** - Assess age and developmental level. - Monitor color, consistency of hematemesis, melena, or rectal bleeding. - Obtain history of use/abuse of substances known to predispose to GI bleeding: Aspirin Aspirin-containing drugs Nonsteroidal antiinflammatory drugs Ibuprofen-containing drugs Steroids - Monitor BP changes. - Assess for signs and symptoms of fluid volume deficit. - Monitor coagulation profile. - Monitor Hgb and Hct. - Monitor liver function studies. - Obtain diet history. **THERAPEUTIC INTERVENTIONS** - Start one or more large-bore IVs. *Rapid volume expansion is necessary to prevent/treat complications of hypovolemia, and IV medication and/or blood component administration is likely.* - Insert nasogastric tube *for lavage of the stomach, to closely monitor continuing blood loss, and for the administration of medications.* - Lavage stomach until clots are no longer present and return is clear, using room temperature saline solution. *Use of iced saline solution may cause undesirable ischemic changes in the gastric mucosa.* - Provide volume resuscitation with crystalloids or blood products as ordered; monitor cardiopulmonary response to volume expansion. - Assist with/coordinate diagnostic procedures performed *to identify site of bleeding:* Endoscopy: *provides direct visualization of esophagus, stomach, and duodenum. This procedure must be done before x-rays that require barium ingestion to maximize visualization by endoscopist.* Sigmoidoscopy/proctoscopy/colonoscopy: *provides direct visualization of rectum and colon.* Barium studies: Barium swallow: *indirect visualization of esophagus, stomach, and small intestine.* Barium enema: *indirect visualization of colon.* Small bowel follow-through: *indirect visualization of small intestine.* Angiography *(may be diagnostic or performed for arterial line placement to infuse vasoconstrictive medications locally; will be inconclusive diagnostically unless bleeding is >0.5 ml/min).* After angiography, dress site with pressure dressing for at least 8 hours. Connect arterial line to pressure/flush system or to vasopressin drip. - Administer vitamin K as ordered *to enable production of coagulation factors.* - Administer antacids and H_2-receptor antagonists (i.e., cimetidine, Zantac) *to suppress gastric/duodenal secretions.* - Arrange/assist with transfer of child to monitored area if hemodynamically unstable. - Guard against inadvertent administration of drugs that may potentiate further bleeding.	Optimal fluid volume will be maintained.

Continued.

Gastrointestinal bleeding cont'd

NURSING DIAGNOSES/ DEFINING CHARACTERISTICS	NURSING INTERVENTIONS / *RATIONALES*	EXPECTED OUTCOMES
DEFINING CHARACTERISTICS cont'd Change in level of consciousness Thirst Dry mucous membranes		
Anxiety/Fear **RELATED TO** Blood loss Hurried activity/care Uncertain outcome **DEFINING CHARACTERISTICS** Tense facial appearance Multiple questions No questions Restlessness Crying Requests for constant attendance by health care personnel	**ONGOING ASSESSMENT** ▪ Assess level of anxiety/fear. ▪ Solicit expression(s) of cause(s) of anxiety/fear. ▪ Assess presence and helpfulness of social support system in managing anxiety/fear. **THERAPEUTIC INTERVENTIONS** ▪ Encourage verbalization/or expressions of anxiety. ▪ Keep child/family informed about his/her status and related information. *Parent may perceive pending transfer from one area to another as a sign of deterioration in child's condition.* ▪ Answer questions honestly and simply; repeat information when necessary. ▪ See Anxiety, p. 4 and Fear, p. 18.	Anxiety/fear will be reduced.
High Risk for Pain/ Discomfort **RELATED TO** Invasive therapies Vomiting Diarrhea Diagnostic procedures **DEFINING CHARACTERISTICS** Verbalizes pain/discomfort Facial grimacing Restlessness	**ONGOING ASSESSMENT** ▪ Assess specific sources of discomfort. ▪ Ask child/parent what measure(s) they believe might provide comfort. **THERAPEUTIC INTERVENTIONS** ▪ Tape/stabilize all tubes, drains, and catheters *to minimize movement that causes discomfort.* ▪ Provide frequent oral hygiene *to remove blood/emesis and moisten mucous membranes.* ▪ Provide meticulous perineal care after all bowel movements. ▪ For child with any type of indwelling nasogastric tube, moisten external nares with water-soluble lubricant at least once per shift *to reduce adherence of mucus, which can dry and cause irritation.* ▪ Change linens as necessary *to minimize discomfort and reduce unpleasant melanic odor.* ▪ Use analgesics with caution *so that changes in level of consciousness related to fluid volume deficit may be carefully evaluated.* ▪ See Pain, p. 35.	Pain/discomfort will be relieved.
High Risk for Impaired Skin Integrity **RELATED TO** Bed rest Frequent stooling Hypovolemia leading to skin ischemia Poor nutritional status	**ONGOING ASSESSMENT** ▪ Assess condition of skin at least every 2 hours.	Skin will remain intact.

Gastrointestinal bleeding cont'd

NURSING DIAGNOSES/ DEFINING CHARACTERISTICS	NURSING INTERVENTIONS / *RATIONALES*	EXPECTED OUTCOMES
DEFINING CHARACTERISTICS Red, irritated skin Poor capillary refill Broken epidermis	**THERAPEUTIC INTERVENTIONS** • Turn child side-to-side as hemodynamic status allows. • Place pressure-relief device(s) beneath child. • Do not allow child to sit on bedpan for long periods of time. • Clean perianal skin with soap and water after each bowel movement; dry well. • Apply a liquid film barrier to perianal area *so that skin is not in direct contact with stool.* • Minimize the use of plastic linen protectors, *which harbor moisture and enhance maceration.* • See Impaired skin integrity, p. 39.	

High Risk for Decreased Level of Consciousness
 RELATED TO
 Elevated levels of cerebral toxins
 Altered metabolic function of the liver
 Increased cerebral sensitivity
 	
 DEFINING CHARACTERISTICS
 Lethargy
 Confusion
 Somnolence
 Fever
 Acid-base imbalance
	ONGOING ASSESSMENT
	 • Assess for changes in LOC.
	 • Monitor ammonia levels.
	 • Monitor acid-base balance.
	 • Monitor temperature.
	
	 THERAPEUTIC INTERVENTIONS
	 • Reduce toxins available to the cerebral circulation by:
	   Use of stomach lavage *to remove blood.*
	   Use of enemas *to remove blood.*
	   Administration of nonabsorbable antibiotics as ordered *to reduce intestinal bacteria count, which will in turn reduce ammonia production.*
	 • Administer antipyretics as ordered.
	 • Correct acid-base balance.
	 • See Decreased level of consciousness, p. 173.
		Normal level of consciousness will be maintained.

Knowledge Deficit
 RELATED TO
 First GI bleeding
 Unfamiliar environment
 	
 DEFINING CHARACTERISTICS
 Multiple questions
 Lack of questions
 Verbalized misconceptions
	ONGOING ASSESSMENT
	 • Assess child's/parent's understanding of cause and treatment of GI bleeding.
	
	 THERAPEUTIC INTERVENTIONS
	 • Explain procedures necessary for diagnosis and/or treatment before they are performed. *Understanding need for unpleasant procedures may help child to comply/participate and increase yield/effectiveness of treatment or procedure.*
	 • Encourage/stress importance of avoidance of substances containing:
	   Aspirin
	   Nonsteroidal antiinflammatory agents
	   Ibuprofen
	   Steroids
	 • Teach child/parent the dose, administration schedule, expected actions, and possible adverse effects of medications that may be prescribed for long periods of time. *Drugs given to decrease gastric acid production may be prescribed indefinitely; child/parent must understand that cessation of bleeding or other symptoms does not mean the need for medication has ended.*
		Child/parent will state an understanding of GI bleeding, diagnosis, and treatment.

Audrey Klopp, RN, PhD, CS, ET

Inflammatory bowel disease

CROHN'S DISEASE; ULCERATIVE COLITIS;
REGIONAL ENTERITIS

Inflammatory bowel disease (IBD) refers to two specific bowel conditions whose symptoms are often so similar that diagnosis is difficult and treatment empirical. Crohn's disease is associated with involvement of all four layers of the bowel and may occur anywhere in the GI tract, although it is most common in the small bowel. Crohn's disease typically occurs in children between 10 and 19 years of age. Ulcerative colitis, which typically occurs between 15 and 30 years of age, involves the mucosa and submucosa only, and occurs only in the colon. The cause is unknown for both diseases. Both diseases are treated medically. If medical management fails or complications occur, surgical resection and possible fecal diversion (ileostomy, colostomy) will be necessary.

NURSING DIAGNOSES/ DEFINING CHARACTERISTICS	NURSING INTERVENTIONS / *RATIONALES*	EXPECTED OUTCOMES
Pain (Abdominal, Joint Pain) **RELATED TO** Bowel inflammation, and contractions of diseased bowel or colon Systemic manifestations of IBD **DEFINING CHARACTERISTICS** Reports of intermittent colicky abdominal pain associated with diarrhea and chronic joint pain Abdominal rebound tenderness Chronic pain in the joints Hyperactive bowel sounds Pallor Diaphoresis Anxiety Restlessness Fatigue Malaise Abdominal distention Pain and cramps associated with eating Food intolerances	**ONGOING ASSESSMENT** • Assess age and developmental level. • Assess pain: Duration Location Frequency Occurrence/onset Severity (scale 1-10, 10 most severe) • Solicit child's perception of relief measures used to control pain. • Auscultate bowel sounds. • Check abdomen for rebound tenderness. • Evaluate child's perception of dietary impact on abdominal pain. *Many children with IBD cannot tolerate dairy products.* **THERAPEUTIC INTERVENTIONS** • Use techniques child/parent have found to be helpful in relieving discomfort. • Provide adequate rest periods *to facilitate sleep, comfort, and relaxation.* • Administer medications as ordered; evaluate and document effectiveness, and observe for signs of untoward effects. • Use diversional activities, hobbies, play, relaxation techniques, and psychosocial support systems *to facilitate comfort and relaxation.* • Make necessary alterations in diet.	Pain will be relieved.
Altered Nutrition: Less Than Body Requirements **RELATED TO** Malabsorption Zinc deficiency Protein nitrogen loss with diarrhea Decreased intake Poor appetite	**ONGOING ASSESSMENT** • Document child's actual weight on admission (do not estimate). • Obtain nutritional history from parent. • Assess for skin lesions, skin breaks, tears, decreased skin integrity, and edema of the extremities. • Assess serum electrolytes, calcium, vitamins K and B_{12}, folic acid, and zinc levels *to determine actual or potential deficiencies.* • Assess patterns of elimination: color, amount, consistency, frequency, odor, and for presence of steatorrhea. • Monitor I&O.	Optimal nutritional state will be maintained.

NURSING DIAGNOSES/ DEFINING CHARACTERISTICS	NURSING INTERVENTIONS / *RATIONALES*	EXPECTED OUTCOMES
DEFINING CHARACTERISTICS Small for age Delayed development of sexual maturity Nausea Diarrhea Decreased/normal serum calcium, potassium, vitamins K and B$_{12}$, folic acid, and zinc Muscle wasting Edema Skin lesions Poor wound healing	**THERAPEUTIC INTERVENTIONS** • Consult dietician to review nutritional history, monitor calorie count, and assist child or parent with menu selection. • Encourage active/passive ROM to child's tolerance. • Keep room as odor free as possible. • Administer vitamin/mineral supplements as ordered *to compensate for deficiencies.* • Encourage family members to bring food child enjoys, within limits of restrictions, *to enhance social nature of mealtime.*	
High Risk for Fluid Volume Deficit **RELATED TO** Presence of excessive diarrhea/nausea/vomiting Blood loss from inflamed bowel mucosa Poor oral intake **DEFINING CHARACTERISTICS** Weight loss Decreased skin turgor Hypotension Concentrated urine Bloody stools Sunken orbits Flat or scaphoid abdomen	**ONGOING ASSESSMENT** • Assess hydration status: tissue around eyes, contour of abdomen, skin turgor, mucous membranes. Monitor I&O, weight, and vital signs. • Document hemoccult-positive stools or obvious presence of bloody diarrhea. • Monitor Hgb and Hct if child is bleeding. **THERAPEUTIC INTERVENTIONS** • Administer medications as ordered, noting possible reactions. *Azulfidine (sulfasalazine) affects inflammatory response; corticosteroids may be used both for antiinflammatory and immunosuppressive benefits.* • Administer IV fluids if child is unable to maintain adequate oral intake. • See Fluid volume deficit, p. 19, GI bleeding, p. 235, and Diarrhea, p. 15.	Normal fluid volume will be maintained.
High Risk for Impaired Skin Integrity **RELATED TO** Decreased nutritional status Frequent loose stools **DEFINING CHARACTERISTICS** Excoriated perianal skin Reddened or irritated areas over bony prominences	**ONGOING ASSESSMENT** • Assess perianal skin after each bowel movement. • Assess skin integrity, noting color, texture, moisture, and temperature. **THERAPEUTIC INTERVENTIONS** • Keep perianal area clean and protect with a zinc-based or petroleum-based product. • Consider use of liquid skin barrier film on perianal region *for protection from diarrheal stool.* • Use prophylactic pressure-relieving devices on bed, chairs.	Perianal skin will remain intact.

Continued.

Inflammatory bowel disease cont'd

NURSING DIAGNOSES/ DEFINING CHARACTERISTICS	NURSING INTERVENTIONS / *RATIONALES*	EXPECTED OUTCOMES
High Risk for Infection **RELATED TO** Poor nutritional status Immunosuppression from steroid therapy **DEFINING CHARACTERISTICS** Decreased total lymphocyte count Poor wound healing Fever or lack of fever with other signs of infection present	**ONGOING ASSESSMENT** ▪ Monitor vital signs. ▪ Monitor WBC. ▪ Assess frequency of infectious episodes. ▪ Assess any wounds for signs of healing. **THERAPEUTIC INTERVENTIONS** ▪ Maintain good handwashing and encourage parent/child to do same *to prevent nosocomial infection.* ▪ Encourage well-balanced diet as tolerated. ▪ Discourage visitation from individuals with colds, flu, sore throat, or fever.	Risk of infection in immunocompromised child will be reduced.
Knowledge Deficit **RELATED TO** Need for continuous and long-term management of chronic disease Change in health care needs related to remission/exacerbation of disease Possible need for surgery **DEFINING CHARACTERISTICS** Multiple questions by child/parent related to disease process and management Noncompliance with earlier therapy Depression Anxiety	**ONGOING ASSESSMENT** ▪ Assess child's/parent's understanding of IBD and necessary management. **THERAPEUTIC INTERVENTIONS** ▪ Set aside a specific uninterrupted time to spend with child/parent *to enhance communication and facilitate learning.* Discuss disease process and management. Encourage child/parent to verbalize the disease process, management, concern, fears, and feelings. Document understanding. ▪ Make appropriate referrals: Dietary Psychiatric counseling Ostomy association	Child/parent will verbalize understanding of disease and management.
Disturbance in Social Functioning **RELATED TO** Delayed growth and development Frequent loss of time from school Frequent need to use bathroom	**ONGOING ASSESSMENT** ▪ Assess level of growth and development. ▪ Assess child's apparent social functioning: Friends Activities School ▪ Explore impact of stool frequency on social functioning. *It is common for children with IBD to have as many as 10-15 bowel movements per day.*	Age-/disease-appropriate socialization will be fostered.

Inflammatory bowel disease cont'd

NURSING DIAGNOSES/ DEFINING CHARACTERISTICS	NURSING INTERVENTIONS / *RATIONALES*	EXPECTED OUTCOMES
DEFINING CHARACTERISTICS Verbal description of social difficulties Poor school attendance record Little or no participation in usual activities for age	**THERAPEUTIC INTERVENTIONS** • Contact teacher to arrange for independent and frequent use of bathroom. • Explore with child activities that could be performed. • Help child/parent contact the National Foundation for Colitis and Ileitis.	

Vivian Jones, RN; Audrey Klopp, RN, PhD, CS, ET

Pyloric stenosis

Hypertrophic pyloric stenosis is a thickening of the pyloric muscle that develops in the first month of life in 1 out of 500 infants. It is familial in 5% to 20% of cases, and boys are affected four times as frequently as girls. Surgical treatment, a pyloroplasty, relieves the obstruction.

NURSING DIAGNOSES/ DEFINING CHARACTERISTICS	NURSING INTERVENTIONS / *RATIONALES*	EXPECTED OUTCOMES

High Risk for Fluid Volume Deficit
RELATED TO
Dehydration
Hypochloremia
Hypokalemic alkalosis
 	
DEFINING CHARACTERISTICS
Nonbilious vomiting
Decreased urine output
Reduced frequency of stools
Weight loss
	ONGOING ASSESSMENT
	• Assess age and developmental level.
	• Assess infant's history for vomiting after feedings, size and frequency of stools, and irritability/lethargy.
	• Assess hydration status:
	  Weigh preoperatively and postoperatively on the same scale in the same clothing at the same time each day *to assess degree of dehydration and success at rehydration.*
	  Check urine specific gravity every 8 hours *to assess hydration.*
	  Maintain strict I&O monitoring.
	  Monitor for signs of dehydration:
	    Dry mucous membranes
	    Increased heart rate
	    Decreased blood pressure
	    Sunken fontanels/eyes
	• Assess the birth history and prior physical status.
	• Assess the physical findings and radiologic studies if done:
	  "Olive" felt in the midepigastrium just cephalad to the umbilicus near the spine. *It is mobile. If the "olive" is felt, no further studies are needed before surgery.*
	  If the "olive" is felt, then review:
	    Ultrasound *to determine size of pyloric shadow (must be at least 1.2 cm with a wall thickness of 0.4 cm to meet the diagnostic criteria).*
	    Upper GI series *to identify a "track" sign (elongation of pyloric channel, indentation of thick muscle, and failure of gastric emptying).*
	• Assess current laboratory data (especially electrolytes).
		A balanced intake and output will be maintained.

Continued.

Pyloric stenosis cont'd

NURSING DIAGNOSES/ DEFINING CHARACTERISTICS	NURSING INTERVENTIONS / *RATIONALES*	EXPECTED OUTCOMES
	THERAPEUTIC INTERVENTIONS - Maintain patent nasogastric tube (if present) by irrigating tube with 2 to 4 ml normal saline solution; remember to subtract amount of irrigation from total output of tube. - Replace nasogastric output with intravenous fluid as ordered *to replace ongoing losses from the GI tract.* - Maintain patent IV line at ordered rate.	
Pain **RELATED TO** Operative incision **DEFINING CHARACTERISTICS** Irritability Crying Inability to sleep Changes in vital signs	**ONGOING ASSESSMENT** - Assess what comforts the infant. - Assess the effects of analgesia on the infant's behavior. - Observe incision for signs of infection (inflammation, drainage), bleeding, and wound healing. - Listen to parents' concerns. **THERAPEUTIC INTERVENTIONS** - Encourage parent to hold and touch child; offer infant pacifier; use soft voice or music *to soothe infant.* - Provide for uninterrupted rest/sleep periods. - Position infant to decrease stress in the incision line.	Pain will be relieved.
Altered Nutrition: Less Than Body Requirements **RELATED TO** Vomiting NPO status Gradual reintroduction of feeding postoperatively **DEFINING CHARACTERISTICS** Weight loss Ketonuria Inadequate wound healing	**ONGOING ASSESSMENT** - Assess preoperative and postoperative weight. - Assess wound for progressive healing. **THERAPEUTIC INTERVENTIONS** - Begin small, frequent feedings when oral intake is ordered *so the infant ingests adequate amounts of feeding without vomiting* (usually glucose water, progressing to dilute formula, and then full-strength formula). - Feed infant in upright position. - Burp infant frequently *to prevent abdominal distention caused by gulping of air.* - Handle infant gently during and after feeding. - Position infant on right side with head elevated *to promote passage of feeding from the stomach to the duodenum.* - Maintain IV fluids until feedings are tolerated.	Adequate nutrition will be maintained.
Knowledge Deficit **RELATED TO** Recent surgery **DEFINING CHARACTERISTICS** Questions or concerns voiced by family	**ONGOING ASSESSMENT** - Assess the family's understanding of the disease, their level of knowledge, and willingness to learn. **THERAPEUTIC INTERVENTIONS** - Encourage parent to assume care for the infant before discharge. - Demonstrate and have parent return demonstrate the feeding procedure and wound care. - Provide phone numbers and the names of persons to contact if questions or concerns arise. - Provide information on a return appointment.	The parent will understand the home care and follow-up needs.

Nedra Skale, RN, MS, CNA

Abdominal wall defect: preoperative

OMPHALOCELE; GASTROSCHISIS

Results from failure in the development of the abdominal contents to return to the abdomen when the wall begins to close during embryonic development. This may constitute a surgical emergency that requires prompt intervention. Defects include: Omphalocele—anomaly noted antepartally or at birth when there is herniation of the abdominal contents through the umbilical cord. A membranous covering may or may not be present. Gastroschisis—congenital defect in which the abdominal contents have herniated through the abdominal wall adjacent to the umbilical cord. There is no membrane present. The umbilical cord is intact.

NURSING DIAGNOSES/ DEFINING CHARACTERISTICS	NURSING INTERVENTIONS / *RATIONALES*	EXPECTED OUTCOMES
Ineffective Breathing Pattern/ Impaired Gas Exchange **RELATED TO** Decreased lung expansion Prematurity **DEFINING CHARACTERISTICS** Increased respiratory rate Abnormal arterial blood gas levels Cyanosis Nasal flaring Altered chest excursion	**ONGOING ASSESSMENT** • Monitor vital signs, especially respiratory rate, noting quality of respiration. • Observe for flaring of nares, grunting, and retractions. • Auscultate all lung lobes and compare breath sounds. • Observe skin color and perfusion. • Monitor blood gas results. **THERAPEUTIC INTERVENTIONS** • Maintain patent airway. • Suction every 2-4 hours. • When moving infant, lift in one motion, holding abdomen lower than lungs. • Elevate head of bed *to decrease diaphragmatic pressure.* • Maintain orogastric tube to low Gomco suction as ordered *to decompress stomach.* • Maintain respiratory support as ordered.	Effective breathing pattern will be maintained.
High Risk for Fluid Volume Deficit **RELATED TO** Excessive losses through skin and urine Loss of fluid through abdominal defect and orogastric tube Low-birth-weight infant **DEFINING CHARACTERISTICS** Increased pulse rate Increased urine specific gravity Increased serum sodium Abnormal weight loss Dry skin and mucous membranes Increased Hct Decreased skin turgor Hypotension	**ONGOING ASSESSMENT** • Assess hydration status using defining characteristics. **THERAPEUTIC INTERVENTIONS** • Maintain parenteral therapy as ordered, taking into consideration infant's weight, I&O, and electrolytes. • Administer volume expanders as ordered. • Provide high-humidity tent for infants treated with radiant warmers. • Place infants in isolettes if condition warrants *to prevent insensible water loss.* • Report abnormal electrolytes, total serum solute to physician. *This may indicate dehydration.* • Replace total orogastric losses as ordered *to prevent fluid and electrolyte imbalances.* • If abdominal sac is intact, cover with sterile gauze. For ruptured sac, use sterile technique, moisten gauze in warmed saline solution, and place over defect. Cover defect with plastic *to prevent evaporative heat and fluid loss.*	Hydration will be optimized.

Continued.

Abdominal wall defect: preoperative cont'd

NURSING DIAGNOSES/ DEFINING CHARACTERISTICS	NURSING INTERVENTIONS / *RATIONALES*	EXPECTED OUTCOMES
High Risk for Infection **RELATED TO** Open abdominal defect Altered immune response **DEFINING CHARACTERISTICS** Lethargy Temperature instability Irritability Cyanosis Redness and swelling around open wound Apnea and bradycardia Drainage	**ONGOING ASSESSMENT** ▪ Note activity and subtle symptoms of infection using defining characteristics. **THERAPEUTIC INTERVENTIONS** ▪ For ruptured abdominal defects, always maintain sterile technique when applying dressings. *Infants with ruptured abdominal sacs are prone to infection.* ▪ Do not unwrap or attempt to reinspect the defect once it has been wrapped *to prevent infection and unnecessary heat loss.* ▪ Administer prophylactic antibiotics as ordered.	Risk for infection will be reduced.
High Risk for Hypothermia **RELATED TO** Open abdominal defect Exposed abdominal organs **DEFINING CHARACTERISTICS** Body temperature <37° C (98.6° F) Skin pale or blue Loss of or failure to gain weight Apneic spells Hypoxia Hypoglycemia Fluid and electrolyte imbalance Irritability	**ONGOING ASSESSMENT** ▪ Maintain normal body temperature between 36.5° C (97.7° F) and 37.0° C (98.6° F). ▪ See Thermoregulation in the low-birth-weight infant, p. 379. **THERAPEUTIC INTERVENTIONS** ▪ Place newborn in warmed isolette, at least 35° C. ▪ Wrap defect in warm normal saline solution dressings. ▪ Cover defect with plastic or bowel bag *to decrease heat loss.*	Potential for hypothermia will be reduced.
High Risk for Injury Secondary to Intestinal Obstruction **RELATED TO** Adhesions Volvulus Paralytic ileus	**ONGOING ASSESSMENT** ▪ Note signs and symptoms of intestinal obstruction using defining characteristics. ▪ Document stooling pattern and characteristics. *Stool and stooling patterns are good indicators of gastrointestinal function.* ▪ Auscultate bowel sounds *to detect intestinal obstruction.*	Risk for injury will be reduced.

Abdominal wall defect: preoperative cont'd

NURSING DIAGNOSES/ DEFINING CHARACTERISTICS	NURSING INTERVENTIONS / *RATIONALES*	EXPECTED OUTCOMES
DEFINING CHARACTERISTICS Presence of persistent vomiting Hematest-positive stools Increase in gastric drainage Presence of abdominal cramping as evidenced by crying and restlessness Changes in bowel sounds	**THERAPEUTIC INTERVENTIONS** ▪ Maintain NPO status. ▪ Maintain oral-gastric tube to low Gomco suction as ordered.	
Altered Parenting RELATED TO Separation and hospitalization of infant **DEFINING CHARACTERISTICS** Parent's reluctance to look at infant Parent verbalizes that infant may be in pain or staff is hurting infant Parent blames self for infant's condition Parent verbalizes guilt feelings for having a "less than perfect" baby	**ONGOING ASSESSMENT** ▪ Assess defining characteristics. **THERAPEUTIC INTERVENTIONS** ▪ If defining characteristics are present, see Parenting in special care nursery, p. 72.	Parent/infant bonding will be initiated.

Ruby Rotor-Cajindos, RN, BSN

Breastfeeding the infant requiring special care

The decision to breastfeed a premature or sick newborn infant is complex. Initiating and maintaining lactation in absence of suckling requires education and support before the initiation of a breast milk expression and collection program.

NURSING DIAGNOSES/ DEFINING CHARACTERISTICS	NURSING INTERVENTIONS / *RATIONALES*	EXPECTED OUTCOMES
Altered Nutrition: Less Than Body Requirements (Maternal) **RELATED TO** Mother's anxiety and stress over infant's condition Physical separation from infant Incomplete or irregular emptying of breasts Engorged breasts Delayed or absent let-down Lack of rest Poor diet **DEFINING CHARACTERISTICS** Weight loss Irritability Decreased milk supply	**ONGOING ASSESSMENT** ▪ Ascertain whether mother consumes adequate fluid and calories. ▪ Evaluate mother's sleep and rest patterns. ▪ Measure quantity of milk being produced. ▪ Note condition of mother's breasts and nipples. ▪ Chart maternal weight weekly. **THERAPEUTIC INTERVENTIONS** ▪ Explain caloric and fluid requirements of nursing mother. ▪ Explain role of stress/emotions in reducing milk production and let-down response. ▪ Encourage mother to handle infant and participate in care as much as possible *to promote bonding.* ▪ Explain need for adequate rest. ▪ Reassure mother that milk supply increases and let-down occurs more quickly when infant begins nursing. ▪ Provide information on nutrition, and obtain dietary consultation if necessary. ▪ Obtain social work consultation. *The social worker may be able to assist in obtaining supplemental food, utilizing resources such as the WIC program.*	Maternal nutritional status will be optimized.
Ineffective Breastfeeding **RELATED TO** Prematurity Low birth weight Medications CNS damage Congenital heart disease Respiratory problems Congenital anomalies Initial oral feedings taken from bottle Poor sucking and swallowing reflexes Failure to coordinate breathing and sucking **DEFINING CHARACTERISTICS** Weight loss Infant falls asleep at breast Duskiness or bradycardia in infant with feeding	**ONGOING ASSESSMENT** ▪ Evaluate infant's ability to nurse: Respiratory rate Color during feeding Ability to maintain temperature Gestational age Weight Tolerance of feeding by bottle Anatomical abnormalities **THERAPEUTIC INTERVENTIONS** ▪ Provide nonnutritive sucking opportunities for infant, using orthodontic pacifier. ▪ Use orthodontic nipples on bottles *to facilitate transition to breast.* ▪ Schedule first nursing attempts between feedings *to avoid frustration in a hungry infant.* ▪ Provide frequent, short opportunities to nurse. ▪ Recognize signs and symptoms that indicate infant is unable to tolerate breastfeeding. *Premature infants may need to nurse for shorter periods of time.* Temperature instability Weight loss or decreased weight gain Refusal to suck at subsequent feedings ▪ Reassure mother that a "get acquainted" period is necessary before nursing will progress. ▪ Encourage mother to spend as much time as possible on unit, *so she is available when infant is hungry.*	Infant will nurse to the best of his or her ability.

NURSING DIAGNOSES/ DEFINING CHARACTERISTICS	NURSING INTERVENTIONS / *RATIONALES*	EXPECTED OUTCOMES

	THERAPEUTIC INTERVENTIONS cont'd
	• Instruct mother on ways to encourage sucking:
	   Attempt nursing during alert periods.
	   Pump/express small amount of milk before putting infant to breast:
	     To ensure that let-down has occurred
	     To draw out nipple
	     To soften full, hard breast so that premature infant can grasp nipple
	   Position infant to easily reach nipples.
	• Gently stroke infant's lower lip with nipple.
	• Put drop of milk or glucose water on infant's lips *to stimulate infant's interest.*
	• Stimulate sucking *by stroking infant's feet.*
	• Change position *to wake sleepy infant.*
	• Unwrap infant *to increase wakefulness (if condition permits).*
	• Hold infant upright *to facilitate swallowing.*
	• Assess infant's tolerance of feeding, and take pauses if needed.
	• Burp infant frequently *to avoid abdominal distention and subsequent pressure on diaphragm.*
	• Administer oxygen during feeding, as indicated.
	• Schedule medications that affect alertness *so they are least likely to cause drowsiness at feeding time.*
	• Explain how the special implications of the infant's disease/condition will influence nursing.	

Altered Nutrition: Less Than Body Requirements (Infant)
 	
RELATED TO
 	
Inadequate intake
Caloric expenditure greater than caloric intake
 	
DEFINING CHARACTERISTICS
 	
Inadequate weight gain
Dry mucous membranes
Decreased urine output with specific gravity >1.010
	ONGOING ASSESSMENT
	• Assess fluid balance:
	   Maintain urine output >48 ml/kg/day.
	   Maintain specific gravity between 1.003 and 1.010.
	   Evaluate skin turgor.
	• Assess adequacy of weight gain:
	   Weigh once daily.
	   Compare weight gain to Dancis curve.
	• Observe quality and duration of sucking.
	• Note length of time infant is satisfied between feedings.
	
	THERAPEUTIC INTERVENTIONS
	• Check creamatocrit of mother's milk *to assess fat content.*
	• Suggest maternal diet improvements *to maintain adequate caloric content of milk.*
	• Notify physician of insufficient weight gain.
	• Feed by nasogastric tube until infant can nurse without excessive caloric usage, and supplement nursing with nasogastric feeding as necessary.
	• Minimize infant's caloric expenditure by maintaining temperature within normal limits.
		Adequate nutrition will be maintained.

Knowledge Deficit **RELATED TO** Lack of knowledge on breastfeeding process Assumption that preterm infant cannot be breastfed Lack of knowledge with mechanical/manual methods of expressing breast milk	**ONGOING ASSESSMENT** • Assess knowledge of breastfeeding the premature infant. • Assess manual/mechanical means of expressing breast milk **THERAPEUTIC INTERVENTIONS** • Discuss the contribution breast milk makes to the infant's recovery. *Mother's milk, especially colostrum, contains antibodies against infection and is more easily digested by the premature baby.* • Reassure parent with explanations of infant's care and condition, *to decrease anxiety regarding breastfeeding.*	Parents will demonstrate an understanding of the breastfeeding process.

Continued.

NURSING DIAGNOSES/ DEFINING CHARACTERISTICS	NURSING INTERVENTIONS / *RATIONALES*	EXPECTED OUTCOMES

DEFINING CHARACTERISTICS
 	
Verbalizes misconceptions
Relates incorrect information
Lack of questions
	THERAPEUTIC INTERVENTIONS cont'd
	• Instruct mother in techniques for hand expression and use of manual/ electric breast pump:
	    Mother should pump breast for no longer than 15 minutes on each side. If pain is experienced, cease pumping immediately, and gradually increase pumping time as tolerated.
	• Suggest activities to enhance milk flow:
	    Comfortable position
	    Nap before pumping
	    Breast massage
	    Back rub with or during pumping *to facilitate relaxation*
	    Looking at picture of baby while pumping
	    Applying heat to breasts *to promote let-down* (heating pad, bath, shower)
	    Soft music
	    If all above measures fail, obtain an order for oxytocin nasal drops *to help initiate the letdown reflex.*
	• Explain proper care of breasts.
	• Refer to the La Leche League or a lactation consultant who will provide support to breastfeeding mothers.	

Laura L. Rybicki, RN, BSN

Choanal atresia

AIRWAY OBSTRUCTION

A congenital condition characterized by blockage of the posterior nares, which can be unilateral or bilateral.

NURSING DIAGNOSES/ DEFINING CHARACTERISTICS	NURSING INTERVENTIONS / *RATIONALES*	EXPECTED OUTCOMES
Ineffective Breathing Pattern RELATED TO Complete or partial obstruction of the nares, caused by a bony structure, cartilage, or membrane coverage **DEFINING CHARACTERISTICS** Failure to pass a nasogastric tube through one or both nares Cyanosis Dyspnea Increased PCO_2 Absence of air exchange on auscultation at the external nares Thick mucus in the nose Mouth breathing	**ONGOING ASSESSMENT** • Closely monitor for signs and symptoms of respiratory distress as listed under defining characteristics. • Assess by auscultation presence of air exchange at the external nares. • Note general skin and mucous membrane color. • Monitor blood gas results. **THERAPEUTIC INTERVENTIONS** • Maintain patent airway by suctioning as needed *to prevent pooling of secretions and possible aspiration.* • Insert oral airway *to accommodate mouth breathing pending surgical correction.* • Administer oxygen as needed *to maintain PaO_2 at prescribed level to maximize oxygenation.* • Place child in semi-Fowler's position *to improve air exchange.* • Notify physician of abnormal blood gas results, *as choanal obstruction may interfere with exhaling carbon dioxide and result in an elevated PCO_2.*	Adequate breathing pattern and gas exchange will be achieved.

NURSING DIAGNOSES/ DEFINING CHARACTERISTICS	NURSING INTERVENTIONS / *RATIONALES*	EXPECTED OUTCOMES
Altered Nutrition: High Risk for Less Than Body Requirements **RELATED TO** Inability to feed orally as a result of respiratory distress **DEFINING CHARACTERISTICS** Increased tachypnea, retractions, nasal flaring, and cyanosis Weight loss Documented inadequate caloric intake Increased urine specific gravity	**ONGOING ASSESSMENT** • Assess infant's ability to tolerate feedings by: Observing respiratory status before, during, and after feedings Evaluating weight gain with Dancis curve and growth chart Checking residual gastric contents and abdominal circumference before each feeding. *Abdominal distention is an early symptom of feeding intolerance.* • Monitor accurate I&O. • Check urine specific gravity every shift. • Weigh infant daily. **THERAPEUTIC INTERVENTIONS** • Notify physician of any signs and symptoms of respiratory distress as listed under defining characteristics. • Maintain gavage feedings *as infant is prone to aspiration if bottle feedings are given.* • If NPO status is necessary because of feeding problems, administer IV fluids *to provide adequate ml/kg/day.* • If gastric residuals are >2-3 ml, notify physician before giving next feeding. • Notify physician of a rising urine specific gravity, *which may be indicative of dehydration.*	Nutritional deficit will be reduced.
High Risk for Infection **RELATED TO** Surgical procedure **DEFINING CHARACTERISTICS** Inflammation of and/ or drainage from incision Increased or decreased WBC count Lethargy Temperature instability	**ONGOING ASSESSMENT** • Note activity and symptoms of infection using defining characteristics. • Assess suture line for drainage and inflammation. • Culture suspicious drainage. • Monitor antibiotic levels *to prevent toxic or subtherapeutic level.* • Monitor vital signs with temperature every 1-2 hours. • Obtain CBC and differentials. **THERAPEUTIC INTERVENTIONS** • Maintain strict handwashing by all individuals handling infant, *as handwashing is the most effective way of preventing spread of infection.* • Use aseptic technique when changing surgical dressings/IV lines. • Administer antibiotics as ordered. • See Thermoregulation in the low-birth-weight infant, p. 379.	Risk of infection will be reduced.
Parental Anxiety **RELATED TO** Hospitalization Fear of infant's death Surgery **DEFINING CHARACTERISTICS** Parent afraid to touch infant Excessive and uncontrollable crying Withdrawal Grief Excessive questions Silence Infrequent or excessive telephone calls	**ONGOING ASSESSMENT** • Assess coping mechanisms of family. • Assess family-infant interaction. • Evaluate maternal support system: Husband or significant other Friends, peers, and clergy • Assess parental need for referrals to other support services. **THERAPEUTIC INTERVENTIONS** • Facilitate open lines of communication between parent and health care team about infant's condition *to help alleviate anxiety.* • Encourage parent to touch and hold infant as physical condition permits *to promote infant bonding.* • Provide psychosocial support for the family, using appropriate resources. • Encourage parent to express feelings, *as parent should not feel responses will be judged as "good" or "bad."* • See Parenting in special care nursery, p. 72.	Parental anxiety will be reduced.

Cynthia R. Wilson, RN, BSN

Cleft lip and palate

MIDLINE DEFECTS

Congenital malformation involving a fissure or split (cleft) of the lip, or of the hard and soft palate, or a combination of both.

NURSING DIAGNOSES/ DEFINING CHARACTERISTICS	NURSING INTERVENTIONS / *RATIONALES*	EXPECTED OUTCOMES
Ineffective Family Coping **RELATED TO** Temporary preoccupation by parent trying to manage the emotional conflict of having an infant with a visible defect Temporary disorganization of the family **DEFINING CHARACTERISTICS** Parental expression of concern about others' response to infant's defect Parental preoccupation with personal reactions (e.g., shock, disbelief, inability/reluctance to look at and interact with infant, guilt feelings, and feelings of loss of the perfect child)	**ONGOING ASSESSMENT** • Assess the following: Understanding/knowledge by parent/family of the nature of cleft and palate Degree of the family's anxiety and level of discomfort Interpersonal relationship among family members The family's reaction to the infant • Identify the existing support systems within the family. **THERAPEUTIC INTERVENTIONS** • Support the open visiting policy. • Encourage parent to: Verbalize feelings Participate in the support group of parents with infants in the neonatal ICU Participate in caretaking activities (e.g., diapering, feeding, bathing, and holding infant). *Caretaking activities will decrease anxiety and provide parent with a sense of purpose.* • Explore potential use of other support systems (e.g., parent-to-parent referral or use of other family members).	The family's coping ability will be maximized.
Knowledge Deficit of Parent/Family **RELATED TO** Lack of previous exposure to this problem **DEFINING CHARACTERISTICS** Inappropriate or exaggerated behaviors (e.g., verbalization of fear that the "baby might die," lowered self-esteem, and hesitancy in bonding with infant) Request for information	**ONGOING ASSESSMENT** • Assess understanding/knowledge of parent/family of the nature of the cleft lip and palate. **THERAPEUTIC INTERVENTIONS** • Let parent see and hold infant as soon as possible after the birth. With infant present, discuss the problems, as well as the infant's normal attributes. • In conjunction with the appropriate physician, provide information regarding: Occurrence of cleft lip and palate Cause and nature of the defect Needs of the infant Available support group systems • Encourage questions. *Concrete information allows parent time to conceptualize problem.* • Give parent the booklet, "Your Cleft Lip and Palate Child" (Mead Johnson & Co.).	Parent will verbalize an understanding of the nature and sequela of the defect.

NURSING DIAGNOSES/ DEFINING CHARACTERISTICS	NURSING INTERVENTIONS / *RATIONALES*	EXPECTED OUTCOMES

Altered Nutrition: Less Than Body Requirements
RELATED TO
Difficulty ingesting food
Inability to form an adequate nutritive seal for sucking
 	
DEFINING CHARACTERISTICS
Failure to gain weight according to the growth curve
Documented inadequate caloric intake
	ONGOING ASSESSMENT
	- Assess fluid and caloric intake daily.
	- Assess weight pattern according to the Dancis curve.
	- Observe the following during the feeding:
	   Respiration
	   Color
	   Nutritive sucking ability
	
	THERAPEUTIC INTERVENTIONS
	- Provide 100-120 cal/kg/day and 100-130 ml/kg/day.
	- Facilitate breastfeeding (see Breastfeeding the infant requiring special care, p. 246).
	   Encourage the mother to massage the breast before nursing to bring milk to the surface. *This will make the breast full and hard, which will help the infant hold the nipple in his or her mouth.*
	   Hold the infant in a semisitting or upright position *to make swallowing easier and to reduce the amount of milk that may come out of the nose because of the defect.*
	   If the infant has difficulty holding the nipple in his or her mouth, have the mother apply pressure to the areola with her fingers. It may be necessary for the mother to guide the nipple to the side of the mouth and hold it there during the entire feeding. *The infant will then be able to "milk" the nipple with his or her gums.*
	   Burp the infant frequently, *since infants with clefts swallow more air during feeding.*
	   Contact the La Leche League for the name of support person for the mother.
	   Give the mother information on breastfeeding an infant with a cleft of the soft palate.
	   If the infant is unable to breastfeed because of the defect, consider using a LactAid until the defect is surgically repaired.
	- Initiate bottle feeding adjustments:
	   Hold infant in an upright or semisitting position.
	   Place the nipple against the inside cheek toward the back of the tongue. If a regular nipple is inadequate, use a nipple designed for premature infants, and enlarge the hole. *A cleft palate nurser may even be necessary.* If the infant is still having problems, use a soft plastic bottle *to squeeze the formula into infant's mouth.*
	   Feed small amounts slowly.
	   Burp infant frequently, as often as after each 10-15 ml of milk.
	   If infant is not able to take all feedings orally, consider a combination of oral and nasogastric feedings.
		Optimal weight gain as indicated per Dancis growth curve will be achieved.

High Risk for Infection **RELATED TO** Accumulated formula in the oral cavity **DEFINING CHARACTERISTICS** Tender, reddened areas on the lip and palate	**ONGOING ASSESSMENT** - Assess the general hygiene, nutrition, and feeding techniques used. - Assess oral cavity (see Defining Characteristics). **THERAPEUTIC INTERVENTIONS** - Cleanse the cleft areas by giving 5-10 ml of water after each feeding. - If a crust has already formed, use a cotton-tipped applicator or swab to apply a peroxide solution (1:1 water and peroxide) *to loosen the crust.* - If the cleft area becomes dry, keep it moist with mineral oil, glycerine, or petrolatum. - If the cleft or lip areas become infected or irritated, contact the physician for further treatment orders.	Risk of infection will be reduced.

Continued.

Gastrointestinal Care Plans (Neonatal)

NURSING DIAGNOSES/ DEFINING CHARACTERISTICS	NURSING INTERVENTIONS / *RATIONALES*	EXPECTED OUTCOMES
High Risk for Ineffective Airway Clearance **RELATED TO** Aspiration of breast milk/formula or mucus because of the anatomical defect **DEFINING CHARACTERISTICS** Abnormal breath sounds Tachypnea/dyspnea Nasal flaring Retractions Cyanosis	**ONGOING ASSESSMENT** • Assess the following: Respiratory rate Presence of nasal flaring or retractions Skin color and capillary refill Breath sounds • Monitor vital signs every 2-3 hours. **THERAPEUTIC INTERVENTIONS** • Suction oropharynx and nasopharynx as needed. • Maintain adequate airway by positioning the infant on his or her abdomen during periods of sleep. • Burp infant frequently during feeding with the infant in an upright position *to minimize possibility of aspiration.* • Pace activities (feeding, bathing, handling) *to avoid distress.* • Provide high-humidity or oxygen therapy as ordered by physician.	A patent airway will be maintained.
High Risk for Impaired Home Maintenance Management **RELATED TO** Defect of infant Inadequate community resources **DEFINING CHARACTERISTICS** Parental expression of difficulty in preparing home for infant Parental request for delay in discharge Decrease in parental calls/visits as discharge date approaches	**ONGOING ASSESSMENT** • Assess general home conditions and availability of any necessary equipment. • Assess other family members' reactions to, acceptance of, and willingness to participate in infant's care. **THERAPEUTIC INTERVENTIONS** • Encourage parent to verbalize degree of preparation: Psychologically Physically Financially • With the social worker and visiting nurse, assist in parental preparation of home for the infant. • Have parent assume total care-taking responsibilities for an extended period before discharge. *Maximizing parental involvement will ensure comfort level.* • Provide the telephone number of the physician or clinic for follow-up care. • Advise parent of potential problems that necessitate professional evaluation before the scheduled follow-up visit.	Appropriate home care activities will be demonstrated.

Cynthia R. Wilson, RN, BSN

Hyperbilirubinemia

JAUNDICE; PHYSIOLOGIC JAUNDICE;
PATHOLOGIC JAUNDICE; BREAST MILK
JAUNDICE

Abnormal elevation of serum bilirubin associated with alterations of bilirubin metabolism. This condition is characterized by jaundice of the skin, the sclera of the eyes, and mucous membranes. Common causes are: physiologic jaundice caused by the neonate's developmental limitations in clearing bilirubin from the plasma; and pathologic jaundice, which includes Rh isoimmunization, ABO incompatibility, sepsis, and breast milk jaundice.

NURSING DIAGNOSES/ DEFINING CHARACTERISTICS	NURSING INTERVENTIONS / *RATIONALES*	EXPECTED OUTCOMES
High Risk for Injury Secondary to Onset of Jaundice Within 24 Hours of Life **RELATED TO** Intravascular hemolysis Infection **DEFINING CHARACTERISTICS** Hct ≤40% Serum bilirubin level of 5-10 mg% Reticulocyte count elevated Total serum solute ≤4.0 Metabolic acidosis Apnea Cardiac failure Hepatomegaly Hypovolemia Massive generalized edema Bruising Hematoma	**ONGOING ASSESSMENT** ▪ Note age of infant at onset of increased serum bilirubin level. ▪ Review maternal/fetal history and clinical data to determine cause. ▪ Obtain initial blood studies: Type and Coombs' test, using cord blood if possible CBC with reticulocyte count and differential Cultures as ordered ABGs as needed ▪ Obtain serum bilirubin every 4 hours. Fractionate bilirubin every 4 hours if bilirubin rise is >5.0-1.0 mg/hr and close to exchange level *to determine the amount of unconjugated bilirubin that presents the danger for kernicterus.* ▪ Check Hct every 4-6 hours *to determine the extent of hemolysis.* ▪ Check Chemstrip every 6 hours. *Erythroblastic infants tend to have islet cell hyperplasia and elevated insulin levels.* ▪ Check total serum solute every 12 hours. *Bilirubin binds with albumin for excretion.* ▪ Assess presence and extent of hematoma and bruising. ▪ Monitor vital signs with BP closely every 2 hours *to determine early signs of:* Cardiac failure Hypovolemia Respiratory failure ▪ Note skin color/sclera. ▪ Maintain accurate I&O. ▪ Record specific gravity every void *to determine early signs of dehydration.* ▪ Observe for signs/symptoms of encephalopathy (kernicterus): *Early signs:* Poor feeding Vomiting Lethargy High-pitched voice Hypotonia Decreased Moro's reflex *Later signs:* Opisthotonos posturing Apnea Irritability Seizures **THERAPEUTIC INTERVENTIONS** ▪ Record specific gravity every void *to determine early signs of dehydration.* ▪ Assist with partial exchange transfusion as ordered. ▪ Initiate phototherapy as ordered. ▪ Provide good skin care *to prevent break in skin integrity.*	Potential for kernicterus will be reduced.

Continued.

Gastrointestinal Care Plans (Neonatal)

NURSING DIAGNOSES/ DEFINING CHARACTERISTICS	NURSING INTERVENTIONS / *RATIONALES*	EXPECTED OUTCOMES
High Risk for Injury Secondary to Onset of Jaundice on the Second to Seventh Day of Life **RELATED TO** Perinatal asphyxia Respiratory distress syndrome Infant of diabetic mother Prematurity Physiologic jaundice Hemolysis resulting from birth trauma (bruising) Polycythemia Increased enterohepatic circulation Delayed stooling pattern **DEFINING CHARACTERISTICS** Jaundice noted on the second day Indirect serum bilirubin: ≥12 mg/dl Rate of bilirubin increase: 5 mg/dl/ day (for bilirubin considered high, refer to protocol manual) Peak bilirubin level of term infant: 6 mg/ dl by 48-72 hours *Premature infant:* 10-15 mg/dl peaking by 4-6 days Lethargy Poor feeding pattern Dark stools Dark, amber, concentrated urine	**ONGOING ASSESSMENT** ▪ See High risk for injury secondary to onset of jaundice within 24 hours of life in preceding diagnosis. ▪ Record stooling pattern. Perform rectal stimulation if no stool for 2-3 days *to promote stooling and bilirubin excretion.* **THERAPEUTIC INTERVENTIONS** ▪ Follow therapeutic interventions for High risk for injury secondary to onset of jaundice within 24 hours of life in preceding diagnosis. ▪ Provide early feedings as tolerated *to stimulate peristalsis/stooling to enhance bilirubin excretion via the gut. Meconium can contain over 1 mg of bilirubin/g.* ▪ Withhold intralipids while infant is undergoing phototherapy as ordered. *Indirect bilirubin is lipid soluble and therefore bilirubin excretion can be altered.*	Potential for kernicterus will be reduced.
High Risk for Injury Secondary to Jaundice Related to Use of Breast Milk **RELATED TO** Breastfeeding	**ONGOING ASSESSMENT** ▪ Correlate the presence of jaundice and the use of breast milk. ▪ Obtain fractionated serum bilirubin as ordered. ▪ Repeat serum bilirubin on the fifth day. **THERAPEUTIC INTERVENTIONS** ▪ Initiate phototherapy as ordered. ▪ Interrupt feeding of breast milk for 2-5 days *to establish differential diagnosis.* ▪ Resume offering breast milk on the fifth or ninth day if serum bilirubin level decreases to 8-10 mg/dl. ▪ Provide good skin care *to prevent break in skin integrity.*	Risks of kernicterus will be reduced.

NURSING DIAGNOSES/ DEFINING CHARACTERISTICS	NURSING INTERVENTIONS / *RATIONALES*	EXPECTED OUTCOMES

DEFINING CHARACTERISTICS

Jaundice occurring on fourth to seventh day
Indirect bilirubin of 15-25 mg/dl
Serum bilirubin declines 2.4 mg/dl after milk is discontinued

---

High Risk for Injury Secondary to Late Onset or Failure to Resolve Jaundice

RELATED TO

Organic causes:
Red cell deficiency and biliary obstruction
Liver damage secondary to total parenteral nutrition
Metabolic and endocrine disturbances

DEFINING CHARACTERISTICS

Absence of glucose 6-phosphate dehydrogenase
Elevated liver enzyme tests
Bilirubin levels >15 mg/dl

ONGOING ASSESSMENT

- Assess infant's clinical course.
- Assess and review all available laboratory data.
- Obtain fractionated serum bilirubin daily and prn. Send specimen for adult biochemistry profile.

THERAPEUTIC INTERVENTIONS

- Discontinue total parenteral nutrition and intralipids until further orders *to establish differential diagnosis. Prolonged use of parenteral nutrition may be toxic to the liver.*
- Initiate phototherapy as ordered.
- Provide good skin care *to prevent break in skin integrity.*

Risks of kernicterus will be reduced.

High Risk for Fluid Volume Deficit

RELATED TO

Use of radiant warmers
Use of phototherapy
Loose stools

DEFINING CHARACTERISTICS

Urine output <1-1.5 ml/kg/hr
Urine specific gravity >1.010-1.012
5% weight loss per 24-hour period
Dry skin and mucous membranes
Thick secretions
Serum Na$^+$ >145 mEq/L
Polycythemia
Rise of bilirubin despite other treatment

ONGOING ASSESSMENT

- Assess hydration status based on:
Daily weights
Skin turgor
Fontanels
Electrolytes every 12 hours
Specific gravity every void with Labstix
Urine output every void
Recorded I&O every 2-4 hours

THERAPEUTIC INTERVENTIONS

- Maintain adequate fluid intake to provide 80-120 ml/kg/day:
Infants receiving phototherapy need 1½ × maintenance fluid *to compensate for water loss by evaporation.*
Infants with low birth weight may require higher fluid requirement (a maximum of 180-200 mg/kg/day) *because of increased water content in the skin, thinner epidermis, and increased skin permeability.*
- Observe closely for signs of fluid overload.

Optimal hydration will be attained.

Continued.

Gastrointestinal Care Plans (Neonatal)

NURSING DIAGNOSES/ DEFINING CHARACTERISTICS	NURSING INTERVENTIONS / *RATIONALES*	EXPECTED OUTCOMES

High Risk for Altered Nutrition: Less Than Body Requirements
RELATED TO
Nothing by mouth
Total parenteral nutrition
Poor oral feeding
Increased peristaltic activity
 	
DEFINING CHARACTERISTICS
Weight loss
Sunken orbits
Hypoglycemia
Restlessness
Irritability
Emesis
Diarrhea
Documented inadequate caloric intake
	ONGOING ASSESSMENT
	• Assess patterns of weight loss/weight gain based on daily weights. Compare to Dancis curve.
	• Assess caloric intake compatible for weight gain.
	• Assess feeding tolerance by:
	  Recording abdominal girth every 3 hours
	  Testing stools by Hematest and reducing substance every 6-8 hours
	  Recording type of stools, frequency, and amount
	
	THERAPEUTIC INTERVENTIONS
	• Provide approximately 90-120 cal/kg/day with formula or breast milk feedings, *which should prompt a weight gain of 10-30 g/day.*
	• Evaluate infant's ability to be fed orally:
	  Use bolus nasogastric feeding for infants weighing <1000 g. *Suck-swallow coordination is not well established before 34 weeks' gestation.*
	  Feed via nasogastric tube if infant is unable to complete oral feeding *to minimize caloric expenditure.*
	  Implement alternate oral and nasogastric feedings until suck-swallow reflex is well established.
		Caloric requirement of infant will be attained with documented weight gain.

Knowledge Deficit of Parents
RELATED TO
Unfamiliarity with hyperbilirubinemia and hospital routines
Breastfeeding withheld
Infant returned to NPO status
Subsequent exchange transfusion needed
 	
DEFINING CHARACTERISTICS
Withdrawn and unable to verbalize understanding of infant's condition
Anxious and extremely worried
	ONGOING ASSESSMENT
	• Assess level and educational background.
	• Assess parental:
	  Resources for information
	  Acceptance of infant's present condition
	  Comprehension of information given
	
	THERAPEUTIC INTERVENTIONS
	• Provide parent with information regarding infant's:
	  Diagnosis and treatment
	  Current condition by means of:
	    Literature on neonatal jaundice
	    Explanation of specific cause and management plan
	• Encourage parent to ask questions *as this will allow verbalization or ventilation.*
	• Encourage attendance at parents' class or support group.
		Parent's ability to comprehend infant's illness will be optimal.

Altered Parenting
RELATED TO
Separation of parent and infant because of:
  Critically ill infant
  Critically ill mother
  Transfer of infant to another hospital
	ONGOING ASSESSMENT
	• Evaluate mother's emotional state. Signs of tension include:
	  Rapid breathing
	  Muscle tension; arms stiff; tires easily
	  Perspiration
	  Rapid or stilted conversation
	• Observe and evaluate parent-infant interactions.
	• Evaluate and document in appropriate chart forms:
	  Frequency of calls
	  Family members who visit
		Optimal parent-infant bonding will be achieved.

Hyperbilirubinemia cont'd

NURSING DIAGNOSES/ DEFINING CHARACTERISTICS	NURSING INTERVENTIONS / *RATIONALES*	EXPECTED OUTCOMES

DEFINING CHARACTERISTICS
 	
Infrequent visits and telephone calls
Delayed display of interactive and fondling behavior
Display of discomfort in handling infant
Display of hostile and demanding behavior in terms of infant care and information
Questions that focus on equipment instead of infant
	THERAPEUTIC INTERVENTIONS
	• Explain visitation and telephone call policies to parents.
	• Encourage early visits.
	• Provide literature on special care unit to the parents.
	• Provide parent with infant's picture.
	• During parental visits:
	    Turn off bili-lite.
	    Remove infant's eye pads.
	    Encourage touching and handling.
	    Allow parents to:
	        Hold and/or feed infant
	        Change infant's diapers and apply lotion
	        Bathe infant as condition permits *to enhance parent-infant bonding*
	• Encourage parent to discuss support system.
	• Request social work referral as needed.	

Rosetonia G. Sapaula, RN, BSN

Low birth weight and total parenteral nutrition

Total parenteral nutrition (TPN) via a central venous catheter is provided for low-birth-weight infants with enteral feeding intolerance. The infant weighing less than 1200 g has an immature alimentary tract with decreased ability to absorb adequate nutrients. TPN is necessary to meet the nutritional requirements associated with increased metabolic demands such as respiratory distress syndrome, apnea, and sepsis.

NURSING DIAGNOSES/ DEFINING CHARACTERISTICS	NURSING INTERVENTIONS / *RATIONALES*	EXPECTED OUTCOMES
Altered Nutrition: Less Than Body Requirements **RELATED TO** Extreme prematurity **DEFINING CHARACTERISTICS** Enteral feeding intolerance Weight loss Inadequate weight gain Negative nitrogen balance Loss of liver glycogen stores Loss of trace elements	**ONGOING ASSESSMENT** • Assess infants at risk (<1200 g) for feeding intolerance, apnea, sepsis, ventilator dependence. • Monitor growth, daily weight, daily head circumference, and weekly length. • Calculate fluid and caloric requirements daily. **THERAPEUTIC INTERVENTIONS** • Provide neutral thermal environment *to reduce caloric expenditure.* • Administer hyperalimentation and intralipids as ordered *to provide adequate hydration and enough calories to promote growth.* • Provide ventilatory support *to decrease caloric loss associated with increased work of breathing in infants in respiratory distress.* • Report to physician weight loss of 10%-15% during the first week of life.	Optimal nutritional support will be maintained.

Continued.

NURSING DIAGNOSES/ DEFINING CHARACTERISTICS	NURSING INTERVENTIONS / *RATIONALES*	EXPECTED OUTCOMES

DEFINING CHARACTERISTICS cont'd
 	
Muscle wasting:
  Hypotonia
  Loss of ventilatory drive
  Apnea
  Difficulty weaning from ventilatory support		

High Risk for Fluid Volume Deficit
RELATED TO
Prematurity
Glucose infusion
Hyperosmolar solutions
Increased insensible water loss
Fluid restriction
 	
DEFINING CHARACTERISTICS
Decreased urine output
Hyperglycemia
Glycosuria
Hypernatremia
Metabolic acidosis
Increased BUN
Increased specific gravity
Weight loss
Sunken fontanels
Poor skin turgor
Thick oral secretions
Decreased peripheral pulses
Peripheral vasoconstriction
Hypotension
Hemoconcentration
	ONGOING ASSESSMENT
	• Assess vital signs and BP.
	• Note peripheral perfusion.
	• Assess hydration status:
	  Accurate I&O
	  Specific gravity
	  Urine Labstix
	• Observe for glucose intolerance.
	• Assess weight loss pattern. *Indicative of dehydration. Weight is the most sensitive parameter for determining degree of insensible water loss.*
	
	THERAPEUTIC INTERVENTIONS
	• Adjust fluids per order *to maintain cardiac output, blood pressure, and peripheral perfusion.*
	• Notify physician of capillary refill greater than 3-4 seconds. *Decreased peripheral perfusion indicative of dehydration.*
	• Report weight loss of 10%-15% or greater.
	• Inform physician of rising Hct. *In presence of decreased peripheral perfusion, central Hct provides most accurate information.*
		Risk of fluid volume deficit will be reduced.

High Risk for Fluid Volume Excess **RELATED TO** Excessive administration of fluids Changing fluid requirements Patent ductus arteriosus Bronchopulmonary dysplasia	**ONGOING ASSESSMENT** • Assess for increased respiratory distress, subcostal retractions, substernal retractions, rales or rhonchi, nasal flaring, need for increased ventilatory support. • Assess for congestive heart failure, murmur, bounding pulses, tachypnea, tachycardia. **THERAPEUTIC INTERVENTIONS** • Decrease total fluids *to decrease risk of congestive heart failure.* • Administer furosemide (Lasix) per order *to decrease total body fluid.* • Use infusion pump for fluid administration *to accurately register 1 ml/ hr or less.*	Risk of fluid overload will be reduced.

NURSING DIAGNOSES/ DEFINING CHARACTERISTICS	NURSING INTERVENTIONS / *RATIONALES*	EXPECTED OUTCOMES
DEFINING CHARACTERISTICS Increased urine output Decreased specific gravity Pulmonary edema Increased peripheral pulses Tachycardia Tachypnea		

High Risk for Metabolic Aberrations
 	
RELATED TO
 	
Extreme immaturity
Inappropriate amounts of parenteral nutrients
Prolonged TPN therapy
Increased mineral requirements during convalescent period
 	
DEFINING CHARACTERISTICS
 	
Metabolic acidosis
Electrolyte imbalance
Trace mineral deficiencies: zinc, copper
Calcium and phosphorous deficiencies
	ONGOING ASSESSMENT
	
	▪ Assess for lethargy or irritability.
	▪ Observe for poor wound healing.
	▪ Note skin rash adjacent to body orifices and on extremities.
	▪ Observe for hair loss.
	▪ Assess for decreased bone density:
	    Serial knee x-rays
	    Rising alkaline phosphatase
	▪ Monitor labs: pH and bicarbonate data base.
	
	THERAPEUTIC INTERVENTIONS
	
	▪ Maintain appropriate TPN concentrations *to provide adequate nutrients for maintenance of skin integrity and promotion of wound healing.*
	▪ Use caution when performing chest physical therapy *to prevent rib fractures.*
	▪ See Altered glucose and calcium metabolism, p. 372.
		Metabolic aberrations will be reduced.

High Risk for Infection (Bacteremia, Fungicemia) **RELATED TO** TPN solution supportive of organism growth Colonization of catheter with subsequent organism invasion of intracutaneous tract Undernourished state Antibiotic therapy Steroid therapy	**ONGOING ASSESSMENT** ▪ Assess for early signs of sepsis using defining characteristics. ▪ Note peripheral perfusion. ▪ Observe for enteral feeding intolerance. ▪ Assess for glucose intolerance. ▪ Monitor CBC and blood culture results. ▪ Monitor labs: serum electrolytes, BUN, creatinine. ▪ Report hypothermia, hyperthermia, or apnea. *Apnea and temperature instability may be first signs of sepsis.* **THERAPEUTIC INTERVENTIONS** ▪ Use aseptic technique when changing IV tubing, handling new bag of solution. ▪ Use in-line 0.22 μm membrane filter that *traps bacteria and fungi (although not endotoxin).* ▪ Avoid breaks in IV line: no stopcocks, no blood drawing, and no additives to bag after it leaves the pharmacy *to decrease infectious contamination.* ▪ Notify physician of blood culture results. *Blood cultures may be negative in fungicemia.* ▪ Administer antibiotics per order.	Risk for infection will be reduced.

Continued.

Low birth weight and total parenteral nutrition cont'd

NURSING DIAGNOSES/ DEFINING CHARACTERISTICS	NURSING INTERVENTIONS / *RATIONALES*	EXPECTED OUTCOMES
DEFINING CHARACTERISTICS Apnea Increased respiratory distress Pulmonary infiltrates Temperature instability Lethargy CBC changes Feeding intolerance Hyperglycemia Glycosuria Hypoperfusion Hypotension		
High Risk for Injury Related to Superior Vena Cava Syndrome (SVCS) **RELATED TO** Irritation of vessel intima from hyperosmolar TPN solution Injury of intima by catheter tip Turbulence around catheter favoring platelet aggregation with subsequent fibrin formation Septic thrombus **DEFINING CHARACTERISTICS** Thoracic duct obstruction Pitting edema of face or head, neck, thorax, upper extremities (generalized) Pulmonary edema Pulmonary infiltrates Pulmonary effusion Intravascular fluid depletion Intravascular fluid overload Hypoproteinemia Renal insufficiency Inappropriate weight gain	**ONGOING ASSESSMENT** - Document dry weight, weigh every 12 hours. - Assess for fluid shifts. Monitor I&O. - Note location of edema. - Assess for cardiorespiratory deterioration, increased respiratory effort, tachypnea, retractions, rales/rhonchi, cyanosis, point of maximal impulse shift, tachycardia, need for increased ventilatory support. - Monitor vital signs after thoracentesis; document pleural fluid output. - Document chest tube output. - Monitor total protein, albumin, BUN, creatinine, and electrolytes. **THERAPEUTIC INTERVENTIONS** - Provide ventilatory support per order. - Elevate head of bed *to decrease cardiorespiratory compromise.* - Infuse albumin or fresh frozen plasma per order *to decrease fluid leakage from vascular to extravascular space.* - Administer furosemide (Lasix) per order *to decrease total body fluid, thus decreasing the work of the heart.* - Avoid placing IVs in scalp or upper extremities. - Restrict IV rate to 2 ml/hr if scalp or upper extremity site is unavoidable *to reduce cardiorespiratory compromise.*	Potential for injury will be reduced.
High Risk for Injury: Impaired Gas Exchange **RELATED TO** Too rapid infusion of lipids	**ONGOING ASSESSMENT** - Assess for vasospasm in periphery: pallor, cyanosis, mottling, blanching, temperature changes. - Note sudden increase in respiratory distress. - Observe for change in activity.	Optimal gas exchange will be maintained.

NURSING DIAGNOSES/ DEFINING CHARACTERISTICS	NURSING INTERVENTIONS / *RATIONALES*	EXPECTED OUTCOMES
DEFINING CHARACTERISTICS Vasospasm Impaired peripheral perfusion Increased respiratory distress Cyanosis Lethargy Irritability Visible serum lactescence	**ONGOING ASSESSMENT cont'd** • Draw serum triglycerides and cholesterol samples *to measure the serum content of fat.* • Monitor blood gases. **THERAPEUTIC INTERVENTIONS** • Stop infusion *to prevent respiratory compromise.* • Provide ventilatory support as ordered. *Intralipids may be found in pulmonary capillaries and may interfere with gas exchanges.* • Report tubid serum from spun Hct to physician. *Most lipids diffuse into adipose tissues. Very-low-birth-weight infant with decreased adipose tissue may have delayed clearance of intralipids.*	
High Risk for Systemic Injury **RELATED TO** Prolonged lipid therapy **DEFINING CHARACTERISTICS** Hepatomegaly Splenomegaly Elevated liver enzymes Jaundice Leukopenia Thrombocytopenia Disposition of brown pigment throughout body Fat disposition in intima of major blood vessels	**ONGOING ASSESSMENT** • Mark edge of liver and spleen. • Assess liver enzymes. • Observe for icterus: skin, sclera, serum, urine. • Observe for brown patches on skin. • Assess for decreased WBCs and decreased platelets. • Monitor data base weekly. **THERAPEUTIC INTERVENTIONS** • If signs of complications occur, discontinue lipids per physician order. *Abnormalities reversible if lipids stopped.* • Advance enteral feedings *to minimize liver damage.*	Potential for injury will be reduced.
Altered Parenting **RELATED TO** Unfamiliarity with TPN therapy Separation of parents and infant **DEFINING CHARACTERISTICS** Asking frequent or repetitive questions Manipulative behavior Anxiety Silence Anger Inconsistent visitation/phone calls	**ONGOING ASSESSMENT** • Assess parent's level of understanding. • Assess parent's knowledge of illness and condition. • Assess parental support system. • Assess parent's knowledge of procedures and equipment. • Determine if mother plans to breastfeed. **THERAPEUTIC INTERVENTIONS** • Explain why infant's condition necessitates use of TPN. • Teach breastfeeding mother how to use breast pump and store milk. *Mother will be able to participate in infant's care by providing breast milk.* • Encourage parent to hold infant. *Presence of central line may be frightening to parent and result in decreased handling of infant; holding promotes bonding.* • See Parenting in special care nursery, p. 72.	Optimal parenting will be provided.

Deborah Rickard, RN, BSN

Necrotizing enterocolitis

Necrotizing enterocolitis (NEC) is an inflammatory disease of the intestinal tract. Related maternal factors: maternal premature rupture of the membranes; antepartum maternal vaginal hemorrhage, incuding placenta previa; multiple pregnancy; maternal toxemia. Related infant factors: prematurity (<33 weeks gestation); low birth weight (<2500 g); inappropriate weight for gestational age; low Apgar scores; history of fetal distress at birth (hypoxia); history of umbilical vessel catheterization (exchange transfusion, vasospasm).

NURSING DIAGNOSES/ DEFINING CHARACTERISTICS	NURSING INTERVENTIONS / *RATIONALES*	EXPECTED OUTCOMES
High Risk for Injury **RELATED TO** Alteration in bowel integrity **DEFINING CHARACTERISTICS** Lethargic—poor feeding Gastric residuals Vomiting (may be bilious or guaiac positive) Abdominal changes: Distention Tenderness or rigidity Erythema Diarrhea Grossly bloody stools Hematest-positive stools without presence of anal fissure	**ONGOING ASSESSMENT** • Observe the abdomen for changes. *Observation at appropriate intervals is the best means to detect subtle condition changes.* Note skin redness or shininess. Note abdominal distention. Check abdomen measurement every 2-3 hours. Note presence of bowel sounds *to evaluate bowel activity.* Note if abdomen is rigid, tense, or has distended loops of bowel. • Assess categorically the stage of: • NEC scare (Stage 1): Evaluate the history of maternal- and/or infant-related factors predisposing to the NEC onset. Assess for nonspecific systematic manifestations of apnea, bradycardia, lethargy, and/or temperature instability. Evaluate gastrointestinal manifestations of poor feeding, increased residuals, emesis, and/or mild distention. Review radiographs for intestinal distention or mild ileus. • Definite NEC (Stage 2): Assess for occult or gross gastrointestinal bleeding. Review radiographs for significant intestinal distention with ileus, small bowel separation, and/or pneumatosis intestinalis. • Advanced NEC (Stage 3): Evaluate for deterioration of vital signs. • Refer to High risk for altered fluid volume, excess, p. 21, or Deficit, p.19. **THERAPEUTIC INTERVENTIONS** • Minimize abdominal handling *to decrease trauma to area:* Limit abdominal palpation. Keep abdomen exposed, avoid diapering. • Decrease bowel activity: Maintain NPO status. Start peripheral IV if necessary. • Assist with obtaining routine radiographs of abdomen every 12-24 hours: A-P, supine, lateral, and upright x-ray positions	Risk of injury will be reduced.
High Risk for Infection **RELATED TO** Prematurity Decreased immunologic state: Decreased WBCs Decreased platelets	**ONGOING ASSESSMENT** • Obtain lab work as needed for septic workup: Blood cultures Stool cultures according to NEC protocol Urine culture CBC with differential and platelet count Serum glucose and/or Chemstrip BUN and creatinine • Note any bleeding tendencies: oozing at heel-stick or IV insertion sites, petechiae, decreased platelet count. *The presence of any of these is suggestive of disseminating intravascular disease (DIC).* • Observe for subtle signs of infection: Temperature variability Pallor	Risk of infection will be reduced.

NURSING DIAGNOSES/ DEFINING CHARACTERISTICS	NURSING INTERVENTIONS / *RATIONALES*	EXPECTED OUTCOMES
DEFINING CHARACTERISTICS Any positive culture suggestive of NEC: Blood Stool Urine	**THERAPEUTIC INTERVENTIONS** • Administer antibiotics as ordered *to improve inflammatory status.* Calculate mg/kg/day. • Utilize enteric bedside precautions *to minimize cross-contamination:* Good handwashing Separate diaper disposal Care of infants with like organisms together Cohort nursing as needed	
High Risk for Fluid Volume Excess or Deficit **RELATED TO** NPO status Nasogastric tube/or-ogastric tube to gravity Insensible losses (radiant warmer, ventilator tubing, etc.) Loose stools **DEFINING CHARACTERISTICS** *Fluid deficit:* Dry skin and mucous membranes Reduced skin turgor Sunken anterior fontanels, overlapping sutures Decreased urine output Weight loss Increased serum sodium ($\geq$145 mEq/L) Increased urine specific gravity Poor perfusion Hypotension Increased heart rate Lethargy High hematocrit Bounding peripheral pulses Evidence of third spacing *Fluid excess:* Low hematocrit Increased heart rate Low urine specific gravity Edema	**ONGOING ASSESSMENT** • Assess daily weights. • Assess daily serum electrolytes and osmolarity. • Assess skin turgor. • Note volume status: Monitor vital signs, especially BP. Check capillary refill. Monitor accurate I&O. Report urine output of <1 ml/kg/1 hr for two consecutive hours. Follow Hct changes. • Observe for third spacing: Edema—periorbital, pedal, or pitting edema; decreased serum protein Decreased total serum solute or total protein Serum oozing with heel-sticks or IV sticks • Assess nature and amount of secretions. • Assess activity level changes. **THERAPEUTIC INTERVENTIONS** • Maintain parenteral therapy as ordered *to achieve 140-150 ml/kg/day to provide adequate hydration.* • Insert nasogastric or orogastric tube *to decompress the abdomen.* Place nasogastric tube either to gravity or low intermittent suction. Replace nasogastric tube drainage if ordered (1:1 with desired solution). • Correct fluid volume needs *to maintain electrolyte and fluid balance:* Correct hypotension with albumin 5%, saline solution, or fresh frozen plasma as indicated. Use vasopressor drugs as indicated. Administer fresh frozen plasma every 8-24 hours *for volume expansion.*	Optimal fluid/volume balance will be achieved.

Continued.

Gastrointestinal Care Plans (Neonatal)

NURSING DIAGNOSES/ DEFINING CHARACTERISTICS	NURSING INTERVENTIONS / *RATIONALES*	EXPECTED OUTCOMES
DEFINING CHARACTERISTICS cont'd Decreased total serum solute or total protein Weight gain		

Impaired Gas Exchange
RELATED TO
Increased abdominal distention affecting respiratory status
Sepsis
Shock
 	
DEFINING CHARACTERISTICS
 	
Frequent apnea and/ or bradycardia
Need for respiratory support
Rales
Retractions
Cyanosis
Presence of acidosis
	ONGOING ASSESSMENT
	• Assess for presence of respiratory distress:
	    Increased or decreased respiratory rate
	    Nasal flare
	    Grunting
	    Retractions (mild-severe, costal-substernal)
	    If child is treated with intermittent mandatory ventilation, note spontaneous respirations.
	• Auscultate breath sounds in all lung fields. Note:
	    Aeration
	    Rales
	    Chest expansion
	• Evaluate for cyanosis:
	    Assess skin color.
	    Note color of mucous membranes.
	    Note nailbed color.
	• Monitor blood gases *to evaluate metabolic/respiratory status.*
	• Observe infant for early signs and symptoms of superimposed infection:
	    Temperature instability (hypothermia or hyperthermia)
	    Peripheral vasoconstriction
	    Requires increased amount of oxygen and/or increased ventilator support
	
	THERAPEUTIC INTERVENTIONS
	• Maintain patent airway:
	    Initiate endotracheal/oral/nasal suction as needed.
	    Assist with ventilation as needed (intermittent mandatory ventilation [IMV], nasal continuous positive airway pressure, hood, nasal cannula).
	    Perform chest physical therapy and postural drainage as needed.
	    Reposition every 2-3 hours.
	• Provide oxygen as needed *to maintain PO_2 at prescribed level.*
	• Correct acidosis through use of sodium bicarbonate, IVs, or fresh frozen plasma, as needed and directed by physician.
	• Organize care *to minimize handling and avoid agitation with subsequent hypoxia.*
		Adequate gas exchange will be achieved.

Altered Glucose and Calcium Metabolism **RELATED TO** Prematurity	**ONGOING ASSESSMENT** • Assess for defining characteristics. **THERAPEUTIC INTERVENTIONS** • If alterations in glucose calcium metabolism are observed, see Altered glucose and calcium metabolism, p. 372.	Normal glucose and calcium blood levels will be maintained.

NURSING DIAGNOSES/ DEFINING CHARACTERISTICS	NURSING INTERVENTIONS / *RATIONALES*	EXPECTED OUTCOMES
DEFINING CHARACTERISTICS *Hypoglycemia:* Chemstrip <40 Jitteriness Lethargy Refusal to suck Hypotonia Apnea or cyanosis High-pitched cry Abnormal eye movements Temperature instability *Hyperglycemia:* Jitteriness Glycosuria greater than trace Chemstrip >120 *Hypocalcemia:* Irritability Jitteriness Seizures Cyanosis Feeding intolerance Calcium level <7 mg/dl		
Altered Nutrition: Less Than Body Requirements **RELATED TO** Inability to feed secondary to suspected or definite diagnosis of NEC NPO status Total parenteral nutrition **DEFINING CHARACTERISTICS** Weight loss Sunken orbits Abdominal distention Vomiting Diarrhea Documented inadequate caloric intake Restlessness Irritability Fluid volume problems	**ONGOING ASSESSMENT** • Assess patterns of weight loss/gain based on daily weights plotted on the Dancis curve/growth chart. • During NPO status: Evaluate for the use of total parenteral nutrition and intralipids during NPO state. Assess enteric feeding history. Record stools—type, frequency, amount. Record and check all stools for Hematest and reducing substance. • After resumption of feedings, assess infant's ability to tolerate feedings. Check residuals before feeding. **THERAPEUTIC INTERVENTIONS** • Once feeding intolerance has been exhibited: Discontinue enteric feedings *to provide rest for the GI tract.* Maintain NPO status for desired length of time. • During NPO status, provide peripheral (or central) parenteral alimentation with intralipids as ordered *to provide best nutritional status possible.* Calculate adequate fluid and caloric intake. • After completion of predetermined NPO period, restart enteric feedings as ordered: Increase feedings as indicated. Decrease IV accordingly *to maintain total fluids.*	Nutritional deficit will be reduced.

Continued.

265

■ **Necrotizing enterocolitis cont'd**

NURSING DIAGNOSES/ DEFINING CHARACTERISTICS	NURSING INTERVENTIONS / *RATIONALES*	EXPECTED OUTCOMES
High Risk for Altered Parenting **RELATED TO** Infant's hospitalization Knowledge deficit **DEFINING CHARACTERISTICS** Excessive questions Increased anxiety Excessive or infrequent telephone calling patterns Verbal or nonverbal expressions regarding infant's condition	**ONGOING ASSESSMENT** ▪ Assess for defining characteristics. **THERAPEUTIC INTERVENTIONS** ▪ If signs of altered parenting are observed, see Parenting in special care nursery, p. 72.	Positive parenting behaviors will be observed.

Phyllis Lawlor-Klean, RN, MS

Percutaneous central venous catheter

Premature and sick infants often need stable venous access for prolonged periods of time for delivery of parenteral nutrition and intravenous medication. Although the delivery of enteral feedings is desirable, it is often contraindicated because of gastrointestinal immaturity, surgical problems, or circulatory compromise. Use of repeated venipunctures for maintaining access compromises the peripheral circulation and is stressful for the infant. This stress may aggravate any preexisting problems and cause disruptions in both feeding and sleep cycles, as well as adversely affect temperature control and oxygenation. An alternative to repeated venipunctures is the insertion of a percutaneous central venous catheter (PCVC) into arm, leg, head, or neck veins. The procedure is done at the child's bedside and eliminates the problems associated with surgically placed central venous catheters, specifically the need for central anesthesia, an incision, or surgical equipment and surgical personnel.

NURSING DIAGNOSES/ DEFINING CHARACTERISTICS	NURSING INTERVENTIONS / *RATIONALES*	EXPECTED OUTCOMES
High Risk for Infection: Catheter Colonization and/ or Sepsis **RELATED TO** Skin insertion site puncture Breaks in closed central venous system Reduced host defenses	**ONGOING ASSESSMENT** ▪ Inspect insertion site and area around dressing each shift. ▪ Assess for changes in vital signs (especially temperature) every 2 hours. ▪ Assess for changes in circulation, activity level, and respiratory efforts. ▪ Draw peripheral and central blood cultures as ordered. ▪ Obtain cultures from any infectious sites.	Risk of infection will be reduced.

NURSING DIAGNOSES/ DEFINING CHARACTERISTICS	NURSING INTERVENTIONS / *RATIONALES*	EXPECTED OUTCOMES
High Risk for Infection: Catheter Colonization and/ or Sepsis cont'd Hematogenous seeding from alternate infectious sites, including wounds, stomas, shunts, grafts, catheters, and endotracheal tubes Prolonged use of catheter **DEFINING CHARACTERISTICS** Temperature fluctuations Lethargy or other changes in activity level Need for increased oxygenation and ventilation Alterations in blood pressure and peripheral perfusion	**THERAPEUTIC INTERVENTIONS** • Change IV tubing, cassette, in-line filter, Buretrol per policy *to reduce possibility of contamination.* • Do not use stopcocks with PVC line *as they can be reservoirs for infection.* • If total parenteral nutrition (hyperalimentation) is infused, change IV tubing every 24 hours or per policy. • If medications need to be administered per PCVC, ensure that strict aseptic technique is followed. • Change PCVC dressing using sterile technique per unit policy/certification. Secure second nurse to restrain infant during procedure *to decrease risk of contamination.* • Minimize infant handling. • If signs of infection are evident, start antibiotic administration through PCVC, as ordered. • If PCVC is thought to be source of infection, discontinue per policy/procedure. • Alleviate parental fear/anxiety by answering questions and providing information about the infant's condition.	

High Risk for Injury: Impaired Catheter Function
 	
RELATED TO
 	
Mechanical impairment (e.g., clotting or kinking of catheter)
Malpositioning
 	
DEFINING CHARACTERISTICS
 	
Resistant or sluggish infusion of parenteral solutions
Leakage of fluids from catheter or exit site
Inability to obtain blood return
Pump alarm indicating "occlusion"
Edema in chest, neck, back
Phlebitis along extremity used for cannulation
	ONGOING ASSESSMENT
	
	• Check continuity of catheter.
	• Check for patency.
	• Verify on x-ray that catheter tip is in right atrium. If tip is in the *thorax,* inspect chest, neck, and back for edema. If tip lies in an *extremity,* inspect for phlebitis and edema.
	
	THERAPEUTIC INTERVENTIONS
	
	• Use mechanical IV pumps *to prevent "dry" IVs and backing up of blood into catheter.* Maintain IV rate between 1-26 ml/hr. *Rates <1 ml/hr are prone to clotting and rates >26 ml/hr can "break" the fragile catheter (1.9 diameter).*
	• Use no larger than a 23-gauge needle to start piggyback infusions, *as this will reduce potential for leakage from the rubber port when needle is removed.*
	• Flush catheter per established policy/procedure *to prevent catheter clotting. Standard flush solution (for rates >1 ml/hr) is 1 ml fluid/1 U heparin.*
	• Apply armboard to cannulated extremity (brachial, femoral, axillary) *to prevent catheter displacement.*
	• If alarm indicates "occlusion" from PCVC, investigate immediately *to prevent loss of line. Clotting can occur within a matter of minutes:*
	   Check position of catheter.
	   Flush per procedure.
	   Remove catheter as ordered.
		Catheter patency will be maintained.

Mary Kay Chathas, RN, MSN; Tracy Lin, RN, MS

Small-for-gestational-age neonate

A small-for-gestational-age (SGA) infant is one whose weight is less than the third percentile for that specific gestational age.

SMALL FOR DATES; INTRAUTERINE GROWTH RETARDATION

NURSING DIAGNOSES/ DEFINING CHARACTERISTICS	NURSING INTERVENTIONS / *RATIONALES*	EXPECTED OUTCOMES
High Risk for Injury: SGA Birth **RELATED TO** Altered fetal growth support (a reduction of fetal growth support provided by the mother transplacentally) Altered fetal growth potential (reduction in fetal growth secondary to genetic disorders and/or infections) **DEFINING CHARACTERISTICS** Body tissue changes—thin, loose, dry skin or poor development of subcutaneous tissue Decreased muscle mass Head larger in proportion to body Sparse hair Wide skull sutures "Old man-like" appearance Open, worried eyes Breast nodule development (depends on gestational age and extent of growth retardation) Scaphoid abdomen Yellow, thin umbilical cord with rapid drying Mature genitalia	**ONGOING ASSESSMENT** • Assess accurate gestational age by Dubowitz exam. • Examine infant for clinical characteristics indicative of SGA infant. • Evaluate via physical exam symmetrical (altered growth potential) versus asymmetrical (impaired support for growth) growth retardation. • Assess neurological status according to age rather than weight. Note neurological activity that is more mature than the infant's actual weight. *Signs of increased maturity are diagnostic of SGA.* • Note behavior of loud cry, strong coordinated suck, good head control, and maximal recoil. **THERAPEUTIC INTERVENTIONS** • Review Dubowitz findings when child is neurologically stable. *Waiting for neurologic stability allows more accurate Dubowitz scoring.*	Risk for injury secondary to being small for gestational age will be identified.
High Risk for Injury: Meconium Aspiration **RELATED TO** SGA specific: Perinatal asphyxia Meconium aspiration	**ONGOING ASSESSMENT** • Assess for defining characteristics. **THERAPEUTIC INTERVENTIONS** • If potential for meconium aspiration is present, refer to Meconium aspiration syndrome, p. 161.	Risk of injury will be reduced.

NURSING DIAGNOSES/ DEFINING CHARACTERISTICS	NURSING INTERVENTIONS / *RATIONALES*	EXPECTED OUTCOMES
DEFINING CHARACTERISTICS Tachypnea Grunting Nasal flaring Retractions Cyanosis Rales Chest hyperexpanded and barrel-shaped		

High Risk for Injury: Polycythemia
RELATED TO
SGA specific:
Chronic asphyxia in utero stimulating erythropoiesis and increased RBC production
 	
DEFINING CHARACTERISTICS
Venous hematocrit 65% or above
Neurological signs:
Lethargic
Hypertonic or hypotonic muscle tone
Seizures
Difficult to arouse
Irritable
Poor feeder
Ruddy skin color
Cyanosis with cry
Jaundice
Signs of respiratory distress syndrome, especially tachypnea
Signs of congestive heart failure especially increased liver size
Hypocalcemia
Hypokalemia
	ONGOING ASSESSMENT
	▪ Assess venous or central Hct every shift. *Venous hematocrit is a more accurate assessment of Hct than heel-stick.*
	▪ Assess for defining characteristics of polycythemia.
	▪ Check Chemstrip (test for glucose on whole blood) every shift if 80% or above; check more frequently if ≤80% (every 1-2 hours). *Hypoglycemia is common to SGA infants as well as in polycythemia.*
	▪ Note alterations in neurological status. *Neurological changes can occur as a result of altered oxygenation with polycythemia.*
	▪ Note changes in respiratory status:
	  Tachypnea
	  Cyanosis
	  Congestive heart failure symptomatology
	
	THERAPEUTIC INTERVENTIONS
	▪ Prepare for partial exchange transfusion if venous Hct is >65%. *Partial exchange may be necessary to decrease Hct to more acceptable levels.*
		A venous Hct level <65% will be achieved and maintained.

Continued.

Gastrointestinal Care Plans (Neonatal)

NURSING DIAGNOSES/ DEFINING CHARACTERISTICS	NURSING INTERVENTIONS / *RATIONALES*	EXPECTED OUTCOMES
High Risk for Ineffective Thermoregulation in Low-Birth-Weight Infant **RELATED TO** *SGA specific:* Increased metabolic rate and increased heat Loss due to decreased subcutaneous fat, illness, decreased glucose stores, and altered heat production	**ONGOING ASSESSMENT** ▪ Assess for defining characteristics. **THERAPEUTIC INTERVENTIONS** ▪ If ineffective thermoregulation is present, see Thermoregulation in the low-birth-weight-infant, p. 379.	Normothermia will be maintained.
DEFINING CHARACTERISTICS *Hyperthermia:* Body temperature greater than 37.4° C (99.4° F) Tachycardia Fluid/electrolyte imbalance Tachypnea Sweating Confusion Irritability *Hypothermia:* Skin pale or blue Body temperature less than 37° C (98.6° F) Loss of or failure to gain weight Apneic spells Hypoxia Hypoglycemia Carbon dioxide retention Confusion Irritability Fluid/electrolyte imbalance		
Altered Calcium Metabolism **RELATED TO** History of asphyxia **DEFINING CHARACTERISTICS** Irritability Jitteriness Seizures Cyanosis Feeding intolerance Calcium level <7 mg/dl	**ONGOING ASSESSMENT** ▪ Assess for defining characteristics. **THERAPEUTIC INTERVENTIONS** ▪ If alteration in calcium metabolism is present, see Altered calcium metabolism, p. 372.	Normal calcium levels will be maintained.

NURSING DIAGNOSES/ DEFINING CHARACTERISTICS	NURSING INTERVENTIONS / *RATIONALES*	EXPECTED OUTCOMES
Altered Glucose Metabolism **RELATED TO** SGA specific: *Hyperglycemia:* Persistent endogenous hepatic glucose production Decreased utilization of glucose peripherally *Hypoglycemia:* Lack of liver glycogen stores Increased utilization of glucose Reduced hepatic and adrenal cortical function Insufficient intake of glucose Hyperinsulinemia Low glucose level (<45 mg/dl) lasting 48-72 hours **DEFINING CHARACTERISTICS** *Hyperglycemia:* Jitteriness Glycosuria greater than trace Chemstrip >120 *Hypoglycemia:* Chemstrip <40 Jitteriness Lethargy Refusal to suck Hypotonia Apnea or cyanosis High-pitched cry Abnormal eye movements Temperature instability	**ONGOING ASSESSMENT** ▪ Evaluate for adequate calories of 100 cal/kg/day. ▪ Assess for defining characteristics. **THERAPEUTIC INTERVENTIONS** ▪ If altered glucose metabolism is present, see Altered glucose metabolism, p. 372.	Normal glucose levels will be maintained.

Altered Nutrition **RELATED TO** Prematurity (SGA) Inadequate intrauterine nutrition	**ONGOING ASSESSMENT**
	 ▪ Assess infant's clinical status.
	 ▪ Determine infant's ability to feed based on:
	     Gestational age (weight should not be a factor because of SGA status)
	     Respiratory status
	     Ability to coordinate suck and swallow
	     Level of activity/neurological status
	 ▪ Plot infant's daily weights on growth curve.
		Adequate caloric intake will be maintained.

Continued.

Gastrointestinal Care Plans (Neonatal)

NURSING DIAGNOSES/ DEFINING CHARACTERISTICS	NURSING INTERVENTIONS / *RATIONALES*	EXPECTED OUTCOMES

DEFINING CHARACTERISTICS
Minimal weight loss
Gains weight rapidly
May not maintain growth spurt
Always seems hungry
	ONGOING ASSESSMENT cont'd
	• Observe for feeding intolerance:
	  Altered Chemstrip (test for glucose on whole blood)
	  Glucosuria
	  Emesis
	  Increased abdominal girth by 0.5 to 1 cm
	  Gastric residual >2 ml
	  Lethargy
	  Apnea and/or bradycardia with oral feeding
	• Monitor I&O *to evaluate hydration and renal status.*
	• Check urine specific gravity and Labstix (pH, protein, glucose, ketones, and blood) every 4-6 hours *to evaluate hydration and renal status.*
	
	THERAPEUTIC INTERVENTIONS
	• Provide adequate hydration of 140-150 ml/kg/day.
	• When suck reflex is well established and feedings are all taken orally, provide a caloric intake of 100-120 cal/kg/day. *This caloric value should provide the desired weight gain of 10-20 g a day.*
	• Caution parent not to overfeed *since these infants act as if they are always hungry.*
	• Provide a neutral thermal environment.	

High Risk for Altered Parenting
RELATED TO
Infant's hospitalization
Knowledge deficit
 	
DEFINING CHARACTERISTICS
Excessive questions
Increased anxiety
Excessive or infrequent telephone calling patterns
Verbal/nonverbal expressions regarding infant's condition
	ONGOING ASSESSMENT
	• Assess degree of parental understanding.
	• Assess parental support system:
	  Two-parent family
	  Other family members
	  Friends/peers
	• Assess growth and development of infant.
	• Assess degree of parental involvement with infant.
	
	THERAPEUTIC INTERVENTIONS
	• Encourage parent to express feelings.
	• Provide parent with information on SGA and the impact this has on the child.
	• Provide explanations appropriate to the parent's level of understanding. *Facilitation of open communication between the parent and the health care team promotes parenting and decreases anxiety.*
	• Encourage parent to visit and phone. Document visits and calls.
	• Make social service referrals as needed.
	• Encourage parent to participate in the infant's care as the physical condition permits.
	• Emphasize the infant's positive aspects.
		Positive parental behaviors will be observed.

High Risk for Impaired Home Maintenance/ Management **RELATED TO** Infant's hospitalization for prematurity or sick newborn	**ONGOING ASSESSMENT** • Assess parent's willingness and ability to handle infant in the hospitalized setting. • Assess weight gain patterns. *SGA infants (< 1800 g) are candidates for discharge because of gestational maturity not reflected by actual weight.* • Assess parental progress in the discharge process.	Parental home maintenance/management skills will be enhanced.

Small-for-gestational-age neonate cont'd

NURSING DIAGNOSES/ DEFINING CHARACTERISTICS	NURSING INTERVENTIONS / *RATIONALES*	EXPECTED OUTCOMES
DEFINING CHARACTERISTICS Inappropriate weight gain patterns Inability to achieve all oral feedings Parent's inability to manage all aspects of care	**THERAPEUTIC INTERVENTIONS** ▪ Initiate early discharge teaching *since infant's skills are not reflected by weight but by ability.* ▪ Encourage parental participation and input into plan of care. ▪ Instruct parent regarding specific handling behaviors of the SGA infant. *Alert, active infant may cry more frequently and require more swaddling and holding.* ▪ Encourage and/or arrange for developmental follow-up because of potential impact of SGA on development process. *Active, alert states may not be indicative of hunger; caution against overfeeding.* ▪ Ensure that appropriate pediatric and/or any consulting services follow-up is arranged.	

Phyllis Lawlor-Klean, RN, MS

Tracheoesophageal fistula with esophageal atresia: preoperative care

TEF

This is the most common esophageal anomaly found in the newborn. During the first trimester of pregnancy, the foregut fails to divide into separate digestive and respiratory systems. There is an abnormal connection (fistula) between the esophagus and trachea. There is also a portion of the esophagus that ends in a blind pouch (atresia).

NURSING DIAGNOSES/ DEFINING CHARACTERISTICS	NURSING INTERVENTIONS / *RATIONALES*	EXPECTED OUTCOMES
High Risk for Ineffective Airway Clearance/ Breathing Pattern **RELATED TO** Accumulation of excessive mucus and saliva in the nose, mouth, and blind pouch Bronchial infection Decreased lung expansion Atelectasis **DEFINING CHARACTERISTICS** Constant drooling of secretions Intermittent cyanosis Tachypnea Nasal flaring	**ONGOING ASSESSMENT** ▪ Assess and document amount, color, and odor of secretions. ▪ Assess respiratory status using defining characteristics. ▪ Assess and document changes in vital signs: heart rate, respiratory rate, BP, and temperature. ▪ Monitor blood gases. ▪ Assess ease of nasogastric tube insertion. ▪ Note pattern of serial chest x-ray examination. *Chest films will reveal the blind pouch filled with air. If air is also present in the intestinal tract and esophageal atresia has been demonstrated, this will confirm the fistula.* **THERAPEUTIC INTERVENTIONS** ▪ Report to physician an excessive accumulation of secretions in the mouth. *The infant is unable to swallow because of the esophageal atresia.* ▪ Perform oral, nasal, and endotracheal suctioning every hour and prn *to maintain patent airway.* ▪ Place a 10-French sump tube in the blind pouch, and attach it to continuous low suctioning with Gomco drainage pump as ordered *to prevent aspiration.*	Optimal breathing pattern will be maintained.

Continued.

Tracheoesophageal fistula with esophageal atresia: preoperative care cont'd

NURSING DIAGNOSES/ DEFINING CHARACTERISTICS	NURSING INTERVENTIONS / *RATIONALES*	EXPECTED OUTCOMES
DEFINING CHARACTERISTICS cont'd Retractions Coarse breath sounds Increased respiratory rate and heart rate Diminished breath sounds Abnormal blood gases Abnormal chest x-ray examination	**THERAPEUTIC INTERVENTIONS cont'd** • Irrigate the sump tube with 1 ml of normal saline every 2 hours *to maintain patency.* • Position the infant on his/her abdomen as tolerated or with the head of bed elevated 45 degrees *to prevent aspiration.* • Maintain ventilatory assistance as ordered. • Administer antibiotics as ordered. *Aspiration pneumonia may occur because of the reflux of acidic gastric juices into the lungs.*	
Altered Nutrition: Less Than Body Requirements RELATED TO NPO status **DEFINING CHARACTERISTICS** Weight loss Restlessness Irritability Documented inadequate caloric intake	**ONGOING ASSESSMENT** • Assess weight pattern in comparison to the Dancis growth curve. • Determine infant's caloric/fluid requirements based on age, weight, intake/output and electrolyte status. • Monitor blood gas Chemstrips. **THERAPEUTIC INTERVENTIONS** • Administer parenteral fluids as ordered *to provide the appropriate caloric and fluid requirements.* • Maintain Chemstrips between 40 and 120 mg/dl *to prevent hypoglycemia.*	Caloric requirements will be attained.
High Risk for Fluid Volume Deficit RELATED TO Use of radiant warmer Loss of fluid through sump tube Inadequate amount of maintenance fluids for infant's weight and gestational age **DEFINING CHARACTERISTICS** Low urine output Elevated urine specific gravity Thick secretions Increased sodium Poor tissue turgor Weight loss Depressed fontanels	**ONGOING ASSESSMENT** • Assess hydration status using defining characteristics. • Assess thermal environment. • Monitor I&O. • Weigh daily. • Report urine output of <2 ml/kg/hr to physician. *This may signify dehydration.* **THERAPEUTIC INTERVENTIONS** • Administer parenteral fluids as ordered. • Provide humidity for an infant under a radiant warmer *to decrease insensible water loss.* • See Thermoregulation in low-birth-weight infant, p. 379.	Fluid balance will be maintained.
Knowledge Deficit of Parents RELATED TO Unfamiliarity with infant's condition	**ONGOING ASSESSMENT** • Assess parent's knowledge of disease entity. • Assess readiness of parent to receive information.	Parent will verbalize an understanding of the nature and sequelae of the infant's problem.

NURSING DIAGNOSES/ DEFINING CHARACTERISTICS	NURSING INTERVENTIONS / *RATIONALES*	EXPECTED OUTCOMES

DEFINING CHARACTERISTICS
 	
Verbal and nonverbal expressions of fear/anxiety with intensive care environment
Unrealistic view of infant's illness
Inappropriate response to infant
Requests for information
	THERAPEUTIC INTERVENTIONS
	• Encourage parent to:
	  Visit and call frequently
	  Verbalize concerns and feelings
	  Participate in infant's care by demonstrating simple tasks (such as diapering and applying lotion)
	  Attend parent's group sessions
	• Provide information about the diagnosis, treatment, and evaluation as appropriate, *to give facts and dispel any fallacies the parent may have.*
	• Facilitate interdisciplinary conferences with other ancillary staff concerning the infant, *so that consistent information is given to the parent.*
	• Refer parent to social worker.	

Altered Parenting RELATED TO Separation/hospitalization of infant Inability of parent to visit **DEFINING CHARACTERISTICS** Expresses verbal/nonverbal fear or anxiety with intensive care environment Exhibits reluctance to look at infant Verbalizes that infant may be in pain or staff is hurting infant Asks inappropriate questions Holds unrealistic view of infant's condition/illness Parent blames self for infant's condition Absence of parental attachment behaviors Verbalizes resentment toward infant Verbalizes guilt feelings for having a "less than perfect" infant Does not visit or call regularly Delays naming infant	**ONGOING ASSESSMENT** • Assess for presence of defining characteristics. **THERAPEUTIC INTERVENTIONS** • See Parenting in special care nursery, p. 72.	Alteration in parenting will be reduced.

Margaret Bell, RN; Olga A. Lazala, RN, BSN

7

Integumentary/ Musculoskeletal Care Plans

Arthritis: juvenile rheumatoid

A chronic inflammatory disease of childhood that presents in one of three subsets: systemic onset—high spiking fevers, rash, pericarditis, pleuritis, serositis, lymphadenopathy, hepatospleno-megaly, and arthritis (number of joints is variable); pauciarticular onset—arthritis (four joints or less), absence of systemic manifestations, and uveitis/iridocyclitis (especially with a positive ANA); polyarticular onset—arthritis (five or more joints), possibility of minor systemic features as outlined in systemic onset, may continue into adult rheumatoid arthritis if rheumatoid factor is positive.

NURSING DIAGNOSES/ DEFINING CHARACTERISTICS	NURSING INTERVENTIONS / *RATIONALES*	EXPECTED OUTCOMES

Joint Pain **RELATED TO** Inflammation associated with increased disease activity **DEFINING CHARACTERISTICS** Child's/parent's report of pain Guarding on motion of affected joints Refusal to participate in self-care or play activities Crying or other sounds associated with pain	**ONGOING ASSESSMENT**
	 • Assess age and developmental level.
	 • Solicit child's/parent's description of pain:
	  Quality
	  Severity
	  Location
	  Onset
	  Duration
	  Aggravating and alleviating factors
	 • Assess for signs of joint inflammation (redness, warmth, swelling, decreased motion).
	 • Determine past measures to alleviate pain.
	 • Assess effect on developmental milestones (walking, balance, bathing, dressing, feeding, toileting).
	 • Assess ability to participate in school activities.
	
	 THERAPEUTIC INTERVENTIONS
	 • Administer antiinflammatory medication as prescribed on a full stomach. *(Can be very irritating to stomach lining and lead to ulcers.)*
	 • Use alternate method of pain control: distraction, guided imagery, relaxation, play therapy as age-appropriate.
	 • Assist child to maintain anatomically correct position (neutral or maximum joint extension).
	 • Encourage the child to wear splints/use ambulation devices as ordered.
	 • Instruct both the child and parent in the proper use of equipment.
	 • Encourage the use of a warm bath or cool packs for inflamed joints. *Some children prefer heat to cold or vice versa.*
		Pain will be at a tolerable level so that the child can participate in self-care activities.

Joint Stiffness **RELATED TO** Inflammation associated with increased disease activity Periods of immobility **DEFINING CHARACTERISTICS** Child's/parent's report of joint stiffness Guarding on motion of affected joints Refusal to participate in self-care or play activities	**ONGOING ASSESSMENT**
	 • Solicit child's/parent's description of stiffness:
	  What joints are affected?
	  When does stiffness occur?
	  How long does stiffness last?
	 • Monitor for changes in location/duration of stiffness.
	 • Determine past measures to alleviate stiffness.
	 • Assess affect on developmental milestones (walking, balance, bathing, dressing, feeding, toileting).
	 • Assess ability to participate in school activities.
	
	 THERAPEUTIC INTERVENTIONS
	 • Assist child to take a 15-minute warm bath on rising for multiple joint stiffness.
	 • Use localized heat for stiffness in only a few joints (paraffin bath, heating pad, hot packs).
	 • Assist child to perform ROM exercises after using heat therapy to affected joint(s).
	 • Allow sufficient time for self-care activities and assist as necessary.
		Stiffness will be at a tolerable level so that child can participate in self-care activities.

Continued.

Arthritis: juvenile rheumatoid cont'd

NURSING DIAGNOSES/ DEFINING CHARACTERISTICS	NURSING INTERVENTIONS / *RATIONALES*	EXPECTED OUTCOMES
	THERAPEUTIC INTERVENTIONS cont'd	
	▪ Avoid scheduling tests/procedures during early morning hours or immediately after napping. *Stiffness will be most problematic after rest periods.*	
	▪ Encourage child to participate in activities that require joint movement.	
	▪ Administer antiinflammatory medication as prescribed on a full stomach. *(Can be very irritating to stomach lining and lead to ulcers.)*	
	▪ Attempt to continue home medication schedule while hospitalized.	
Fatigue **RELATED TO** Increased disease activity Anemia of chronic illness **DEFINING CHARACTERISTICS** Child's/parent's report of lethargy, exhaustion, listlessness Sleeping longer than is developmentally appropriate Decreased attention span Inability to perform regular activities	**ONGOING ASSESSMENT** ▪ Solicit child's/parent's description of stiffness: Joints affected Time stiffness occurs Aggravating and alleviating factors ▪ Determine sleep patterns (nighttime/day naps) and if amount of sleep is appropriate for age. ▪ Assess interference with lifestyle and ability to attend school and extracurricular activities. **THERAPEUTIC INTERVENTIONS** ▪ Provide two or three periods of 60-minute uninterrupted rest daily. ▪ Encourage afternoon naptime. ▪ Provide familiar toys from home during rest periods. ▪ Encourage child to pace activities *to conserve energy.*	Fatigue will be reduced to a level that child can participate in self-care activities.
Impaired Physical Mobility **RELATED TO** Pain Stiffness Fatigue Altered joint function Muscle weakness **DEFINING CHARACTERISTICS** Child's/parent's description of difficulty performing purposeful movement Decreased ability to perform ADL, ambulate, or achieve developmental milestones Decreased muscle strength Decreased ROM	**ONGOING ASSESSMENT** ▪ Solicit child's description of: Aggravating and alleviating factors Joint pain and stiffness (especially in AM) Ability to perform ADL at home and in school ▪ Observe child's ability to: Ambulate Perform ADL ▪ Assess achievement of age-appropriate developmental milestones (walking, balance, bathing, dressing, feeding, toileting). **THERAPEUTIC INTERVENTIONS** ▪ Allow adequate time for all activities, considering not only physical deficit(s) but also age of child. ▪ Consult with occupational therapist/clinical specialist if child cannot perform self-care skills appropriate for age. ▪ Assist with ambulation/ADL as identified in ongoing assessment. ▪ Reinforce proper use of adaptive equipment/ambulatory devices as taught by occupational/physical therapist. ▪ Ask parents to bring equipment/ambulatory devices from home if applicable. ▪ Encourage child to wear footwear with nonskid bottoms and that provides good support. ▪ Reinforce ROM and muscle strengthening exercises as taught by occupational/physical therapist. ▪ Reinforce principles of joint protection taught by occupational therapist, if age appropriate. ▪ Reinforce proper body alignment during both rest and activity. *Improper body alignment can lead to contractures.*	Impaired physical mobility will not restrict child from performing ADL.

NURSING DIAGNOSES/ DEFINING CHARACTERISTICS	NURSING INTERVENTIONS / *RATIONALES*	EXPECTED OUTCOMES

Delayed Motor Development **RELATED TO** Joint stiffness Joint pain Joint contractures Impaired mobility **DEFINING CHARACTERISTICS** Inability to achieve developmental milestones within standard time frame	**ONGOING ASSESSMENT**
	• Assess achievement of following milestones:
	  Sitting alone
	  Crawling
	  Standing
	  Walking
	  Drinking from cup
	  Self-feeding
	  Toileting
	• Assess parent's understanding of normal motor development.
	• Solicit child's/parent's description of current physical disabilities or functional difficulties.
	
	THERAPEUTIC INTERVENTIONS
	• Provide activities to promote motor development as appropriate to age/condition.
	  Provide opportunity to sit with assistance.
	  Provide opportunity/space for crawling.
	  Use playpen for daily recreation time.
	  Encourage child to pull to stand.
	  Assist to practice walking/doing stairs.
	  Provide toys that can be pushed.
	  Encourage use of tricycle.
	  Include use of clay in playtime.
	  Encourage music/games that synchronize hand and foot movement.
	• Consult occupational/physical therapist to provide a program to assist in developing motor skills.
	• Involve parent/siblings in a daily program of developing motor skills.
		Child will achieve motor development skills within 6 months of standard milestone time frame.

Self-Care Deficit **RELATED TO** Pain Stiffness Fatigue Altered joint function Muscle weakness Age (chronological/ developmental) **DEFINING CHARACTERISTICS** Child's/parent's description of difficulty with self-care activities Decreased ability to participate with self-care activities, as age-appropriate	**ONGOING ASSESSMENT**
	• Observe child's level of functioning with:
	  Bathing
	  Personal hygiene
	  Dressing
	  Toileting
	  Feeding
	• Assess impact of self-care deficit on life-style and ability to function at school.
	• Assess need for assistive devices to perform self-care activities.
	• Assess whether parent can provide appropriate care after discharge; consider need for home health care.
	
	THERAPEUTIC INTERVENTIONS
	• Encourage independence; assist child only when necessary. *Child's self-image improves when he/she can perform personal care independently.*
	• Consult occupational therapist for adaptive equipment (dressing/eating aids); request parent to bring equipment from home as appropriate.
	• Allow child adequate time for self-care activities, considering not only ability, but also age.
	• Allow child to decide on shower versus bath for daily care; discourage bed bath. *Allowing input in decision making fosters sense of independence.*
	• Provide child with guidance in choosing and pacing activities.
	• Reinforce self-care techniques taught by occupational therapist.
	• Encourage an assertive attitude (using cues) when child cannot perform activities independently. *The use of cues for assistance helps the child maintain a feeling of control over his or her environment.*
		Self-care activities will be performed independently or with assistance as cued by child.

Continued.

Integumentary/Musculoskeletal Care Plans (Pediatric)

NURSING DIAGNOSES/ DEFINING CHARACTERISTICS	NURSING INTERVENTIONS / *RATIONALES*	EXPECTED OUTCOMES

Knowledge Deficit

RELATED TO

New disease/ symptoms
Unfamiliarity with treatment regimen
Cognitive limitations
Lack of interest to learn (denial)

DEFINING CHARACTERISTICS

Many similar questions
Lack of questions
Verbalized misconceptions
Verbalized lack of knowledge
Inaccurate follow-through of previous instructions

ONGOING ASSESSMENT

- Assess child's/parent's:
  Level of knowledge of juvenile rheumatoid arthritis
  Treatment
  Prognosis
- Identify priorities for child's education. *Child's and parent's priorities may differ.*
- Assess child's:
  Ability to focus on task
  Attention span
  Readiness to learn
- Determine to what extent discomfort will interfere with learning.

THERAPEUTIC INTERVENTIONS

- Provide a private, quiet environment for education.
- Schedule educational sessions with parent, allowing some time to be separated from child. *Allows parent to mention issues they do not wish to discuss in front of child.*
- Schedule educational sessions with child during time of maximal comfort. *Pain will distract child and may lead to inability to concentrate.*
- Keep duration of sessions appropriate to attention span of the audience—child versus parent (accommodate the shortest attention span).
- Use educational techniques in accordance with child's/parent's cognitive level.
- Refrain from using the word "drug"; instead use "medication." *The word* drug *is used negatively at schools for drug prevention programs—"Say No to Drugs!" Children receive a mixed message about their juvenile rheumatoid arthritis drugs.*
- Introduce/reinforce disease process information:
  Unknown cause
  Chronicity of juvenile rheumatoid arthritis throughout childhood/ adolescence
  Inflammatory process
  Joint involvement
  Organ involvement (polyarticular/systemic)
  Uveitis/iridocyclitis (pauciarticular)
  Remissions/exacerbations
  Control versus cure issues
- Introduce/reinforce medication therapy information:
  Name of drug
  Purpose/use of drug
  Dose and route
  Time of administration (home/school)
  Potential side effects
- Introduce/reinforce self-care strategies:
  Home exercise program (ROM and muscle strengthening)
  Pain management
  Joint protection
  Appropriate play activities
  Adequate rest
  Nutritionally sound diet
  Splinting/assistive devices, when appropriate
- Acknowledge that there are current nontraditional treatments and encourage child/parent to discuss these with a member of health care team *before* trying them.
- Instruct child/parent to discuss use of over-the-counter medications with a health care team member before using.
- Provide written information of above items to child and parent.

Child/parent will verbalize increased awareness of juvenile rheumatoid arthritis, its treatment, and prognosis as it relates to disease process.

NURSING DIAGNOSES/ DEFINING CHARACTERISTICS	NURSING INTERVENTIONS / *RATIONALES*	EXPECTED OUTCOMES
High Risk for Sleep Pattern Disturbance **RELATED TO** Pain Stiffness Inactivity Family stress **DEFINING CHARACTERISTICS** Child's/parent's report of inability to fall asleep or frequent nighttime awakening Increasing irritability/ restlessness Reduction in performance in school and play activities	**ONGOING ASSESSMENT** • Solicit child's/parent's description of sleep pattern: Number of hours asleep per 24 hours Ability to fall asleep Nighttime awakening/inability to remain in bed Aggravating/alleviating factors • Determine child's usual ritual of preparing for bed. • Assess need for familiar objects/toys to accompany child to bed. **THERAPEUTIC INTERVENTIONS** • Encourage same ritual of preparing for bed when possible. • Provide special object/toy or ask parent to bring them from home. *Familiar surroundings relax and give a sense of security.* • Encourage parent to "room in" with child during hospitalization, when possible. • Suggest use of warm bath/shower before bed. *Warm water relaxes muscles, facilitates relaxation.* • Assist child in changing positions frequently during night when needed. • Provide quiet environment; discuss a mutually acceptable awakening pattern for routine care (vital signs). • Avoid stimulating foods (caffeine), and activities before bedtime. • Consult clinical specialist if sleep pattern disturbance may be related to psychological factors.	Number of hours asleep (per 24-hour period) will be at least two thirds appropriate amount for child's age.
High Risk for Ineffective Family Coping **RELATED TO** Inadequate support system Developmental age of child Knowledge deficit Parental grieving of loss of perfect child **DEFINING CHARACTERISTICS** Child/parent/sibling expresses concern about family's response to illness Parent displays protective behavior disproportionate to child's ability to be independent Child/parent/sibling refusing to discuss changes imposed by juvenile rheumatoid arthritis (limitations, altered body function, etc.) Child/family expresses feelings of hopelessness/ helplessness Routine family life is disrupted	**ONGOING ASSESSMENT** • Identify behaviors that suggest grieving. • Assess behavioral patterns that suggest altered self-concept or ineffective individual/family coping. • Identify defense mechanisms and determine if appropriate. **THERAPEUTIC INTERVENTIONS** • Recognize family's need to use appropriate defense mechanisms. • Allow child time to make personal adjustments to changes in body image. • Preschedule time each day for child/family to discuss current concerns. • Encourage expression of feelings. • Involve family in setting realistic long- and short-term goals. • Avoid unpleasant surprise situations. • Assist family to develop problem-solving techniques. • Introduce child/family to other children with juvenile rheumatoid arthritis (similar age and type of juvenile rheumatoid arthritis). • Refer child/family to social service department if needed.	The family will exhibit positive expressions, feelings, and actions.

Continued.

Integumentary/Musculoskeletal Care Plans (Pediatric)

NURSING DIAGNOSES/ DEFINING CHARACTERISTICS	NURSING INTERVENTIONS / *RATIONALES*	EXPECTED OUTCOMES
Altered Nutrition: Less Than Body Requirements **RELATED TO** Loss of appetite related to chronic illness and medication side effects Psychosocial factors **DEFINING CHARACTERISTICS** Loss of weight with or without adequate caloric intake Below 15th percentile of weight for height on growth curve, or a decline in 2 percentile lines Inadequate caloric intake Caloric intake inadequate to maintain metabolic state during time of increased disease activity	**ONGOING ASSESSMENT** ▪ Document child's actual weight on admission and reassess every week. ▪ Obtain nutritional history from both parent and child, when possible. ▪ Obtain medication history. ▪ Assess child's feeding skills, including setup needs. **THERAPEUTIC INTERVENTIONS** ▪ Assist child with meal setup and feeding, as needed. ▪ Provide finger foods for children with poor dexterity. ▪ Encourage family to visit at mealtimes. ▪ Encourage frequent small meals/snacks of high-calorie/high-protein foods. ▪ Consult dietitian as needed. ▪ Reinforce dietary teaching to child and parents.	Optimal caloric intake will be maintained with no further weight loss during hospitalization.
Altered Nutrition: More Than Body Requirements **RELATED TO** Inactivity Psychosocial factors **DEFINING CHARACTERISTICS** Above 85th percentile of weight for height on growth curve Reported or observed dysfunctional eating behavior	**ONGOING ASSESSMENT** ▪ Document child's actual weight on admission and reassess every week. ▪ Obtain a nutritional history from both child and parent. ▪ Obtain medication history. ▪ Assess level of activity and estimated energy expenditure per day. **THERAPEUTIC INTERVENTIONS** ▪ Instruct child/parent in nutritionally sound diet. ▪ Assist child to choose menu items from each food group. ▪ Consult dietitian as needed. ▪ Discuss eating behaviors: actual physical need for food versus habitual eating. ▪ Discuss situations that lead to overeating. ▪ Encourage a daily exercise program that will not cause undue stress to joints. (Consult with physician and physical therapist to set up a program.) ▪ Reinforce formal dietary teaching to child and parent.	Optimal nutrition will be maintained without an increase in weight during hospitalization.
Fever **RELATED TO** Active disease (seen with systemic onset)	**ONGOING ASSESSMENT** ▪ Solicit child's/parent's description of fever patterns before admission: Time of occurrence Febrile temperature Duration of temperature elevation Presence/absence of rash with fever ▪ Assess whether febrile symptoms interfere with child's daily activities and ability to attend school. ▪ Assess temperature every 2 hours.	Fevers will be manageable and not interfere with daily activities.

NURSING DIAGNOSES/ DEFINING CHARACTERISTICS	NURSING INTERVENTIONS / *RATIONALES*	EXPECTED OUTCOMES
DEFINING CHARACTERISTICS Episodic fevers of 38° C (100.4° F) or greater Return of temperature to baseline between episodes One to two fever episodes/day Diaphoresis	**THERAPEUTIC INTERVENTIONS** • Administer antipyretic as ordered. If aspirin is used, monitor for elevated liver enzymes. *Aspirin use in systemic onset juvenile rheumatoid arthritis may cause transient liver toxicity.* • Document all temperatures on a graph-type form. *This will assist in determining fever patterns.* • Encourage adequate hydration.	
High Risk for Decreased Cardiac Output **RELATED TO** Pericarditis Myocarditis (seen with systemic onset, possibly polyarticular) **DEFINING CHARACTERISTICS** Child's/parent's report of fatigue, chest pain, or shortness of breath Tachycardia Hypoxia	**ONGOING ASSESSMENT** • Solicit child's/parent's description of ability to keep up with peers during normal daily activities. • Monitor heart rate and rhythm every shift. • Assess fluid status. • Assess interference with ability to perform self-care activities and attend school. **THERAPEUTIC INTERVENTIONS** • Document and report significant changes in heart rate or rhythm. • Instruct child to pace activities *to maximize energy conservation.* See Fatigue, p. 278. • Administer steroids (intravenously/orally) as ordered. • Instruct child/parent regarding side effects of steroid therapy and how to minimize them.	Optimal cardiac rhythm and output will be maintained.
High Risk for Actual Visual Impairment **RELATED TO** Inflammation of the iris and/or ciliary body known as uveitis/iridocyclitis, seen in pauci-articular **DEFINING CHARACTERISTICS** Positive slit lamp exam Insidious onset of decreased vision Posterior synechiae causing irregular or poorly reactive pupil Secondary cataracts, glaucoma (late manifestations)	**ONGOING ASSESSMENT** • Solicit child's/parent's description of change in visual capacity. **THERAPEUTIC INTERVENTIONS** • Educate child and parent of potential eye condition and lack of prodromal overt symptoms such as redness/itching. *When visual acuity has presented as a problem, irreversible damage has already occurred.* • Reinforce need for regular prophylactic exams by an ophthalmologist (not optometrist). • Administer eyedrops for active disease as indicated. *May be as frequently as every 60 minutes.*	Potential: Visual capacity will be unchanged. Actual: No further decrease in vision.

Reneé Zubay Fife, RN, MSN

Burns

SKIN LOSS—PARTIAL THICKNESS/FULL-THICKNESS

Burns in children are unfortunately a common occurrence. Scald, electrical, chemical, and flame burns are all seen. Recovery depends on cause, extent, severity, and age of the child, with infants at highest risk. First-degree burns involve only the epidermis, as in sunburn, and are painful. Second-degree burns involve partial-thickness skin loss, including all epidermal and partial corium layers. Second-degree burns typically blister and are very painful. Third-degree burns involve full-thickness skin loss, causing obvious depth to the wound and discoloration without blistering. Because of nerve destruction, third-degree burns are not usually painful.

NURSING DIAGNOSES/ DEFINING CHARACTERISTICS	NURSING INTERVENTIONS / *RATIONALES*	EXPECTED OUTCOMES
Impaired Skin Integrity **RELATED TO** Burns Thrombocytopenia purpura Anaphylaxis **DEFINING CHARACTERISTICS** Blanching of skin Redness Leathery appearance Skin color changes: brown to black Blistering, weeping skin Pain/absence of pain Skin loss	**ONGOING ASSESSMENT** ▪ Assess age and developmental level. ▪ Assess percentage of body surface burned. Use age-appropriate body surface chart. *The child with severe, large burns may require treatment at a burn center.* ▪ Identify and document location of burns. Check color, texture, turgor, and depth of wounds. Check for blisters, large open wounds, blanching. Assess degree of pain. Assess for any odors. Assess for adherent debris/hair. Take photos for later comparison. ▪ Avoid trauma to area that could increase tissue destruction. **THERAPEUTIC INTERVENTIONS** ▪ Use burn pack or nonadherent sheeting *to prevent sticking.* ▪ Use hydrotherapy tub as ordered *to aid in cleansing and loosening slough, exudate, eschar.* ▪ Apply topical bacteriostatic substances as directed. *Use extreme care when removing topical ointments during dressing change to prevent removal of granulating skin.* ▪ Elevate extremities, if possible, *to reduce swelling.* ▪ Dress wounds to prevent burn-to-burn contact; keep body, limbs in correct anatomical position *to decrease improper healing and contractures.* ▪ Do not bandage facial burns. Apply topical ointments and leave wound open to air.	Optimal skin integrity will be maintained.
High Risk for Infection **RELATED TO** Altered skin integrity Invasive therapies **DEFINING CHARACTERISTICS** Elevated WBCs Elevated temperature Presence of positive cultures Wound sepsis: abdominal distention, ileus, disorientation	**ONGOING ASSESSMENT** ▪ Monitor and record vital signs; notify physician if abnormal. ▪ Observe potential sites of infection. Assess odor and wound appearance at each dressing change. ▪ Obtain and monitor wound cultures. ▪ Monitor WBC for sudden changes. *Initial WBC may be low because of cell destruction and inflammatory response and should increase gradually. Sudden increase may indicate infection.* ▪ Routinely assess IV line sites, Foley catheter, and other invasive sites for infection. ▪ Monitor topical agent's effectiveness via wound cultures as ordered. ▪ Observe for disorientation, fever and ileus; *may indicate impending septic shock.* **THERAPEUTIC INTERVENTIONS** ▪ Maintain aseptic technique; wear mask and sterile gloves for physical contact *to prevent iatrogenic contamination.* ▪ Keep area clean.	The risk for infection will be reduced.

NURSING DIAGNOSES/ DEFINING CHARACTERISTICS	NURSING INTERVENTIONS / *RATIONALES*	EXPECTED OUTCOMES

THERAPEUTIC INTERVENTIONS cont'd
- Assist child with personal hygiene.
- Implement isolation if needed, limit visitors.
- Trim hair around wound *to decrease contamination.*
- Leave blisters intact *to form natural barrier. Blisters that affect movement or that are infected require surgical drainage.*
- Apply topical antimicrobials as ordered (*Silvadene, Sulfamylon, Betadine, silver nitrate, gentamicin*).
- Administer IV antibiotics, which may be ordered prophylactically, but should be specific to cultured organism when identified.

High Risk for Fluid Volume Deficit

RELATED TO

NOTE: Fluid volume deficit directly proportional to extent, depth of "burn" injury because of inflammatory response, protein shift followed by fluid shifts and evaporation

Massive fluid shifting and circulating volume loss *result in fluid accumulation in tissue with blister formation*

Hemorrhage; stress ulcer (Curling's ulcer)

DEFINING CHARACTERISTICS

Altered mental status
Tachycardia
Hypotension
Thirst
Skin pale and cool, dusky-looking in dark-skinned child
Oliguria
Restlessness
Hypoxia
Alteration in acid-base balance
Catabolism (outpouring of K^+ and nitrogen)
Coffee-ground emesis via nasogastric tube
Melena stools
Altered electrolytes, especially hyperkalemia

ONGOING ASSESSMENT
- Assess for signs/symptoms of fluid volume deficit (see Defining Characteristics).
- Monitor vital signs and hemodynamic status; report to physician if out of range. May require central venous pressure line placement.
- Monitor urine specific gravity every 4 hours.
- Monitor I&O every 2 hours; report urine output <0.5 ml/kg/hr.
- Obtain daily weight.
- Observe for cardiac dysrhythmias associated with hyperkalemia.
- Observe for coffee-ground emesis, bloody emesis, melena stools, abdominal distention, and epigastric pain.
- Evaluate Hgb and Hct, *which will be affected by hemodilution or hemoconcentration.*

THERAPEUTIC INTERVENTIONS
- Apply cardiopulmonary monitor.
- Assist with IV and central line placements. *Multiple lines or a central line may be required for rapid fluid rescue to prevent circulatory collapse.*
- Administer IV fluids, electrolytes (Na^+, K^+), plasma or plasma expanders as ordered.
- Administer albumin and diuretic (mannitol) as ordered *to reverse fluid shifts and decrease edema.*
- Administer antacids/H_2-receptor antagonist prophylactically *to minimize potential for gastric bleeding (cimetidine, ranitidine). Duodenal stress ulcers are seen more frequently in children than in adults, but develop later in the course of treatment and recovery (approximately 4 weeks).*

Fluid volume deficit will be reduced.

Continued.

Burns cont'd

NURSING DIAGNOSES/ DEFINING CHARACTERISTICS	NURSING INTERVENTIONS / *RATIONALES*	EXPECTED OUTCOMES
High Risk for Ineffective Breathing Pattern **RELATED TO** Massive injury Acidosis **DEFINING CHARACTERISTICS** Dyspnea Shortness of breath Tachypnea Use of accessory muscles Cough Cyanosis Alterations in ABGs Restlessness Anxiety Confusion	**ONGOING ASSESSMENT** ▪ Assess respiratory rate, rhythm, and depth; breath sounds. ▪ Assess for dyspnea, shortness of breath, use of accessory muscles, cough, and presence of cyanosis. ▪ Monitor ABGs. ▪ Assess pulse oximetry readings. ▪ Observe for confusion, anxiety, and/or restlessness. ▪ Assess hemodynamic pressures if available. *Increasing pulmonary pressures may indicate pulmonary edema.* ▪ Review chest x-ray results. **THERAPEUTIC INTERVENTIONS** ▪ Raise head of bed and maintain good body alignment for optimal breathing and lung expansion. ▪ Apply cardiopulmonary monitor. ▪ Maintain humidified oxygen delivery system. ▪ Provide chest physical therapy if burns are not to chest. ▪ Encourage use of incentive spirometer.	Optimal breathing pattern will be maintained.
High Risk for Altered Peripheral Tissue Perfusion **RELATED TO** Blockage of micro-circulation Blood loss Compartment syndrome (edema restricting circulation) Decreased platelets **DEFINING CHARACTERISTICS** Weak, thready pulses Pallor Extremities cool to touch Pain Numbness Prolonged PT/PTT	**ONGOING ASSESSMENT** ▪ Check pulses of all extremities. Use Doppler if necessary. ▪ Monitor vital signs (BP, heart rate, and respiratory rate) for abrupt changes. ▪ Assess color and temperature of extremities. ▪ Check for pain, numbness, or swelling of extremities. ▪ Monitor laboratory data; report findings (e.g., platelets, PT/PTT) to physician. **THERAPEUTIC INTERVENTIONS** ▪ Maintain good alignment of extremities *to allow adequate blood flow without compression on arteries.* ▪ Notify physician immediately of noted alteration in perfusion. ▪ Administer blood products as ordered. ▪ Perform passive range of motion (PROM) if needed *to increase circulation.* ▪ Prepare for and assist with fasciotomy/escharotomy *to relieve compression of nerves/blood vessels. Burns of chest may cause restriction/constriction that decreases chest expansion; escharotomy will be needed to alleviate constricted movement.*	Optimal tissue perfusion will be maintained.
High Risk for Altered Nutrition **RELATED TO** Prolonged interference in ability to ingest or digest food Increased basal metabolic rate **DEFINING CHARACTERISTICS** Increased ketones Decreased albumin Generalized weakness	**ONGOING ASSESSMENT** ▪ Obtain base weight; weigh daily if possible. ▪ Measure I&O. ▪ Closely monitor caloric intake. ▪ Monitor urine, serum glucose, and ketone levels. ▪ Assess for muscle weakness. ▪ Monitor serum and urine electrolytes and BUN. ▪ Check for bowel sounds. *Paralytic ileus is common in first few days after burn.* ▪ Monitor IV infusions and tube feedings. ▪ Monitor gastric pH. **THERAPEUTIC INTERVENTIONS** ▪ Consult dietitian *to assist in meeting nutritional needs.* ▪ Maintain peripheral and/or central lines. ▪ Provide total parenteral nutrition as ordered.	Adequate nutrition will be maintained.

NURSING DIAGNOSES/ DEFINING CHARACTERISTICS	NURSING INTERVENTIONS / *RATIONALES*	EXPECTED OUTCOMES

DEFINING CHARACTERISTICS cont'd

Negative nitrogen balance (hypoproteinemia)

Increased BUN

Alteration in fluid and electrolyte status

THERAPEUTIC INTERVENTIONS cont'd

- Place feeding tube and provide feedings/supplements as needed. *Even if child is able to eat or bottle feed, supplemental TPN or tube feedings may be required to meet metabolic demands of healing and growth.*
- Do not use bolus tube feedings.
- Provide child with preferred foods in small, frequent portions.
- Provide high-protein, high-calorie diet. *Infants may require high-calorie formula.*

Pain

RELATED TO

Injury

DEFINING CHARACTERISTICS

Complaints of pain

Increased restlessness

Alterations in sleep pattern

Irritability

Facial grimaces

Guarding

ONGOING ASSESSMENT

- Assess pain characteristics while considering child's age and developmental level. *The young child and infant cannot verbalize pain.*
- Obtain parent's assistance in evaluating pain and pain control.
- Assess vital signs. *Increasing pain can cause transient increases in respiratory and cardiac rates and BP.*
- Evaluate and document effectiveness of chosen pain control methods. *Changing effectiveness is expected. First- and second-degree burns are very painful; pain will decrease over time and healing. Third-degree burns do not cause pain because of nerve destruction, but as nerves regenerate, pain will increase.*

THERAPEUTIC INTERVENTIONS

- Administer sedatives and analgesics prescribed for pain (via IV while child is critical).
- Consider patient-controlled analgesia use for older child.
- Apply topical anesthetics as ordered.
- Avoid pressure on injured tissues; use bed span.
- Position child *to promote comfort.*
- Alleviate all unnecessary stressors or discomfort sources.
- Allay fears and anxiety.
- Turn *to help relieve pressure points,* obtain pressure-relieving mattress or beds as needed.
- Premedicate for dressing changes; allow sufficient time for medication to take effect.
- Saturate dressings with sterile normal saline solution before removal. *This will ease dressing removal by loosening adherents and decrease pain.*
- Use distraction/relaxation techniques as indicated.

Pain will be relieved or reduced.

Anxiety/Fear

RELATED TO

Change in body image

Anticipation of pain

Questionable outcome

Isolation

Circumstance of injury

Age

DEFINING CHARACTERISTICS

Restlessness

Combativeness

Tachypnea

Tachycardia

Hypoxia

ONGOING ASSESSMENT

- Observe for signs of anxiety.
- Identify normal level of coping.
- Assess level of development.

THERAPEUTIC INTERVENTIONS

- Display confident, calm manner.
- Encourage ventilation of feedings and concerns.
- Reduce distracting stimuli *to maintain quiet environment.*
- Hold infant/child if possible.
- Encourage parent participation.
- Discuss parental feelings (guilt, grief) *to help parent care for the child.*

Anxiety will be maintained.

Continued.

Burns cont'd

NURSING DIAGNOSES/ DEFINING CHARACTERISTICS	NURSING INTERVENTIONS / *RATIONALES*	EXPECTED OUTCOMES
Knowledge Deficit: Child/Family **RELATED TO** Injury Treatments **DEFINING CHARACTERISTICS** Multiple questions Noncommunication Staring Change in behavior Guarding	**ONGOING ASSESSMENT** • Assess readiness to learn. • Assess baseline knowledge of injury and treatment, prognosis. • Assess child's developmental level. **THERAPEUTIC INTERVENTIONS** • Explain all procedures and tests. • Explain need for sterile technique and isolation *to prevent infection.* • Explain reason for frequent assessment/orientation to environment. • *To alleviate fears,* explain reason for gloves and masks during sterile procedures. • Explain home care requirements. • Teach dressing change procedure if needed. • Provide safety/accident prevention information. • Provide follow-up consultations as needed (psychological, plastic surgery, social work).	Child and family will understand necessity for treatments and procedures.

Linda M. St. Julien, RN, MS; Michele Knoll Puzas, RNC, MHPE

Extremity fracture

CLOSED REDUCTION; OPEN REDUCTION;
INTERNAL FIXATION; EXTERNAL FIXATION

A fracture is a break or disruption in the continuity of a bone. Fractures occur when a bone is subjected to more stress than it can absorb. Fractures are treated by one or a combination of the following: closed reduction—alignment of bone fragments by manual manipulation without surgery; open reduction—alignment of bone fragments by surgery; internal fixation—immobilization of fracture site during surgery with rods, pins, plates, screws, wires, or other hardware; immobilization through use of casts, splints, traction, posterior molds, etc.; external fixation—immobilization of bone fragments.

NURSING DIAGNOSES/ DEFINING CHARACTERISTICS	NURSING INTERVENTIONS / *RATIONALES*	EXPECTED OUTCOMES

Pain **RELATED TO** Fracture Soft tissue injury **DEFINING CHARACTERISTICS** Guarding behavior Muscle spasm Diaphoresis Increased pulse rate Increased blood pressure Increased or decreased respirations Pallor Crying, moaning Grimacing Anxiety	**ONGOING ASSESSMENT**
	 • Assess age and developmental level.
	 • Assess for pain or discomfort. Use a pain scale appropriate to child's age/development.
	 • Assess pain characteristics:
	     Location
	     Quality/character
	     Severity
	     Onset
	     Duration
	     Precipitating factors
	     Relieving factors
	 • Determine past experience with pain and pain relief measures.
	
	 THERAPEUTIC INTERVENTIONS
	 • Maintain immobilization and support of affected part. *Immobility prevents further tissue damage and muscle spasm.*
	 • Reposition and support unaffected parts as permitted *to promote general comfort.*
		Pain will be reduced.

NURSING DIAGNOSES/ DEFINING CHARACTERISTICS	NURSING INTERVENTIONS / *RATIONALES*	EXPECTED OUTCOMES
DEFINING CHARACTERISTICS cont'd Restlessness Withdrawal Irritability Verbalized complaint of pain	**THERAPEUTIC INTERVENTIONS** cont'd • Elevate affected part *to decrease vasocongestion.* • Apply cold *to decrease swelling* (for first 24-48 hours). Apply for 20-30 minutes every 1-2 hours. • Anticipate need for analgesia. • Respond immediately to request for analgesia. • Medicate 30 minutes before wound/pin care or physical therapy *to decrease pain of movement.* • Teach relaxation techniques to older child. • Administer muscle relaxants as necessary.	
High Risk for Fluid Volume Deficit **RELATED TO** Multiple fractures Long bone fractures Blood vessel damage with bleeding Third spacing of fluids caused by trauma **DEFINING CHARACTERISTICS** Weak, rapid pulse Cool, clammy skin Rapid, shallow respirations Decreased blood pressure Slow capillary refill Decreased urinary output Anxiety Altered level of consciousness	**ONGOING ASSESSMENT** • Assess for symptoms of hypovolemia. • Assess amount of bleeding from external wounds. • Assess for third spacing or bleeding around fracture site. • Obtain a circumference measurement of injured area every 8 hours *to assess for further bleeding/third spacing fluid.* • Note amount of bleeding on cast. **THERAPEUTIC INTERVENTIONS** • Administer IV fluids and blood products as ordered. • Maintain alignment and immobility of fracture site *to prevent disruption of the bone healing process.* • Administer humidified oxygen as ordered.	Risk of fluid volume deficit will be reduced.

High Risk for Altered Tissue Perfusion
RELATED TO
Trauma
Surgery
Compartment syndrome
Neurovascular compromise
 	
DEFINING CHARACTERISTICS
Distal to fracture site:
Skin cool, cyanotic
Diminished or absent pulse
Slow/absent capillary refill
Edema
Hematoma
	ONGOING ASSESSMENT
	• Assess distal to fracture site every 2-4 hours for 48 hours until stable, then every 8 hours. Observe for:
	    Color
	    Sensation
	    Movement
	    Capillary refill
	    Swelling
	    Pulses (presence and quality)
	    Pain
	• Compare to opposite extremity.
	
	THERAPEUTIC INTERVENTIONS
	• Remove restrictive clothing and/or jewelry from affected part.
	• Elevate affected part above level of heart on pillows or by suspension traction if ordered *to promote venous return and decrease edema.* Do not elevate *above* level of heart if compartment syndrome is suspected; arterial pressure should be maintained by keeping limb at heart level. *This will promote arterial blood flow.*
	• Encourage exercise of unaffected parts distal to site as allowed *to promote circulation.*
		Risk for alteration in tissue perfusion and neurovascular compromise will be reduced.

Continued.

Extremity fracture cont'd

NURSING DIAGNOSES/ DEFINING CHARACTERISTICS	NURSING INTERVENTIONS / *RATIONALES*	EXPECTED OUTCOMES
DEFINING CHARACTERISTICS cont'd Paresis Hyperesthesia Numbness, tingling Pain (progressive and disproportional to injury) Pain on passive stretching of muscle Tightness of muscle compartment	**THERAPEUTIC INTERVENTIONS cont'd** • Report any neurovascular compromise to physician immediately. • Document all findings completely. • Have cast cutter available for splitting, bivalving, or removal of cast if necessary. • Prepare child for surgical intervention (i.e., fasciotomy) if compartment syndrome is probable. *Severe tissue swelling that decreases blood flow causes ischemia and may result in permanent motor and/or sensory damage.*	

High Risk for Infection
RELATED TO
Open fracture
External fixation pins
Surgical intervention
 	
DEFINING CHARACTERISTICS
Local:
Pain/tenderness
Redness
Swelling
Excess warmth
Purulent drainage
Delayed healing
Loosening of pins
Systemic:
Increased pulse rate
Fever
Change in level of consciousness
Decreased urinary output
Increased WBCs
	ONGOING ASSESSMENT
	• Assess wound and/or pin site for:
	    Local signs of infection
	    Skin tension around pins
	    Signs of developing gangrene (vesicles filled with red, watery fluid and gas bubbles coming from tissue)
	• Assess for systemic signs of infection.
	• Monitor vital signs every 2-4 hours for 48 hours until stable, then every 8 hours.
	• Assess for odors or drainage through immobilization devices that are not removed (i.e., casts, splints).
	
	THERAPEUTIC INTERVENTIONS
	• Maintain adequate hydration and nutritional status *to promote wound healing.*
	• Use sterile technique when changing wound dressings. *This is necessary in absence of intact first line of defense.*
	• Keep dressing dry and intact. Give wound care as ordered.
	• Initiate wound precautions if purulent drainage is present.
	• Document appearance of wound.
	• Administer antibiotics as ordered.
	• Administer tetanus toxoid and/or hypertet as indicated.
	• Perform appropriate pin site care:
	    Provide care to all pin sites every 8-24 hours.
	    Provide pin care as ordered or use standard protocol (e.g., cleanse each pin site with hydrogen peroxide with sterile applicator and rinse with normal saline to remove crusting from pin site).
	    Apply sterile dressing and/or ointment as ordered. Wipe off fixator with alcohol.
	    Document observations.
		Risk of infection will be reduced.

Altered Nutrition: Less Than Body Requirements **RELATED TO** Increased nutritional needs for wound and fracture healing **DEFINING CHARACTERISTICS** Poor dietary selection Poor wound and fracture healing	**ONGOING ASSESSMENT** • Monitor dietary intake and calorie count if indicated. • Assess child's food preferences. • Assess lab values. **THERAPEUTIC INTERVENTIONS** • Encourage and teach importance of diet with adequate amounts of protein; calcium; vitamins C, D, and A; iron and calories, *which are essential for bone and tissue healing. Healing increases metabolism; need for calories is increased to prevent protein breakdown.* • Refer to clinical dietitian as needed. • Provide for adequate rest periods. *Rest conserves energy for cellular metabolism, which is necessary for tissue and bone repair and growth.*	Adequate nutrition will be maintained.

Extremity fracture cont'd

NURSING DIAGNOSES/ DEFINING CHARACTERISTICS	NURSING INTERVENTIONS / *RATIONALES*	EXPECTED OUTCOMES
DEFINING CHARACTERISTICS cont'd Delayed bone repair Decreased total protein, albumin, transferrin, lymphocyte levels		
Impaired Physical Mobility **RELATED TO** Cast Fixation device Pain Surgical procedure Immobilizer **DEFINING CHARACTERISTICS** Reluctance to attempt movement Limited ROM Mechanical restriction of movement Decreased muscle strength and/or control Impaired coordination Inability to purposefully move within physical environment, including bed mobility, transfer, ambulation	**ONGOING ASSESSMENT** - Assess ROM of unaffected parts proximal and distal to immobilization device. - Assess ability to perform basic ADL. - Assess ability to ambulate. - Assess present and preinjury level of mobility. - Assess muscle strength to all extremities. **THERAPEUTIC INTERVENTIONS** - Encourage isometric, active, and resistive ROM exercises to all unaffected joints four times a day and as tolerated *to prevent muscle atrophy and maintain adequate muscle strength required in mobility.* - Apply splint to support foot in neutral position (applied to lower extremity frames and traction) *to prevent foot drop.* - Perform flexion and extension exercises to proximal and distal joints of affected extremity when indicated. - Assist up to chair or wheelchair when ordered; teach transfer technique. - Lift extremity by external fixation frame if stable; avoid handling of injured soft tissue. - Reinforce crutch ambulation taught by physical therapist using appropriate weight-bearing status. Assist with gait belt until gait becomes stable. - Obtain occupational therapy consultation as needed.	Maximum mobility within prescribed restrictions will be achieved.
High Risk for Ineffective Breathing Pattern **RELATED TO** Fat embolism Pulmonary embolus Type of immobilization device/site of fracture **DEFINING CHARACTERISTICS** Tachycardia Tachypnea Precordial chest pain Rales, wheezing Cough Dyspnea Shortness of breath Cyanosis Petechiae Altered level of consciousness Abnormal blood gas values	**ONGOING ASSESSMENT** - Assess for symptoms of breathing pattern abnormality (see Defining Characteristics). **THERAPEUTIC INTERVENTIONS** - Encourage cough and deep breathing exercises *to promote adequate lung expansion.* - Position child for maximum lung expansion. - Provide adequate hydration (IVs, oral fluids) *to mobilize secretions.* - Administer humidified oxygen as ordered. - Alleviate anxiety (explain procedures, provide emotional support) caused by respiratory distress *to decrease oxygen demands.*	Normal breathing pattern will be maintained.

Continued.

Integumentary/Musculoskeletal Care Plans (Pediatric)

NURSING DIAGNOSES/ DEFINING CHARACTERISTICS	NURSING INTERVENTIONS / *RATIONALES*	EXPECTED OUTCOMES
High Risk for Impaired Skin Integrity **RELATED TO** Presence of immobilization device Improper immobilization device **DEFINING CHARACTERISTICS** Pain/tenderness/ burning Redness Swelling Skin breakdown Foul smell, drainage, or warm area under cast	**ONGOING ASSESSMENT** ▪ Assess immobilized extremity for redness/breakdown. ▪ If casted, check edges of cast for roughness. ▪ Assess bony prominences for redness/breakdown. **THERAPEUTIC INTERVENTIONS** ▪ Use antipressure devices (i.e., flotation devices, eggcrate mattress, air mattress), as appropriate. ▪ Maintain adequate hydration and nutritional status. *Good nutrition is necessary for tissue growth and repair.* ▪ Reposition every 2 hours. ▪ Prevent pressure on toes from sheets; use bed cradle if necessary. ▪ Trim and petal tape rough edges of a cast *to prevent irritation.* ▪ Massage skin around cast with alcohol *to toughen skin.* ▪ Pad pin edges *to protect injury to other areas.* ▪ Turn and provide skin care every 2-4 hours. ▪ See Impaired skin integrity, p. 39.	Risk for impairment of skin integrity will be reduced.
High Risk for Body Image Disturbance **RELATED TO** Change or loss of body part **DEFINING CHARACTERISTICS** Refusal to participate in care Unrealistic perception of course of treatment	**ONGOING ASSESSMENT** ▪ Assess child's/family's feelings and level of acceptance about injury and method of treatment. **THERAPEUTIC INTERVENTIONS** ▪ Perform preoperative teaching if time permits; use pictures of devices if necessary. ▪ Explain procedures and treatment modalities (show x-rays *to aid teaching*). ▪ Encourage and give permission to verbalize feelings. *Ventilation of feelings supports honesty and objectivity of the situation and promotes realistic perception.* ▪ Encourage/support a realistic assessment of the situation. ▪ Avoid false reassurances. ▪ Consult occupational therapist for modification of clothing. ▪ See Body image disturbance, p. 7.	Risk for disturbance in body image will be reduced.
Self-Esteem Disturbance **RELATED TO** Loss of body function Inability to perform role responsibilities Loss of control Hospitalization **DEFINING CHARACTERISTICS** Withdrawal behavior Demanding behavior Inability to solve problems Anger Denial Hostility Noncompliance	**ONGOING ASSESSMENT** ▪ Assess coping mechanism used by child or family. ▪ Assess effect of injury on self-esteem. **THERAPEUTIC INTERVENTIONS** ▪ Help child identify previous stress situations and ways of dealing with them. ▪ Identify and reinforce child's strengths. ▪ Support continued significant roles with family and friends—provide for visits, phone calls, written work, etc. as tolerated. ▪ Encourage child to plan and participate in activities of care. Adapt care to child's routines and needs. ▪ Provide opportunities for independent activities. *Independence facilitates coping.* Consult child life therapist. ▪ Arrange the environment to promote independent use of materials needed for ADL. *To develop self-esteem, child and family must be active participants in the rehabilitation process.* ▪ Continually teach and inform child and family about physical status, treatment plan, etc. ▪ Make social service referral early in hospitalization for financial and resource counseling as needed.	Disturbance in self-esteem will be reduced.

Extremity fracture cont'd

NURSING DIAGNOSES/ DEFINING CHARACTERISTICS	NURSING INTERVENTIONS / *RATIONALES*	EXPECTED OUTCOMES
High Risk for Injury RELATED TO Loss of continuity of cast **DEFINING CHARACTERISTICS** Pain Malalignment on x-rays Skin breakdown under cast Neurovascular impairment	**ONGOING ASSESSMENT** • Assess cast for cracks, weakened areas, indentations, softened or wet areas. **THERAPEUTIC INTERVENTIONS** • Leave cast open to air until completely dry. *Drying of plaster cast takes 24-48 hours. Air drying promotes drying from inside out to ensure a stable cast. A fiberglass cast will dry in just a few hours.* • Prevent indenting cast by moving it with palms of hands and supporting it on nonplastic pillows until dry. *Plastic traps heat released during application.* • Reposition child and cast every 2 hours *to allow for drying of cast.* • Keep cast clean and dry. Prevent soiling from urine/feces.	Risk for injury will be reduced.

Knowledge Deficit RELATED TO
 New procedures/ treatment
 New condition
 Home care needs
 	
 DEFINING CHARACTERISTICS
 Child and/or family verbalizes lack of adequate knowledge regarding care/use of immobilization device, mobility limitations, complications, and follow-up care
 Confusion; asking many questions
 Lack of questions
 Inaccurate follow-through of instruction
 Improper performance
 Inappropriate or exaggerated behaviors (i.e., hostile, agitated, hysterical, apathetic)
	ONGOING ASSESSMENT
	 • Encourage child/parent to verbalize questions.
	 • Solicit current understanding of diagnosis, treatment, follow-up, etc.
	 • Assess readiness and ability of child and family to assume responsibility for care.
	
	 THERAPEUTIC INTERVENTIONS
	 • Instruct child/parent to:
	   Elevate extremity above level of heart with pillows while in reclining position *to prevent swelling;* prop affected leg on footstool or chair while sitting.
	   Do prescribed exercises several times a day *to maintain muscle tone.*
	   Use appropriate assistive device (walker, crutches) and maintain prescribed weight-bearing status.
	   Identify and report to physician signs of neurovascular compromise of extremity—pain, numbness, tingling, burning, swelling, or discoloration.
	   Use pain relief measures safely.
	   Obtain proper nutrition *to promote bone/wound healing and prevent constipation.*
	   Arrange for follow-up care.
	 • For a child in a cast, instruct to:
	   Notify physician:
	     If cast cracks or breaks
	     Of foul odor under cast
	     Of any fresh drainage through cast
	     Of foreign body under cast
	     Of broken areas of skin around cast
	     Of pain or burning under cast
	     Of warm areas on cast
	   Keep cast clean and dry; tub bathing permitted only if cast is protected and not immersed.
	   Inspect skin around edges of cast for irritation. Rub skin around cast with alcohol *to help toughen it.* Do not use oil; *this will soften the cast.*
	   Do *not* put anything under cast, poke under cast, or put powder or lotion under cast. *This may abrade skin and cause an infection.*
	 • For child with surgical incision, instruct to observe incision for signs of infection and notify physician if they develop.
	 • For child with an external fixation device:
	   Instruct child/parent to:
	     Perform pin care
	     Perform wound care
	     Observe for loosening of pins
	     Cleanse device
	   Involve child/parent in procedures.
	   Supervise persons performing procedures.
	   Provide with own supplies as needed.
		Parent and/or child will verbalize understanding of treatment modalities, possible complications, and follow-up care.

Michele Knoll Puzas, RNC, MHPE; Marilyn R. Magafas, RN, MBA

Maxillary osteotomy

FRACTURED JAW; WIRED JAW; LEFORT PROCEDURE

An intraoral surgical procedure involving intentional fracture of the maxilla with the aid of bone cuts to correct jaw deformities or repair traumatic injuries.

NURSING DIAGNOSES/ DEFINING CHARACTERISTICS	NURSING INTERVENTIONS / *RATIONALES*	EXPECTED OUTCOMES
Ineffective Breathing Pattern **RELATED TO** Wired jaws Possible nasal or pharyngeal swelling/bleeding Possible laryngeal edema caused by prolonged endotracheal intubation Excessively tight pressure dressing Anxiety-induced difficulty related to sensation of wire fixation **DEFINING CHARACTERISTICS** Elevated respiratory rate Labored respirations Nasal breathing Change in depth of respirations Use of accessory muscles Nasal flaring	**ONGOING ASSESSMENT** • Assess age and developmental level. • Assess rate and rhythm of respirations. • Assess nasal airway for patency. • Auscultate breath sounds. **THERAPEUTIC INTERVENTIONS** • Keep head of bed elevated at all times *to prevent aspiration and minimize edema.* • Have wire cutters or scissors taped to wall at head of bed. *Scissors can be used to release elastic fixator.* • Have aspirator with Yankauer suction at bedside. • Instruct child/parent on oral suctioning with Yankauer suction tube. Use careful positioning near incision sites. • Clean nasal airway with normal saline solution as ordered. • Maintain humidified air or oxygen via face tent *to moisten nasal mucosa and soothe pharynx after intubation.* • Administer decongestants as ordered. • Instruct child who feels nauseated to sit up and turn head to side. *Nurse should be prepared to suction secretions to prevent aspiration.* • Reassure anxious child that breathing is normal even with fixation of jaw. • Notify physician immediately of any respiratory distress.	Normal breathing pattern will be maintained.
Altered Nutrition: Less Than Body Requirements **RELATED TO** Wired jaws Change in dietary habits Nausea **DEFINING CHARACTERISTICS** Weight loss Documented inadequate caloric intake Decreased fluid intake	**ONGOING ASSESSMENT** • Obtain baseline weight. • Assess weight every day. • Monitor I&O every shift. • Determine dietary preferences. • Observe for sedative effects of antiemetics. • Observe for signs of dehydration. **THERAPEUTIC INTERVENTIONS** • Arrange for dietary consultation. • Keep head of bed elevated *to minimize risk of aspiration during feeding.* • Instruct on proper use of feeding syringes, especially near incisions. • Instruct child not to attempt to open mouth. • Provide with antiemetics as ordered. • Provide child with a diet of preferred items that are high in calories, protein, and vitamin C. • Provide child with liquids and soft or blended foods that require no chewing. • Have dietary supplements at bedside. • Maintain IV fluids as ordered. • Encourage fluids. • Explain that while some weight loss is expected (up to 10 pounds in normal adolescent), *loss can be minimized with adequate diet.* • See Fluid volume deficit, p. 19.	Optimal nutrition will be achieved.

NURSING DIAGNOSES/ DEFINING CHARACTERISTICS	NURSING INTERVENTIONS / *RATIONALES*	EXPECTED OUTCOMES

High Risk for Infection
RELATED TO
Inadequate oral hygiene
Presence of intraoral drains
 	
DEFINING CHARACTERISTICS
Elevated temperature
Excessive oral secretions
Foul odor from mouth
Increased facial swelling
Excessive drainage on head and face dressing
	ONGOING ASSESSMENT
	• Check head and face dressing for excessive drainage; note color, amount, presence of foul odor.
	• Monitor temperature.
	• Observe for increased facial swelling; loosen dressing as needed.
	
	THERAPEUTIC INTERVENTIONS
	• Administer IV antibiotics as ordered.
	• Administer corticosteroids as ordered. *May not be ordered for immunocompromised child.*
	• Apply ice packs to both sides of face for first 24 hours postoperatively *to minimize edema.*
	• Instruct parent and child on proper mouth care *to remove particles of food, which provide medium for bacterial growth:*
	   Normal saline solution or Peridex oral rinses after each meal and at bedtime
	   Brushing teeth with a child-size, soft toothbrush after meals and at bedtime, beginning 48 hours after surgery
		Potential for intraoral infection will be reduced.

Impaired Verbal Communication **RELATED TO** Wired jaws Increased facial swelling Poor control of oral secretions **DEFINING CHARACTERISTICS** Difficulty understanding child's speech	**ONGOING ASSESSMENT** • Assess child's ability to communicate before surgery if possible. • Determine whether child can speak postoperatively so he/she is understood by others. • Identify alternate methods of communication. • Assess neurological status, especially if communication impairment is new/sudden. **THERAPEUTIC INTERVENTIONS** • Have call light within reach. • Provide older child with paper and pen at bedside. • Provide picture board for young child. • Inform child/parent that the wires/elastics will usually be removed in 6-8 weeks. • Inform child/parent that opening the mouth is not possible if wires are used as fixator. If guiding elastics are used to fix jaw, then some mandibular ROM is allowed. • Offer support and reassurance. • See Impaired communication, p. 11.	Alternate means of communication will be established.

Knowledge Deficit
RELATED TO
Lack of previous, similar experiences
 	
DEFINING CHARACTERISTICS
Repeated questions
Lack of questions
Child/parent unable to perform return demonstrations on proper use of feeding syringes and proper oral hygiene maintenance
	ONGOING ASSESSMENT
	• Determine if child or family has any questions.
	• Determine if child or parent can use feeding syringes and perform proper oral hygiene with ease.
	
	THERAPEUTIC INTERVENTIONS
	• Inform parent and child of the following:
	   Wire cutters or scissors provided *for emergency wire or elastics removal*
	   Correct way to cut wires or elastics
	   Dietary instructions to be provided per dietitian, along with syringes and suction catheters for home use
	   Proper cleaning of feeding syringes after each use
	   Need for teens to avoid alcohol *to minimize risk of vomiting and/or loss of control of secretions*
	   Best position to assume for vomiting
	   Importance of maintaining proper oral hygiene
	   Significant degree of facial swelling will usually be gone in 1 week; preoperative appearance will return in 3 to 6 months
	   Liquid diet supplements as needed
	   Social service/other consultations as needed
		Child and family will demonstrate and verbalize adequate, safe self-care.

Victoria Malone, RN, BSN, FNP; Frank Hohn, DDS

Muscular dystrophies

MUSCULAR ATROPHY; DUCHENNE; WERDNIG-
HOFFMANN; FSH; KUGELBERG-WELANDER

Muscular dystrophy (MD) is an inherited disorder characterized by muscle weakening and atrophy.

Duchenne MD is the most common form of the disease that affects males almost exclusively. Onset of muscle weakness is seen between the ages of 3 to 5 years; children exhibit both pseudohypertrophy of the calf muscles and Gowers' sign in the early stages. Progressive to the point of profound atrophy, ambulation becomes impossible by the early teen years and death usually occurs before 20 years.

Werdnig-Hoffmann paralysis in the most severe form becomes visible before age 2. The affected infant is floppy, moves very little, and is chronically dyspneic. Life expectancy is less than 5 years.

Facioscapulohumeral (FSH) paralysis begins with weakening of the muscles of the face and shoulders. Late progression involves the pelvic girdle and lower extremities. Onset is between 7 and 20 years of age; life expectancy is between 15 and 30 years of age.

Signs of Kugelberg-Welander disease appear between 5 and 15 years of age. Muscle weakness in the extremities is the prominent symptom. Progression is slow; in many cases, allowing for a normal life expectancy.

NURSING DIAGNOSES/ DEFINING CHARACTERISTICS	NURSING INTERVENTIONS / *RATIONALES*	EXPECTED OUTCOMES
Ineffective Airway Clearance **RELATED TO** Muscle weakness Pooled secretions Spinal collapse **DEFINING CHARACTERISTICS** Poor cry Poor cough efforts Retractions Diminished lung sounds	**ONGOING ASSESSMENT** • Assess age and developmental level. • Assess respiratory function, breathing pattern, evidence of retractions, quality of cry/cough, evidence of pooled secretions. • Evaluate muscle strength, using blowing games/bubbles, and incentive spirometer. • Assess body alignment. **THERAPEUTIC INTERVENTIONS** • Position for ease in respirations. • Suction as necessary. *Respiratory failure and pneumonia are frequent causes of death.* • Provide small, slow feedings *to decrease risk of aspiration.* • Obtain physical therapy consultation. *A trunk support may be necessary to keep body aligned for ease in respiration. Progression of spinal collapse may necessitate surgical intervention (spinal fusion) to support cardiopulmonary function.*	Optimal airway clearance will be maintained.
Impaired Physical Mobility **RELATED TO** Inherited disorder Muscle fiber necrosis Muscle weakness Muscle atrophy **DEFINING CHARACTERISTICS** Limited ROM Decreased muscle strength, control Inability to move purposefully within physical environment	**ONGOING ASSESSMENT** • Assess muscle strength. • Assess body alignment. *Spinal deformities/collapse occur in children with severe disease.* • Assess independent mobility and endurance. • Monitor changes in CPK (creatinine phosphokinase) and myopathic muscle biopsy, which denote further muscle deterioration. *Muscle and cardiac changes will limit endurance as disease progresses.* • Identify limitations and safety issues. **THERAPEUTIC INTERVENTIONS** • Obtain physical and occupational therapy consultations as needed. • Encourage independence in as many activities as possible *to maintain optimal function and inhibit deterioration.* • Maintain prescribed stretching exercises or ROM program *to deter atrophy and contractures.*	Optimal physical mobility will be maintained.

Muscular dystrophies cont'd

NURSING DIAGNOSES/ DEFINING CHARACTERISTICS	NURSING INTERVENTIONS / *RATIONALES*	EXPECTED OUTCOMES
DEFINING CHARACTERISTICS cont'd Reluctance to attempt movement	**THERAPEUTIC INTERVENTIONS** cont'd • Provide physical supports as needed (limb braces, orthotic jacket, reach extenders, night splints, lifts, ADL aids, walkers, wheelchair) *to maintain as much mobility as possible.* • Provide a safe environment.	
High Risk for Impaired Skin Integrity **RELATED TO** Immobility **DEFINING CHARACTERISTICS** Reddened areas Pallor Poor capillary refill Blisters Open lesions Necrosis	**ONGOING ASSESSMENT** • Assess child's ability for independent movement. • Assess skin, especially bony prominences, for defining characteristics. **THERAPEUTIC INTERVENTIONS** • Encourage movement by child. *Independent movement inhibits ischemia and tissue breakdown.* • Change child's position frequently if independent mobility is limited. • Provide prophylactic mattress and wheelchair pad. • Maintain nutrition and hydration. • Keep skin clean and dry.	Risk for impaired skin integrity will be reduced.

Altered Nutrition: More Than Required/Less Than Required
RELATED TO
Overeating
Poor intake
GI disturbance
Muscle weakness (facial/jaw)
 	
DEFINING CHARACTERISTICS
Weight above or below average for age and height
Poor food choices
Poor appetite
	ONGOING ASSESSMENT
	• Assess weight/height.
	• Assess dietary habits, food choices, frequency of eating.
	• Assess chewing, swallowing ability. *Muscle weakness may inhibit satisfactory chewing and ability to swallow.*
	• Assess dental status in the older child. *Poor dentition can affect food choice and intake. Dentition suffers as a result of inability to provide adequate self-hygiene.*
	• Assess for gastric dilatation, rectal prolapse, impaction, constipation.
	
	THERAPEUTIC INTERVENTIONS
	• Assist child/parent in choosing foods, especially snack foods. *Food is sometimes a respite from boredom or a reward; choices should be of low-fat, high-nutritive value.*
	• Obtain dietary consultation. *Caloric intake should be determined considering child's basal requirements and energy expenditure.*
	• Provide tube feedings for infant or child unable to obtain adequate oral nourishment.
	• Notify physician of gastrointestinal disturbance and treat as needed:
	    Remove impactions.
	    Increase dietary fiber.
	    Administer medications as ordered.
	• Request dental consultation if needed; provide dental hygiene.
	• Allow sufficient time for meals. Assist child if needed; try to keep foods at desired temperatures.
		Nutritional balance will be maintained.

Impaired Verbal Communication **RELATED TO** Muscle weakness (face, jaw) **DEFINING CHARACTERISTICS** Unintelligible speech Apparent frustration	**ONGOING ASSESSMENT** • Assess current and past communication strategies. • Identify changing needs. • Assess family's ability to interact with child. *Family may perceive communication as understandable and acceptable.* **THERAPEUTIC INTERVENTIONS** • Provide alternate methods of communication if desired, and appropriate to age. • Use signs/strategies successfully used by child/family. • Obtain speech therapy consultation when needed. • See Impaired verbal communication, p. 11.	Adequate communication will be maintained.

Continued.

Muscular dystrophies cont'd

NURSING DIAGNOSES/ DEFINING CHARACTERISTICS	NURSING INTERVENTIONS / *RATIONALES*	EXPECTED OUTCOMES
Body Image Disturbance **RELATED TO** Progressive disease Physical deterioration Increasing disability **DEFINING CHARACTERISTICS** Self-deprecation Careless behavior Unkempt appearance Hopeless/powerless demeanor	**ONGOING ASSESSMENT** ▪ Assess for defining characteristics. ▪ Assess child's ability to care for self and participate in activities. ▪ Obtain parent's perceptions of child's body image and/or changes in attitude/behaviors. **THERAPEUTIC INTERVENTIONS** ▪ Encourage verbalization of feelings. ▪ Assist in identifying and implementing methods to improve appearance/level of activity. ▪ Obtain psychiatric consultation *to assist child and family in adapting to chronic and possibly terminal disease.* ▪ See Body image disturbance, p. 7.	Body image disturbance will be reduced.
Knowledge Deficit: Family **RELATED TO** New phenomena New needs **DEFINING CHARACTERISTICS** Multiple questions Stated lack of understanding Hesitant behavior Incorrect statements or performance	**ONGOING ASSESSMENT** ▪ Assess family's understanding of diagnosis/prognosis/child's future needs. ▪ Assess readiness to learn. ▪ Assess family's support systems. **THERAPEUTIC INTERVENTIONS** ▪ Obtain social service consultation *to assist with learning, emotional, and economic requirements.* ▪ Explain all treatments and procedures; involve parent in child's care. *Parent will have to care for child at home.* ▪ Allow parent to teach staff what works best for child at home. ▪ Advise genetic counseling. ▪ Provide information on self-help groups where available (Muscular Dystrophy Association). ▪ Arrange home health assistance when needed.	Family will understand nature of disease process, progress, and necessary home care.

Michele Knoll Puzas, RNC, MHPE

Osteomyelitis

Inflammation of the bone, especially the marrow, caused by a pathogenic organism, usually Staphylococcus, Streptococcus, Salmonella, or Haemophilus flu, and introduced via soft tissue trauma.

NURSING DIAGNOSES/ DEFINING CHARACTERISTICS	NURSING INTERVENTIONS / *RATIONALES*	EXPECTED OUTCOMES

Infection: Bone
RELATED TO
Infection that has migrated to bone tissue
 	
DEFINING CHARACTERISTICS
Local inflammation of involved bone as characterized by:
Pain/guarding
Edema
Warmth
Redness
	ONGOING ASSESSMENT
	▪ Assess age and developmental level.
	▪ Assess affected area for signs and symptoms of infection:
	  Pain
	  Edema
	  Warmth
	  Redness (describe in detail)
	▪ Assess lab values, especially WBC and sedimentation rate.
	▪ Assess x-ray or bone scan findings.
	
	THERAPEUTIC INTERVENTIONS
	▪ Obtain appropriate cultures and sensitivities:
	  Blood
	  Aspirate from bone abscess if present
	▪ Administer IV antibiotics as ordered.
	▪ Administer antipyretics.
	▪ Provide fluids *to prevent dehydration in a febrile state.*
	▪ Cleanse area. *Sometimes primary soft tissue infection may not be found since it is already healed by time osteomyelitis is evident.*
	▪ Apply warm compress or heating pads *to promote circulation to affected area.*
		Signs and symptoms of infection will be relieved.

Pain **RELATED TO** Infection Inflammation **DEFINING CHARACTERISTICS** Verbalized bone pain with/without movement Nonverbal signs, cries, and grimaces Physical signs (e.g., increased heart rate, increased blood pressure, and diaphoresis)	**ONGOING ASSESSMENT** ▪ Assess affected area for pain with movement. ▪ Assess verbal and nonverbal signs of pain. ▪ Assess analgesic effectiveness. ▪ Monitor vital signs for signs and symptoms of pain. **THERAPEUTIC INTERVENTIONS** ▪ Administer analgesics as ordered. ▪ Immobilize limb. ▪ Apply warm packs to affected area *since heat provides an alternate sensation to pain.* ▪ Encourage child to use previous coping mechanisms. ▪ Provide diversional activities (refer to Diversional activity deficit, p. 16).	Pain will be relieved or reduced.
High Risk for Injury **RELATED TO** Necrosis of bone Fragile bone **DEFINING CHARACTERISTICS** Pain of affected bone with movement Guarded movement of affected limb	**ONGOING ASSESSMENT** ▪ Assess ROM. ▪ Assess x-ray and bone scan findings for bone destruction. **THERAPEUTIC INTERVENTIONS** ▪ Immobilize affected area. ▪ Provide passive ROM as indicated. ▪ Obtain physical therapy consultation.	Chance of injury will be reduced.

Continued.

Integumentary/Musculoskeletal Care Plans (Pediatric)

NURSING DIAGNOSES/ DEFINING CHARACTERISTICS	NURSING INTERVENTIONS / *RATIONALES*	EXPECTED OUTCOMES
High Risk for Altered Nutrition: Less Than Body Requirement **RELATED TO** Decreased intake related to pain or change in dietary provisions Increased nutritional demands for healing **DEFINING CHARACTERISTICS** Poor appetite Decreased weight	**ONGOING ASSESSMENT** • Assess intake. • Assess appetite. **THERAPEUTIC INTERVENTIONS** • Provide desired foods, encourage parent to bring food from home. • Assist child at mealtime as needed. *Poor intake may be caused by inability to feed self.* • Provide pain control before meals; *appetite will improve if child is pain free.* • Refer to Altered nutrition: less than body requirements, p. 33.	Adequate nutrition will be maintained.
Knowledge Deficit **RELATED TO** Hospitalization and treatment Lack of experience **DEFINING CHARACTERISTICS** Verbalized lack of understanding Questioning	**ONGOING ASSESSMENT** • Assess parent and child for readiness to learn and cognitive level. • Assess current status and ability to learn (e.g., *a febrile or uncomfortable child is not able to listen and comprehend*). **THERAPEUTIC INTERVENTIONS** • Provide explanation concerning: Development of osteomyelitis Importance of long-term IV therapy: IV maintenance Side effects of prescribed antibiotic • Explain necessity for tests (e.g., aspirations, blood culture and sensitivity, x-rays, and scans). • Stress importance for continued oral antibiotic after discharge. • Provide follow-up appointments, prescriptions, and home health services if home treatment is necessary. *Long-term IV antibiotic therapy can be provided in home if this service is available from home health agencies in area.*	Parent and child will understand importance of tests, therapy, and follow-up.

Susan Geoghegan, RN, BSN; Michele Knoll Puzas, RNC, MHPE

Scoliosis repair: spinal instrumentation

CORTEL DUBOUSSET; H-ROD; LUQUE RODS;
DWYER PROCEDURE

Spinal instrumentation for severe scoliosis refers to the surgical fixation and correction of scoliosis that is progressive and not responsive to bracing and exercise. Adolescents are the primary age group seen for scoliosis repair. Correction is accomplished with the Cortel Dubousset, Harrington, Luque, or Dwyer instrumentation, each of which uses a different kind of fixator. Differences in fixator dictate postoperative care. The Harrington rod is somewhat less stable and requires a longer period of postoperative immobility. Immediate postoperative care is often provided in an ICU setting.

NURSING DIAGNOSES/ DEFINING CHARACTERISTICS	NURSING INTERVENTIONS / *RATIONALES*	EXPECTED OUTCOMES
Anxiety/Fear **RELATED TO** Anticipation of physical harm or psychological threat (e.g., impending surgery) Forced adaptation to change in health status	**ONGOING ASSESSMENT** • Assess age and developmental level. • Recognize level of anxiety/fear (mild, severe). Note any signs/symptoms, especially nonverbal communication. • Assess normal coping patterns (interview child/family/significant others/physician). • Assess knowledge levels, reason for hospitalization, scoliosis, body image, anatomy involved, and postoperative expectations (i.e., ICU, frame).	Anxiety/fear will be reduced.
DEFINING CHARACTERISTICS *Mild:* Restlessness Increased awareness Increased questioning *Moderate-severe:* Avoidance of looking at equipment Very little movement in bed Withdrawal Tense/anxious appearance	**THERAPEUTIC INTERVENTIONS** • Introduce parent/child to ICU staff and visit ICU preoperatively. • Practice aspects of anticipated therapy such as deep breathing, spirometer, leg exercises, fracture bedpan. *Sometimes knowing what to expect lessens fear and anxiety and facilitates postoperative compliance.* • Display confident, calm manner and understanding attitude. • Establish rapport through continuity of care. • Explain preoperative and postoperative procedures/routines. • Encourage ventilation of feelings. • Provide a quiet environment; reduce distracting stimuli. • Encourage questions to clear up misconceptions. • Encourage family to visit. • Use other supportive measures (e.g., medications and psychiatric liaison). • Provide diversional measures.	

Impaired Physical Mobility
RELATED TO
Required immobilization related to nature of surgery
Prolonged immobilization
Surgery proximal to spinal cord and nerve roots
Development of edema, infection, hematoma at surgical site with nerve root/cord compression
	ONGOING ASSESSMENT
	• Assess for impaired mobility, cord compression.
	  Use verbal commands: ask to do simple tasks (e.g., wiggle toes and dorsiflex feet) *to assess motor function.*
	  Use light touch and pain to check sensations.
	
	THERAPEUTIC INTERVENTIONS
	• Maintain child's body in good alignment.
	• Log roll from side to side every 2 hours.
	• Use antipressure devices prophylactically as ordered/indicated.
	• Perform passive ROM while on bed rest or frame *to minimize risk of injury that may be related to active ROM.*
	• Explain progressive physical activity.
	• Encourage appropriate use of assistive devices.
	• Encourage early ADL when possible.
		The consequences of immobility will be reduced.

Continued.

Integumentary/Musculoskeletal Care Plans (Pediatric)

NURSING DIAGNOSES/ DEFINING CHARACTERISTICS	NURSING INTERVENTIONS / *RATIONALES*	EXPECTED OUTCOMES

DEFINING CHARACTERISTICS
Inability to purposefully move within physical environment
Weakness in leg, foot, or toes
Reluctance to attempt mobility, limited ROM, decreased muscle strength and control
Increased back pain
Signs and symptoms of cord compression:
  Radiating pain in distal nerve root (thigh, calf, foot)
  Asymmetric lower extremity reflexes
  Change in sensory function		

Pain **RELATED TO** Surgical procedure Immobility Bone harvesting (rib or iliac) **DEFINING CHARACTERISTICS** Guarding behavior Self-focus, withdrawal Crying Moaning Restlessness Irritability Facial mask of pain Altered muscle tone Changes in vital signs, respiration, color Altered sleep pattern Verbalized discomfort	**ONGOING ASSESSMENT** • Assess for signs and symptoms of discomfort. *Postoperative pain is expected, but should diminish over time. Sudden onset or increase in pain should be investigated as a potential symptom of complications.* • Assess neurological status before administering pain medications. **THERAPEUTIC INTERVENTIONS** • Anticipate need for analgesia. Consider patient-controlled analgesic (PCA), around-the-clock injections, or continuous infusion to control pain immediately after surgery.	Pain will be relieved or reduced.
High Risk for Altered Tissue Perfusion **RELATED TO** Immobility with venous stasis (*preventing normal blood flow and facilitating clot formation*)	**ONGOING ASSESSMENT** • Observe skin over extremities for color, pallor, rubor, hair distribution. • Inspect for distention of any superficial vessels of lower extremities. • Monitor vital signs. • Assess circulation, mobility, and sensation of all extremities. Compare temperature of extremities; palpate pulses (radial, femoral, pedal); and compare symmetry. Palpate extremities for edema. • Assess for development of thrombophlebitis: leg swelling, redness, pain on dorsiflexion. Measure calves and thighs if symptoms of deep vein thrombosis are present.	Optimal tissue perfusion will be maintained.

NURSING DIAGNOSES/ DEFINING CHARACTERISTICS	NURSING INTERVENTIONS / *RATIONALES*	EXPECTED OUTCOMES

High Risk for Altered Tissue Perfusion cont'd

Reactions to anesthesia and medications
Blood loss
Lengthy surgical procedure

DEFINING CHARACTERISTICS

Ischemic pain
Increased coldness, numbness, loss of hair, trophic skin changes, pallor, or rubor
Swelling of lower extremities
Delayed healing of lesions
Changes in BP
Venous distention in lower extremities
Pulmonary embolism:
  Dyspnea
  Tachycardia
  Chest pain
  Fever
  Neck vein distention
  Cyanosis
  Restlessness
  Hypoxemia
  Hemoptysis
  Petechiae on chest/shoulders

ONGOING ASSESSMENT cont'd
- Assess for pulmonary embolism (see Defining Characteristics). Encourage patient to report pain, shortness of breath, or hemoptysis.
- Monitor ABGs, especially if signs of embolism are present.

THERAPEUTIC INTERVENTIONS
- Use cardiopulmonary monitor.
- Maintain child's body alignment.
- Apply antiembolic hose or sequential compression devices *to decrease risk of deep vein thrombosis and pulmonary embolism.*
- Turn frequently or as ordered.
- Encourage coughing and deep breathing.
- Demonstrate and encourage leg exercises.
- Administer prophylactic anticoagulant therapy if ordered. *Not all children will require anticoagulants, depending on type of surgery and age and condition of child.*
- If embolus is suspected:
  Position child *to ease respiratory efforts.*
  Provide oxygen by mask or nasal cannula.
  Prepare for emergent intubation.
  Provide anticoagulants.
  Prepare for surgical intervention. *This may be necessary if anticoagulation has failed.*

High Risk for Impaired Gas Exchange

RELATED TO

Hypostatic pneumonia related to prolonged anesthesia
Immobilization in operating room and on frame

DEFINING CHARACTERISTICS

Sudden onset of shaking chills
Fever
Flushed skin
Productive cough (pink-tinged)

ONGOING ASSESSMENT
- Assess respiratory rate, rhythm, amplitude. Auscultate breath sounds.
- Monitor ABGs.
- Obtain sputum for culture and sensitivity *if infection is suspected.*
- Note chest pain, shortness of breath, or hemoptysis.

THERAPEUTIC INTERVENTIONS
- Log roll every 2 hours.
- Demonstrate breathing exercises and encourage use of spirometer (blow bottles, glove) *to prevent hypostatic pneumonia.*
- Administer antibiotics, if ordered.
- Perform chest percussion and postural drainage as necessary.
- Administer humidified air or oxygen as ordered.
- Encourage fluids *to decrease viscosity of secretions.*

Optimal gas exchange will be maintained.

Continued.

Integumentary/Musculoskeletal Care Plans (Pediatric)

NURSING DIAGNOSES/ DEFINING CHARACTERISTICS	NURSING INTERVENTIONS / *RATIONALES*	EXPECTED OUTCOMES
DEFINING CHARACTERISTICS cont'd Sharp chest pain, increased on inspiration Headache Rales/rhonchi Tachypnea Decreased breath sounds over affected lung area Hypoxemia		
High Risk for Fluid Volume Deficit/ Excess **RELATED TO** Rapid blood loss or excess fluid loss (through fever, diarrhea, nasogastric drainage, diaphoresis, and inadequate fluid intake) Aggressive fluid therapy in operating room **DEFINING CHARACTERISTICS** *Deficit:* Specific gravity >1.025 Decreased urine output Sudden weight loss Hypotension Thirst Tachycardia Decreased skin turgor Dry mucous membranes Weakness *Excess:* Specific gravity <1.010 Facial/peripheral edema Increased urine output	**ONGOING ASSESSMENT** • Monitor hydration status: Skin turgor Mucous membranes I&O Urine specific gravity Serum electrolytes NOTE: Expect some facial edema related to positioning in OR. • Monitor vital signs (including central venous pressure during initial postoperative course). • Monitor drainage from Hemovac. **THERAPEUTIC INTERVENTIONS** • Administer IV fluids as prescribed. • Encourage oral liquid intake when able. • Notify physician of changes in hydration or excessive Hemovac/other drainage.	Fluid volume and electroltye balance will be maintained.
High Risk for Urinary Retention **RELATED TO** Obstructive uropathy Recent anesthesia	**ONGOING ASSESSMENT** • Assess for symptoms of urinary retention. • Evaluate medications, especially morphine or derivatives, for possible side effects.	Optimal urinary elimination will be maintained.

NURSING DIAGNOSES/ DEFINING CHARACTERISTICS	NURSING INTERVENTIONS / *RATIONALES*	EXPECTED OUTCOMES
High Risk for Urinary Retention cont'd Medications Obstructed catheter Spinal cord compression, neurogenic bladder **DEFINING CHARACTERISTICS** Complaints of lower abdominal pain or discomfort Desire but inability to urinate Paresthesia Decreased (<30 ml/ hr) or absent urinary output for 2 consecutive hours Frequency Hesitancy Urgency Lower abdomen distention Restlessness	**ONGOING ASSESSMENT cont'd** • Assess for decreased neurological function; paresthesia of lower extremities; decreased bowel sounds. **THERAPEUTIC INTERVENTIONS** • Maintain patency of urinary catheter. • Notify physician if patient does not void within 4 hours after removal of catheter. • If cord compression is suspected, prepare for surgical intervention.	

High Risk for Constipation/ Impaction
RELATED TO
 	
Anesthesia
Inadequate fluid or food intake
Decreased mobility
Emotional tension
Analgesics
Spinal cord or nerve root compression or damage
 	
DEFINING CHARACTERISTICS
 	
Feeling of fullness
Cramping pain
Tender abdomen
Headache
Nausea
Anorexia
Abdominal distention
Gurgling, decreased, or absent bowel sounds
Hard masses of stool on examination or expelled
Flatulence
Dehydration
Vomiting
	ONGOING ASSESSMENT
	• Monitor GI activity and fluid balance:
	  Auscultate bowel sounds in all four quadrants every 4 hours.
	  Monitor child's tolerance to fluids.
	  Check abdominal girth every day.
	  Ask child to inform nurse of nausea, flatulence, or need for bowel movement.
	• Monitor for signs of neurological impairment that may accompany bowel elimination problem:
	  Paresthesia (numbness, tingling of extremities)
	  Absent or decreased reflexes (nerve root) or increased reflexes (spinal cord)
	
	THERAPEUTIC INTERVENTIONS
	• Notify physician of abnormal signs.
	• Encourage fluid intake.
		Optimal bowel elimination will be maintained.

Continued.

Integumentary/Musculoskeletal Care Plans (Pediatric)

NURSING DIAGNOSES/ DEFINING CHARACTERISTICS	NURSING INTERVENTIONS / *RATIONALES*	EXPECTED OUTCOMES

High Risk for Infection
RELATED TO
Surgical incision
 	
DEFINING CHARACTERISTICS
Fever
Increased WBC
Surgical incision:
  Swelling
  Hematoma
  Redness
  Odor
  Burning/itching
  Pain
  Numbness
	ONGOING ASSESSMENT
	• Assess surgical site:
	  Note color, moisture, texture, and temperature.
	  Assess incision line and dressing for drainage.
	  Check incision for cleanliness, approximation, swelling, hematoma, redness, odor.
	  Ask about burning or itching.
	• Assess nutritional status.
	
	THERAPEUTIC INTERVENTIONS
	• Keep dressing dry and intact.
	• Maintain Steri-strips to incision until significant healing, then remove all that have not fallen off before cast is applied.
	• Clean and dry skin with each turning.
	• Report any changes (i.e., redness, swelling, drainage, or heat) at incisional area.
	• *Prevent pressure on incisional area by:*
	  Turning patient as scheduled
	  Using prophylactic antipressure devices
	  Maintaining proper body alignment
	• Encourage adequate nutrition and hydration.
		Risk of infection will be reduced.

High Risk for Injury
RELATED TO
Unstable condition of spine
Equipment failure
 	
DEFINING CHARACTERISTICS
Attempts to get up
Brakes not on bed
Improper lifting
Improper turning
Nausea and vomiting
Wretching actions
	ONGOING ASSESSMENT
	• Assess environment for safety hazards.
	• Assess all equipment for proper working conditions (e.g., safety straps, brakes, screws in place).
	• Assess type of spinal instrumentation for expected limitations.
	• Assess for nausea and vomiting.
	• Assess placement/drainage from nasogastric tube.
	
	THERAPEUTIC INTERVENTIONS
	• Provide safe environment.
	• Avoid sitting up for longer than 15 minutes at one time *to minimize stress on infusion site.*
	• Use proper turning/lifting techniques *to avoid displacement of spinal instrument.*
	  Turn in bed using log roll technique. Obtain assistance when necessary.
	  Ambulate with back brace or corset as ordered. Child may be in bed and have bathroom privileges without wearing brace/corset.
	  Maintain head of bed at or below 30 degrees. Flex knee gatch no greater than 30 degrees.
	• Administer antiemetics as ordered.
	• Reinsert nasogastric tube if necessary.
		Injury will be prevented.

High Risk for Disturbance in Body Image/Self-Concept **RELATED TO** Scoliosis Body brace Lack of privacy Separation from family/peers	**ONGOING ASSESSMENT** • Assess child's perception of self and expectations of surgery and bracing. *Female adolescents are the most frequently seen patients with scoliosis requiring surgical correction and bracing. The adolescent is particularly concerned with self-concept and body image and will require sensitive nursing care.*	Body image/self-concept disturbance will be limited.

Scoliosis repair: spinal instrumentation cont'd

NURSING DIAGNOSES/ DEFINING CHARACTERISTICS	NURSING INTERVENTIONS / *RATIONALES*	EXPECTED OUTCOMES

DEFINING CHARACTERISTICS
Dependence
Depression
Denial/grief
Withdrawal
Restlessness
Regression
Anger
Sadness
Frequent questions
Frequent complaints
Negative attitude
Crying/irritability
Distorted self-image
Expressed self-doubt
Verbalized discontent with body
	THERAPEUTIC INTERVENTIONS
	• Encourage verbalization of concerns.
	• Be sensitive to concerns about body image; intervene appropriately.
	  Provide mirrors so body can be visualized.
	  Assist with self-care activities, especially hair care, makeup.
	  Provide as much privacy as possible, especially during bathing and toileting.
	  Allow to continue as many normal activities as possible (e.g., ADL, schooling).
	  Provide diversional activities (e.g., telephone, television, friends), and establish schedules.	

Knowledge Deficit RELATED TO
New surgical procedure
Unfamiliarity with preoperative and postoperative care
Discharge/home care
Bracing and brace care
 	
DEFINING CHARACTERISTICS
Frequent questions
Frequent complaints
Vague physical complaints
Anxiousness
Restlessness
Withdrawal
Regression
	ONGOING ASSESSMENT
	• Assess current understanding of spinal instrumentation and postoperative care.
	• Assess knowledge of home care needs and ability to perform self-care.
	• Assess readiness for learning.
	
	THERAPEUTIC INTERVENTIONS
	• Provide information appropriate to type of surgery.
	• Provide information concerning:
	  Skin care
	  Cast care (if applicable)
	  Nutrition
	  Physical limitations
	  Medications
	  Back brace/corset
	• Provide discharge teaching:
	  Child may ride home in car with seat reclining *to reduce stress on back*.
	  Recommend a firm mattress; child should not sleep on abdomen; should try to maintain proper body alignment.
	  Activities should be limited to walking with corset/brace; no flexion or extension of back.
	  Child should exercise as directed by physician or physical therapist.
	  No sports, driving, or sexual activity until directed by physician.
	  Child may return to work/school when approved by physician.
	  Arrange follow-up appointments, provide emergency phone numbers. Instruct parent/child to notify physician of persistent lower back pain, leg pain, numbness, weakness, change in gait or bowel/bladder function, fever, or wound changes.
		Child will verbalize understanding of surgery and demonstrate home/self-care measures.

Michele Knoll Puzas, RNC, MHPE; Victoria Malone, RN, BSN, FNP

Systemic lupus erythematosus

LUPUS/SLE

A chronic, systemic inflammatory disease characterized by multi-system involvement. Mild disease can affect joints and skin. More severe disease can affect kidneys, heart, lung, and central nervous system as well as joints and skin. Females are affected six times more often than males.

NURSING DIAGNOSES/ DEFINING CHARACTERISTICS	NURSING INTERVENTIONS / *RATIONALES*	EXPECTED OUTCOMES
Impaired Skin Integrity **RELATED TO** Inflammation Vasoconstriction Overexposure to sun **DEFINING CHARACTERISTICS** Change in skin and/ or mucous membranes Redness Pain Tenderness Itching Skin breakdown/ ulcers Skin rash: Red Nonraised Tender Molar rash Oral/nasal ulcers	**ONGOING ASSESSMENT** ▪ Assess age and developmental level. ▪ Assess skin integrity: Note color, moisture, texture, temperature. Note any redness, swelling, or tenderness. Note size of lesions, including oral, nasal, fingertip, and leg ulcers. ▪ Solicit description of pain: Quality Severity Location Onset Duration Aggravating and alleviating factors ▪ Assess interference with life-style. ▪ Assess interference with ADL and achieving developmental milestones. **THERAPEUTIC INTERVENTIONS** ▪ Clean, dry, and moisturize intact skin with warm (not hot) water, especially over bony prominences, twice daily, using an unscented lotion (Eucerin or Lubriderm). *Scented lotions may contain alcohol, which dries skin.* ▪ Encourage adequate nutrition and hydration. ▪ Assist with ADL as needed while facilitating maximum independence. ▪ Instruct child to avoid ultraviolet light: Wear protective sunscreen (SPF 15) when in sun and reapply every 4 hours. Sunbathing: contraindicated. Wear wide-brim hat and long sleeves *to protect skin (sun can exacerbate disease process).* Wear protective eyewear. Plan outdoor activities that will avoid sun exposure from 10 AM to 2 PM *(sun is at maximum intensity).* Swimming: in early morning or late afternoon if waterproof sunscreen is used and reapplied every 4 hours. ▪ Introduce/reinforce information on use of hydroxychloroquine sulfate (Plaquenil): Purpose Use Potential side effects Other pertinent information (i.e., toxicity to infants and children) ▪ Inform adolescent of availability of special makeup (at large department stores) to cover rash, especially facial rash: Covermark (Lydia O'Leary) Dermablend Marilyn Miglin ▪ Instruct child to rinse mouth with half-strength hydrogen peroxide three times a day when oral ulcers are present. *Hydrogen peroxide helps keep oral ulcers clean.* ▪ Instruct child to avoid irritating foods (e.g., spicy or citric) when oral ulcers are present.	Optimal skin integrity will be maintained.

NURSING DIAGNOSES/ DEFINING CHARACTERISTICS	NURSING INTERVENTIONS / *RATIONALES*	EXPECTED OUTCOMES
Impaired Skin Integrity: Alopecia (Scalp Hair Loss) **RELATED TO** Inflammation Exacerbation of disease process High-dose corticosteroid use **DEFINING CHARACTERISTICS** Diffuse hair loss areas Loss of discrete scalp hair patches	**ONGOING ASSESSMENT** • Assess integrity of scalp hair: Note scalp hair loss amount and distribution. Note scarring in the areas of scalp hair loss. • Assess degree to which this symptom interferes with child's ability to attend school and participate in extracurricular activities. **THERAPEUTIC INTERVENTIONS** • Instruct child/parent to avoid scalp contact with harsh chemicals (e.g., hair dye, permanent, curl relaxers, etc.): Use a mild shampoo (e.g., P&S). Decrease frequency of shampooing. Avoid use of rubberbands or tight braids. • Instruct the child/parent that scalp hair loss occurs during an exacerbation of disease activity: Scalp hair loss may be the first sign of an impending disease exacerbation. Scalp hair loss may not be permanent. *As the disease activity subsides, scalp hair begins to regrow.* A short haircut is useful during times of scalp hair loss. Regrown hair may have different texture, often finer. Hair will not regrow in areas of scarring. • Encourage child/parent to investigate ways (scarves, hats) to conceal scalp hair loss, if interfering with life-style. • Discuss parent's feelings and concerns regarding child's hair loss. • Discuss methods to deal with teasing from other children.	Child/parent will be able to cope with hair loss.
Fever **RELATED TO** Inflammation **DEFINING CHARACTERISTICS** Temperature greater than 38.4° C (101° F) Chills Shaking chills (rigor) Diaphoresis Dehydration	**ONGOING ASSESSMENT** • Assess vital signs at least every 2 hours. • Assess for chills, shaking, and diaphoresis. • Assess for signs of dehydration: Decreased skin turgor Dry mucous membranes Decreased urine output • Monitor I&O. **THERAPEUTIC INTERVENTIONS** • Administer antipyretics as ordered. Avoid aspirin (*in general aspirin for antipyretic use is avoided in pediatrics*). • Administer steroids in divided dose as ordered. • Encourage hydration. • See Hyperthermia, p. 28.	Optimal body temperature will be maintained below 38.4° C (101° F).
Altered Peripheral Tissue Perfusion **RELATED TO** Vasospasm of digits **DEFINING CHARACTERISTICS** Pain, numbness, cold sensation Triphasic color (Raynaud's) changes— white, blue, red Digital ulcers	**ONGOING ASSESSMENT** • Assess hands and feet for color, temperature, and skin integrity. • Solicit description of pain, numbness, cold sensations, change in color, and factors that cause Raynaud episodes. • Assess interference with ADL, developmental milestones, and ability to attend school and participate in activities. **THERAPEUTIC INTERVENTIONS** • Keep extremities warm (socks, blankets, gloves, mittens). • Remove vasoconstricting factors when possible. • Administer vasodilating medications (e.g., nifedipine) as ordered.	Episodes of Raynaud's will be reduced.

Continued.

NURSING DIAGNOSES/ DEFINING CHARACTERISTICS	NURSING INTERVENTIONS / *RATIONALES*	EXPECTED OUTCOMES
	THERAPEUTIC INTERVENTIONS cont'd	

	▪ Instruct child/parent to avoid undue cold exposure:
	    Wear multiple layers of clothing (hat/cap, ear muffs, nose protector, mittens/gloves, socks) in cold environment.
	    Use gloves in school.
	    Avoid swimming in physical education class.
	    Avoid winter sports if Raynaud episodes cannot be prevented.
	    Suggest wearing items made of wool, cotton, down, or thinsulate *(provide the most protection from cold exposure).*
	 ▪ Instruct child/parent to avoid caffeine and nicotine *(cause vasoconstriction).*
	 ▪ Instruct child/parent in stress management; *stress can precipitate vasospasm:*
	    Identify stressful situations.
	    Identify past coping mechanisms.
	    Identify new coping mechanisms.
	    Instruct child in techniques of progressive muscle relaxation and imagery.
	 ▪ Refer for instruction in biofeedback techniques if child is old enough.	

Joint Pain **RELATED TO** Inflammation **DEFINING CHARACTERISTICS** Child's/parent's report of pain Refusal to perform activities with affected joint Guarding on motion of affected joints Crying or other sounds associated with pain	**ONGOING ASSESSMENT** ▪ Solicit child's/parent's description of pain (quality, severity, location, onset, duration). ▪ Assess for signs of joint inflammation (redness, warmth, swelling, decreased motion). ▪ Determinate past measures used to alleviate pain. ▪ Assess effect on developmental milestones (walking, balance, bathing, dressing, feeding, toileting). ▪ Assess child's ability to participate in school activities. **THERAPEUTIC INTERVENTIONS** ▪ Administer antiinflammatory medication as prescribed on a full stomach. *Antiinflammatory drugs can be very irritating to stomach lining and lead to ulcer disease.* ▪ Encourage use of warm bath for inflamed joints. ▪ Encourage child to wear splints/use ambulation devices as ordered. ▪ Encourage child to assume anatomically correct position. Do not use knee gatch or pillows to prop knees. Use small flat pillow under head. ▪ Encourage use of ambulation aid(s) when pain is related to weight bearing. ▪ Consult occupational therapist for proper splinting of affected joints. ▪ Use alternate methods of pain control (distraction, guided imagery, relaxation, play therapy), as age appropriate.	Pain will be at a tolerable level so that child can participate in self-care activities.

Joint Stiffness
 RELATED TO
 Inflammation
 Movement
 	
 DEFINING CHARACTERISTICS
 Verbalized complaint of joint stiffness
 Inability to move easily after extended periods of rest
	ONGOING ASSESSMENT
	 ▪ Solicit child's/parent's description of stiffness:
	    Joints affected
	    When stiffness occurs
	    Duration of stiffness
	 ▪ Monitor for changes in location/length of stiffness.
	 ▪ Determine past measures used to alleviate stiffness.
	 ▪ Assess interference with ability to participate in school activities.
	 ▪ Assess affect on developmental milestones.
		Stiffness will be reduced or eliminated.

NURSING DIAGNOSES/ DEFINING CHARACTERISTICS	NURSING INTERVENTIONS / *RATIONALES*	EXPECTED OUTCOMES
	THERAPEUTIC INTERVENTIONS • Assist child to take a 15-minute warm shower or bath on rising for multiple joint stiffness. • Use localized heat for stiffness in only a few joints (paraffin bath, heating pad, hot packs). • Assist child to perform ROM exercises after heat therapy. • Allow sufficient time for self-care activities and assist as necessary. • Avoid scheduling tests or treatment during early morning hours or immediately after napping. • Administer antiinflammatory medication as prescribed on full stomach. • Attempt to maintain child's home medication schedule while hospitalized. • Encourage child to participate in activities that require joint motion. • Remind child to avoid prolonged periods of inactivity.	

High Risk for Injury
 RELATED TO
 Altered renal function
 Inflammation and sclerosis of glomeruli
 Side effects of connective tissue disease
 	
 DEFINING CHARACTERISTICS
 Increased BUN and creatinine
 Hematuria
 Proteinuria
 Peripheral edema
 Altered levels of consciousness
 Hypertension
 Decreased cardiac output
 Nausea
 Vomiting
	ONGOING ASSESSMENT
	 • Assess urinary output at least every 2 hours (weigh diapers if applicable).
	 • Monitor intake of fluids.
	 • Obtain nutritional history from child/parent.
	 • Monitor electrolyte levels as drawn.
	 • Assess for edema, especially of lower extremities.
	 • Assess vital signs at least every 2 hours.
	 • Assess for level of consciousness changes.
	 • Weigh child daily.
	
	 THERAPEUTIC INTERVENTIONS
	 • Obtain dietary consultation as needed.
	 • Administer immunosuppressant medications as ordered:
	     Methylprednisolone
	     Cyclophosphamide
	 • Instruct child/parent of potential side effects of immunosuppressant medications in this care plan.
	 • See Renal failure, acute, p. 358, and Cardiac output, decreased, p. 10.
		Optimal renal function will be maintained.

Altered Central Nervous System: Severe Headaches, Seizures, Organic Psychosis, Organic Brain Syndrome
 RELATED TO
 Inflammation
 Severe, active SLE (usually occurs early in disease course, often combined with increased disease activity in other organ systems)
	ONGOING ASSESSMENT
	 • Assess for the presence or history of headaches:
	     Location
	     Onset
	     Duration
	     Severity
	     Quality
	     Aggravating and alleviating factors
	 • Assess for presence or history of seizure activity:
	     Aura
	     Type
	     Onset
	     Duration
		Optimal central nervous system function will be maintained.

Continued.

Systemic lupus erythematosus cont'd

NURSING DIAGNOSES/ DEFINING CHARACTERISTICS	NURSING INTERVENTIONS / *RATIONALES*	EXPECTED OUTCOMES

Altered Central Nervous System: Severe Headaches, Seizures, Organic Psychosis, Organic Brain Syndrome cont'd
 	
Organic psychosis (may be caused by high-dose cortico-steroids)
 	
DEFINING CHARACTERISTICS
 	
Headaches, often severe and throbbing
Seizures, most often grand mal
Organic psychosis (see ongoing assessment)
Difficulty concentrating
	ONGOING ASSESSMENT cont'd
	▪ Assess for presence of organic psychosis:
	    Impaired judgment
	    Inappropriate speech
	    Disorganized behavior
	    Disorientation
	    Impaired reality testing
	    Impaired comprehension
	    Decreased attention
	    Hallucinations
	▪ Assess effect on cognitive developmental milestones.
	▪ Assess ability to maintain age-appropriate scholastic achievement.
	
	THERAPEUTIC INTERVENTIONS
	▪ Provide quiet, restful environment when headaches are present.
	▪ Administer nonnarcotic analgesics and corticosteroids as ordered for headaches.
	▪ Instruct child/parent of potential immunosuppressant side effects.
	▪ Provide a quiet, safe environment during seizures (including padded side rails).
	▪ Inform other members of health care team of potential for seizures (occupational and physical therapists, child life specialist).
	▪ Administer neuroleptics, corticosteroids, and immunosuppressants as ordered.
	▪ Instruct child/parent in use and potential side effects of neuroleptic(s), prednisone, and/or immunosuppressants.
	▪ Provide safe, structured, predictable environment when symptoms of organic psychosis are present:
	    Provide continuity of caregivers; one-to-one care may be necessary. Encourage parents to stay with child.
	    Decrease environmental stimuli; keep child in private room if necessary.
	    Remove potentially dangerous objects from room, but allow child to keep at least one safe toy at bedside.
	    Orient to person, place, and time as necessary. Keep clock and calendar in room if child is age appropriate.
	    Provide clear, concise instructions at level child can comprehend.
	    Administer antipsychotic, corticosteroid, and/or immunosuppressant drugs as ordered.
	    Offer parental support and allow time to vent feelings.
	    Decrease ambiguity and confusion by offering limited choices.	

High Risk for Impaired Gas Exchange
RELATED TO
Inflammation
Pleuritis
Pleural effusion
Pulmonary infection
Pleuritic chest pain
	ONGOING ASSESSMENT
	▪ Assess respiratory rate and depth by listening to breath sounds a minimum of once every shift.
	▪ Assess for:
	    Dyspnea (quantify and relate to exacerbating events)
	    Use of accessory muscles (sternocleidomastoid, abdominal, diaphragmatic)
	    Changes in orientation, restlessness
	    Changes in activity tolerance
	    Position needed for normal/easy breathing
	▪ Monitor changes in vital signs, especially breathing pattern/respiratory rate.
	▪ Assess ability to participate in school and extracurricular activities.
		Optimal respiratory status within limits of disease will be achieved.

NURSING DIAGNOSES/ DEFINING CHARACTERISTICS	NURSING INTERVENTIONS / *RATIONALES*	EXPECTED OUTCOMES
DEFINING CHARACTERISTICS Shortness of breath Tachypnea Nasal flaring Respiratory depth changes Altered chest excursion Dyspnea on exertion Chest pain	**THERAPEUTIC INTERVENTIONS** • Pace and schedule activities and tests/procedures *to prevent dyspnea caused by fatigue.* • Provide reassurance, allay anxiety by staying with child during acute respiratory distress episodes; encourage parent to stay with child during hospitalization. • Provide oxygen as ordered and as needed. • Instruct child/parent in environmental factors that may worsen pulmonary conditions (e.g., pollen, smoking). • Instruct child/parent of "cold" symptoms and associated problems. • Encourage child/parent to receive influenza vaccine every year and pneumococcal vaccine at some point. *CDC encourages all individuals with chronic illness or lung disease to be immunized against flu.* • Provide quiet play activities that can be done in bed.	
High Risk for Decreased Cardiac Output **RELATED TO** Effusions Cardiac dysrhythmias (atrial and ventricular) **DEFINING CHARACTERISTICS** Child's report of palpitations or "funny feeling" in chest area Child's/parent's report of fatigue or shortness of breath Irregular heart rate Tachycardia/bradycardia Hypoxia	**ONGOING ASSESSMENT** • Monitor heart for rate, rhythm, and ectopy every shift. • Assess fluid status. • Assess mentation. • Assess energy level and ability to participate in daily care activities. **THERAPEUTIC INTERVENTIONS** • Administer antiarrhythmic medications as ordered. • If dysrhythmia occurs, determine child's response. Document and report if significant or symptomatic. • Instruct child/parent in principles of energy conservation. See Fatigue, p. 314.	Optimal cardiac rhythm and output will be maintained.

Self-Care Deficit
RELATED TO
Pain
Stiffness
Fatigue
Muscle weakness
Age (chronological/ developmental)
Organic psychosis
 	
DEFINING CHARACTERISTICS
Child's/parent's report of difficulty with self-care activities
Decreased functional ability of upper/ lower extremities
	ONGOING ASSESSMENT
	• Observe child's level of functioning with:
	    Bathing
	    Personal hygiene
	    Dressing
	    Toileting
	    Feeding
	• Assess impact of self-care deficit on life-style and ability to function at school.
	• Determine if parents can provide appropriate care after discharge; consider need for home health care.
	• Assess need for assistive devices to perform self-care activities.
	
	THERAPEUTIC INTERVENTIONS
	• Encourage independence; assist child only as necessary. *Child's self-image improves when he/she can perform personal care independently.*
	• Consult occupational therapist for adaptive equipment (dressing aids, eating aids) or ask parent to bring from home as appropriate.
		Self-care activities will be performed independently or with assistance as needed by child, and as age-appropriate.

Continued.

Systemic lupus erythematosus cont'd

NURSING DIAGNOSES/ DEFINING CHARACTERISTICS	NURSING INTERVENTIONS / *RATIONALES*	EXPECTED OUTCOMES
	THERAPEUTIC INTERVENTIONS cont'd • Allow child adequate time for self-care activities, considering not only ability, but also age. • Allow child to choose shower or bath for daily care; discourage bed bath. *Allowing input in decision making fosters sense of independence.* • Do not schedule tests/activities during self-care time. • Provide child with guidance in choosing and pacing activities. • Reinforce self-care techniques taught by occupational therapist.	

Fatigue
RELATED TO
Increased disease activity
Anemia of chronic disease
 	
DEFINING CHARACTERISTICS
Lack of energy, exhaustion, listlessness
Decreased attention span
Sleeping longer than developmentally appropriate
Inability to keep up with regular activities
	ONGOING ASSESSMENT
	• Solicit child's/parent's description of fatigue:
	    Time of occurrence
	    Relationship to activities
	    Aggravating and alleviating factors
	• Determine sleep pattern (nighttime/day naps) and if amount is appropriate for age.
	• Assess interference with life-style and child's ability to attend school and extracurricular activities.
	• Determine past measures used to alleviate fatigue.
	
	THERAPEUTIC INTERVENTIONS
	• Provide two or three periods of 60 minutes of uninterrupted rest daily. *Patients often have limited energy supply.*
	• Encourage afternoon naptime.
	• Provide familiar toys from home during rest periods.
	• Encourage child to pace activities *to conserve energy.*
	• If fatigue is related to interrupted sleep, see Sleep pattern, disturbance, p. 318.
		Fatigue will be reduced to a level that child can participate in self-care activities as age-appropriate.

Knowledge Deficit
RELATED TO
New disease/symptoms/procedures
Unfamiliarity with treatment regimen
Lack of interest to learn (denial)
Cognitive limitations
 	
DEFINING CHARACTERISTICS
Many similar questions
Lack of questions
Verbalized misconceptions
Verbalized lack of knowledge
Inaccurate follow-through of previous instructions
	ONGOING ASSESSMENT
	• Assess child's/parent's:
	    Level of knowledge of lupus
	    Treatment
	    Prognosis
	• Identify priorities for child's education. *Child's/parent's priorities may differ.*
	• Assess child's:
	    Ability to focus on task at hand
	    Attention span
	    Readiness to learn
	• Determine extent discomfort will interfere with learning.
	• Assess the cognitive learning style of both parent and child (visual/verbal).
	
	THERAPEUTIC INTERVENTIONS
	• Provide a private, quiet environment for education.
	• Schedule educational sessions with parent, allowing some time to be separated from child. *Allows parent to address issues he/she does not wish to discuss in front of child.*
	• Schedule educational sessions with child during time of maximal comfort. *Pain will distract child and may lead to inability to concentrate.*
	• Keep duration of sessions appropriate to the attention span of audience-child versus parent (accommodate the shortest attention span).
	• Use educational techniques in accordance with child's/parent's cognitive level.
	• Refrain from using the word "drug"; instead use "medication." *The word drug is used negatively at schools for drug prevention programs—"Say No to Drugs!" Children receive a mixed message about their lupus medications.*
		Child/parent will verbalize increased awareness of lupus, its treatment, and prognosis as it relates to child's current disease activity.

NURSING DIAGNOSES/ DEFINING CHARACTERISTICS	NURSING INTERVENTIONS / *RATIONALES*	EXPECTED OUTCOMES

THERAPEUTIC INTERVENTIONS cont'd

- Introduce/reinforce disease process information:
    Unknown cause
    Chronicity of lupus throughout childhood/adolescence
    Inflammatory process
    Joint involvement
    Organ involvement
    Uveitis/iridocyclitis (pauciarticular)
    Remissions/exacerbations
    Control versus cure issues
- Introduce/reinforce medication therapy information:
    Name of drug
    Purpose/use of drug
    Dose and route
    Time of administration (home/school)
    Potential side effects
- Introduce/reinforce self-care strategies:
    Home exercise program (ROM and muscle strengthening)
    Pain management
    Joint protection
    Appropriate play activities
    Adequate rest
    Nutritionally sound diet
    Splinting/assistive devices, when appropriate
- Acknowledge that there are current nontraditional treatments and encourage child/parent to discuss these with a member of health care team *before* trying them.
- Instruct child/parent to discuss use of over-the-counter medications with a health care team member before using.
- Provide written information of above items to child and parent.

High Risk for Injury: Side Effects Related to Prednisone and Immunosuppressant Medications

RELATED TO

Long-term use
High dosage

DEFINING CHARACTERISTICS

Prednisone:
Facial puffiness
"Buffalo" hump
Hypertension
Diabetes mellitus
Osteoporosis
Avascular necrosis
Addisonian crisis
Acne
Impaired growth
Glaucoma
Immunosuppressants:
Bone marrow
  suppression
Sterility
Cancer

ONGOING ASSESSMENT

- Assess for cushingoid facial appearance/acne.
- Assess for fat pads on back (buffalo hump).
- Assess blood pressure at least every shift.
- Assess for lower extremity edema.
- Monitor urine for sugar and acetone or monitor blood glucose at least once a day.
- Monitor for spontaneous bone fractures.
- Monitor for bone and joint pain, especially of hips and shoulders. *Avascular necrosis most prominent in femoral and humeral heads.*
- Assess child's past and present growth pattern(s) using a standard growth chart.
- Assess child's/parent's perception of current side effects.
- Monitor CBC.
- Monitor for blood in urine or pain, burning with urination (*signs of hemorrhagic cystitis*).

THERAPEUTIC INTERVENTIONS

- Instruct child/parent in potential side effects of long-term use of prednisone:
    Facial puffiness
    Buffalo hump
    Diabetes mellitus
    Osteoporosis
    Avascular necrosis
    Increased appetite
    Increased infection risk
    Stunted growth
    Acne
    Glaucoma

Child/parent will understand the risk of injury related to medications.

Continued.

Systemic lupus erythematosus cont'd

NURSING DIAGNOSES/ DEFINING CHARACTERISTICS	NURSING INTERVENTIONS / *RATIONALES*	EXPECTED OUTCOMES
	THERAPEUTIC INTERVENTIONS cont'd	

- Instruct in potential side effects of immunosuppressant medications:
  Increase infection risk *caused by bone marrow suppression*
  Nausea/vomiting
  Sterility
  Hemorrhagic cystitis
  Cancer
- Reinforce that side effects are potential and each child does not suffer every side effect.
- Instruct child to wear Medic Alert tag stating use of prednisone and/or immunosuppressant.
- Instruct parent/child to never alter prednisone dose. Steroids must be tapered slowly after high-dose or long-term use. *Body produces the hormone cortisol in adrenal glands. After high-dose/long-term use of extraneous forms of steroids, body no longer produces cortisol. Increased cortisol levels needed in times of stress. Without supplementation, steroid-dependent person will enter Addisonian crisis.*
- Discuss child's coping mechanisms regarding unwanted side effects of medication (especially facial puffiness, acne, increased weight, stunted growth).
- Instruct child/parent that a single early morning dose of prednisone will help reduce potential side effects, *but* physician must determine when dose may be consolidated to a single dose. As disease activity increases, prednisone may need to be given more frequently throughout the day—three or four times daily.

Altered Nutrition: Less Than Body Requirements **RELATED TO** Loss of appetite related to chronic illness and medication side effects Psychosocial factors **DEFINING CHARACTERISTICS** Loss of weight with/ without adequate caloric intake Below 15th percentile of weight for height on growth curve, or a decline in 2 percentile lines Inadequate caloric intake Caloric intake inadequate to maintain metabolic state during times of increased disease activity	**ONGOING ASSESSMENT** • Document child's actual weight on admission and reassess every week. • Obtain nutritional history from both parent and child, when possible. • Obtain medication history. • Assess child's feeding skills, including setup needs. **THERAPEUTIC INTERVENTIONS** • Assist child with meal setup and feeding, as needed. • Provide finger foods for children with poor dexterity/joint pain in fingers. • Encourage family to visit at mealtimes. • Encourage frequent small meals/snacks of high-calorie/high-protein foods. • Consult dietitian as needed. • Reinforce dietary teaching to child and parents.	Optimal caloric intake will be maintained.

NURSING DIAGNOSES/ DEFINING CHARACTERISTICS	NURSING INTERVENTIONS / *RATIONALES*	EXPECTED OUTCOMES
Altered Nutrition: More Than Body Requirements **RELATED TO** Inactivity Psychosocial factors Increased appetite from steroid therapy **DEFINING CHARACTERISTICS** Above the 85th percentile of weight for height on growth curve Reported or observed dysfunctional eating behavior	**ONGOING ASSESSMENT** ▪ Document child's actual weight on admission and reassess every week. ▪ Obtain a nutritional history from both child and parent. ▪ Obtain medication history. ▪ Assess level of activity and estimated energy expenditure per day. **THERAPEUTIC INTERVENTIONS** ▪ Instruct child/parent in a nutritionally sound diet. ▪ Assist child to choose menu items from each food group. ▪ Consult dietitian as needed. ▪ Discuss eating behaviors: actual physical need for food versus habitual eating. ▪ Discuss situations that lead to overeating. ▪ Encourage daily exercise program that will not cause undue stress to joints or cause excessive fatigue (consult with physician and physical therapist to set up a program). ▪ Reinforce formal dietary teaching to child and parent. ▪ Assure child/parent that appetite will decrease as steroid dose is decreased.	Optimal nutrition will be maintained without an increase in weight during hospitalization.
High Risk for Ineffective Family Coping **RELATED TO** Inadequate support system Developmental age of child Knowledge deficit Grieving loss of perfect child Grieving loss of body image **DEFINING CHARACTERISTICS** Child/parent/sibling expresses concern about family's response to the illness Parent displays protective behavior disproportionate to child's ability to be independent Child/parent/sibling refusing to discuss changes imposed by lupus (limitations, altered body function, etc.) Child/family expresses feelings of hopelessness/helplessness Routine family life is disrupted	**ONGOING ASSESSMENT** ▪ Identify behaviors that suggest grieving. ▪ Assess behavioral patterns that suggest altered self-concept or ineffective individual/family coping. ▪ Identify defense mechanisms and determine appropriateness. **THERAPEUTIC INTERVENTIONS** ▪ Recognize family's need to use appropriate defense mechanisms. ▪ Allow child time to make personal adjustments to changes in body image. ▪ Preschedule time each day for child/family to discuss current concerns. ▪ Encourage expression of feelings. ▪ Involve family in setting realistic long- and short-term goals. ▪ Avoid unpleasant surprise situations. ▪ Encourage shared responsibilities within family. ▪ Assist family to develop problem-solving techniques. ▪ Introduce child/parent to other children with lupus (similar age, sex, and symptoms). ▪ Refer child/family to social service department if needed.	The family will express positve feelings and actions.

Continued.

Systemic lupus erythematosus cont'd

NURSING DIAGNOSES/ DEFINING CHARACTERISTICS	NURSING INTERVENTIONS / *RATIONALES*	EXPECTED OUTCOMES
High Risk for Sleep Pattern Disturbance **RELATED TO** Pain Stiffness Inactivity Family stress **DEFINING CHARACTERISTICS** Child's/parent's report of inability to fall asleep or frequent nighttime awakening Increasing irritability/ restlessness Reduction in performance in school and play activities	**ONGOING ASSESSMENT** ▪ Solicit child's/parent's description of sleep pattern: Number of hours asleep per 24 hours Ability to fall asleep Nighttime awakening/inability to remain in bed Aggravating/alleviating factors ▪ Determine child's usual bedtime ritual. ▪ Assess need for familiar objects/toys to accompany child to bed. **THERAPEUTIC INTERVENTIONS** ▪ Encourage same ritual of preparing for bed when possible. ▪ Provide special object/toy or ask parent to bring them from home. *Familiar surroundings relax and give a sense of security.* ▪ Encourage parent to "room in" with child during hospitalization, when possible. ▪ Suggest use of warm bath/shower before bed. *Warm water relaxes muscles, facilitates relaxation.* ▪ Assist child to change positions frequently during night when needed. ▪ Provide quiet environment; discuss mutually acceptable awakening pattern for routine care (vital signs). ▪ Avoid stimulating foods (caffeine) and activities before bedtime. ▪ Consult clinical specialist if sleep pattern disturbance may be related to psychological factors.	Number of hours asleep (per 24 hour period) will be at least two thirds the appropriate amount for child's age.

Reneé Zubay Fife, RN, MSN; Linda Ehrlich Muzio, RN, MSN, CS

Traction

Traction is the application of a pulling force to an area of the body or to an extremity. Skeletal traction is applied directly through the bone via Steinmann pins or Kirschner wires. Traction can also be applied through the use of balanced suspension or skin traction.

NURSING DIAGNOSES/ DEFINING CHARACTERISTICS	NURSING INTERVENTIONS / *RATIONALES*	EXPECTED OUTCOMES
Knowledge Deficit **RELATED TO** Lack of experience with traction New diagnosis **DEFINING CHARACTERISTICS** High anxiety level Multitude of questions Lack of questions Verbalized lack of knowledge of traction	**ONGOING ASSESSMENT** ▪ Assess age and developmental level. ▪ Assess previous hospital experiences. ▪ Assess knowledge regarding traction. ▪ Assess child's/parent's readiness for learning. **THERAPEUTIC INTERVENTIONS** ▪ Encourage parent/child to verbalize questions and concerns. ▪ Explain purpose of traction as related to injury and healing process. *Providing information helps alleviate anxiety and enables child to absorb and retain further information and instructions.* ▪ Explain traction apparatus. ▪ Teach preventative measures related to possible complications of injury of traction (e.g., pain, malalignment). ▪ Explain procedure of pin insertion/boot/elastic application. ▪ Explain traction removal and application of cast brace as appropriate.	Child will verbalize understanding of purpose and application of traction.

NURSING DIAGNOSES/ DEFINING CHARACTERISTICS	NURSING INTERVENTIONS / *RATIONALES*	EXPECTED OUTCOMES

Pain
RELATED TO
Fractured limb
Skeletal pins (pain at insertion site)
Muscle spasms
 	
DEFINING CHARACTERISTICS
Verbalized pain
Irritability
Restlessness
Crying/moaning
Facial grimaces
Altered vital signs: increased pulse, increased blood pressure, increased respirations
Withdrawal
Unwilling to change position
Inability to sleep
	ONGOING ASSESSMENT
	■ Solicit subjective information regarding pain.
	■ Assess for signs and symptoms of pain. Use a pain scale adjusted for age.
	■ Assess pain characteristics:
	  Location
	  Quality
	  Severity
	  Onset
	  Duration
	  Precipitating factors
	■ Assess past experience with pain and pain relief measures.
	■ Assess effectiveness of present pain relief measures.
	■ Assess for correct positioning of traction and alignment of affected extremity. *Incorrect positioning and malalignment can be a source of pain.*
	■ Assess types of activity that increase pain.
	
	THERAPEUTIC INTERVENTIONS
	■ Instruct child/parent to request analgesics at early sign of pain.
	■ Respond immediately to child's complaint of pain.
	■ Anticipate need for analgesics.
	■ Give analgesics as ordered and evaluate effectiveness *to determine if comfort has been provided or if another relief approach is needed. Dosage, drug, or route may also need to be revised.*
	■ Eliminate additional stressors or sources of pain/discomfort by providing these comfort measures:
	  Relaxation techniques
	  Diversionary activity: provide age-appropriate activities—toys, books, games, television, sewing, radio
	  Heat or cold application
	  Position changes
	  Verbal and physical reassurance
	  Touch (backrubs, holding). *Directing attention away from pain or to other body areas decreases perception of pain.*
	■ Explain pain management regimen to child/family.
	■ Explore other possible causes of pain.
	■ Explain that traction decreases muscle spasms and will help lessen pain.
	■ See Pain, p. 35.
		Pain will be reduced or relieved.

High Risk for Altered Tissue Perfusion
RELATED TO
Fractured limb
Immobility imposed by traction
Insertion of skeletal pin
Edema with neurovascular compromise
Compartment syndrome
	ONGOING ASSESSMENT
	■ Assess neurovascular status immediately after injury, following traction application, and then every 2-4 hours for 48 hours; every shift when stable:
	  Color
	  Capillary refill
	  Pulses above and below injury
	  Temperature
	  Sensation
	  Motion
	  Edema
	Baseline data is useful in determining absence, presence, or extent of neurovascular compromise.
	■ Assess amount of pain and pain with passive motion.
	■ Assess for positive Homans' sign.
	■ Compare affected extremity to unaffected and to previous assessments.
	■ Perform assessments of muscular strength with neurovascular checks.
		Risk for altered tissue perfusion and resultant complications will be reduced.

Continued.

Traction cont'd

NURSING DIAGNOSES/ DEFINING CHARACTERISTICS	NURSING INTERVENTIONS / *RATIONALES*	EXPECTED OUTCOMES
DEFINING CHARACTERISTICS Edema Pale and cool extremity Sluggish or absent capillary refill Numbness and tingling Diminished or absent pulses distal to injury Cyanosis Pain Altered sensation *Compartment syndrome:* Pain on passive stretch of muscles involved Progressive pain disproportionate to expectations Pallor or cyanosis distal to injury site Edema of limb distal to injury Decreased active and passive muscle movement to injury site Numbness/tingling Tightness of compartment	**THERAPEUTIC INTERVENTIONS** • Elevate extremity by suspension traction. *Elevation enhances venous blood return, which in turn enhances circulation to area.* • Provide footboard or wrist splints as needed. • Instruct and encourage exercises for affected and unaffected extremity as allowed. • Apply antiembolic stockings or sequential compression devices as ordered and remove on a regular basis for skin inspection. • Report increasing pain or neurovascular compromise to physician. • Instruct child/family on complications/warning signs of impaired circulation and methods to prevent complications. • Remove constrictive dressings, straps, or equipment as indicated. *Constrictive forces may be source of or worsen existing compartment syndrome.*	
High Risk for Fluid Volume Deficit **RELATED TO** Multiple fractures Blood vessel damage **DEFINING CHARACTERISTICS** Weak, rapid pulse Cool, moist skin Decreased blood pressure Anxiety Slow capillary refill Decreased urinary output	**ONGOING ASSESSMENT** • Assess amount of bleeding. • Assess for symptoms of hypovolemia. *Amount of bleeding should be evaluated in relation to child's blood pressure, pulse rate, and other signs of hemorrhage.* • Monitor vital signs. • Monitor lab values: Hgb/Hct. • Record I&O. *Urinary output is sensitive indicator of fluid volume status.* **THERAPEUTIC INTERVENTIONS** • Apply pressure to area bleeding. • Administer IV fluids and blood as ordered. • See Fluid volume deficit, p. 19.	Risk of fluid volume deficit will be reduced.

High Risk for Infection
RELATED TO
Interrupted first line of defense
Interruption of bone structure
	ONGOING ASSESSMENT
	• Assess pin sites and/or open wounds for signs of infection every shift:
	  Drainage
	  Odor
	  Warmth
	  Excessive pain/tenderness
	• Assess for skin tension at pin sites.
	• Assess vital signs (especially temperature) every 4 hours.
	• Monitor lab values (WBC).
		Risk of infection will be reduced.

NURSING DIAGNOSES/ DEFINING CHARACTERISTICS	NURSING INTERVENTIONS / *RATIONALES*	EXPECTED OUTCOMES
DEFINING CHARACTERISTICS Redness Swelling Purulent drainage Odor Tenderness/pain Warmth at affected site Elevated temperature Increased WBCs	**THERAPEUTIC INTERVENTIONS** • Perform pin care every 8 hours as ordered. • Use aseptic technique in performing pin care and changing dressings. • Document appearance of pin sites and any wounds. • Administer antibiotics as ordered. • Instruct child/family on purpose of pin care and signs and symptoms of infection. • Encourage foods high in protein and vitamin C. *Vitamin C facilitates wound healing.* • Notify physician of infection or skin tension at pin sites.	
Impaired Physical Mobility **RELATED TO** Fractured limb Imposed restrictions related to traction and injury **DEFINING CHARACTERISTICS** Reluctance to move Inability to move Limited ROM and muscle strength	**ONGOING ASSESSMENT** • Assess ability to perform ADL. • Assess present and preinjury level of mobility. • Assess ROM of unaffected extremity. • Assess muscle strength. **THERAPEUTIC INTERVENTIONS** • Encourage independence within limitation. • Instruct in use of assistive devices (overhead trapeze and side rails). • Teach isometric and other exercises to affected extremity as appropriate. • Teach strengthening exercises to affected extremities as appropriate. *Quad sets, ankle pumps, straight leg raises, gluteal sets, push ups, heel slides, and abductor sets help prevent development of stiff joints and muscle atrophy.* • Assist with repositioning. Maintain body in functional alignment. • Initiate consultation for exercise program. • Instruct child/family on complications of immobility and measures to decrease occurrence. • Obtain occupational therapy and child life specialist consultations.	Optimal mobility will be maintained.

High Risk for Injury
RELATED TO
Improper positioning of traction
Malalignment of bone ends
 	
DEFINING CHARACTERISTICS
Verbalized pain or discomfort at traction site
	ONGOING ASSESSMENT
	• Assess traction apparatus every shift:
	   Weight
	   Knots
	   Ropes
	• Assess child's position in traction.
	• Assess that ropes are not frayed or stretched.
	• Assess that spreader bars, foot plate, or splints do not touch foot of bed.
	• Assess that bed linens do not interfere with traction.
	• Assess child's whole body alignment. *Weight of traction is often enough to pull child's body out of alignment.*
	
	THERAPEUTIC INTERVENTIONS
	• Maintain affected extremity in functional traction.
	• Tighten all traction equipment.
	• Secure all knots with tape.
	• Keep weights hanging freely. *Deviations alter amount of traction applied, as well as therapeutic effect.*
	• Maintain continuous traction if ordered.
	• Maintain rope in center of pulley.
	• Maintain adequate countertraction. (Avoid elevating head of bed >30 degrees except during meals, for children in lower extremity skeletal traction.) *Countertraction is necessary for effective traction.*
	• Anchor child's upper body to the bed as needed *to prevent sliding toward traction.*
	• Provide foot plate or wrist splint *to maintain proper position of affected extremity.*
		Risk for injury to alignment will be reduced.

Continued.

Integumentary/Musculoskeletal Care Plans (Pediatric)

NURSING DIAGNOSES/ DEFINING CHARACTERISTICS	NURSING INTERVENTIONS / *RATIONALES*	EXPECTED OUTCOMES

High Risk for Impaired Skin Integrity
RELATED TO
Immobility
Prolonged bed rest
Contact with traction apparatus
Countertraction (child's body weight)
 	
DEFINING CHARACTERISTICS
Redness
Blanching
Irritation
Excoriation
	ONGOING ASSESSMENT
	• Examine skin for preexisting breakdown or potential problem areas.
	• Assess for preexisting risk factors for skin breakdown:
	    Physical conditions
	    Age
	    Mental state
	    Mobility
	• Inspect skin at least every 8 hours (especially affected extremity maintained in traction).
	
	THERAPEUTIC INTERVENTIONS
	• Clean, dry, and moisturize skin daily. Remove traction boot if possible.
	• Massage bony prominences. (Never massage reddened areas.)
	• Maintain correct padding for affected extremity in traction. *Pressure areas and skin irritation can develop under or at edge of traction device and/or other equipment.*
	• Keep bed linen wrinkle free and dry.
	• Apply prophylactic pressure-relieving mattress to bed if needed.
	• Encourage adequate hydration and teach importance of balanced diet.
	• For actual skin breakdown see Impaired skin integrity, p. 39.
		Skin integrity will be maintained with no evidence of breakdown.

High Risk for Ineffective Breathing Pattern **RELATED TO** Immobility Pulmonary embolus Fat embolism Pneumonia **DEFINING CHARACTERISTICS** Tachypnea Tachycardia Wheezing, rales Cough Dyspnea Shortness of breath Pleuritic chest pain Anxiety Restlessness and irritability Petechiae Altered level of consciousness Hemoptysis Productive cough	**ONGOING ASSESSMENT** • Assess respiratory rate and depth at least once/shift. • Assess breathing pattern. • Assess past history of breathing problems. • Assess present history for preexisting problems that may lead to breathing difficulties. • Assess mental status. • Monitor ABG results. **THERAPEUTIC INTERVENTIONS** • Encourage child to perform cough and deep breathing exercises. *Coughing and deep breathing are effective means of bronchial hygiene.* • Encourage frequent use of incentive spirometer. • Use antiembolic devices as ordered. • Administer humidified oxygen as ordered. • Report any signs or symptoms of ineffective breathing pattern immediately. • See Ineffective breathing pattern, p. 8.	Risk of ineffective breathing pattern will be reduced.
High Risk for Constipation **RELATED TO** Immobility Medications Unusual position	**ONGOING ASSESSMENT** • Assess bowel patterns before hospitalization. • Assess dietary habits. • Assess passage of flatus/stool. • Record bowel movements. • Assess medications and their contribution to constipation.	Risk for constipation will be reduced.

NURSING DIAGNOSES/ DEFINING CHARACTERISTICS	NURSING INTERVENTIONS / *RATIONALES*	EXPECTED OUTCOMES
DEFINING CHARACTERISTICS Straining at stool Passage of hard stool Distended abdomen Nausea/vomiting Complaint of no stool in several days Decreased appetite Complaint of abdominal pain or fullness	**THERAPEUTIC INTERVENTIONS** • Encourage diet high in roughage and bulk. *Bulk encourages regularity and facilitates easy evacuation.* • Encourage fluids. • Give stool softeners and laxatives as ordered. • Provide privacy during elimination. *Voluntary overriding of the defecation reflex can result in severe constipation and/or impaction.* • Assist with use of fracture bed pan; provide pain relief medications. *Child may be hesitant to use bed pan because of pain on motion.*	
High Risk for Altered Urinary Elimination **RELATED TO** Immobility Presence of catheter **DEFINING CHARACTERISTICS** *Retention:* Bladder distention Frequency Decreased output Inability to urinate Dribbling *Urinary tract infection:* Burning/pain on urination Increased temperature Increased WBC	**ONGOING ASSESSMENT** • Assess previous patterns of voiding. • Palpate bladder for distention. • Evaluate time intervals between voiding. *Establishment of routine pattern minimizes risk of complications.* • Assess frequency, amount, and character of urine. • Assess for signs or symptoms of retention. • Assess for signs or symptoms of urinary tract infection. **THERAPEUTIC INTERVENTIONS** • Initiate methods to encourage voiding. • Encourage fluids. Offer fluids of preference, or food with high water content. • Encourage cranberry/prune juice to keep urine acidic. *(Bacteria less active in acidic environment.)* • Provide privacy. • Record I&O. • Remove Foley catheter as soon as possible. • Medicate with antibiotics as ordered *for urinary tract infection prophylaxis and treatment.*	Normal urinary elimination pattern will be maintained.
High Risk for Injury **RELATED TO** Pin migration **DEFINING CHARACTERISTICS** Pain at pin sites Movement at pin sites	**ONGOING ASSESSMENT** • Assess pin sites every shift for migration. • Assess skin around pin for tears. • Assess for pain at pin sites. **THERAPEUTIC INTERVENTIONS** • Report any signs of pin migration to physician. • Cover pin with cork or adhesive tape *to protect from accidental injuries.*	Risk for injury related to pin migration will be reduced.

Diversional Activity Deficit
RELATED TO
Restricted activity
	ONGOING ASSESSMENT
	• Assess developmental and psychosocial status before hospitalization and application of traction:
	  Age
	  Level of consciousness
	  School
	• Assess level of independence.
	• Assess for evidence of change in behavior.
	• Assess support systems (i.e., family, peers, etc.).
		Acceptance of limitations that result from prolonged bed rest and traction will be verbalized.

Continued.

Traction cont'd

NURSING DIAGNOSES/ DEFINING CHARACTERISTICS	NURSING INTERVENTIONS / *RATIONALES*	EXPECTED OUTCOMES
DEFINING CHARACTERISTICS Verbalized frustration Anger High anxiety level Lack of expression Complaints of boredom and loneliness Increase in daytime sleep periods	**THERAPEUTIC INTERVENTIONS** • Provide time for talking and listening to child's concerns. *Ventilation of feelings supports honesty and objectivity of situation and promotes realistic perception.* • Listen in supportive manner. • Provide privacy as needed. • Allow child as much control as possible over his/her environment. *Independence facilitates coping.* • Provide diversionary activities compatible to situation. • Allow child to personalize environment. • Provide compatible roommate, same age group, if possible. • Stress positive aspects of cure and condition. • Initiate social service, child life referrals as needed. • Introduce child to other children who have successfully dealt with similar situations. • Allow for flexibility in visiting hours *to facilitate contact with support systems.* • Encourage family, sibling, friends to visit, bring favorite toys, games, food. • See Diversional activity deficit, p. 16.	

Catherine Brown, RN, BAN; Michele Knoll Puzas, RNC, MHPE

Circumcision

Circumcision is the surgical removal of the foreskin of the glans penis. The parental decision to have the newborn circumcised is usually based on one or more of the following factors: concern about hygiene, religious convictions, tradition, culture, or social norms.

NURSING DIAGNOSES/ DEFINING CHARACTERISTICS	NURSING INTERVENTIONS / *RATIONALES*	EXPECTED OUTCOMES

High Risk for Injury RELATED TO
 	
Surgical procedure
Circumcision in presence of undiagnosed penile anomaly—hypospadias, epispadias
	ONGOING ASSESSMENT
	
	• Check operative site for bleeding, lacerations, edema, and discoloration.
	• Assess for signs of sepsis:
	    Unusual discharge
	    Foul odor
	    Poor feeding
	    Temperature instability
	• Monitor I&O. *Document first voiding; edema of urinary meatus may cause urinary retention and decrease urine output.*
		Potential for injury will be reduced.

Circumcision cont'd

NURSING DIAGNOSES/ DEFINING CHARACTERISTICS	NURSING INTERVENTIONS / *RATIONALES*	EXPECTED OUTCOMES
DEFINING CHARACTERISTICS Hemorrhage Irritation of glans penis Incomplete removal of foreskin Nicking or cutting urethral meatus Ureteral stenosis Denuding shaft of penis Sepsis	**THERAPEUTIC INTERVENTIONS** • If bleeding is noted from circumcision, apply gentle pressure on site of bleeding with sterile gauze pad and notify physician. • Gently clean penis *to remove urine and feces.* • Place petrolatum gauze around glans after each diaper change *to soothe inflammation and ease removal.* • If gauze adheres to penis, use sterile water to soak dressing loose. *It can then be removed gently.*	

Pain/Discomfort
RELATED TO
Interruption of integument
Surgical procedure performed with mild sedation
 	
DEFINING CHARACTERISTICS
Crying
Irritability
Short periods of sleep or restless sleep
Decreased appetite
Emesis
Flushing of skin
	ONGOING ASSESSMENT
	• Assess for pain/discomfort with defining characteristics.
	
	THERAPEUTIC INTERVENTIONS
	• Use following comfort measures:
	  Offer pacifier.
	  Rock, cuddle, and talk to infant.
	  Ascertain appropriate analgesia order.
	• Prevent infant from disrupting catheterization site *to avoid discomfort and bleeding.*
	• Instruct parent on comfort techniques.
		Discomfort will be reduced.

Parental Knowledge Deficit
RELATED TO
Inexperience with circumcision
 	
DEFINING CHARACTERISTICS
Parent unaware that circumcision is an elective surgical procedure
Erroneous parental assumption that circumcision is required for hygiene, or by physician or hospital
Prevention of: balanitis, phimosis, carcinoma of glans or cervix
	ONGOING ASSESSMENT
	• Assess parental desire for circumcision.
	• Assess parental knowledge of rationale for performing circumcision.
	• Assess parental knowledge of risks/benefits.
	
	THERAPEUTIC INTERVENTIONS
	• *Before procedure:*
	Explain rationale, risk/benefits and alternatives; *because of parental need for adequate information to make informed decisions.*
	Ascertain that consent has been signed.
	• *After procedure:*
	Explain care of circumcision and instruct parent to report the following:
	  Bleeding
	  Foul odor
	  Unusual discharge
	  Decreased urine output
	Inform parent that glans penis, normally dark red in appearance during healing, becomes covered with a yellow exudate in 24 hours, which persists for 2-3 days. *This is part of the normal healing process and is not a sign of infection.*
	Discuss various comfort measures with parent.
		Parental knowledge deficit will be reduced.

Deborah Rickard, RN, BSN

Diaphragmatic hernia

HERNIA OF BOCHDALEK

A diaphragmatic hernia is the herniation of the abdominal contents into the thoracic cavity through an opening that most often involves the left diaphragm. This constitutes one of the most urgent of neonatal surgical emergencies. If not immediately identified and treated, the hernia may progressively lead to fatal respiratory distress.

NURSING DIAGNOSES/ DEFINING CHARACTERISTICS	NURSING INTERVENTIONS / *RATIONALES*	EXPECTED OUTCOMES
Ineffective Breathing Pattern/ Impaired Gas Exchange **RELATED TO** Decreased lung expansion Ineffective diaphragmatic excursion Hypoplastic lung **DEFINING CHARACTERISTICS** Cyanosis Tachypnea Chest retractions Diminished or absent breath sounds Increased chest diameter with asymmetry Mediastinal and point of maximal impulse (PMI) shift to the unaffected side Abdomen flat or scaphoid	**ONGOING ASSESSMENT** ▪ Monitor apical pulse, blood pressure, temperature, and respirations. ▪ Assess breath sounds in all lung fields; note bilateral equality. ▪ Observe for nasal flaring, grunting, and retracting. ▪ Monitor skin color and perfusion. ▪ Monitor blood gas results. ▪ Assess infant's tolerance to handling. **THERAPEUTIC INTERVENTIONS** ▪ Suction every 1 to 2 hours *to maintain patent airway.* ▪ Report sudden or deteriorating changes in respiratory status to physician. *This could suggest pneumothorax and could require insertion of chest tube.* ▪ Position on affected side *to maximize lung expansion.* ▪ Elevate head of bed *to allow gravitational descent of abdominal contents into abdominal cavity.* ▪ Maintain nasogastric suction *for bowel decompression.* ▪ Provide neutral thermal environment *to prevent acidosis.* ▪ Provide respiratory support as ordered. ▪ Administer sedation or muscle relaxants as ordered *to allow for controlled ventilation.* ▪ Maintain water-seal chest suction *to allow for lung reexpansion.* ▪ Strip chest tubes every hour *to prevent occlusion.* ▪ If unable to maintain adequate oxygenation levels with previous interventions, refer to Pulmonary hypertension: persistent, p. 164. *Adequate oxygenation levels are difficult to maintain with right to left shunting.*	An effective breathing pattern will be maintained.
High Risk for Fluid Volume Deficit **RELATED TO** Abnormal fluid loss Inadequate fluid replacement **DEFINING CHARACTERISTICS** Decreased blood pressure Poor perfusion Decreased skin turgor Dry mucous membranes Tachycardia Increased specific gravity Decreased urine output Increased or stable Hct despite blood loss	**ONGOING ASSESSMENT** ▪ Assess for fluid volume deficit with defining characteristics. ▪ Monitor I&O closely. ▪ Check Hct. ▪ Weigh infant daily. ▪ Monitor electrolytes. **THERAPEUTIC INTERVENTIONS** ▪ Administer parenteral fluids appropriate for infant's weight, output, and electrolyte status. ▪ Report high or low specific gravity values >1.010 or <1.003 *to determine hydration status.* ▪ Notify physician of abnormal urine dipstick, such as glucose or protein present. *This could indicate altered renal function and electrolyte shifts.* ▪ Administer blood products as ordered. ▪ Provide IV fluid replacement *to replace nasogastric drainage.* ▪ Provide humidity if infant is under radiant warmer *to prevent insensible water loss.*	Optimal hydration status will be maintained.

NURSING DIAGNOSES/ DEFINING CHARACTERISTICS	NURSING INTERVENTIONS / *RATIONALES*	EXPECTED OUTCOMES
Pain **RELATED TO** Diaphragmatic hernia repair Numerous invasive procedures **DEFINING CHARACTERISTICS** Restlessness Crying Agitation Irritability Grimacing	**ONGOING ASSESSMENT** • Assess infant's comfort level with defining characteristics. • Assess need for pain medication. **THERAPEUTIC INTERVENTIONS** • Give pain medication as ordered *to relieve discomfort.* • Limit invasive procedures as much as possible. • Use pacifier *to satisfy sucking desire.* • Provide quiet environment *to reduce stimulation and promote rest.*	Pain will be relieved.
High Risk for Infection **RELATED TO** Surgical procedure **DEFINING CHARACTERISTICS** Temperature instability Increased or decreased WBC count Redness and swelling around open wound Foul-smelling drainage	**ONGOING ASSESSMENT** • Assess for infection with defining characteristics. • Monitor CBC results. • Note color, type, and amount of drainage from surgical site. • Send sample of drainage for culture and sensitivity. **THERAPEUTIC INTERVENTIONS** • Place dressings around site *to maintain sterility and prevent infection.* • Administer prescribed antibiotics immediately after culture results are obtained. *Prompt administration of antibiotics will lessen incidence of infection.*	Risk for infection will be reduced.
Knowledge Deficit: Parental **RELATED TO** Unfamiliarity with infant's condition **DEFINING CHARACTERISTICS** Asking same question of different members of health team Apparent confusion over events Inappropriate response to infant	**ONGOING ASSESSMENT** • Assess parental knowledge of disease/surgery. • Assess parental experience with well and ill infants. **THERAPEUTIC INTERVENTIONS** • Encourage parent to: Visit and call frequently Verbalize concerns and feelings Participate in infant's care by demonstrating simple tasks, such as diapering and applying lotion • Reinforce information given by other members of health team. • Provide explanations appropriate for parent's level of understanding *to decrease anxiety.*	Knowledge deficit will be reduced.

Margaret Bell, RN; Olga A. Lazala, RN, BSN

Osteogenesis imperfecta

BRITTLE BONE DISEASE

A congenital condition characterized by abnormal brittleness of the bones.

NURSING DIAGNOSES/ DEFINING CHARACTERISTICS	NURSING INTERVENTIONS / *RATIONALES*	EXPECTED OUTCOMES

High Risk of Injury RELATED TO Altered neuromuscular/skeletal development related to effects of osteogenesis imperfecta **DEFINING CHARACTERISTICS** Frequent and/or easily caused fractures Wasted and/or underdeveloped muscles Rapid, but inefficient healing of fractures	**ONGOING ASSESSMENT**
	• Review obstetric/delivery history.
	• Review family history.
	• Review physical assessment data.
	• Observe for signs of previous fractures whenever handling infant:
	    Excessive or prolonged crying
	    Swelling or redness
	    Misalignment of body
	
	THERAPEUTIC INTERVENTIONS
	• Handle infant carefully, avoiding sharp or forceful movements *that may cause fractures.*
	• Use infant seat or pillow for moving infant *to avoid any bending pressure on bones.*
	• Use flexible diaper rolls *to facilitate positioning; these are less likely to cause pressure.*
	• Line crib and bath tub with diapers *to minimize contact trauma.*
	• Use lightweight, nonrestrictive clothing.
	• Avoid thick diapers; lift buttocks rather than legs when diapering.
		Prevention of new fractures will be achieved.

High Risk for Nutritional Deficiency RELATED TO Crowding of small stomach into chest cavity, irritability related to pain **DEFINING CHARACTERISTICS** Weight loss Inability to feed	**ONGOING ASSESSMENT**
	• Determine appropriate feeding route based on:
	    Gestational age
	    Sensitivity of gag reflex
	    Level of irritability
	    Respiratory rate
	    Level of activity/alertness
	• Assess infant's ability to tolerate feedings:
	    Observe for vomiting.
	    Observe amount of residual per nasogastric tube before feedings.
	    Assess abdominal circumference *to observe for distention.*
	• Assess weight daily.
	
	THERAPEUTIC INTERVENTIONS
	• Encourage oral feedings when appropriate, using assessment data and the following criteria:
	    Gestational age ≥32 weeks
	    Respiratory rate of 40-60
	    Tolerance of 5-10 ml at first feeding
	• Offer pacifier with nasogastric feedings *to satisfy sucking reflex.*
	• Hold feedings and notify physician if residual is ≥3-4 ml; *large residuals are a symptom of feeding intolerance.*
	• Offer small, frequent feedings; *these are more easily digested by the small stomach.*
	• Elevate infant's head slightly with infant seat or pillow during feedings *to facilitate digestion and to minimize regurgitation.*
	• Use nasogastric tube or position to burp infant; do not pat or rub back.
		Nutritional deficit will be reduced.

NURSING DIAGNOSES/ DEFINING CHARACTERISTICS	NURSING INTERVENTIONS / *RATIONALES*	EXPECTED OUTCOMES
High Risk for Fluid Volume Deficit **RELATED TO** Idiopathic hyperthermia, profuse diaphoresis **DEFINING CHARACTERISTICS** Excessive weight loss Poor skin turgor Decreased urine output Increased urine specific gravity Lethargy Electrolyte imbalance Sunken fontanels Poor perfusion Hypotension Increased heart rate	**ONGOING ASSESSMENT** <ul><li>Assess weight pattern; weigh every 24 hours. *Excessive weight loss is symptom of dehydration.*</li><li>Observe skin turgor.</li><li>Assess I&O. *Urine output should be 1-2 ml/kg/hr.*</li><li>Assess nature and amount of secretions.</li><li>Observe activity level.</li><li>Assess fontanels (are fontanels sunken, do sutures overlay?).</li><li>Monitor vital signs, including blood pressure, every 2-4 hours.</li><li>Check urine specific gravity every 4-8 hours. *Should be <1.006 to 1.008.*</li><li>Monitor serum electrolytes every 24-48 hours.</li></ul> **THERAPEUTIC INTERVENTIONS** <ul><li>Adjust IV or feedings to provide 80-100 ml/kg/day on first day of life; 100-120 ml/kg/day thereafter. Add 10%-20% based on severity of dehydration.</li></ul>	Optimal fluid balance will be achieved.
High Risk for Impaired Skin Integrity **RELATED TO** Decreased handling of infant Decreased spontaneous movement of infant Decreased circulation and healing ability **DEFINING CHARACTERISTICS** Skin breakdown Reddened areas over bony prominences	**ONGOING ASSESSMENT** <ul><li>Observe infant's skin for reddened areas.</li><li>Assess environment for any potential sources of pressure or trauma.</li><li>See High risk for impaired skin integrity, p. 41.</li></ul> **THERAPEUTIC INTERVENTIONS** <ul><li>Use sheepskin under infant.</li><li>Massage infant gently with a cloth (particularly bony prominences) every 3-4 hours.</li><li>Reposition infant gently every 2-4 hours *to redistribute pressure.*</li><li>Maintain adequate nutritional intake.</li></ul>	Prevention of skin breakdown will be achieved.
High Risk for Parental Knowledge Deficit **RELATED TO** Denial Unfamiliarity with terms Inability to comprehend explanations	**ONGOING ASSESSMENT** <ul><li>Observe parental attitude as expressed by comments and behavior.</li><li>Assess parental level of knowledge as expressed by appropriateness of questions.</li><li>Observe parental reactions to changes in infant's condition or treatment.</li></ul> **THERAPEUTIC INTERVENTIONS** <ul><li>Encourage parental discussion of feelings and concerns regarding infant and condition.</li><li>Offer information and ask for feedback regarding: Infant's condition Unit policies Roles/responsibilities of unit personnel</li><li>Contact social service department if indicated.</li></ul>	Knowledge deficit will be reduced.

Continued.

Osteogenesis imperfecta cont'd

NURSING DIAGNOSES/ DEFINING CHARACTERISTICS	NURSING INTERVENTIONS / *RATIONALES*	EXPECTED OUTCOMES
DEFINING CHARACTERISTICS Inappropriate or negative questions Hostility or suspicion toward staff Anxiety Disbelief or denial		
High Risk for Altered Parenting **RELATED TO** Fear of infant's response to parental handling Depression over prognosis Anxiety over how others will view parent **DEFINING CHARACTERISTICS** Inconsistency or disinterest in visiting or calling Disinterest or uneasiness in handling infant Nonverbal/verbal expression of concern for infant's condition Guilt, hostility, or suspicion	**ONGOING ASSESSMENT** • Observe frequency of visits or calls. • Observe parental interaction with infant. • Assess parental developmental stages. • Assess parental support system: 　Family members 　Friends 　Religious beliefs • Assess parental emotional response to reason for infant's hospitalization. **THERAPEUTIC INTERVENTIONS** • Initiate calls to parent if necessary and encourage visits. *Contact with infant is important in establishing bonding.* • Encourage parent to hold infant and provide as much care as possible. • Encourage parental expression of feelings regarding infant's condition. • Stress positive aspects of infant's condition. • Make referrals as indicated: 　Social service 　Parent support group in the neonatal ICU	Initiation and development of parent-infant bonding will be observed.

Christine Todd, RN, BS, BGS

8

Renal/Endocrine/ Metabolic Care Plans

PEDIATRIC PATIENT
Diabetes insipidus
Diabetes: insulin-dependent
Diabetic ketoacidosis
Dialysis
Glomerulonephritis: acute
Hemolytic uremic syndrome
Hyperglycemic hyperosmotic nonketotic
  coma
Hypertension
Nephrotic syndrome
Renal failure: acute
Renal transplant: postoperative
Syndrome of inappropriate antidiuretic
  hormone

NEONATAL PATIENT
Glucose and calcium metabolism, altered
Infant of a diabetic mother
Thermoregulation in the low-birth-weight
  infant

Diabetes insipidus

DI; NEUROGENIC DIABETES

Diabetes insipidus (DI) is a disturbance of water metabolism caused by a failure of vasopressin (antidiuretic hormone [ADH]) synthesis or release resulting in the excretion of a large amount of dilute urine. Diabetes insipidus may also have a nephrogenic or psychogenic etiology.

NURSING DIAGNOSES/ DEFINING CHARACTERISTICS	NURSING INTERVENTIONS / *RATIONALES*	EXPECTED OUTCOMES
Actual Fluid Volume Deficit **RELATED TO** Compromised endocrine regulatory mechanism Neurohypophyseal dysfunction Hypopituitarism Hypophysectomy **DEFINING CHARACTERISTICS** Polyuria Polydypsia Sudden weight loss Urine specific gravity <1.005 Hypernatremia (Na$^+$ >145 mEq/L) Depressed fontanel Absent tears Change in mental status Urine osmolality: <300 mOsm/L Thirst Requests for cold/ice water Output exceeds intake	**ONGOING ASSESSMENT** • Assess age and developmental level. • Monitor I&O. Report urine volume >200 ml in each of 2 consecutive hours or >500 ml in a 2-hour period. • Monitor for increased thirst *(a preference for cold or iced water is a hallmark of DI).* • Weigh daily *to detect excessive fluid loss, especially in incontinent children with inaccurate I&O.* • Monitor urine specific gravity every shift *(may be as low as 1.000).* • Monitor for serum Na$^+$ levels >145 mEq/L. *Dehydration is hyperosmolar state in which serum Na$^+$ rises.* • Monitor for signs of hypovolemic shock (e.g., tachycardia, tachypnea, hypotension). • Monitor serum and urine osmolality. • Monitor mental status; *infants should be awake or easily aroused and recognize parents.* • Monitor other electrolytes: K$^+$, BUN, creatinine; also Hgb and Hct. Report abnormal values. **THERAPEUTIC INTERVENTIONS** • Allow child to drink at will. • Provide a source of easily accessible fluids, as desired. • If child has decreased LOC or impaired thirst mechanism, obtain parenteral fluid orders. • Administer medication as ordered. If vasopressin is given, monitor for water intoxication and/or rebound hyponatremia. • See Fluid volume deficit, p. 19. • Administer IV electrolyte replacement *because critical electrolyte losses occur with water loss.* Avoid replacement of losses with dextrose solutions *because of increased risk of water intoxication.*	Normal fluid volume will be achieved.
High Risk for Constipation **RELATED TO** Fluid volume deficit **DEFINING CHARACTERISTICS** Frequency and amount less than usual pattern Straining at stool Hard, formed stools	**ONGOING ASSESSMENT** • Assess usual bowel patterns and habits. • Assess for deviation from normal. • Assess characteristics of stool (i.e., color, consistency, amount). **THERAPEUTIC INTERVENTIONS** • See Constipation, p. 12.	Normal pattern of bowel elimination will be maintained.

NURSING DIAGNOSES/ DEFINING CHARACTERISTICS	NURSING INTERVENTIONS / *RATIONALES*	EXPECTED OUTCOMES
High Risk for Impaired Skin Integrity **RELATED TO** Urinary frequency with potential incontinence **DEFINING CHARACTERISTICS** Red, excoriated skin Urinary incontinence	**ONGOING ASSESSMENT** • Inspect skin every shift; document condition and changes in status. *Early detection and intervention may prevent progression of impaired skin integrity.* • Assess for continence. • Assess other risks to child's skin integrity (e.g., immobility, nutritional status). **THERAPEUTIC INTERVENTIONS** • Provide easy access to bathroom/urinal/bedpan. • Change infant's diapers frequently; apply ointment *to prevent breakdown.* • Teach parent skin care. • See High risk for impaired skin integrity, p. 39.	Skin will remain intact.
Fear/Anxiety **RELATED TO** Unquenchable thirst Excessive urination Medications and treatments **DEFINING CHARACTERISTICS** Restlessness Increased questioning Withdrawal Excessive demands Difficulty sleeping Expressed concern about health changes	**ONGOING ASSESSMENT** • Assess level of fear/anxiety. • Assess usual coping strategies. **THERAPEUTIC INTERVENTIONS** • Encourage child/parent to verbalize feelings *(aids assessment of anxiety, and allows child to be aware of feelings).* • See Fear, p. 18/Anxiety, p. 4.	Fear/anxiety will be reduced.
Knowledge Deficit **RELATED TO** Disease process Medications and treatments **DEFINING CHARACTERISTICS** Requests for information Verbalized misconceptions/misinterpretations	**ONGOING ASSESSMENT** • Assess level of knowledge of disease process. • Assess level of understanding of medications and treatments. **THERAPEUTIC INTERVENTIONS** • Explain condition and treatment(s) in simple, brief terms to child/ family. • Ask child/family to verbalize explanations of conditions/treatments *(to indicate any misconceptions or misinterpretations).*	Family and/or child will verbalize correct understanding of medications and treatments.

Mary Ann Naccarato, RN, BSN; Kim Johnson, RN, BSN

333

Diabetes: insulin-dependent

TYPE II DIABETES; JUVENILE DIABETES; DIABETES MELLITUS

A pancreatic disorder in which the β cells of the islets of Langerhans do not secrete enough insulin, if any. Insulin, a hormone usually secreted after meals, facilitates glycogen storage in the liver, transport of glucose into muscle and fat cells, and maintains blood glucose at normal levels. Inadequate insulin causes hyperglycemia and glycosuria, which lead to fluid and electrolyte imbalance. Gluconeogenesis (use of protein and fat stores) causes ketoacidosis, muscle wasting, and weight loss.

NURSING DIAGNOSES/ DEFINING CHARACTERISTICS	NURSING INTERVENTIONS / *RATIONALES*	EXPECTED OUTCOMES
Altered Nutrition: Less Than Body Requirements **RELATED TO** Decreased number or function of pancreatic islet cells Increased blood glucose level by poor cell uptake Glycosuria caused by exceeding renal tubular capacity limits **DEFINING CHARACTERISTICS** Polydipsia Polyphagia Polyuria Weight loss Increased blood glucose/abnormal glucose tolerance test	**ONGOING ASSESSMENT** • Assess age and developmental level. • Assess for signs and symptoms of hyperglycemia or diabetic ketoacidosis. Assess vital signs every 4 hours. Monitor strict I&O. Check urine for sugar and acetone at least every shift. Monitor blood lab results: Glucose (70-110 mg/dl) Na (136-147 mEq/L) Cl (95-110 mEq/L) Co_2 (21-32 mEq/L) **THERAPEUTIC INTERVENTIONS** • Administer insulin as ordered (progressively): Insulin drip (if condition warrants) Regular insulin subcutaneously preprandially Regular/NPH AM and PM split-mixed dose when indicated. *Lifelong daily injections are necessary.* • Rotate injection sites and document site with each injection. *Sites are rotated for optimal insulin absorptions.* • Provide appropriate diet: Obtain dietary consultations. Reinforce need for child to consume all foods on tray and not save for later use. Check each meal tray for proper identification and proper number of calories. • Give all meals and snacks on time. *When individual cannot utilize insulin, metabolic state is altered.* • Observe child for "cheating" or snacking between meals.	Nutritional requirements will be adequate while diabetic state is controlled.
Ineffective Individual Coping **RELATED TO** Diagnostic and treatment course New problem Chronic disease **DEFINING CHARACTERISTICS** Regressive behavior Anger/noncompliance with regimen Refusal to attempt procedures independently	**ONGOING ASSESSMENT** • Assess coping mechanisms for diagnosis and treatment. • Assess for noncompliance, anger, regressive behavior. • Assess child/family relationship and family dynamics. Identify primary caretaker. • Assess past coping strategies. • Assess hobbies; identify potential stressors. **THERAPEUTIC INTERVENTIONS** • Perform all procedures, calmly and unhurriedly. *Coping with chronic disease and mastering managerial skills are directly related to initial instruction.* • Encourage verbalization of feelings about diagnosis and chronicity. Encourage drawing or role-playing to deal with feelings. • Reinforce that anger and "mourning" loss of freedom are normal coping mechanisms. *Parent should know that regression and acting out are normal.*	Coping behaviors will be maximized.

NURSING DIAGNOSES/ DEFINING CHARACTERISTICS	NURSING INTERVENTIONS / *RATIONALES*	EXPECTED OUTCOMES
	THERAPEUTIC INTERVENTIONS cont'd ▪ Support and reinforce progress toward independence. ▪ Answer any and all questions. ▪ Obtain support services as needed: diabetes teaching service, psychiatric liaison.	

Knowledge Deficit
RELATED TO
Initial diagnosis of chronic disease
Multifaceted treatment involved in controlling diabetes and its potential complications
 	
DEFINING
CHARACTERISTICS
Anxiety
Fear
Anger about chronicity
Many questions
Lack of questions
Noncompliance with dietary restrictions
Failure to attempt insulin injections or blood glucose chemistry
	ONGOING ASSESSMENT
	▪ Assess willingness to learn.
	▪ Assess cognitive abilities (as age-appropriate).
	▪ Assess physical abilities. *Physical limitations (e.g., lack of motor control and poor vision) necessitate changes in teaching plan.*
	▪ Assess retention from one class session to next.
	
	THERAPEUTIC INTERVENTIONS
	▪ Contact diabetes teaching service.
	▪ Explain definition of diabetes, including signs and symptoms. *Explanation should be age-appropriate; use pictures if needed. All teaching should be toward parent/child (primary caretaker).*
	  Reinforce fact that diabetes is chronic incurable condition that can be controlled by diet, insulin, and exercise.
	  Explain need for diet-controlled exchange system and importance of strict adherence.
	  Explain that daily exercise is important to lower blood sugar and also allows for normal socialization. *Exercise increases body's sensitivity to insulin and decreases serum cholesterol and triglyceride levels, decreasing risk factors for developing cardiovascular complications of diabetes. Children should be allowed to maintain all normal activities (playground, sporting activities).*
	▪ Reinforce and encourage progress toward independence at blood glucose monitoring and insulin techniques:
	  Define insulin; discuss different types, action, duration, especially split-mixed insulin regimen.
	  Demonstrate accurate method of drawing up and administering insulin; explain rationale for rotating injection sites.
	  Explain that blood glucose monitoring is necessary for diabetic control; normal glucose level is 70-110 mg/dl.
	  Demonstrate accurate method of obtaining and interpreting blood glucose Chemstrips or Accu-Chek system (or other electronic device).
	  Define hypoglycemia (blood glucose <40 mg/dl) and possible causes.
	  Discuss signs and symptoms of hypoglycemia:
	    Mild: child cool, sweaty, shaky, irritable, tired, weak, hungry, has personality changes; headache.
	    Moderate: child experiences nausea, sleepiness, disorientation, fainting, decreased LOC.
	    Severe: child is convulsive or comatose.
	  Instruct in treatment for hypoglycemia symptoms (e.g., 4 oz. orange juice, hard candy, sugar, candy bar).
	  Discuss use of glucagon for hypoglycemic coma.
	  Define hyperglycemia (serum glucose >140 mg/dl) and possible causes.
	  Teach signs and symptoms of hyperglycemia: glycosuria, polyuria (bed-wetting), polydipsia, polyphagia, acetone breath.
	  Discuss/define diabetic ketoacidosis and need for immediate medical attention. *Child/family must learn basic survival skills of diabetes mellitus (DM) management to prevent complications (see Diabetic ketoacidosis, p. 336).*
	  Discuss need for careful blood sugar monitoring during illness (may require insulin adjustment). Provide emergency phone numbers.
		Child/parent will demonstrate knowledge of and compliance with treatment regimen.

Continued.

Renal/Endocrine/Metabolic Care Plans (Pediatric)

NURSING DIAGNOSES/ DEFINING CHARACTERISTICS	NURSING INTERVENTIONS / *RATIONALES*	EXPECTED OUTCOMES

THERAPEUTIC INTERVENTIONS cont'd

- Reinforce need for regular follow-up care (e.g., of eyes, feet, and teeth) *to prevent microvascular complications of diabetes (e.g., reduced vision, blindness, foot problems, and renal failure).*
- Encourage questioning, *for clarification and evaluation of effectiveness of teaching.*
- Assist child/adolescent in maintaining perceptions of normal behaviors/ activities by individualizing plans for activity/meals/insulin/blood glucose testing. *Children do not want to feel different from their peers.*

Linda Walsh, RN, BSN; Michele Knoll Puzas, RNC, MHPE

Diabetic ketoacidosis

HYPERGLYCEMIA; DIABETES MELLITUS; DKA

Diabetic ketoacidosis (DKA) is an acute, potentially life-threatening complication of diabetes mellitus. Normally the body metabolizes glucose for energy needs. In the diabetic, glucose metabolism does not occur because of absent or ineffective insulin that is necessary for migration of glucose into cells. Diabetic ketoacidosis results from cellular metabolism of fat to produce energy. By-products of this metabolic process are ketone bodies (organic acids) that cause metabolic acidosis. Children admitted to a PICU have usually progressed to shock with respiratory and cardiac changes as a result of severe electrolyte imbalance.

NURSING DIAGNOSES/ DEFINING CHARACTERISTICS	NURSING INTERVENTIONS / *RATIONALES*	EXPECTED OUTCOMES
High Risk for Injury RELATED TO Ketoacidosis resulting from: Omission/ reduction of insulin Inability of cells to recognize/use available insulin Initial onset of diabetes Infection/ intercurrent illness Acute pancreatitis Stress **DEFINING CHARACTERISTICS** *Clinical:* Polydipsia, polyuria Weakness, anorexia Abdominal pain Kussmaul's respirations Acetone breath	**ONGOING ASSESSMENT** - Assess age and developmental level. - Monitor and record urine ketone. *Presence of ketone denotes ketoacidotic state.* - Monitor blood glucose as necessary. *Serum glucose levels will decrease with appropriate IV fluid and insulin therapy.* - Monitor potassium level once therapy has begun. *With metabolic and fluid correction, K^+ returns intracellularly, and serum hypokalemia may result from K^+ loss with diuresis.* - Auscultate for bowel sounds. Assess for abdominal pain, checking intensity of pain and location. Document and notify physician of any changes. *Abdominal pain, nausea, vomiting result from ketoacidosis.* - Monitor and record respiratory rate, depth, and presence of Kussmaul's respirations and notify physician of deviations. *Deep, rapid respirations indicate increase in acidic state. Carbon dioxide and acetone are being blown off with each breath, in an attempt to compensate for acidosis.* - Monitor ABGs as ordered. Notify physician if abnormal and maintain oxygen as ordered. - Monitor for hypoglycemia. *Signs and symptoms include confusion, tremors, pallor, weakness, diaphoresis, serum glucose <60 mg/dl.* **THERAPEUTIC INTERVENTIONS** - Administer and record IV fluids and additives as ordered. - Use normal saline solution to correct volume depletion. *Restriction of glucose solutions is desired until blood glucose drops to 250 mg/dl.* - Initiate K^+ therapy if indicated.	Risk of injury caused by ketoacidosis will be reduced.

NURSING DIAGNOSES/ DEFINING CHARACTERISTICS	NURSING INTERVENTIONS / *RATIONALES*	EXPECTED OUTCOMES
DEFINING CHARACTERISTICS cont'd Blurred vision Nausea, vomiting Pallor, diaphoresis, dehydration *Laboratory:* Serum glucose >300 mg/dl and <900 mg/dl Serum ketones Decreased serum pH, phosphate, bicarbonate Normal/low/elevated serum potassium Urine glucose: 2% Urine acetone: large	**THERAPEUTIC INTERVENTIONS** cont'd ▪ Administer sodium bicarbonate only in cases of severe, life-threatening acidosis. *Early or overzealous use of NaHCO₃ often results in rebound metabolic alkalosis once rehydration has occurred.* ▪ Administer and record insulin injection, drip as ordered. Follow hospital/unit procedure for preparation of insulin drip. *Short-acting insulin (IV infusion) enables transport of glucose to cells and promotes fat/protein storage.* ▪ If signs of hypoglycemia present, administer IV dextrose bolus as ordered. Administer sugar under tongue if NPO or offer orange juice if child tolerates oral fluids. Document and notify physician. *With decrease of blood glucose and with IV infusion, child is at risk for hypoglycemia and cerebral edema.* ▪ Document consistency and amount of emesis. Elevate head of bed 30 degrees and prepare for possible nasogastric tube placement. ▪ Administer antiemetics as ordered.	
Fluid Volume Deficit **RELATED TO** Osmotic diuresis from hyperglycemia Vomiting Kussmaul's respirations **DEFINING CHARACTERISTICS** Abdominal pain Hypotension, tachycardia Dilute urine Output greater than intake Increased serum values: WBC, Hgb, Hct, glucose, BUN Increased sodium, creatinine Oliguria or anuria possible in severe dehydration and shock	**ONGOING ASSESSMENT** ▪ Monitor vital signs every 2 hours; notify physician of any abnormalities, especially heart rate, BP. *Severe hypotension and tachycardia precede hypovolemic shock.* ▪ Assess skin turgor. ▪ Monitor and record I&O. Notify physician if urine output is <30 ml for 2 consecutive hours. *Urinary output should be at least 30 ml/hr. Lower output indicates decreased renal perfusion.* ▪ Monitor and record urine specific gravity. *This parameter is an early indicator of dehydration and/or electrolyte imbalance.* ▪ Weigh child daily; record. ▪ Monitor serum Hct, Hgb, serum osmolality, BUN, glucose, and urine laboratory values; *values will be increased because of hemoconcentration.* **THERAPEUTIC INTERVENTIONS** ▪ Administer isotonic IV fluid (saline solution) followed by glucose IV fluid when glucose levels drop. *Isotonic saline solution is administered to increase volume quickly and maintain sodium balance. Restrict glucose only until serum glucose begins to drop to prevent hypoglycemia.* ▪ Reassure child during episodes of abdominal pain and vomiting. *These symptoms are thought to be related to severe dehydration and electrolyte imbalance and should subside when fluid volume is corrected.*	Fluid volume deficit will be reduced.
Altered Levels of Consciousness **RELATED TO** Acid-base imbalance Ineffective breathing pattern Dehydration	**ONGOING ASSESSMENT** ▪ Assess LOC by use of coma scale on neurological flow sheet. ▪ Assess serum electrolytes, glucose, pH levels. ▪ Monitor respiratory rate, tidal volume, quality. *Change in quality of respirations may lead to decreased sensorium and ultimately, respiratory arrest.*	Normal LOC will be restored and maintained.

Continued.

Renal/Endocrine/Metabolic Care Plans (Pediatric)

NURSING DIAGNOSES/ DEFINING CHARACTERISTICS	NURSING INTERVENTIONS / *RATIONALES*	EXPECTED OUTCOMES
DEFINING CHARACTERISTICS Change in alertness, orientation, ability to respond verbally, decreased motor response, decreased pupillary reaction Kussmaul's respirations Agitation Impaired judgment Lethargy Drowsiness Coma	**THERAPEUTIC INTERVENTIONS** • Maintain serial documentation on neurological flow sheet. *Flow sheet documentation quickly identifies immediate changes and trends in child's neurological status.* • Correct serum electrolytes, fluid, glucose, and pH imbalance. • Provide for safety as necessary: side rails, restraints. • Explain all procedures as they are performed. • Prepare for intubation. *Severely compromised child may need respiratory support before respiratory arrest occurs.*	

High Risk for Decreased Cardiac Output
RELATED TO
Cardiac dysrhythmias secondary to hyperkalemia/hypokalemia
 	
DEFINING CHARACTERISTICS
Dysrhythmias observed per ECG or cardiac monitor
Irregular pulse
Bradycardia
Low blood pressure
Change in mentation
Dizziness
Cool skin
	ONGOING ASSESSMENT
	• Monitor ECG for early signs of potassium imbalance. *Electrolyte abnormalities exhibit specific effects on ECG. Recognition of hyperkalemia/hypokalemia can alert nurse of life-threatening situation.*
	   Progressive signs of hyperkalemia:
	     High-peaked T waves
	     Flat P waves
	     Prolonged PR interval
	     Atrial arrest
	     Prolonged QRS, slow ventricular rate
	     Ventricular fibrillation, asystole
	   Signs of hypokalemia:
	     Prolonged low-amplitude T waves
	     Prominent U waves
	     Ectopic beats
	• Monitor for changes in cardiac output; check BP and pulses regularly. *BP and pulses reflect cardiac output.*
	
	THERAPEUTIC INTERVENTIONS
	• Place child on cardiac monitor.
	• Provide accurate administration of fluids and electrolytes to correct fluid, acid-base imbalance. *Acidosis is associated with hyperkalemia, which causes slowed conduction. In contrast, aggressive treatment can result in hypokalemia, which causes ectopic cardiac rhythms.*
	• Prepare for placement of central line for cardiodynamic monitoring.
	• Notify physician of abnormal ECG. Record ECG for future reference.
	• Place patient on cardiac monitor if indicated. *Children in mild DKA may not require monitoring if clinically stable.*
		Risk of cardiac complication will be reduced.

Altered Nutrition: Less Than Body Requirements **RELATED TO** Lack of glucose metabolism caused by absence of effective insulin Use of fat/protein for energy needs Protein loss caused by diuresis	**ONGOING ASSESSMENT** • Obtain weight; compare with usual weight if possible. • Assess skin condition, turgor. • Assess for muscle wasting, weakness. • Assess dietary habits, especially for new onset diabetic. • Monitor I&O. • Monitor urine for sugar and protein. • Monitor blood sugar routinely once DKA resolved.	Optimal nutrition will be maintained.

NURSING DIAGNOSES/ DEFINING CHARACTERISTICS	NURSING INTERVENTIONS / *RATIONALES*	EXPECTED OUTCOMES

DEFINING CHARACTERISTICS
Weight loss
Ketoacidosis
Hyperglycemia
Abdominal discomfort
Flushed skin
Nausea/vomiting
Diuresis
	THERAPEUTIC INTERVENTIONS
	• Administer insulin (short-acting) *to enable glucose transport to cells. Glucose metabolism for energy requirements spares fat and protein for cell growth and maintenance and allows fat/protein storage.*
	• Notify physician when serum glucose has dropped to 250 to 300 mg/dl. *At this time glucose IV should be administered and insulin therapy halted to prevent hypoglycemia and cerebral edema.*
	• After critical stage:
	  Provide oral intake when nausea and vomiting have abated and LOC has stabilized.
	  Obtain dietary consultation.
	  Provide parent and child instruction on American Dietetic Association meal planning once oral nutrition is tolerated and IV maintenance has been discontinued.
	  Continue to administer subcutaneous insulin on routine, daily basis to prevent reoccurrence of DKA.
	  Allow child to test own blood sugar, self-administer insulin, and make menu selections when able.	

Knowledge Deficit RELATED TO
Unfamiliarity with disease process and treatment
Noncompliance with medications, testing urine and blood, and follow-up care
 	
DEFINING CHARACTERISTICS
Unawareness of factors leading to ketoacidosis
Verbalized lack of knowledge
Questions about ketoacidosis
	ONGOING ASSESSMENT
	• Assess child's/parent's understanding of causes and consequences of diabetic ketoacidosis.
	• Assess other factors that may be contributing to child's inability to understand or comply with explanations:
	  Anxiety
	  Denial of illness, etc.
	  Developmental level: *Adolescents in particular have difficulty dealing with this chronic disease, as it forces them to be different from their peers.*
	
	THERAPEUTIC INTERVENTIONS
	• Explain to child and parent:
	  Symptoms of early acute diabetic ketoacidosis (drowsiness, nausea, vomiting, flushed skin, thirst, excessive urination, glycosuria, ketonuria). *Child and family need to identify signs and symptoms of impending hyperglycemia/ketoacidosis to avoid complications and future hospitalizations.*
	  Factors that predispose child to diabetic ketoacidosis (illness, stress, infection, insufficient insulin, decreased activity, and exercise).
	  Importance of balanced diet, routine exercise, weight control, accurate medication administration, regular urine ketone and blood testing, and follow-up care.
	  Management of diabetes during other illness:
	    Importance of taking insulin even if feeling ill and not eating
	    Appropriate diet and insulin dosage modifications
	    Keeping physician informed of status
	    Frequent testing for ketonuria and hypoglycemia/hyperglycemia
	• Refer for psychological counseling if needed.
	• Refer to diabetes teaching service.
		Child and parent will demonstrate knowledge of disease process and the importance of medications, urine and blood testing.

Michele Knoll Puzas, RNC, MHPE

Dialysis

PERITONEAL DIALYSIS/HEMODIALYSIS; VASCULAR
ARTERIOVENOUS ACCESS; EXTERNAL CATHETERS
(SUBCLAVIAN, INTERNAL JUGULAR, FEMORAL,
QUINTON PERMCATH)

Dialysis is the diffusion of solute molecules and fluids across a semipermeable membrane. Dialysis is often necessary to sustain life in people with no, or very little, kidney function. The purpose of dialysis is to remove excess fluids, toxins, and metabolic wastes from the blood and control BP during renal failure.

There are two types of dialysis: peritoneal dialysis and hemodialysis. Peritoneal dialysis uses the patient's own peritoneum as the semipermeable membrane; hemodialysis uses a man-made artificial membrane as the semipermeable membrane. Dialysis requires the presence of an osmotic gradient. This gradient enhances the movement of solute molecules from the side of higher concentration to the side of lower concentration and causes water to move from the side of low concentration to the side of high concentration.

Both types of dialysis require an access to the dialysis system. Peritoneal dialysis requires surgical insertion of a peritoneal dialysis catheter. These catheters are made of Silastic material and are either straight or curled with one or two Dacron cuffs. The most well-known peritoneal catheter is the Tenckoff; however, there are currently several different designs and manufacturers of catheters. The type of catheter used is usually related to the surgeon's preference.

Hemodialysis requires a vascular access. This can be accomplished by surgically creating an arteriovenous (A-V) fistula or graft (man-made material used to connect an artery and a vein) or by insertion of an external catheter into the subclavian, internal jugular, or femoral vein. External A-V shunts are currently considered obsolete and are rarely used today. Adaptation of the port-a-cath for hemodialysis use is currently under investigation.

NURSING DIAGNOSES/ DEFINING CHARACTERISTICS	NURSING INTERVENTIONS / *RATIONALES*	EXPECTED OUTCOMES
Altered Fluid Volume **RELATED TO** *Excess:* Renal insufficiency Malfunctioning peritoneal catheter Inadequate ultrafiltration Noncompliance with fluid restrictions *Deficit:* Overdialysis/ultrafiltration Presence of infection with fever or vomiting, diarrhea Inadequate fluid replacement (especially in peritoneal dialysis patients) **DEFINING CHARACTERISTICS** *Excess:* Abdominal pain Complaints of fullness Shortness of breath Nausea Decreased urinary output	**ONGOING ASSESSMENT** • Assess age and developmental level. • Obtain baseline vital signs and dry weight. • Monitor BP every 4 hours during peritoneal dialysis and every hour during hemodialysis. • Record fluid I&O. • Weigh twice a day (at beginning and end of dialysis). • Measure abdominal girth daily at end of drain time. • Monitor child for tachypnea, retractions, nasal flaring. • Auscultate breath sounds at least every 4 hours; more often as indicated. • Monitor electrolytes, especially K⁺. • Observe for nausea, vomiting, edema, disorientation, sunken fontanel, dry mucous membranes, absence of tears. Check fontanel and mucous membranes of infants every 4 hours during peritoneal dialysis. **THERAPEUTIC INTERVENTIONS** • Change position at least every 2 hours *to maximize drainage.* Elevate head of bed to 45 degrees; turn child on side. • Stop or slow dialysis if signs of hypokalemia are present. Consult with physician or peritoneal dialysis nurse on addition of K⁺. • Notify physician, and change dialysate concentrate when child reaches dry weight *to prevent dehydration.* • Stop dialysis if drainage is inadequate. *Overinfusion causes pain, dyspnea, nausea, and electrolyte imbalance. Rapid shifts in fluid and chemical status during hemodialysis can cause rapid changes in child's status. Dialysate can be adjusted to compensate for increases or decreases in electrolyte imbalances.*	Fluid and electrolyte balance will be maintained while continuing to remove toxins and wastes from blood.

NURSING DIAGNOSES/ DEFINING CHARACTERISTICS	NURSING INTERVENTIONS / *RATIONALES*	EXPECTED OUTCOMES

DEFINING CHARACTERISTICS cont'd

Increased abdominal girth
Weight gain
Periorbital and peripheral edema

Deficit:
Weight loss beyond dry weight
Diarrhea
Dry skin (poor turgor)
Sunken eyes and fontanels
Absence of tears
Dry mucous membranes
Lethargy
Abdominal pain
Nausea

High Risk for Altered Peripheral Tissue Perfusion

RELATED TO

Interruption in arteriovenous (A-V) access blood flow

DEFINING CHARACTERISTICS

Pain over access area
Absence of pulse above venous site
Absence of thrill over anastomosis area
Absence of bruit over access
Decreased temperature of affected limb
Cyanosis of nailbeds of affected limb
Mottled skin

ONGOING ASSESSMENT

- Assess A-V access for signs and symptoms of inadequate blood flow:
  Palpate for pulse and thrill.
  Auscultate for bruit; "swishing" sound should be audible. *When artery is connected to vein, blood is shunted from artery into vein, causing turbulence. This may be palpated above venous side of access for "thrill" or buzzing.*
  Check for blanching of nailbeds of affected limb.
  Check for mottling of skin of affected limb.

THERAPEUTIC INTERVENTIONS

- Promote following preventive measures to ensure adequate blood flow:
  Do not take BP in access limb.
  Do not draw blood specimens from access limb.
- Instruct child/parent to *avoid* devices and activities that endanger access patency, including:
  Sleeping on access limb
  Wearing tight clothing over limb with access
  Carrying school bags, purses, or packages over access arm
  Participating in activities or sports that involve active use of and/or trauma to access limb. *Thrombosis is a common complication of vascular access. Causes include thrombi (caused by venipuncture), extrinsic pressure (BP cuff, tourniquet, sleeping on limb or tight clothes), or trauma to access limb (related to activities or sports that involve active use of limb).*
- Maintain proper positioning of access limb. Consider elevating limb postoperatively *to reduce dependent edema.* Consider arm sling for support when child is ambulatory. Encourage normal use of access limb *as this also promotes healing and reduced edema.*

Patency of A-V access will be maintained.

High Risk for Infection

RELATED TO

Contamination to entry site of peritoneal catheter

ONGOING ASSESSMENT

- Assess peritoneal drainage with each exchange *(normal is clear).*
- Assess area around catheter site. *Catheter site should be clean with no signs of inflammation.*

Risk for infection will be reduced.

Continued.

Renal/Endocrine/Metabolic Care Plans (Pediatric)

NURSING DIAGNOSES/ DEFINING CHARACTERISTICS	NURSING INTERVENTIONS / *RATIONALES*	EXPECTED OUTCOMES

DEFINING CHARACTERISTICS

Complaints of abdominal pain, tenderness, feeling warm, and having chills

Infants:

Irritability; poor feeding; vomiting and/or diarrhea; decreased or lack of bowel sounds, ileus

Rigid abdominal wall

Pericatheter site reddened with discharge

Fever

Cloudy effluent

Positive culture and sensitivity

Cell count >100; differential >70% polys even without positive culture

ONGOING ASSESSMENT cont'd

- Assess tunnel; palpate along tunnel to evaluate tenderness, swelling, and expressed drainage.
- Assess child for complaint or signs of abdominal tenderness (*an infant or small child will not be able to verbalize*).
- Assess vital signs every 4 hours unless child is febrile, then every 2 hours.
- Ask child to describe how he/she feels during exchanges. *Early detection and treatment of infection will minimize complications resulting from infection.*

THERAPEUTIC INTERVENTIONS

- Use strict aseptic technique when setting up dialysis and hooking up; *poor hygiene and improper technique during connect and disconnect procedures are the no. 1 cause of peritonitis, the most common complication of peritoneal dialysis.*
- Maintain drainage receptacle below level of peritoneum *to avoid backflow of dialysate.*
- Maintain closed system at all times. Do not break closed system without permission from dialysis staff or nephrologist.
- Notify nephrologist and/or dialysis staff for any signs of infection. *Treatment can be instituted quickly and more serious complications can be avoided.*

High Risk for Infection

RELATED TO

A-V access cannulation

Frequent cannulation

Improper cleaning before cannulation

Poor hygiene

DEFINING CHARACTERISTICS

Pain over access site

Fever

Red, swollen, warm area around site

Drainage from access site

Red streaks up arm or leg

ONGOING ASSESSMENT

- Assess A-V access for signs and symptoms of infection.
- Obtain specimen for culture when infection is suspected.

THERAPEUTIC INTERVENTIONS

- Maintain asepsis with A-V access during dialysis:
   3-minute surgical scrub of access area (povidone-iodine scrub or Hibiclens). Wipe area with antiseptics. *Povidone-iodine is recommended agent.*
   Apply povidone-iodine ointment to cannulation sites.
   Cover cannulation sites with sterile bandages.
   Allow only dialysis staff to cannulate A-V access. *This is child's lifeline and is not for general use.*
   Stress good hygiene.
   Remove bandages 4 to 6 hours after dialysis.
- Explain to child/parent importance of maintaining asepsis with external catheter. *Infection is almost an inevitable complication of external vascular device. Infection may be localized cellulitis, but septicemia can occur. Meticulous daily care and avoidance of trauma to area prevent risk of infection.*
- Instruct child/parent to keep dressing clean and dry at all times:
   Protect catheter dressing while bathing (tub and sponge baths only); no swimming; no showers.
   Keep entire catheter under occlusive dressing; reinforce as necessary.
   Instruct child/parent of signs of infection and importance of reporting observations immediately.

Risk for infection will be reduced.

NURSING DIAGNOSES/ DEFINING CHARACTERISTICS	NURSING INTERVENTIONS / *RATIONALES*	EXPECTED OUTCOMES
High Risk for Infection **RELATED TO** Hemodialysis catheter External devices subject to contamination from skin Improper aseptic technique Integrity of dressing not maintained Child picking or pulling at dressing and catheter **DEFINING CHARACTERISTICS** Pain around catheter site Fever Red, swollen, warm area around catheter exit site Drainage from exit site	**ONGOING ASSESSMENT** • Assess hemodialysis catheter for signs and symptoms of infection. • Obtain blood and catheter exit site culture if there is any evidence of infection. • Visually inspect and palpate areas around and over intact dressing each shift for phlebitis, tenderness, inflammation, and infiltration. • Assess perfusion of affected lower limb every 4 hours. Check for proper blanching and absence of cyanosis. **THERAPEUTIC INTERVENTIONS** *Subclavian and internal jugular:* • Maintain asepsis with subclavian/internal jugular catheters during dialysis: Clean area with antiseptic. *Povidone-iodine (Betadine) solution before and after use is recommended agent.* Change the sterile dressing over catheter exit site before each dialysis treatment. Use sterile technique when initiating or discontinuing dialysis. Instill heparin into catheter *to prevent catheter clotting between use* and secure placement of catheter and caps after dialysis. *Do not* use catheter for any other purpose than hemodialysis. *This is a lifeline.* • Explain to child/parent importance of maintaining asepsis and to recognize when asepsis is compromised and seek assistance appropriately. *Because of location and long-term use of catheter, infection is almost inevitable. Infection may be localized at exit site but septicemia can occur.* • Instruct child/parent to keep dressing clean and dry at all times. *Meticulous care of catheter site and maintaining a dry and intact dressing will lower risk of infection.* Protect catheter dressing while bathing; no showers. Advise against swimming. If dressing becomes loose, reinforce with tape as necessary. If dressing comes off or becomes *wet*, go to dialysis unit of emergency room as soon as possible for sterile catheter site care if incapable of performing at home. Instruct child/parent of signs of infection. *Femoral catheters:* • Maintain asepsis with femoral catheter during dialysis: Use sterile technique when initiating or discontinuing dialysis. Instill heparin into catheter *to prevent interdialytic clotting of catheter* and secure placement of catheter and caps after dialysis. If intravenous line cannot be started in peripheral vessel, femoral catheter may be used with extreme caution. • Maintain femoral catheter: Change *all* dressings every 48 hours or more often if soiled. Inspect insertion site at time of dressing change for phlebitis, tenderness, inflammation, infiltration, purulent drainage, or other signs of infections. Notify physician if infection is suspected. Anticipate need to change femoral catheter every 24-72 hours *to lower risk of infection.* Maintain strict bed rest. *It is necessary to keep child on bed rest with cannulated leg flat to prevent kinking and malfunction of intravenous catheter. Compromised femoral catheter may also compromise blood flow to leg.* Notify physician of any signs of decreased perfusion to affected limb. *Catheter may have to be removed or changed to smaller lumen.*	Risk of infection will be reduced.

Continued.

Renal/Endocrine/Metabolic Care Plans (Pediatric)

NURSING DIAGNOSES/ DEFINING CHARACTERISTICS	NURSING INTERVENTIONS / *RATIONALES*	EXPECTED OUTCOMES
Pain **RELATED TO** Length of procedure Actual infusion of dialysate Distended abdomen Catheter insertion **DEFINING CHARACTERISTICS** Complaints of abdominal pain during procedure Tossing about in bed Complaints of feeling full Crying Restless and irritable Verbal report of pain Guarding pain site	**ONGOING ASSESSMENT** • Assess continually for signs of discomfort. • Assess need for pain medications. • Evaluate effectiveness of medications. • Refer to Pain, p. 35. **THERAPEUTIC INTERVENTIONS** • Remain at bedside during initiation of dialysis. Do not allow air to inflow; always use warm fluids. • Allow/encourage family involvement during dialysis *to provide comfort.* • Change child's position *to relieve discomfort during inflow.* • Allow ambulation if permitted. • Lessen or eliminate source of discomfort if possible. May need to reduce flow. • Explain reasons for inflow pain: *pH of fluid lower than body—causes discomfort until equilibration; air in cavity causes discomfort; pressure on organs and diaphragm causes discomfort until patient becomes accustomed to procedure; cold or hot solution.* • Provide diversional activities *to direct focus away from pain/procedure.* • See Diversional activity deficit, p. 16.	Pain will be reduced.
Fear **RELATED TO** New procedures Unknown outcome Fear of dying Surgery Needle sticks Access failures **DEFINING CHARACTERISTICS** Anxious Withdrawn Procrastination with procedures Combative with procedures Unprovoked crying or combativeness Denial of health problem	**ONGOING ASSESSMENT** • Assess current levels of knowledge and ability/willingness to learn. • Assess family support systems and interactions. • Assess stage of grieving. **THERAPEUTIC INTERVENTIONS** • Review diagnosis and treatments available so child and family will be more familiar with diagnosis and treatment, thus less fearful. • Review rationale for dialysis. • Encourage child/family to vocalize concerns. • Be nonjudgmental but supportive of fears. • Encourage child/family to participate in care, comfort measures. • Use behavior modification as indicated to elicit cooperative patient behavior. • Use diversional activities. • Review causes of access failures and preventive measures. • Be honest with patient. Never lie or try to "trick" child; *this only leads to more fear (untrustworthy professionals) and undermines goal.*	Child's and family's fears will be reduced/managed.

NURSING DIAGNOSES/ DEFINING CHARACTERISTICS	NURSING INTERVENTIONS / *RATIONALES*	EXPECTED OUTCOMES
Knowledge Deficit RELATED TO New procedure New diagnosis Home management **DEFINING CHARACTERISTICS** Anxiety Restlessness Withdrawal Regression Frequent questions Frequent complaints Vague physical complaints Confusion	**ONGOING ASSESSMENT** · Assess current knowledge levels of diagnosis and treatment. · Assess ability to learn. · Assess family interactions. **THERAPEUTIC INTERVENTIONS** · Review diagnosis. · Review dialysis and rationale. · Discuss dietary/fluid requirements and restrictions: low sodium, low potassium, adequate protein, high calories, free fluids. · Arrange dietary consultation if necessary. · Discuss medications and use. · Demonstrate and request return demonstration of access care before discharge. · Discuss return appointments, follow-up care, emergency numbers. · Arrange social service consultation if necessary. · Encourage child/parent to ask questions. · Teach child/parent to check for adequate blood flow through shunt/ fistula: Arrange teaching sessions when participants are ready. Demonstrate how to feel for pulses and thrill. Designate specific areas to feel for pulses and thrill. *Absence of pulses and thrill may indicate clotting of access; inform nephrologist or dialysis staff immediately.* *Waiting to declot access may result in inability to "save access" and require surgery to establish new vascular access.* Allow adequate time for return demonstration. · Instruct child/parent to inform nephrologist or dialysis staff immediately for any signs and symptoms of infection: Pain over access site Fever Red, swollen, and warm access site Drainage from access Red streaks along access area · Teach how to manage accidental separation or dislodgement of external access connections. *Information given to the child/parent of child's medical condition and proper care of external access will increase child's awareness of his/her condition and decrease anxiety concerning ADL with renal failure.* · Instruct child/parent in care of dressings if applicable.	Child/parent will be able to verbalize diagnosis, treatment, and home management.

Agnes Jones-Perry, RN, BSN; Wilma J. Hunter, RN, MS, CPNP, CNN

Glomerulonephritis: acute

POSTSTREPTOCOCCAL GLOMERULONEPHRITIS

Acute glomerulonephritis (AGN) is caused by an immune response to a streptococcal infection. It is believed that streptococci-generated immune complexes become trapped in the glomerular capillary loop, resulting in a decreased plasma filtration rate. Acute glomerulonephritis is most often related to types 4, 12, and 49 of group A β-hemolytic streptococcus, which causes both pharyngitis and impetigo. Symptoms of AGN appear in 10 to 14 days after the initial streptococcal illness.

NURSING DIAGNOSES/ DEFINING CHARACTERISTICS	NURSING INTERVENTIONS / *RATIONALES*	EXPECTED OUTCOMES
Infection **RELATED TO** Group A β-hemolytic streptococcus Pharyngitis Impetigo Upper respiratory infection **DEFINING CHARACTERISTICS** Pain Redness Skin rash Fever Lethargy Positive culture	**ONGOING ASSESSMENT** • Assess age and developmental level. • Assess for physical evidence of infection. • Review results of specimen cultures. • Obtain recent history for signs and symptoms of infection or exposure to infected individuals. **THERAPEUTIC INTERVENTIONS** • Provide comfort measures as needed. • Administer antibiotics (*usually will not be ordered unless cultures are positive*).	Infection will be detected and treated.
Fluid Volume Excess **RELATED TO** Diminished glomerular filtration Increased Na$^+$ retention **DEFINING CHARACTERISTICS** Periorbital edema Facial puffiness Generalized edema Dark urine, dysuria Decreased output— oliguria Hematuria Proteinuria Specific gravity ≥1.020 Serum electrolytes within normal limits Anorexia Mild/moderate hypertension	**ONGOING ASSESSMENT** • Assess for facial/periorbital edema in AM. *Generalized edema appears later in disease course and late during day.* • Measure I&O. *Child may become oliguric; persistent anuria/oliguria may indicate acute renal failure. A slight increase in output usually indicates increasing kidney function with diuresis following in 3 to 4 days.* • Evaluate temperature, pulse, respiration, and BP. • Weigh daily. • Evaluate lab results: urinalysis, serum electrolytes, BUN, creatinine, ESR, and ASO titer. *ESR (erythrocyte sedimentation rate) reflects acute inflammation and can be used to follow disease course. ASO titer (antistreptolysin O) can be used to detect streptococcal antibodies 4 to 6 weeks after infection. Urinalysis may reveal 3+ to 4+ hematuria and proteinuria with increasing specific gravity.* **THERAPEUTIC INTERVENTIONS** • Restrict fluid intake to equal urinary and insensible loss when signs of hypertension, renal, or cardiac failure are present. • Provide a no-added-salt diet. Restrict K$^+$ only if child is oliguric. • Restrict protein if child becomes azotemic and oliguric. *Because of anorexia, dietary restrictions are seldom needed.* • Administer antihypertensives and in severe cases furosemide (Lasix) as ordered, *to control blood pressure and fluid volume. Other diuretics have not been useful.*	Complications related to fluid volume excess will be reduced.
High Risk for Decreased Cardiac Output **RELATED TO** Hypervolemia Cardiac decompensation	**ONGOING ASSESSMENT** • Monitor for defining characteristics. • Evaluate chest x-rays, lung sounds for pulmonary edema. • Monitor ABGs. • Evaluate I&O, weight changes.	Risk for decreased cardiac output will be reduced.

NURSING DIAGNOSES/ DEFINING CHARACTERISTICS	NURSING INTERVENTIONS / *RATIONALES*	EXPECTED OUTCOMES
DEFINING CHARACTERISTICS Variation in hemodynamic parameters Dysrhythmias, ECG changes Rales, tachypnea, dyspnea Abnormal ABGs, frothy sputum Weight gain, edema, oliguria Anxiety, restlessness Weakness, fatigue Abnormal heart sounds Decreased peripheral pulses Cold, clammy skin Decreased mentation	**THERAPEUTIC INTERVENTIONS** • Place child on cardiopulmonary monitor. • Position for comfort and ease of respiration. • Restrict fluids as ordered. • Administer humidified oxygen and restrict activity *to decrease cardiac demands.* • Keep emergency drugs nearby. • See Cardiac output, decreased, p. 10.	
High Risk for Seizure Activity **RELATED TO** Hypertensive encephalopathy **DEFINING CHARACTERISTICS** Headache Dizziness Vomiting Diminished vision Hemiparesis Disorientation Convulsions	**ONGOING ASSESSMENT** • Assess for defining characteristics. • Assess for history of seizure activity. **THERAPEUTIC INTERVENTIONS** • Administer anticonvulsants as ordered. • Administer antihypertensives *to control blood pressure and decrease risk for encephalopathic changes.* • See Seizure activity, p. 200.	Risk for seizure activity will be reduced.
Knowledge Deficit **RELATED TO** New diagnosis Hospitalization **DEFINING CHARACTERISTICS** Stated lack of understanding Many questions Appearance of confusion Hesitant behaviors Irritability	**ONGOING ASSESSMENT** • Assess child/parent for current knowledge of disease process and child's current status. • Assess developmental level of child. • Assess readiness for learning. **THERAPEUTIC INTERVENTIONS** • Provide information about course of disease and all treatments, procedures. • Explain home care measures: I&O, BP measurement. • Explain need for follow-up. *Although most children recover completely, there may be persistent hematuria and above-average BUN for some weeks. A small percentage of children may progress to acute renal failure.*	Parent/child will understand disease process and follow-up required.

Michele Knoll Puzas, RNC, MHPE

Hemolytic uremic syndrome

ACUTE RENAL FAILURE

Hemolytic uremic syndrome (HUS) is a life-threatening disorder affecting infants and children (2 months to 8 years) characterized in the acute phase by severe hemolytic anemia, severe gastroenteritis, oliguria, purpura, and CNS changes. Although the cause is unknown, onset is usually preceded by a viral or bacterial infection. Damage to endothelial tissue (cause unknown) results in excessive fibrin and platelet deposits in the blood vessels. The fibrin deposits damage RBCs as they flow through the vessel resulting in RBC fragmenation and destruction.

The early phase of the disorder may last from 1 to 7 days and causes what appears to be flulike symptoms (pallor, irritability, low-grade fever, vomiting and diarrhea, and abdominal pain). The acute phase is seen by the tenth day of illness. Other symptoms seen in the acute phase are hepatosplenomegaly, hypertension, and rarely cardiac failure.

NURSING DIAGNOSES/ DEFINING CHARACTERISTICS	NURSING INTERVENTIONS / *RATIONALES*	EXPECTED OUTCOMES
Impaired Gas Exchange **RELATED TO** Anemia (RBCs fragmented by fibrin are destroyed in liver/spleen) **DEFINING CHARACTERISTICS** Negative Coombs Decreased Hgb, increased reticulocytes Pallor/jaundice Hypoxia Hypoxemia Ischemia Tachypnea	**ONGOING ASSESSMENT** <ul><li>Assess age and developmental level.</li><li>Assess CBC, especially Hgb.</li><li>Assess WBC with differential.</li><li>Assess color, activity level.</li><li>Assess vital signs. *Heart and respiratory rates will increase in initial effort to prevent hypoxia, hypoxemia, ischemia, and tissue necrosis.*</li></ul> **THERAPEUTIC INTERVENTIONS** <ul><li>Apply cardiopulmonary monitor.</li><li>Maintain IV access.</li><li>Administer oxygen as ordered.</li><li>Transfuse packed RBCs.</li></ul>	Adequate gas exchange will be maintained.
Actual Injury: Bleeding **RELATED TO** RBC destruction Thrombocytopenia **DEFINING CHARACTERISTICS** Thrombocytopenic purpura Petechiae Ecchymoses Bloody diarrhea Rare: increased PT, PTT	**ONGOING ASSESSMENT** <ul><li>Assess skin surface for purpura, petechiae, and ecchymoses.</li><li>Inspect diarrhea for blood; *this is a fairly common occurrence and increases morbidity, especially in infants.*</li><li>Monitor vital signs for signs of shock.</li><li>Monitor neurological status; *central nervous system changes may be attributed to intracranial bleeding and can cause permanent damage.*</li></ul> **THERAPEUTIC INTERVENTIONS** <ul><li>Protect infant/child from trauma that may further precipitate bleeding.</li><li>Notify physician of overt blood loss.</li><li>Administer blood transfusion as ordered. (See Blood and blood product transfusion therapy, p. 389.)</li></ul>	Risk for injury related to bleeding will be reduced.

NURSING DIAGNOSES/ DEFINING CHARACTERISTICS	NURSING INTERVENTIONS / *RATIONALES*	EXPECTED OUTCOMES
Altered Urinary Elimination **RELATED TO** Impaired renal function RBC destruction and sequelae **DEFINING CHARACTERISTICS** Oliguria or anuria Increased BUN Increased serum creatinine Hypertension Proteinuria Hematuria	**ONGOING ASSESSMENT** • Monitor I&O. • Evaluate serum electrolytes, especially BUN and creatinine. • Monitor urine for protein and blood. • Monitor serial BP for signs of hypertension. **THERAPEUTIC INTERVENTIONS** • Notify physician of signs of renal insufficiency. • Prepare infant/child for peritoneal catheter placement and dialysis. *Peritoneal dialysis performed early in disease course improves prognosis. Although most children recover completely, at least 5% will have permanent renal impairment related to cortical necrosis/glomerular sclerosis.* • See Dialysis, p. 340 and Acute renal failure, p. 358.	Urinary elimination will be maintained.
Knowledge Deficit: Family **RELATED TO** New diagnosis Emergent procedure **DEFINING CHARACTERISTICS** Asks many questions or asks no questions Hesitant involvement Confused appearance	**ONGOING ASSESSMENT** • Assess family's understanding of current diagnosis and treatments. • Assess readiness to learn. • Assess child's developmental level and ability to understand. **THERAPEUTIC INTERVENTIONS** • Explain all treatments and procedures. • Explain at a time and in a manner most suited to learning. • Describe hemolytic uremic syndrome and causes. *Parent may feel guilt over lack of control.* • Teach parent and child about necessary home care: Medications BP measurement • Provide consultations and follow-up as needed.	Family will understand hemolytic uremic syndrome and its treatment.

Michele Knoll Puzas, RNC, MHPE

Hyperglycemic hyperosmotic nonketotic coma

DIABETIC COMA; NONKETOTIC HYPEROSMOLAR COMA

Hyperglycemic hyperosmotic nonketotic coma (HHNC) can be a complication of diabetes but may also result from hyperalimentation, dialysis, IV fluids, steroid therapy, diuretic administration, pancreatitis, diabetes insipidus, and severe burns. The severe hyperglycemia persists because of ineffective or inadequate insulin levels and results in osmotic diuresis and severe dehydration.

NURSING DIAGNOSES/ DEFINING CHARACTERISTICS	NURSING INTERVENTIONS / *RATIONALES*	EXPECTED OUTCOMES
Fluid Volume Deficit **RELATED TO** Hyperglycemia Osmotic diuresis **DEFINING CHARACTERISTICS** Increased urine output Sudden weight loss Hemoconcentration Increased BUN/creatinine Hypotension Thirst/dry skin and mucous membranes Poor skin turgor Decreased cardiac output Hypokalemia Hypernatremia Change in LOC Ventricular dysrhythmias	**ONGOING ASSESSMENT** • Assess age and developmental level. • Assess for defining characteristics. • Monitor electrolytes, glucose, I&O, weight, and central venous pressure. • Monitor vital signs, Hgb, Hct, serum osmolarity, BUN, creatinine *to determine hemoconcentration and renal clearance.* • Auscultate lungs for rhonchi, and rales that may result from circulatory overload related to aggressive fluid therapy. • Monitor cardiac function. **THERAPEUTIC INTERVENTIONS** • Administer isotonic IV fluids *to increase cardiac output and tissue perfusion along with correcting fluid imbalance.* • Administer insulin according to blood glucose levels. *Insulin therapy is essential to decrease serum glucose and osmolarity. This will allow extracellular fluid to shift to intracellular fluid, alleviating intracellular dehydration.* • Apply cardiopulmonary monitor.	Optimal fluid level will be maintained.

Altered Nutrition: Less Than Body Requirements **RELATED TO** Insulin deficiency Ineffective metabolism of available glucose **DEFINING CHARACTERISTICS** Weight loss Muscle weakness Hyperglycemia Abdominal pain	**ONGOING ASSESSMENT**
	• Monitor blood glucose levels.
	• Observe for abdominal pain. *Nausea and vomiting may result from fluid/electrolyte imbalance as well as ketonemia. Ketonemia is not necessarily present until later in disease course.*
	
	THERAPEUTIC INTERVENTIONS
	• Administer continuous low-dose insulin infusion. *Microinfusion will be necessary for small children/infants. Rapid infusion of insulin could result in hypoglycemia.*
	• Promote nutrition. *Once electrolyte and glucose imbalances are corrected, appetite will be restored.*
	  Provide fluids and progress diet as tolerated.
	  Obtain dietary consult if needed.
		Optimal nutrition will be maintained.

Hyperglycemic hyperosmotic nonketotic coma cont'd

NURSING DIAGNOSES/ DEFINING CHARACTERISTICS	NURSING INTERVENTIONS / *RATIONALES*	EXPECTED OUTCOMES

Altered LOC
RELATED TO
Dehydration
Electrolyte imbalance
 	
DEFINING CHARACTERISTICS
Change in orientation, verbal response, motor response, pupillary action
Agitation
Impaired judgment
Seizure activity
Positive Babinski's sign
	ONGOING ASSESSMENT
	• Monitor LOC. Maintain neurological flow sheet.
	• Monitor vital signs, fluid volume, and electrolyte balance.
	• Assess for potential for injury secondary to seizure activity.
	
	THERAPEUTIC INTERVENTIONS
	• Protect from injury caused by impaired neurological function.
	    Keep side rails up and bed in low position at all times.
	    Maintain oral airway.
	    Reorient child to surroundings as needed. *Child may be unaware of past events and limitations.*
	• Restore fluid volume. *As dehydration and hyperglycemia resolve, LOC will improve.*
	• Allow parent unlimited access. *Will enhance child's reorientation and ease parental fears.*
		Optimal LOC will be maintained.

Knowledge Deficit **RELATED TO** Cognitive limitations Lack of interest New condition **DEFINING CHARACTERISTICS** Verbalized interest, questions Statement of misconception Request for information	**ONGOING ASSESSMENT** • Assess for predisposing factors and most current cause. • If child has diabetes, assess level of knowledge and home care practices *to identify factors that interfere with health maintenance.* **THERAPEUTIC INTERVENTIONS** • Describe HHNC, its cause, and treatment. Explain all procedures. • If child is diabetic, review effective self-care practices and introduce new information/skills as necessary when child is stable. *Detailed instruction will be best received after critical stage is passed and parent is less stressed.*	Parent/child will understand current condition, treatment, and preventive measures.

Michele Knoll Puzas, RNC, MHPE

Hypertension

HIGH BLOOD PRESSURE; INCREASED SYSTEMIC
PRESSURE

Sustained elevation of arterial blood pressure above the normal upper limit of 140/90 mm Hg or 20 points above that considered normal for one's age. This care plan focuses on the child with mild to moderate hypertension.

NURSING DIAGNOSES/ DEFINING CHARACTERISTICS	NURSING INTERVENTIONS / *RATIONALES*	EXPECTED OUTCOMES
Decreased Cardiopulmonary, Renal, or Peripheral Tissue Perfusion **RELATED TO** Diminished blood flow caused by increased vascular resistance Hypervolemia **DEFINING CHARACTERISTICS** Tachypnea Labored respirations Adventitious breath sounds Angina, palpitation Urine output less than 30 ml/hr Increasing BUN/creatinine Hematuria or proteinuria Mental status changes Restlessness/agitation/apathy Cool, clammy skin Pallor, cyanosis Mottled skin Decreased/absent peripheral pulses	**ONGOING ASSESSMENT** • Assess age and developmental level. • Assess for evidence of decreased tissue perfusion, as outlined in defining characteristics, every 2-4 hours or more often as appropriate. • Assess vital signs every 2-4 hours or more often as appropriate. Use proper BP equipment with cuff bladder that is two-thirds limb diameter *to ensure more accurate measurements.* • Apply "normals for age" when assessing BP results. • Assess breath sounds and heart sounds every 4 hours to detect changes from baseline that indicate changes in cardiopulmonary status. • Assess and record I&O and daily weight. • Assess for peripheral edema (lower extremities, sacral area, periorbital). • Document findings and notify physician of untoward change(s). • Monitor and document effectiveness of medications. • Monitor for side effects of medications (e.g., hypokalemia, hypovolemia). **THERAPEUTIC INTERVENTIONS** • Implement measures to reduce vascular resistance and improve tissue perfusion: Give antihypertensive drugs, diuretics as ordered. Discourage intake of coffee, tea, colas, and chocolate that are high in caffeine. *Caffeine stimulates sympathetic nervous system.* Maintain physical and emotional rest. Administer sedative prn *to reduce stress and associated vasoconstriction.* Maintain fluid and dietary sodium restrictions *to reduce fluid retention, which contributes to hypertension.* • Ensure adequate fluid intake unless contraindicated. *Volume depletion enhances potency of antihypertensive drugs and will also reduce perfusion to kidneys. Volume depletion stimulates renin-angiotensin release, further complicating hypertension.*	Adequate tissue perfusion will be maintained or attained.
Knowledge Deficit **RELATED TO** Cognitive limitation Lack of interest Lack of information **DEFINING CHARACTERISTICS** Statement of misconceptions, knowledge gaps Request for information	**ONGOING ASSESSMENT** • Assess child's and family's level of knowledge regarding disease and prescribed management. • Assess readiness for learning. **THERAPEUTIC INTERVENTIONS** • Encourage questions about disease and prescribed treatments. • Involve family or significant others *so they can effectively provide support upon discharge.* • Plan teaching in stages considering child/family readiness. Provide information in terms that child and family can understand by using appropriate teaching aides in the following areas: Nature of disease and its effect on target organs (i.e., renal damage, visual impairment, heart failure, stroke) Risk factors (obesity, diet high in saturated fat and cholesterol, smoking, stress; race [more common in blacks]; family history) Rationale for weight reduction (if overweight) and low-salt diet Possible side effects of medications (Interaction with over-the-counter drugs such as cough and cold medicines, and aspirin compounds, *which have vasoconstricting effect*)	Understanding of disease and its long-term effects on target organs will be verbalized.

NURSING DIAGNOSES/ DEFINING CHARACTERISTICS	NURSING INTERVENTIONS / *RATIONALES*	EXPECTED OUTCOMES

THERAPEUTIC INTERVENTIONS cont'd

Encourage potassium-rich foods (e.g., fruit juices, bananas) as appropriate. *Most diuretics are potassium wasting. Be aware of any renal insufficiency that contraindicates K^+ supplements in acute phase.*

Teach relaxation techniques to combat stress, *which can influence physiological responses that aggravate hypertension.*

Role of physical exercise in weight reduction.

Safety measures to observe:

  Avoid sudden changes in position *to reduce severity of orthostatic hypotension.*

  Avoid hot tubs and saunas, *which cause vasodilation and potential hypotension.*

  Avoid prolonged standing, *which can cause venous pooling.*

Signs and symptoms to report to physician:

  Chest pain

  Shortness of breath

  Edema

  Weight gain

  Nosebleeds

  Changes in vision

  Headaches, dizziness

  Lethargy

  Increased crying/irritability

  Increased vomiting

  Changes in activity/disposition *(small children may not be able to verbally express)*

- Instruct child (age appropriate)/family to take own blood pressure *to provide child with sense of control and ability to seek prompt medical attention.*
- Assist in establishing medication routine considering child's school and sleep habits. *This will minimize chance of error and potentiate better compliance with therapy.* Involve school nurses if necessary.
- Provide information about community resources and support groups *that can assist and support child/family in changing life-style* (e.g., American Heart Association, weight loss programs, stop smoking programs).

Altered Nutrition: More Than Body Requirement RELATED TO

Excessive intake in relation to metabolic needs, resulting in overweight or obesity

High sodium intake, which promotes fluid retention, weight gain, and hypertension

DEFINING CHARACTERISTICS

Overweight (10% over ideal weight for age, height, and frame)

ONGOING ASSESSMENT

- Assess child and family attitudes toward food and salt.
- Assess child's need for psychological support in his/her effort to reduce weight and/or sodium intake.
- Weigh daily and record. Notify physician of weight gain.

THERAPEUTIC INTERVENTIONS

- Implement prescribed reducing, no-added-salt diet. *Excess caloric and sodium intake result in obesity and fluid retention, respectively. Both predispose to hypertension and subsequent complications.*
- Communicate with dietitian regarding child's likes and dislikes and cultural preferences.
- Support and reinforce child's effort to adhere to prescribed diet.
- Involve entire family in diet. *Restrictions are usually good for all members. This increases compliance of child.*
- Instruct on and encourage low-fat and cholesterol diet. *Important in children also. Cholesterol level >150 mg/dl in children considered at risk. It predisposes to cardiovascular disease and complications, which may include hypertension.*

Entire family will adopt healthier life-style and eating habits and maintain ideal body weight.

Continued.

Hypertension cont'd

NURSING DIAGNOSES/ DEFINING CHARACTERISTICS	NURSING INTERVENTIONS / *RATIONALES*	EXPECTED OUTCOMES
DEFINING CHARACTERISTICS cont'd Obesity (20% over ideal weight for age, height, and frame) Edema Weight gain		
Pain: Headache and Dizziness **RELATED TO** Headache caused by increased arterial vascular pressure, which causes arterioles to dilate and exert pressure on surrounding tissues Dizziness caused by hypotensive state related to drug therapy **DEFINING CHARACTERISTICS** Complaints of occipital headache, usually on waking Restlessness or irritability; crying, whimpering Facial mask of discomfort Complaints of dizziness or lightheadedness	**ONGOING ASSESSMENT** ▪ Assess for nonverbal signs of discomfort. ▪ Assess occurrence, quality, severity, and location of headache. ▪ Assess precipitating and relieving factors. **THERAPEUTIC INTERVENTIONS** ▪ Administer analgesics as ordered. Child may also need sedative or tranquilizer as adjunct *to reduce stress and discomfort.* ▪ Minimize environmental stimuli. Restrict visitors if necessary. *Stress and anxiety can increase the perception of pain and discomfort. Allow parent to help care for and comfort child if desired; helps relieve child's anxiety and fear.* ▪ Encourage relaxation techniques (deep breathing exercise, imagery, etc.). ▪ Assist with ambulation if necessary *to prevent child from falling if dizziness occurs. Dizziness is associated with both hypertension and hypotension secondary to drug therapy.* ▪ Elevate head of bed 30 degrees to minimize changes in position *that can trigger dizziness or lightheadedness.* ▪ Change position slowly. Sit before standing up from a lying position *to allow the body to adapt to redistribution of blood.* ▪ Allow child to have "familiar items" such as blanket, doll, teddy bear, etc. from home. ▪ Include child in self-care as much as possible *(helps to reduce fear and gain cooperation).*	Maximum level of comfort will be maintained.
Noncompliance **RELATED TO** Financial constraints Difficulty in making life-style changes Lack of knowledge Negative side effects of prescribed treatment	**ONGOING ASSESSMENT** ▪ Assess child's life-style and habits. ▪ Assess child's willingness to be compliant. ▪ Assess previous patterns of compliant/noncompliant behavior. **THERAPEUTIC INTERVENTIONS** ▪ If noncompliance is problem, determine cause; *this will dictate appropriate method of intervention.* If knowledge deficit, see Knowledge deficit, p. 352. If financial constraints, refer parents to social services department. If negative side effects of prescribed treatment, explain that many side effects can be controlled or eliminated. If lack of adequate support in changing life-style, initiate referral to support group (e.g., American Heart Association, weight loss programs, stress management classes, social services).	Optimal compliance with treatment will be achieved.

Hypertension cont'd

NURSING DIAGNOSES/ DEFINING CHARACTERISTICS	NURSING INTERVENTIONS / *RATIONALES*	EXPECTED OUTCOMES
DEFINING CHARACTERISTICS Verbalized noncompliance Elevated BP Evidence of development of complications (i.e., renal failure, visual impairment, heart failure, stroke) Evidence of exacerbation of symptoms (i.e., hypertensive crisis) Failure to keep appointments	**THERAPEUTIC INTERVENTIONS cont'd** • Instruct child (as age appropriate) to take own blood pressure, *which will provide immediate feedback and a sense of control.* • Reinforce compliant behavior *to promote future compliance.* • Include family in explanations and teaching, *to encourage their support and assistance in child's compliance.* • Include child in self-care as much as possible. *This enhances cooperation with treatment, thus compliance.*	

Wilma J. Hunter, RN, MS, CPNP, CNN

Nephrotic syndrome

GLOMERULAR NEPHRITIS; NEPHROSIS; RENAL INSUFFICIENCY

Nephrotic syndrome refers to a group of symptoms (edema, proteinuria, hypoalbuminemia, hyperlipidemia) that result from the dumping of plasma proteins into the urine. This occurs when the glomerular capillary membrane becomes excessively permeable after membrane damage/injury. These symptoms may or may not become chronic, depending on cause.

NURSING DIAGNOSES/ DEFINING CHARACTERISTICS	NURSING INTERVENTIONS / *RATIONALES*	EXPECTED OUTCOMES

Actual Injury: Glomerular Capillary Membrane
RELATED TO
Glomerulonephritis (antigen-antibody reaction):
  Diabetes mellitus
  Systemic lupus erythematosus
  Renal vein thrombosis
  Nephrotoxins
  Congenital
  Idiopathic
 	
DEFINING CHARACTERISTICS
Severe proteinuria
Hypoalbuminemia
Hyperlipidemia
Edema
	ONGOING ASSESSMENT
	• Assess age and developmental level.
	• Obtain historical data that may help in identifying cause (i.e., medications, drug use, recent illness, hereditary illness).
	• Collect urinary specimens for renal function tests.
	• Assess lab results:
	  Serum albumin, triglycerides
	  Urinary protein, WBCs, RBCs
	
	THERAPEUTIC INTERVENTIONS
	• Administer steroids (*used to treat antigen-antibody and inflammatory reactions and decrease edema and protein loss*).
	• Prepare for needle biopsy of kidney. *This is necessary for definitive diagnosis.*
		Effects of injury will be reduced.

Continued.

355

Nephrotic syndrome cont'd

NURSING DIAGNOSES/ DEFINING CHARACTERISTICS	NURSING INTERVENTIONS / *RATIONALES*	EXPECTED OUTCOMES
Fluid Volume Excess **RELATED TO** Decreased renal filtering capacity Fluid loss into interstitial spaces **DEFINING CHARACTERISTICS** Total body edema Low BP Puffy eyelids Elevated BUN and creatinine levels Abnormal electrolytes Decreased Hgb and Hct	**ONGOING ASSESSMENT** • Monitor temperature, pulse, respirations, and postural BP. • Monitor I&O. • Obtain weight; compare with estimated dry weight. • Check urine specific gravity and dipstick for protein, blood, pH. • Measure abdominal girth every day. • Assess for edema. • Monitor lab work: Hgb Hct Electrolytes BUN/creatinine • Assess for signs of anemia: Stools for blood Pallor • Assess for signs of shock. **THERAPEUTIC INTERVENTIONS** • Limit IV and oral fluid intake as prescribed. Use electronic IV infusion device *for accuracy.* Limit free water oral intake *to allow increased intake of nutritious fluids with or between meals.* Provide child's medication with fluids other than water. • Administer electrolytes as ordered. • Administer salt-poor albumin and diuretics as ordered. *Albumin causes shift of fluids into vascular system, enhancing the diuretic effects.*	Optimal fluid balance will be achieved.
High Risk for Impaired Skin Integrity **RELATED TO** Tissue edema **DEFINING CHARACTERISTICS** Poor skin turgor Skin tautness over bony areas Redness over bony areas Taut, shiny, thin skin at points of edema	**ONGOING ASSESSMENT** • Assess dependent areas for skin breakdown. • Assess for pitting edema. • Observe open wounds for proper healing. **THERAPEUTIC INTERVENTIONS** • Change child's position frequently if immobile. • Use pillows for support when positioning *to relieve pressure areas and prevent tissue breakdown.* • Keep skin clean and dry. • Avoid tight clothing. • Elevate edematous extremities. • Provide pressure-relieving devices *as prophylactic measures.*	Optimal skin integrity will be maintained.
Altered Nutrition: Less Than Body Requirements **RELATED TO** Impaired renal function and protein loss Poor appetite	**ONGOING ASSESSMENT** • Monitor food intake. • Monitor proteinuria. • Perform calorie count if needed.	Adequate dietary requirements will be maintained.

NURSING DIAGNOSES/ DEFINING CHARACTERISTICS	NURSING INTERVENTIONS / *RATIONALES*	EXPECTED OUTCOMES

DEFINING CHARACTERISTICS
 Low serum protein
 Proteinuria
 Muscle wasting
 Weight loss
	THERAPEUTIC INTERVENTIONS
	 • Obtain dietary consultation.
	 • Administer vitamin supplements.
	 • Offer small, frequent meals of preferred foods; allow parent to bring favored foods from home if desired.
	 • Provide diet:
	   High in protein, calories (CHO), and potassium
	   Low in sodium, fat. *Protein is required for tissue growth, carbohydrates to spare protein and for energy. Potassium is needed because of high loss with interstitial fluid shift and diuresis.*
	 • Consider tube feeding supplements and/or TPN if child's condition warrants.	

High Risk for Infection **RELATED TO** Immunosuppression of steroid therapy **DEFINING CHARACTERISTICS** Elevated temperature Elevated WBC Malaise Signs and symptoms of infection without fever	**ONGOING ASSESSMENT** • Assess for signs of infection. • Assess vital signs, especially temperature. • Observe visitors for any obvious symptoms of infection. • Assess status of immunization. **THERAPEUTIC INTERVENTIONS** • Screen roommates or consider private room. • Limit visitors and staff contact. • Report signs of infection immediately *to ensure prompt treatment and prevent exacerbation of renal symptoms.*	Risk of infection will be reduced.

Knowledge Deficit
 RELATED TO
 New diagnosis
 Chronicity of disease
 Long-term medical management
 	
 DEFINING CHARACTERISTICS
 Lack of questions
 Overly anxious
 Inability to talk about present status
	ONGOING ASSESSMENT
	 • Assess parent's and child's knowledge base and readiness for learning.
	 • Assess support system and ability to provide home/self-care.
	
	 THERAPEUTIC INTERVENTIONS
	 • Explain nephrotic syndrome, all tests, and procedures.
	 • Instruct to observe for increased edema by:
	   Daily weights
	   Periorbital edema
	   Abdominal distention
	   Ankle edema
	 • Provide instruction:
	   On use of dipsticks for protein
	   On signs of infection
	   On dietary needs/restrictions
	   On medication therapy
	 • Provide follow-up appointments and encourage compliance.
		Parent and child will understand disease process and follow-up care.

Kathy Alexander, RN; Michele Knoll Puzas, RNC, MHPE

Renal failure: acute

ATN; ACUTE TUBULAR NECROSIS; RENAL
INSUFFICIENCY; HEMODIALYSIS; PERITONEAL
DIALYSIS; VASCULAR ACCESSES

In acute renal failure, the kidneys are incapable of clearing metabolic waste products from the blood. This may occur as a single acute event with return of normal renal function, or result in chronic renal insufficiency or chronic renal failure. During the period of loss of renal function, hemodialysis or peritoneal dialysis is used to clear the accumulated toxins from the blood. Renal failure can be divided into three major types: prerenal failure (resulting from a decrease in renal blood flow), postrenal failure (caused by an obstruction), and intrarenal failure (caused by a problem within the vascular system, the glomeruli, the interstitium, or the tubules). "Hospital-acquired" renal failure is most likely acute tubular necrosis (ATN), which can result from nephrotoxins or an ischemic episode.

NURSING DIAGNOSES/ DEFINING CHARACTERISTICS	NURSING INTERVENTIONS / *RATIONALES*	EXPECTED OUTCOMES
Altered Patterns of Urinary Elimination **RELATED TO** Severe renal ischemia secondary to sepsis, shock, or severe hypovolemia with hypotension (usually after surgery or trauma) Nephrotoxic drugs or antibiotics (such as amphotericin and gentamicin) Renal vascular occlusion Hemolytic blood transfusion reaction **DEFINING CHARACTERISTICS** Increased BUN and creatinine Urine specific gravity fixed at or near 1.010 Hematuria, proteinuria Urine output <400 ml/24 hr (in absence of inadequate fluid intake or fluid losses by another route)	**ONGOING ASSESSMENT** • Assess age and developmental level. • Assess for alteration in urinary elimination. • Monitor and record I&O every hour. Include all fluid losses such as stool, emesis, and wound drainage. • Monitor urine specific gravity; check for protein and blood every 4 hours. • Palpate bladder for distention. • Assess for patency of Foley catheter (if present). • Notify physician of urine output <30 ml/hr. • Monitor blood and urine chemistry as ordered: Electrolytes (Na, K⁺, Cl, Ca, P, Mg) BUN, creatinine Urinalysis, urine electrolytes (notify physician of abnormalities). *Smaller incremental changes in children are often more significant than in adults; normal creatinine levels in children are age-related and differ from adult values. Normal phosphorus levels: 4.0-7 <10 yrs. 3.0-5 >10 yrs.* • Obtain daily weights. **THERAPEUTIC INTERVENTIONS** • Administer fluids and diuretics as ordered; document child's response. • Maintain patency of Foley catheter. If urine output decreases, irrigate Foley catheter with sterile saline solution *to ensure patency.* • When administering medications metabolized by the kidneys (such as antibiotics), remember that excretion of these drugs may be altered. Dosages, frequency, or both may require adjustment.	Optimal urine elimination will be maintained.
Excess Fluid Volume **RELATED TO** Inability of body to properly excrete fluid and electrolytes	**ONGOING ASSESSMENT** • Assess for signs of circulatory overload, congestive heart failure, and pulmonary congestion. • Monitor heart rate, BP, CVP, and respiratory rate. *Edematous patients may actually be intravascularly depleted; similarly, when fluids begin to shift, overload can occur quickly, requiring management adjustments.* • Monitor and record I&O. Include all stools, emesis, and drainage. • Weigh child daily (before and after dialysis), and record.	Optimal fluid balance will be maintained.

NURSING DIAGNOSES/ DEFINING CHARACTERISTICS	NURSING INTERVENTIONS / *RATIONALES*	EXPECTED OUTCOMES

Excess Fluid Volume cont'd

Excessive administration of oral/IV fluids during periods of decreased renal function

DEFINING CHARACTERISTICS

Increased central venous pressure (CVP) and BP

Acute weight gain, edema

Signs and symptoms of congestive heart failure (jugular vein distention, rales)

Shortness of breath, dyspnea

Pericarditis, friction rub

ONGOING ASSESSMENT cont'd

- Auscultate breath sounds and heart sounds. Notify physician of any abnormalities.
- Monitor laboratory work (such as serum electrolytes and osmolality) as ordered.

THERAPEUTIC INTERVENTIONS

- Administer oral and IV fluids per physician's orders *to replace sensible and insensible losses.* NOTE: *Not all patients enter oliguria phase of renal failure. If urine output remains high, volume replacement can be considerable.*
- Administer medications (such as diuretics) per physician's orders; document response.
- Prepare child for hemodialysis, ultrafiltration, or peritoneal dialysis if indicated, *to clear body of excess fluid and waste products. Even when child reaches diuretic phase of renal failure, dialysis will still be needed to clear solutes.*
- If peripheral edema present, handle extremities/move child gently *to prevent shearing.*
- Administer IV medications in least amount of fluid possible *to minimize fluid intake during periods of decreased renal function with fluid overload.*

High Risk for Decreased Cardiac Output

RELATED TO

Dysrhythmias caused by electrolyte imbalance from acute renal failure:

Primary hyperkalemia:

Decreased renal elimination of electrolytes: K^+, P, Mg, Na

Metabolic acidosis (present with acute renal failure) exacerbates hyperkalemia by causing cellular shift of H^+ and K^+

Excess H ions traded intracellularly with K ions, causing increased extracellular K^+

Hyponatremia results from excessive extracellular fluid (dilutional effect), edema, and restricted IV or dietary intake

ONGOING ASSESSMENT

- Assess for signs of decreased cardiac output and electrolyte disturbances.
- Monitor vital signs. Notify physician of abnormalities.
- Monitor serum electrolytes as ordered.
- Monitor cardiac rhythm; notify physician of abnormalities.
- Determine child's hemodynamic response to arrhythmias.

THERAPEUTIC INTERVENTIONS

- Administer oral and IV fluids as ordered *to maintain optimal fluid balance;* note effects.
- Administer medications (such as sodium bicarbonate [$NaHCO_3$], calcium salts, glucose/insulin, K^+ exchange resins) per order *to equilibrate electrolyte disturbances temporarily.* Note child's response.
- Maintain hemodynamic parameters as indicated (heart rate, BP, CVP, urine output).
- Administer oxygen as needed.
- Provide calm environment with minimal stressors.
- Restrict activity to conserve oxygen.
- Prepare child for dialysis or ultrafiltration when indicated.
- See Cardiac output, decreased, p. 10.

Optimal cardiac output will be maintained.

Continued.

Renal failure: acute cont'd

NURSING DIAGNOSES/ DEFINING CHARACTERISTICS	NURSING INTERVENTIONS / *RATIONALES*	EXPECTED OUTCOMES

High Risk for Decreased Cardiac Output cont'd

Hypocalcemia can also occur, although exact cause is unknown

DEFINING CHARACTERISTICS

Decreased cardiac output:
Change in BP, heart rate, CVP, peripheral pulses
Decreased urine output
Abnormal heart sounds
Dysrhythmias
Anxiety/restlessness

Hyperkalemia
(K > 5.5 mEq/L)
ECG changes such as:
  Widened QRS complex, increased T waves
  Prolonged PR interval
  Bradycardia, dysrhythmias, cardiac arrest

Hyponatremia
(Na <115 mEq/L)
Nausea/vomiting
Lethargy, weakness
Seizures with severe deficit

Hypocalcemia
(Ca <6.0 mg/dl)
Perioral paresthesia
Twitching, tetany, seizures
Cardiac dysrhythmias

Ineffective Breathing Pattern
RELATED TO

Volume overload leading to congestive heart failure/left ventricular failure
Metabolic acidosis (caused by kidneys' inability to properly excrete hydrogen ions) leading to hyperventilation as compensatory mechanism

ONGOING ASSESSMENT

- Assess rate and depth of respirations every hour.
- Auscultate breath sounds; document findings. Notify physician if adventitious sounds are present.
- Monitor ABGs as ordered and as needed; notify physician of abnormal results.
- Monitor results of chest radiographs.

THERAPEUTIC INTERVENTIONS

- Encourage pulmonary toilet: turning, coughing, and deep breathing exercises every hour.
- Use tracheal suction as needed *to clear airway.*
- Maintain head of bed at angle at least 30 degrees *to promote lung expansion.*
- Administer oxygen as ordered.

Effective breathing pattern will be maintained.

Renal failure: acute cont'd

NURSING DIAGNOSES/ DEFINING CHARACTERISTICS	NURSING INTERVENTIONS / *RATIONALES*	EXPECTED OUTCOMES
DEFINING CHARACTERISTICS Shortness of breath Rales, wheezes Dyspnea Hyperventilation Orthopnea	**THERAPEUTIC INTERVENTIONS cont'd** • Administer medications (e.g., diuretics, bronchodilators) as ordered. • For further interventions/assessment, see Ineffective airway clearance, p. 3, and Ineffective breathing pattern, p. 8.	
Altered Nutrition: Less Than Body Requirements **RELATED TO** Stomatitis Anorexia, decreased appetite Nausea, vomiting Diarrhea Constipation Melena, hematemesis Dietary restrictions **DEFINING CHARACTERISTICS** Loss of weight Documented inadequate caloric intake Caloric intake inadequate to keep pace with abnormal disease/metabolic state	**ONGOING ASSESSMENT** • Assess for possible cause of child's decreased appetite or GI discomfort. • Assess actual oral intake; obtain calorie counts as necessary. • Monitor serum laboratory values (e.g., electrolytes, albumin level). • Record output of emesis and stools. Observe all stools/emesis for gross blood; test for occult blood (guaiac/Hematest). Report results to physician. • Assess weight gain pattern. • Obtain history of food likes and dislikes; include preferences in diet as much as possible. **THERAPEUTIC INTERVENTIONS** • Administer small frequent feedings as tolerated. • Consult dietitian *to assist in providing child with a low-potassium, high-carbohydrate diet as indicated.* • Administer enteral/parenteral feedings as ordered. • Provide frequent oral hygiene *to freshen mouth.* • Offer ice chips/hard candy if not contraindicated. • Offer antiemetics such as diphenhydramine (Benadryl) or dimenhydrinate (Dramamine) as ordered per physician. • See Altered nutrition: less than body requirements, p. 33. • Make meals look appetizing; try to eliminate other procedures at mealtime if possible and focus on eating.	Nutritional state will be maximized.
High Risk for Injury: Anemia **RELATED TO** Bone marrow suppression secondary to insufficient renal production of erythropoietic factor Increased hemolysis leading to decreased life span of red blood cells secondary to abnormal chemical environment in plasma Bleeding tendencies: Decreased platelets and defective cohesion of platelets Inhibition of certain clotting factors	**ONGOING ASSESSMENT** • Observe for signs of fatigue, pallor, bleeding from puncture sites and incisions, and bruising tendencies. Document accordingly. • Monitor laboratory work (Hgb, Hct, platelets, and coagulation studies) as ordered and report results. • Check for guaiac in all stools and emesis. Report results. • Observe for signs of fluid overload and adverse reactions during transfusion. **THERAPEUTIC INTERVENTIONS** • Administer oxygen as ordered *to maintain oxygenation.* • Administer blood transfusions as ordered. • If fluid overload is a problem after transfusion, administer diuretics. • Administer erythropoietin (recombinant human erythropoietin) as ordered *to decrease effects of anemia; greatly reduces need for frequent blood transfusions as near normal Hgb/Hct is maintained.*	Occurrence of anemia will be reduced.

NURSING DIAGNOSES/ DEFINING CHARACTERISTICS	NURSING INTERVENTIONS / *RATIONALES*	EXPECTED OUTCOMES
DEFINING CHARACTERISTICS Fatigue Pallor Dyspnea Hct <30% Prolonged PT/PTT Bleeding tendencies, especially from GI tract		

Actual or High Risk for Decreased Level of Consciousness
RELATED TO
Accumulation of toxic waste products of metabolism
Electrolyte imbalances
Hypoxia
 	
DEFINING CHARACTERISTICS
Decreased concentration
Apathy
Confusion
Lethargy leading to coma
Convulsions
Neuromuscular irritability
Asterixis
	ONGOING ASSESSMENT
	- Assess for alteration in LOC, muscular weakness, and irritability.
	- Document child's neurological status.
	- Check electrolyte/ABG results for abnormalities to determine cause of change in LOC.
	
	THERAPEUTIC INTERVENTIONS
	- Notify physician of any changes in child's LOC.
	- Reorient child to environment as needed.
	- Maintain bed in low position with side rails up at all times *for safety.*
	- Keep call light within easy reach of child.
	- Use seizure precautions for child with decreased LOC:
	    Keep side rails padded.
	    Keep oral airway apparatus at bedside at all times.
	- Prepare for dialysis as necessary *to decrease toxic waste products.*
	- See Decreased level of consciousness, p. 173.
		Optimal state of consciousness will be maintained.

High Risk for Systemic or Local Infection **RELATED TO** Debilitated state with poor nutrition Poor skin integrity and wound healing Use of indwelling catheters, subclavian lines, Foley catheters, ET tubes, etc.	**ONGOING ASSESSMENT** - Assess for potential sites of infection: urinary, pulmonary, wound, or IV line. - Monitor temperature every 4 hours. Notify physician of temperature >38° C (100.4° F). - Monitor WBC count. - Note signs of localized or systemic infection; report promptly. - If infection suspected, obtain specimens of blood, urine, sputum, etc., for culture and sensitivity as ordered.	Potential for systemic/local infection will be reduced.

NURSING DIAGNOSES/ DEFINING CHARACTERISTICS	NURSING INTERVENTIONS / *RATIONALES*	EXPECTED OUTCOMES
DEFINING CHARACTERISTICS Increased temperature Increased WBC count Local inflammation, redness, or abnormal drainage Positive culture results (blood, wound, sputum, or urine)	**THERAPEUTIC INTERVENTIONS** ▪ Provide scrupulous perineal and catheter care. ▪ Provide meticulous sksin care *to avoid skin breakdown over pressure areas.* ▪ Use aseptic technique when performing dressing changes, wound irrigations, catheter care, and suctioning. ▪ Avoid the use of indwelling catheters or IV lines whenever possible. ▪ If use of indwelling catheters or IV lines is mandatory, change them per unit/hospital policy. ▪ Protect child from exposure to other children with infection. ▪ If infection is present, administer antibiotics as ordered.	
Knowledge Deficit RELATED TO New condition New procedures **DEFINING CHARACTERISTICS** Multiple questions Lack of questions Request for information	**ONGOING ASSESSMENT** ▪ Assess current knowledge of illness by child/family. ▪ Encourage verbalization of feelings and questions. **THERAPEUTIC INTERVENTIONS** ▪ Discuss need for monitoring equipment and frequent assessments. ▪ Explain all tests and procedures *before* they occur. Use terms child/ parent can understand; be clear and direct. ▪ Explain purpose of fluid and dietary restrictions. ▪ Explain need for dialysis and what child should expect during procedure. ▪ Instruct child to perform deep breathing and coughing exercises *to promote lung expansion and clearing.* ▪ Involve child's family in care as much as possible (when appropriate). ▪ Encourage family conferences with members of health care team (e.g., physicians, nurses, rehabilitation personnel, social workers) as necessary. *This will facilitate family involvement in multidisciplinary planning.* ▪ Consult appropriate resource persons such as rehabilitation personnel, physicians, social workers, psychologists, clergy, occupational therapists, and clinical specialists as needed. ▪ Provide on-going teaching, clarification regarding illness process, tests, etc. *Many explanations may be required before child/family begins to comprehend all ramifications of related factors.*	Child and family will verbalize understanding of disease process and associated treatments.

Wilma J. Hunter, RN, MS, CPNP, CNN

Renal transplant: postoperative (cadaveric or living related)

Renal transplantation is the surgical implantation of a renal allograft from either a cadaveric or live donor into a child with end-stage renal failure. Most frequently, transplant candidates are on chronic hemodialysis or peritoneal dialysis, exhibiting symptoms of azotemia, anemia, fluid overload, and oliguria. After a successful operative course, the renal transplant recipient recovers in the intensive care unit or stepdown unit to monitor fluid shifts and vital signs.

NURSING DIAGNOSES/ DEFINING CHARACTERISTICS	NURSING INTERVENTIONS / *RATIONALES*	EXPECTED OUTCOMES
High Risk for Fluid Volume Deficit/ Excess **RELATED TO** Immediately after surgery from renal transplantation child may vacillate between fluid depletion and fluid overload within minutes Prolonged ischemic time causing acute tubular necrosis (ATN); child may experience diuresis several days after surgery Pulmonary edema **DEFINING CHARACTERISTICS** *Deficit:* Increased fluid output Polyuria Weight loss Dry mucous membranes Weakness Thirst *Excess:* Edema Weight gain Shortness of breath, orthopnea Intake greater than output Abnormal breath sounds: rales (crackles)	**ONGOING ASSESSMENT** ▪ Assess age and developmental level. ▪ Weigh daily. Use same scale if available *to avoid discrepancies in measuring device.* ▪ Monitor I&O hourly in pediatric ICU and every 4 hours on general unit. ▪ Note and document the presence of peripheral or sacral edema. ▪ Auscultate lungs every 4 hours to assess for rales (crackles). ▪ Assess skin turgor and hydration of mucous membranes. **THERAPEUTIC INTERVENTIONS** ▪ Replace fluids ml per ml plus 30 ml/hr *to account for insensible loss; or replace according to unit protocol. Replacement protocols may vary among institutions. Acute tubular necrosis (ATN) patients may have diuresis several days after surgery, exceeding 200-400 ml/hr. Living related transplant recipients have greater urine volumes early after surgery, which may exceed 400-600 ml/hr. Fluid replacement must match output so that child does not dehydrate.* ▪ Notify physician if urine output <30 ml/hr. ▪ Administer diuretics and restrict fluids as indicated. ▪ Encourage deep breathing, coughing, and turning *to prevent associated respiratory complication.* ▪ Begin progressive ambulation, as ordered, *to facilitate adequate tissue perfusion to edematous body areas.*	Fluid status will be maintained.
High Risk for Urinary Retention **RELATED TO** Blockage caused by clots.	**ONGOING ASSESSMENT** ▪ Obtain preoperative history of child's urination. *If child was oliguric, urinary bladder may be atrophied and/or reduced in size.* ▪ Assess urine for color, amount, sediment, and presence of clots in Foley bag. *Depending on volume of urine, bladder capacity, muscle tone, and degree of hematuria, an indwelling catheter will remain in place for 2-7 days.*	Urinary retention will be prevented.

Renal transplant: postoperative (cadaveric or living related) cont'd

NURSING DIAGNOSES/ DEFINING CHARACTERISTICS	NURSING INTERVENTIONS / *RATIONALES*	EXPECTED OUTCOMES
DEFINING CHARACTERISTICS Bladder distention Small, frequent voiding Absence of urine output Sensation of bladder fullness Dysuria	**ONGOING ASSESSMENT cont'd** ▪ Assess for abdominal/bladder distention resulting from clotted Foley catheter or urine leak. ▪ Keep accurate I&O every hour in ICU or every 4 hours on general unit. ▪ After discontinuing Foley catheter, assess for amount, color, clarity, sediment, and blood in voided urine. **THERAPEUTIC INTERVENTIONS** ▪ Maintain Foley catheter drainage, preventing kinks *which would obstruct flow.* ▪ If gross hematuria evident, strain urine for clots, notify transplant physician, and irrigate Foley catheter with physician approval. *Bleeding from anastomosis can result in clotted Foley catheter.* ▪ After discontinuing Foley catheter, ask child to void every 1-2 hours *to avoid urine retention and overdistention of urinary bladder. If bladder capacity significantly compromised, child will need to empty bladder more frequently. Full bladder causes additional strain on ureteral anastomosis.*	
High Risk for Local/Systemic Infection **RELATED TO** Immunosuppression with antirejection medications decreases circulating lymphocytes and decreases child's ability to fight infectious organisms **DEFINING CHARACTERISTICS** Fever Wound infection Upper respiratory infection Positive cultures	**ONGOING ASSESSMENT** ▪ Monitor temperature 1-3 times/day. ▪ Inspect wound twice daily for local erythema, purulent drainage, or dehiscence; notify transplant physician if any occurs. ▪ Culture wound for aerobic organisms if drainage is purulent, green, or foul-smelling. ▪ Culture urine if child is febrile, dysuric, or if urine turns cloudy. ▪ Monitor all culture reports. **THERAPEUTIC INTERVENTIONS** ▪ Wash hands before and after touching child. *Bacteria, viruses, fungi, and protozoa that are indigenous in nontransplant populations may be infectious in immunosuppressed transplant patient.* ▪ Care for child in private room *(patients do not require isolation).* ▪ Restrict visitors. ▪ Administer antibiotics as ordered. ▪ Teach child and family about avoiding infectious crowds, importance of good hygiene, and signs and symptoms of infection. *Family needs to understand increased risk of infection and importance of calling transplant physician if signs of infection occur.*	Risk for infection will be reduced.
Pain **RELATED TO** Incisional pain Ineffective analgesia Pain exacerbated by straining and early ambulation	**ONGOING ASSESSMENT** ▪ Assess for verbal and nonverbal pain symptoms. ▪ Observe and record vital sign changes indicative of increased pain. ▪ Assess effectiveness of prescribed analgesia. **THERAPEUTIC INTERVENTIONS** ▪ Reinforce relaxation techniques and changes in position *to alleviate incisional or muscular pain, thereby reducing need for narcotic analgesia* (as age appropriate). ▪ Calm infants and small children by holding, cuddling, music. ▪ Encourage child to splint abdominal incision *to reduce pain.* ▪ Titrate prescribed analgesia as needed. ▪ Premedicate child 20 minutes before ambulating, performing ADL, or large dressing changes *to minimize pain induced by movement.* ▪ Assist with ambulation and ADL until child can resume self-care. ▪ Teach parent methods to alleviate child's pain.	Pain will be relieved or reduced.

Continued.

Renal transplant: postoperative (cadaveric or living related) cont'd

NURSING DIAGNOSES/ DEFINING CHARACTERISTICS	NURSING INTERVENTIONS / *RATIONALES*	EXPECTED OUTCOMES
DEFINING CHARACTERISTICS Facial mask of pain Crying/moaning Complaints of pain Guarding behavior Diaphoresis BP and pulse rate change Change in respiratory rate Fussy/irritable (infant)		
Anxiety/Fear **RELATED TO** Change in health status: No longer on dialysis Threat of rejection or infection Fear of death, losing child **DEFINING CHARACTERISTICS** Apprehension Feelings of inadequacy Facial tension Restlessness Scared/frightened Worried	**ONGOING ASSESSMENT** ▪ Assess for signs of anxiety/fear. ▪ Assess child's and family's dependent/independent behaviors. ▪ Assess available support systems. ▪ Assess functional coping mechanisms. ▪ Assess child's ability to accept self-care responsibility. **THERAPEUTIC INTERVENTIONS** ▪ Allow child/family time to ventilate fears and anxiety. *After surgery, parent of transplant child must maintain child's health and cannot rely on dialysis staff. Independence is often frightening, especially with risk of rejection or infection.* ▪ Assist with identifying support systems available. ▪ Offer emotional support and consult social service staff if indicated. ▪ Set limits for regressive and aggressive behavior for patient (and possibly siblings) and assist parents *to maintain consistency.* ▪ Assist parent in dealing with child's anxiety/fear; assist with identifying ways to incorporate child into self-care.	Anxiety/fear will be reduced.
Knowledge Deficit **RELATED TO** New condition **DEFINING CHARACTERISTICS** Questioning Lack of questions Request for information Misconceptions	**ONGOING ASSESSMENT** ▪ Assess child's/family's readiness to discuss transplant surgery, postoperative course, and potential life-style changes. *Teaching begins before surgery. Children often do not understand impact of transplant until several months after surgery. For this reason, teaching begins during dialysis; staff proceeds gradually, taking into account child's learning style, education level, and readiness to learn.* ▪ Assess previous knowledge of transplant and clarify misconceptions. ▪ Identify learning needs.	The child/family will state an understanding of renal transplantation, including postoperative self-care techniques.

NURSING DIAGNOSES/ DEFINING CHARACTERISTICS	NURSING INTERVENTIONS / *RATIONALES*	EXPECTED OUTCOMES

THERAPEUTIC INTERVENTIONS

- Prepare and use visual aids and logs for record keeping (e.g., medication charts, I&O sheets, vital sign log).
- Develop and implement teaching plan to include following:
  Signs and symptoms of graft rejection
  Medication teaching:
  Instruct child to take medication *every day* for life.
  Immunosuppressive medications must be taken daily for as long as child has a kidney transplant, to prevent rejection.
  Instruct child to wear medical alert bracelet *to identify that he/she uses antirejection medications and is transplant patient.*
  Instruct and supervise self-administration of medications at bedside, *in preparation for self-administration at home.*
  Instruct child/parent on reasons for *all* medications, side effects, schedule, complications associated with medications, when to be concerned, and when to report to transplant/nephrology team (i.e., fine tremors associated with cyclosporine A; however, sudden increase may signal toxicity).
  Signs and symptoms of local and systemic infection. *Transplant recipients are at increased risk for developing infection because of immunosuppressive therapy.*
  Dietary restrictions, if any.
  Physical self-examination:
    24-hour I&O
    BP, pulse, temperature (twice daily)
    Daily weight
    Daily self-assessment for graft tenderness
- Instruct child/parent on appropriate course of action if rejection or infection is suspected.

Wilma J. Hunter, RN, MS, CPNP, CNN

Syndrome of inappropriate antidiuretic hormone

DILUTIONAL HYPONATREMIA; SIADH

Syndrome of inappropriate antidiuretic hormone (SIADH) is characterized by the continued synthesis and release of antidiuretic hormone (ADH) unrelated to plasma osmolarity; water retention and dilutional hyponatremia occur. Potential causes include head trauma, brain tumor, subarachnoid hemorrhage, and systemic cancer.

NURSING DIAGNOSES/ DEFINING CHARACTERISTICS	NURSING INTERVENTIONS / *RATIONALES*	EXPECTED OUTCOMES
Fluid Volume Excess **RELATED TO** Compromised endocrine regulatory mechanism Neurohypophyseal dysfunction Inappropriate ADH syndrome Excessive fluid intake Renal failure Steroid therapy **DEFINING CHARACTERISTICS** Intake greatly exceeding output Sudden weight gain Cellular edema Absence of peripheral edema Cerebral edema Water intoxication High specific gravity Serum hyponatremia Serum hypoosmolality Urine hypernatremia Urine hyperosmolality	**ONGOING ASSESSMENT** ▪ Assess age and developmental level. ▪ Carefully monitor I&O and urine specific gravity. ▪ Weigh daily. *A sudden weight gain of 2.2 lb can indicate retention of 1 L water. SIADH patients can retain 3-5 L.* ▪ Assess child for: Apprehension Confusion Muscle twitches Convulsions Nausea/vomiting Abdominal cramps ▪ Assess for signs of cerebral edema: Headache Decreased mental status Seizures Vomiting Bulging fontanels ▪ Check for fingerprint edema over sternum, reflecting cellular edema. *Water diffuses from hypoosmotic intravascular space to intracellular space.* ▪ Monitor for symptoms of increased ICP (e.g., slow bounding pulse, increased pulse pressure, irritability, lethargy, increased BP, vomiting). ▪ Raise head of bed and monitor neurological status every 1-2 hours. ▪ Monitor for symptoms of water intoxication (e.g., change in mentation, confusion, incoordination). *Brain cells are particularly sensitive to increased intracellular H_2O.* ▪ Monitor serum Na^+ and serum osmolality, urine Na^+, and urine osmolality, specific gravity. **THERAPEUTIC INTERVENTIONS** ▪ Restrict fluid to 30%-75% of maintenance requirements according to degree of hyponatremia and hypoosmolality present. ▪ Provide ice chips and frequent mouth care *to alleviate thirst.*	Fluid volume and serum sodium and osmolality will be within normal limits.
High Risk for Injury **RELATED TO** Change in mentation secondary to cerebral edema Seizure activity secondary to hyponatremia **DEFINING CHARACTERISTICS** Confusion Convulsions Lack of coordination	**ONGOING ASSESSMENT** ▪ Assess LOC, orientation, and mental status. ▪ Assess serum Na^+ levels *(normal is 135-145 mEq/L. When serum Na^+ level drops below 118, seizure activity may occur).* **THERAPEUTIC INTERVENTIONS** ▪ Maintain bed in low position, side rails up. Pad side rails. ▪ Maintain padded restraints as indicated. ▪ Provide assistance/supervision with ambulation. ▪ See Seizure activity, p. 200.	Risk for physical injury will be reduced.

NURSING DIAGNOSES/ DEFINING CHARACTERISTICS	NURSING INTERVENTIONS / *RATIONALES*	EXPECTED OUTCOMES
High Risk for Diarrhea **RELATED TO** Fluid volume excess Hyponatremia **DEFINING CHARACTERISTICS** Loose, watery stools Increased stool frequency Increased bowel sounds Urgency	**ONGOING ASSESSMENT** • Assess usual bowel habits and patterns. • Assess for deviations from normal. • Assess characteristics of stool (i.e., color, consistency, amount). • Assess bowel sounds. • Include number of stools on I&O record. • Assess for signs of dehydration (i.e., sunken fontanel, decreased weight, dry mucous membranes). • Observe and report skin condition. *Frequent diarrhea stools may lead to irritation and excoriation.* **THERAPEUTIC INTERVENTIONS** • Change infant's diapers frequently to assess for presence of diarrhea. • Administer medications as ordered and observe and report effectiveness. • See Diarrhea, p. 15.	Stools will be of normal color and consistency for age.
High Risk for Constipation **RELATED TO** Fluid restriction Decreased motility secondary to hyponatremia **DEFINING CHARACTERISTICS** Frequency and volume less than usual pattern Straining at stool Hard, formed stools	**ONGOING ASSESSMENT** • Assess usual bowel habits and patterns. • Assess for deviations from normal. • Assess characteristics of stool (i.e., color, consistency, amount). **THERAPEUTIC INTERVENTIONS** • Administer medications as ordered; observe and report effectiveness. • Provide adequate bulk in diet.	Normal bowel elimination will be achieved.
High Risk for Altered Thought Processes **RELATED TO** Severe hyponatremia **DEFINING CHARACTERISTICS** If serum Na^+ 115-120 mEq/L: Lethargy Personality changes If serum Na^+ <115 mEq/L: Loss of reflexes Coma	**ONGOING ASSESSMENT** • Monitor for changes in LOC and confusion every 2 hours. *This is an early neurological sign. Neurological signs in child with head injury may be related to hyponatremia.* • Assess serum Na^+ levels. • Monitor for disorientation, hostility, decreased deep tendon reflexes, drowsiness, lethargy, headache. **THERAPEUTIC INTERVENTIONS** • Administer hypertonic saline solution as ordered. • Reduce environmental stimuli that child may find confusing. • Explain reasons for altered thought processes to family.	Thought processes will return to normal.

Continued.

Syndrome of inappropriate antidiuretic hormone cont'd

NURSING DIAGNOSES/ DEFINING CHARACTERISTICS	NURSING INTERVENTIONS / *RATIONALES*	EXPECTED OUTCOMES
High Risk for Pain/ Discomfort **RELATED TO** Stomach cramps secondary to hyponatremia Increased thirst secondary to fluid restriction Headache secondary to cerebral edema **DEFINING CHARACTERISTICS** Verbal/nonverbal communication of pain or discomfort Diaphoresis BP/pulse rate increased Pupillary dilation Increased/decreased respirations	**ONGOING ASSESSMENT** • Assess characteristics of pain/discomfort: location, duration, quality, intensity. • Assess effective sources of relief for child's pain/discomfort. **THERAPEUTIC INTERVENTIONS** • Alleviate causes of discomfort: Continue measures to correct fluid volume excess and hyponatremia. Offer ice chips and frequent mouth care. *This will help to alleviate thirst.* • See Pain, p. 35.	Comfort will be obtained.
High Risk for Altered Nutrition: Less Than Body Requirements **RELATED TO** Anorexia Nausea Vomiting Abdominal cramps secondary to hyponatremia Diarrhea **DEFINING CHARACTERISTICS** Body weight 5%- 15% or more below ideal weight for height and frame Inadequate food intake	**ONGOING ASSESSMENT** • Assess nutritional intake. • Assess for nausea/vomiting/diarrhea. • Assess height/weight and dietary needs. • Assess usual dietary pattern. • Assess food preferences. **THERAPEUTIC INTERVENTIONS** • Provide food preferences within limits of prescribed diet. • If vomiting occurs, record amount and characteristics. • Refer to dietitian. *Collaboration increases effectiveness of dietary management.* • Administer medications as ordered. Observe and report effectiveness. • Assist child with eating. • See Altered nutrition, p. 33.	Adequate nutritional intake will be obtained.
High Risk for Impaired Skin Integrity **RELATED TO** Diarrhea Inadequate nutrition Altered neurological status/coma Inadequate access to bedpan or bathroom Use of diapers	**ONGOING ASSESSMENT** • Inspect skin every shift; document condition and changes. *Early detection and intervention may prevent progression of impaired skin integrity.* • Assess frequency of diarrhea, proximity to bedpan or bathroom, need for hygiene. • Assess other risks to child's skin integrity (e.g., immobility, urinary incontinence).	Skin integrity will be maintained.

NURSING DIAGNOSES/ DEFINING CHARACTERISTICS	NURSING INTERVENTIONS / *RATIONALES*	EXPECTED OUTCOMES
DEFINING CHARACTERISTICS Reddened skin Poor capillary refill Blisters Discomfort/pain Partial-thickness skin loss	**THERAPEUTIC INTERVENTIONS** • Provide easy access to bedpan or bathroom. • Provide hygiene after every episode of diarrhea. • Change position every 2 hours. • Change diapers frequently. • Apply skin-protecting ointments/sprays. *Provides a barrier between skin and diarrhea.* • See Impaired skin integrity, p. 39.	
Fear/Anxiety **RELATED TO** Fluid restrictions Changes in mentation GI symptoms Medications and treatments **DEFINING CHARACTERISTICS** Restlessness Increased questioning Withdrawal Excessive demands Tearfulness/crying	**ONGOING ASSESSMENT** • Assess child's level of fear/anxiety. • Assess parent's level of fear/anxiety. **THERAPEUTIC INTERVENTIONS** • Encourage child to verbalize feelings *to aid in assessment and allow child awareness of own feelings.* • Cuddle child/hold. • Decrease stimulation. • Encourage parental participation in child's care and use of coping mechanisms. *Child's fear/anxiety will be reduced if parent is also less anxious and able to attend to child's needs.*	Fear/anxiety will be reduced.
Knowledge Deficit **RELATED TO** New disease process/acute onset Unfamiliarity with medications and treatments **DEFINING CHARACTERISTICS** Request for information Verbalized misconceptions/misinterpretations	**ONGOING ASSESSMENT** • Assess family's level of knowledge of disease process. • Assess family's level of understanding of medications and treatments. **THERAPEUTIC INTERVENTIONS** • Explain child's condition/treatments in simple, brief terms to child/family. • Ask child/family to verbalize explanations of condition/treatments *to indicate any misconceptions or misinterpretations.* • Explain transient nature of disorder. • Provide frequent updates on child's condition/improvement.	Child/family will understand disease process and rationale for medications and treatments.

Kimberly P. Souder, RN, BSN

Glucose and calcium metabolism, altered

HYPOGLYCEMIA; HYPERGLYCEMIA; HYPOCALCEMIA

The neonate emerges from a uterine environment where glucose and calcium had been continuously provided and fetal plasma levels were regulated by placental exchange. The infant who is premature terminates this supply, making homeostasis of metabolism difficult to achieve because of the immature regulatory system.

NURSING DIAGNOSES/ DEFINING CHARACTERISTICS	NURSING INTERVENTIONS / *RATIONALES*	EXPECTED OUTCOMES
Altered Glucose Metabolism **RELATED TO** Intrauterine malnutrition resulting from prematurity, postmaturity or small-for-gestational age Increased use of blood glucose resulting from maternal toxemia, respiratory distress, hypothermia, or infant of diabetic mother Iatrogenic causes Inadequate glucose intake Sepsis Stress **DEFINING CHARACTERISTICS** *Hypoglycemia:* Chemstrip <40 mg/dl Jitteriness Lethargy Refusal to suck Hypotonia Apnea or cyanosis Hct >65 Abnormal eye movements Temperature instability *Hyperglycemia:* Jitteriness Glycosuria greater than trace Chemstrip >120 mg/dl Osmotic diuresis Dehydration	**ONGOING ASSESSMENT** • Assess for presence of defining characteristics: hypoglycemia/hyperglycemia. • Monitor Chemstrip every 15-30 minutes until stable. *Rapid vacillations in serial blood glucose levels make frequent monitoring essential to avoid compromising the neonate.* • Monitor urine pH and glucose every void. If urine glucose is >1+, notify physician. • Note amount of glucose present in IV fluid. • Monitor blood gases prn. • Check Hct *to evaluate possibility of hyperviscosity/polycythemia as underlying factor.* • Monitor CBC and blood cultures. *Hypoglycemia and hyperglycemia have been found to be associated with gram-negative rod infections.* • Monitor I&O closely. • Monitor weight daily. **THERAPEUTIC INTERVENTIONS** • Initiate early feeding if infant is at risk for hypoglycemia. • Administer or change IV dextrose fluids as ordered by physician, when Chemstrip is <20-40 mg/dl or >120 mg/dl. • Support with oxygen therapy as needed. *An infant who may be asphyxiated rapidly dissipates glycogen stores and resorts to anaerobic glycolysis as a major source of energy.* • Maintain neutral thermal environment. *Infant rapidly depletes glucose stores to increase heat production.* See Thermoregulation in the low-birth-weight infant, p. 379. • If polycythemia present, assist physician with partial exchange transfusion using fresh frozen plasma *to decrease blood viscosity associated with hypoglycemia.* • Maintain IV rate *to provide appropriate fluid and electrolyte requirements.*	Chemstrip level will be between 40-120 mg/dl.
Altered Calcium Metabolism: Hypocalcemia **RELATED TO** *Maternal causes:* Diabetes and toxemia Dietary deficiency of calcium Hyperparathyroidism	**ONGOING ASSESSMENT** • Assess for presence of defining characteristics. • Observe infant for jitteriness or irritability. • Monitor blood calcium levels daily. • Check magnesium and phosphorus levels if calcium level is not improved after 24 hours of calcium therapy. *Hypomagnesemia and hyperphosphatemia may precipitate hypocalcemia and should be suspected when clinical response to IV push calcium is not obtained.*	Calcium level will be stable at 8-10 mg/dl.

NURSING DIAGNOSES/ DEFINING CHARACTERISTICS	NURSING INTERVENTIONS / *RATIONALES*	EXPECTED OUTCOMES
Altered Calcium Metabolism: Hypocalcemia cont'd *Intrapartum causes:* Perinatal asphyxia Prematurity *Postnatal causes:* Hypoxia Shock Sepsis Metabolic acidosis treated with sodium bicarbonate Respiratory distress Administration of citrated blood **DEFINING CHARACTERISTICS** Irritability Jitteriness Seizures Cyanosis Feeding intolerance Calcium level <7 mg/dl	**THERAPEUTIC INTERVENTIONS** ▪ Notify physician if blood calcium level is <8.0 mg/dl. *Hypocalcemia is principal metabolic disorder that may produce seizures.* ▪ Ensure placement of umbilical vein catheter or umbilical artery catheter if needed for calcium infusion. ▪ Administer 10% calcium gluconate solution as ordered: Calculate dose: 200 mg/kg dose immediately, then 500 mg/kg/day maintenance. Infuse calcium slowly over 20 minutes. *Rapid infusion may cause bradycardia and cardiac standstill.* Do not infuse calcium with IV solutions containing sodium bicarbonate; *may lead to precipitates within the IV solutions.*	
High Risk for Injury RELATED TO Calcium administration **DEFINING CHARACTERISTICS** Calcium burn Bradycardia or other cardiac dysrhythmias	**ONGOING ASSESSMENT** ▪ Determine patency of IV catheter. ▪ Assess peripheral IV site for redness or blanching during infusion. ▪ Monitor heart rate during calcium infusion; observe for bradycardia. ▪ Observe IV line for presence of precipitant. **THERAPEUTIC INTERVENTIONS** ▪ Place infant on cardiac monitor *to detect bradycardia.* Immediately discontinue calcium administration if heart rate <100 bpm, notify physician. ▪ Discontinue peripheral IV line if redness or blanching occurs during calcium infusion. ▪ Stop infusion if precipitant is present.	Complications from calcium administration will be prevented.
Parental Knowledge Deficit RELATED TO Separation/hospitalization of infant Fear and anxiety over abruptness of illness **DEFINING CHARACTERISTICS** Anxiety Frequent questioning Repetitive questioning Lack of questions Inconsistent visitation patterns	**ONGOING ASSESSMENT** ▪ Assess parent's level of understanding and knowledge of child's condition. ▪ Assess parent's knowledge of procedures and equipment. **THERAPEUTIC INTERVENTIONS** ▪ Explain equipment and nursery routine *to provide parent with information to decrease anxiety.* ▪ Provide parent with unit booklet. ▪ Explain infant's condition specifically (i.e., change in neurological status and plan of care). ▪ Refer parent to physician and other professional resources for further questions as needed. ▪ See Parenting in special care nursery, p. 72.	Parent will be able to verbalize knowledge and understanding of infant's condition.

Digna S. Limjoco, RN

Infant of a diabetic mother

IDM

Maternal hyperglycemia causes fetal hyperinsulinism with subsequent neonatal hypoglycemia in response to the withdrawal of maternal glucose supply. Other associated problems include respiratory distress, hypocalcemia, polycythemia, hyperbilirubinemia, birth trauma secondary to macrosomia, and multiple congenital anomalies.

NURSING DIAGNOSES/ DEFINING CHARACTERISTICS	NURSING INTERVENTIONS / *RATIONALES*	EXPECTED OUTCOMES

High Risk for Impaired Gas Exchange

RELATED TO

Increased risk of insufficient pulmonary surfactant

DEFINING CHARACTERISTICS

Expiratory grunting

Difficult inspirations with substernal/intercostal retractions

Tachypnea

Nasal flaring

Cyanosis

Irritability with "complaining" cry and hoarseness

Brief inspiratory effort with prolonged expiration

Fine crackling rales

Apnea

Respiratory and/or metabolic acidosis

Hypoxemia

Decreased breath sounds

Asymmetrical chest expansion

ONGOING ASSESSMENT

- Determine gestational age *to assess newborn for potential problems common to large-for-gestational-age infant (i.e., respiratory distress secondary to prematurity).*
- Assess abnormal breathing patterns:
  Periodic breathing
  Apnea
  Tachypnea
  Grunting, nasal flaring, retractions
- Assess respiratory pattern, quality of breath sounds, and chest excursion.
- Assess changes in acid-base status.
- Monitor blood gases every 2-6 hours and prn.
- Check oximeter readings every 2 hours and prn.

THERAPEUTIC INTERVENTIONS

- Suction secretions *to maintain open airway.*
- Initiate oxygen therapy as ordered.
- Position infant on side or abdomen, with neck slightly hyperextended *to promote gas exchange.*
- Assist in weaning from oxygen or ventilatory support as per established guidelines.
- Minimize handling *to prevent further irritability.*

Potential for impaired gas exchange will be reduced.

High Risk for Injury

RELATED TO

Transient hyperinsulinism

Depleted glucose stores

DEFINING CHARACTERISTICS

Rapid decline in glucose concentration in first 1½ to 2 hours

Glucose concentration <30 mg/dl in first 6 hours of life

ONGOING ASSESSMENT

- Assess:
  Maternal history
  Respiratory status
  Motor function
  Neurological status
  Vital signs
- Monitor glucose levels closely for the first 24-48 hours:
  Obtain baseline blood glucose and Chemstrip.
  Check Chemstrips every hour for first 6-8 hours, then every 4 hours for next 24 hours until stable at 80-120 mg/dl.
- Check serum glucose if Chemstrip is <40 mg/dl in first 72 hours of life.
- Check urine for acetone, reducing substances, and specific gravity every 2-4 hours.

Potential for hypoglycemia and its related sequela will be reduced.

NURSING DIAGNOSES/ DEFINING CHARACTERISTICS	NURSING INTERVENTIONS / *RATIONALES*	EXPECTED OUTCOMES

DEFINING CHARACTERISTICS cont'd
 	
Transient phase after birth, characterized by fluctuations in glucose levels, lasting 1 to 4 hours
Prolonged initial phase of hypoglycemia; <25 mg/dl associated with:
  Apnea
  Tachypnea
  Cyanosis
  Pallor
  Diaphoresis
  Jitteriness
  Limpness/
    listlessness
  Failure to suck
  Absent Moro reflex
  Convulsions
  Coma
	THERAPEUTIC INTERVENTIONS
	▪ Provide early enteral feedings if condition allows or start IV of $D_{10}W$ *to provide adequate caloric intake and maintain blood sugar.*
	▪ Provide neutral thermal environment *to reduce stress and to provide for minimal heat loss and energy expenditure.*
	▪ Notify physician if Chemstrip <25 mg/dl.
	▪ Notify physician of any significant changes in vital signs or level of responsiveness. *This may be indicative of hypoglycemia.*
	▪ See Glucose and calcium metabolism, altered, p. 372.	

High Risk for Injury
RELATED TO
Depressed fetal parathyroid function
Maternal causes:
Diabetes and toxemia
Dietary deficiency of calcium
Hyperparathyroidism
 	
DEFINING CHARACTERISTICS
Calcium level ≤7 mg/dl
Irritability
Jitteriness
Cyanosis
Seizures
	ONGOING ASSESSMENT
	▪ Assess for presence of defining characteristics.
	▪ Monitor blood calcium levels daily.
	▪ Check magnesium and phosphorous levels if calcium level is not improved after 24 hours of calcium therapy. *Hyperphosphatemia may precipitate hypocalcemia and should be suspected when clinical response to IV calcium maintenance is not obtained.*
	
	THERAPEUTIC INTERVENTIONS
	▪ Notify resident if blood calcium level is <7.0 mg/dl. *Hypocalcemia is principal metabolic disorder, which may produce seizures.*
	▪ Ensure placement of umbilical vein catheter or umbilical artery catheter if needed for calcium infusion *to prevent ischemic compromise.*
	▪ Place infant on cardiac monitor *to detect bradycardia.*
	▪ Administer 10% calcium gluconate solution as ordered:
	  Calculate dose: 200 mg/kg dose immediately, then 500 mg/kg/day maintenance.
	  Infuse calcium slowly over 20 minutes; may use autosyringe if available. *Rapid infusion may cause bradycardia and cardiac standstill.*
	  Do not infuse calcium with IV solutions containing sodium bicarbonate, *which may lead to precipitates within intravenous solutions.*
		Calcium level will be stable at 8-10 mg/dl.

High Risk for Injury **RELATED TO** Polycythemia Hyperviscosity Increased erythropoiesis	**ONGOING ASSESSMENT** ▪ Assess infant for complications of hyperviscosity, based on defining characteristics. ▪ Review maternal/fetal history. ▪ Obtain baseline central venous Hct. ▪ If partial exchange transfusion is necessary, check Hct 3 to 4 hours after its completion. ▪ Assess urine specific gravity and dipstick with each void. ▪ Maintain accurate intake and output.	Potential risks of hyperviscosity syndrome will be reduced.

Continued.

Infant of a diabetic mother cont'd

NURSING DIAGNOSES/ DEFINING CHARACTERISTICS	NURSING INTERVENTIONS / *RATIONALES*	EXPECTED OUTCOMES
High Risk for Injury cont'd Enhanced placental transfusion at delivery Fetal hypoxia Decreased extracellular volume Maternal osmotic diuresis related to hyperglycemia Transient dehydration in the first days of life **DEFINING CHARACTERISTICS** Central venous Hct >65% Plethora Tachypnea Capillary refill over 3 seconds Acrocyanosis/cyanosis Lethargy Vomiting Jaundice, increased bilirubin Respiratory distress Congestive heart failure Convulsions Hypotension Decreased urine output Increased urine specific gravity	**THERAPEUTIC INTERVENTIONS** • Notify physician if central venous Hct >65%. • Maintain parenteral/enteral fluids as ordered. *This will decrease hyperviscosity of blood.* • Assist with partial exchange transfusion per protocol *to reduce Hct between 50% and 55%.* • Notify physician if urine dipstick is positive for hematuria; *may be indicative of renal vein thrombosis.*	
High Risk for Injury: Altered Metabolism of Bilirubin **RELATED TO** Increased likelihood of bruising or development of cephalohematomas related to infant's larger size Polycythemia **DEFINING CHARACTERISTICS** Serum bilirubin >15 mg/dl Jaundice NPO status Hct >65 mg/dl	**ONGOING ASSESSMENT** • Assess presence and extent of hematomas and bruising. • Note skin color/sclera. • Send baseline fractionated serum bilirubin at 18 hours of age. Obtain fractionated bilirubin every 4 hours if bilirubin rise is >0.5-1.0 mg/hr and close to exchange level. Otherwise, obtain serum bilirubin every 12 hours. • Check Hct every 6 hours. • Check serum solute every 12 hours. • Maintain accurate I&O. • Record specific gravity every void *to determine early signs of dehydration.* **THERAPEUTIC INTERVENTIONS** • Initiate phototherapy as ordered. • Provide early feedings as tolerated to stimulate peristalsis/stooling *to enhance bilirubin excretion via gut. Meconium contains large amounts of bilirubin.* • Record stooling pattern. Perform rectal stimulation if no stool for 2-3 days *to promote stooling and bilirubin excretion.*	Risk for kernicterus will be reduced.

NURSING DIAGNOSES/ DEFINING CHARACTERISTICS	NURSING INTERVENTIONS / *RATIONALES*	EXPECTED OUTCOMES

THERAPEUTIC INTERVENTIONS cont'd
- Provide good skin care *to promote skin integrity.*
- Observe for signs/symptoms of encephalopathy. *This may indicate ker-nicterus:*

  Early signs are:
  Poor feeding
  Vomiting
  Lethargy
  High-pitched cry
  Hypotonia
  Decreased Moro reflex
  Late signs are:
  Opisthotonos posturing
  Apnea
  Irritability
  Seizures
- Assist with exchange transfusion as needed.

High Risk for Congenital Abnormalities

RELATED TO

Diabetic mother
Prematurity
Cesarean section

DEFINING CHARACTERISTICS

Cardiorespiratory dis-orders:
Apnea
Bradycardia
Birth injury:
Shoulder dystocia
Fractures of clavicle or humerus
Erb's palsy
Phrenic nerve palsy
Macrosomia
Cardiac defects:
Transposition of great vessels
Ventricular septal defect
Atrial septal defect
Renal defects:
Agenesis
Decreased urine output
Gastrointestinal defects:
Small left colon syndrome
Neurological defects:
Anencephaly
Meningocele syndrome
Skeletal defects:
Caudal regression syndrome
Hemivertebral

ONGOING ASSESSMENT
- Assess infant for congenital anomalies per defining characteristics.
- Assess maternal history for tight control of glucose levels during preg-nancy, particularly during first trimester.
- Assess heart sounds, pulses, and capillary refill.
- Assess for decreased or asymmetrical movement.
- Assess for lower extremity anomalies, *which are known as caudal regression syndrome, specific to infants of diabetic mothers.*

THERAPEUTIC INTERVENTIONS
- Notify physician of any deviations from normal physical findings. *Con-genital anomalies are 2 to 4 times more frequent among infants of dia-betic mothers than general population.*
- Notify physician of any significant changes in respiratory status, neuro-logical status, or sudden drop in Hct; *may indicate intraventricular hem-orrhage.*

  Transfuse infant as ordered.
  Initiate oxygen therapy as ordered.
  Administer anticonvulsant therapy as ordered.
  Assist with diagnostic procedures as ordered.
- Notify physician of any decreased or asymmetrical movements; *may indicate a possible fractured clavicle, brachial palsy, or Bell's palsy re-lated to difficult delivery.*
- Notify physician of abnormal heart sounds *to detect any cardiomyopa-thies.*

  Assist with ECG, echocardiogram, x-rays, or cardiac catheterization as ordered.
- Notify physician if infant has abdominal distention, bile-stained emesis, or if infant fails to pass meconium on second day of life; *may indicate presence of microcolon related to presence of immature ganglion cells in intermyetic plexus.*

  Assist with radiographic studies as ordered.
- Notify physician of unusual physical findings such as macroglossia; un-usual fissures in lobule of external ear; indentations on posterior rim of helix. *Differential diagnosis of Beckwith-Wiedemann versus infant of di-abetic mother must be made:*

  Assist with genetic work-up.
  Obtain blood for chromosome studies as per protocol.

Potential for injury will be reduced.

Continued.

Infant of a diabetic mother cont'd

NURSING DIAGNOSES/ DEFINING CHARACTERISTICS	NURSING INTERVENTIONS / *RATIONALES*	EXPECTED OUTCOMES
Parental Anxiety **RELATED TO** Disease process New environment Hospital procedures and care **DEFINING CHARACTERISTICS** Restlessness Facial tension Extraneous movements: foot shuffling; hand/arm movements Guilt Disbelief Frequent repetitive questions Lack of questions Inconsistent visiting patterns	**ONGOING ASSESSMENT** • Assess parent's experience with well and ill children. • Assess parent's level of understanding of child's condition: large size, preterm infant. • Assess parent's knowledge of procedures and equipment. **THERAPEUTIC INTERVENTIONS** • Orient parent to: 　Unit 　Staff 　Procedures and equipment 　Visiting policy • Provide parent with unit booklet. • Maintain open communication with parent *to decrease anxiety.* • Allow parent to express fears. • Encourage parent to ask questions. • Encourage parent to participate with infant's care. *This will enhance parent/child bonding.* • Provide consistent caregivers *to facilitate trust and teaching/learning process.* • Arrange for follow-up. • See Parenting in special care nursery, p. 72.	Parental anxiety will be reduced.

Rosa Fuentes, RN, BSN

Thermoregulation in the low-birth-weight infant

HYPERTHERMIA; HYPOTHERMIA

Maintenance of an optimal thermal environment for the low-birth-weight infant is achieved when body temperature is maintained between 36.5° C and 37° C (97.7° F to 98.6° F); this range ensures minimal metabolic expenditures and prevents the consequences of thermal stress. Brown-fat metabolism in the newborn is the method for heat production; brown fat is located mainly in the middle to upper thorax.

NURSING DIAGNOSES/ DEFINING CHARACTERISTICS	NURSING INTERVENTIONS / *RATIONALES*	EXPECTED OUTCOMES
Ineffective Thermoregulation RELATED TO Temperature fluctuations caused by prematurity	**ONGOING ASSESSMENT** • Assess infant's axillary temperature, including vital signs every hour until stable. *Temperature fluctuations can cause apnea and bradycardia in preterm infant.* • Assess for signs of hyperthermia/hypothermia as described in defining characteristics. • Monitor blood gases daily. Report abnormal findings to physician. *Acidosis may ensue as glucose is metabolized and lactic acid build-up occurs.*	Temperature fluctuations will be reduced.

DEFINING CHARACTERISTICS *Hyperthermia:* Dehydration Body temperature >37° C (98.6° F) axillary Tachycardia Fluid/electrolyte imbalance Tachypnea Sweating Febrile convulsions Carbon dioxide retention Hypotension Impaired weight gain	• Assess criteria to select appropriate thermal environment:
	  Weight
	  Gestational age
	  Treatment
	 • Monitor serum glucose or Chemstrip. Report to physician glucose levels <40 mg/dl. *Preterm infants are especially susceptible to hypoglycemia caused by limited glycogen stores, which may also lead to neurological damage if not corrected immediately.*
	 • Monitor urine output and electrolytes. Report significant changes to physician:
	  Specific gravity >1.010
	  Urine output <2 ml/kg/hr	

Hypothermia: Body temperature <36.5° C (97.7° F) axillary Pale or cyanotic skin Loss of or failure to gain weight Apneic spells Hypoglycemia Metabolic acidosis	**THERAPEUTIC INTERVENTIONS**
	 Infant's weight <1 kg:
	 • Place infant under radiant warmer.
	 • Attach serum-control probe to infant's skin.
	 • Adjust temperature dial to desired level (36.5° C to 37° C [97.7° F to 98.6° F]). *Infant may safely be rewarmed 1° C every hour.*
	 • Minimize insensible water loss. *Infant's can lose >15% of birth weight within first week of life:*
	  Use humidity hood over body; maintain temperature of hood between 34.0° C and 38° C (94.2° F to 100.3° F).
	  Drape plastic wrap over radiant warmer.
	  Minimize handling.
	  If plastic wrap or body hood must be removed during a procedure, supplement heat source with heat lamp positioned approximately 2-3 feet from infant. *This distance is appropriate to prevent skin burns.*
	 Infant's weight 1-1.5 kg:
	 • Place in isolette.
	 • If close observation is required, use booties, hat, and diaper only; otherwise dress in shirt.
	 • Do not bathe infant who requires external heat source until condition stabilizes.
	 Infant's weight >1.5 kg:
	 • Transfer infant to a bassinet if condition is stable.
	 • Dress in hat, booties, t-shirt, and diapers; cover with 2-3 blankets.	

Continued.

Thermoregulation in the low-birth-weight infant cont'd

NURSING DIAGNOSES/ DEFINING CHARACTERISTICS	NURSING INTERVENTIONS / *RATIONALES*	EXPECTED OUTCOMES

Ineffective Thermoregulation cont'd
RELATED TO
Environmental factors
 	
DEFINING CHARACTERISTICS
Hyperthermia:
Dehydration
Body temperature >37° C (98.6° F) axillary
Tachycardia
Fluid/electrolyte imbalance
Tachypnea
Sweating
Febrile convulsions
Carbon dioxide retention
Hypotension
Impaired weight gain
 	
Hypothermia:
Body temperature <36.5° C (97.7° F) axillary
Pale or cyanotic skin
Loss or failure to gain weight
Apneic spells
Hypoglycemia
Acidosis
	ONGOING ASSESSMENT
	• Assess infant's potential for heat loss in environment based on principles of:
	    Conduction (cold sheets, scale, x-ray). *Conductive heat loss occurs when body loses heat to cooler objects that come into direct contact with skin.*
	    Convection (room temperature, drafts, cold oxygen administration). *Convection involves flow of heat from body surface to cooler surrounding air or air circulating over body surface.*
	    Radiation (assess proximity to cold walls/windows); *involves loss of infant's body heat to cooler, solid objects not directly in contact with skin.*
	    Evaporation (wet linen, wet infant); *involves loss of heat caused by conversion of liquid on infant's skin to vapor.*
	• Assess for heat excess related to:
	    Excessive handling
	    Inappropriate environmental temperature
	• Monitor incubation temperature as well as skin temperature.
	
	THERAPEUTIC INTERVENTIONS
	• Place warm sheet between infant and scale when infant is weighed.
	• If oxygen therapy or ventilation needed, maintain oxygen temperature equal to isolette temperature, but not <34° C to 37° C (94.2° F to 98.6° F).
	• Wean infant as tolerated from isolette:
	    Decrease bed temperature 0.5° C if infant is able to maintain axillary temperature of 36.4° C (97.6° F).
	    Disconnect bed and open portholes when isolette temperature reaches 27° C (80.6° F).
	    Move infant to bassinet if temperature is stable and weight gain satisfactory.
	Care of hypothermic infant:
	• Provide infant with appropriate environmental support:
	    If infant is in bassinet, move to isolette.
	    If infant is in isolette, move to radiant warmer (see Care of infant <1 kg, p. 379) or use heat lamp.
	• Attach skin temperature probe as necessary *to monitor temperature.*
	Care of hyperthermic infant:
	• Alleviate source of hyperthermia (i.e., bed temperature, bundling).
	• Cool infant slowly:
	• Do not use alcohol or cold water.
	• Wipe infant gently with tepid cloth.
	• Adjust radiant warmer temperature; gradually decrease by 0.5° C over 20 minutes.
	• Attach skin temperature probe *to monitor temperature.*
		Temperature fluctuations will be reduced.

Vanida Komutanon, RN

9

Hematologic/Oncologic/ Immunologic Care Plans

PEDIATRIC PATIENT
Acquired immunodeficiency syndrome
  (AIDS)
Aplastic anemia
Blood and blood product transfusion
  therapy
Cancer and chemotherapy
Disseminated intravascular coagulation
Hemophilia
Idiopathic thrombocytopenic purpura
Sickle cell pain crisis

NEONATAL PATIENT
Anemia in the growing premature infant
Care of the infant of a mother at risk
  for AIDS
Polycythemia

Acquired immunodeficiency syndrome (AIDS)

HIV

Human immunodeficiency virus (HIV) causes a spectrum of immunodeficiency diseases that is called acquired immune deficiency syndrome (AIDS) when opportunistic infections (OI) and malignancies (OM) develop. Children may present at any stage of infection. Of the estimated one million Americans infected with HIV, approximately 15,000 are infants or children. HIV is spread by intravenous drug use with shared syringes, sexual intercourse without condoms, and from mother to fetus across the placenta. Most children with AIDS became infected transplacentally. Between 25% and 50% of infants born to HIV-infected mothers will be infected. Early in the epidemic, hemophiliacs and children receiving transfusions became infected from HIV-contaminated blood and blood products. Since the advent of HIV antibody testing in 1985, transfusion-related infections have dramatically decreased. Although adults may have a period of many years before symptoms of AIDS develop, infants who are infected in utero sicken much sooner. Half of infected infants have symptoms of AIDS before their first birthday, and 82% before their third birthday. Because infants with AIDS are frequently cared for by mothers who also have AIDS, patient education and services must be provided for the entire family. Foster care placement may become unavoidable. AIDS in adolescents more closely resembles the course of disease experienced by adults. All adolescents, whether or not they are infected with HIV, need confidential and honest counseling on ways to avoid infection by practicing safe sex and eliminating drug use. It is impossible to detail treatments in this care plan because therapy is rapidly improving to bolster the immune system. It is also impossible to outline local regulations regarding testing and reporting HIV infection.

NURSING DIAGNOSES/ DEFINING CHARACTERISTICS	NURSING INTERVENTIONS / *RATIONALES*	EXPECTED OUTCOMES

Infection
RELATED TO
Presence of HIV
 	
DEFINING CHARACTERISTICS
Decreased number of T_4 helper cells, altered T_4 helper cell function, reversed T_4/T_8 ratio, altered cellular immune response, hypergammaglobulinemia response, decreased response to antigens in skin testing
Positive HIV antibody
Positive HIV culture
	ONGOING ASSESSMENT
	• Assess age and developmental level.
	• Assess for presence of fever, pain, altered activity levels, poor appetite, weight loss, vomiting or diarrhea, skin rashes, difficulty breathing, or loss of developmental milestones.
	• Obtain tuberculosis history.
	• Obtain immunization history. *(Routine immunizations are continued; expect subcutaneous inactivated polio vaccine to be given instead of live oral vaccine. Need vaccines for* Haemophilus influenzae *type b, pneumococcal pneumonia, and influenza virus.)*
	
	THERAPEUTIC INTERVENTIONS
	• Wash hands before entering, after leaving room.
	• Administer antiviral agents and immune-modulating therapies as ordered. *Antiviral agents prevent HIV from replicating and infecting additional cells. Immune modulators improve T-cell numbers/effectiveness and decrease risk of opportunistic infections.*
	• Prevent contact with other diseases:
	   If possible, assign to private room; if not possible, do not allow exposure to anyone with known infection.
	   Advise staff, visitors to avoid contact with child if they suspect cold, influenza, measles, or chickenpox.
		Risk of future infections will be reduced.

NURSING DIAGNOSES/ DEFINING CHARACTERISTICS	NURSING INTERVENTIONS / *RATIONALES*	EXPECTED OUTCOMES
Altered Nutrition: Less Than Body Requirements **RELATED TO** Loss of appetite Fatigue Oral or esophageal candidiasis **DEFINING CHARACTERISTICS** Calorie intake inadequate to meet metabolic requirements Failure to gain weight	**ONGOING ASSESSMENT** • Document child's actual weight on admission. • Obtain nutritional history. • Inspect mouth for *Candida* infection. • Document dietary and fluid I&O. • Obtain weight at least once a week. • Monitor serum/urine electrolytes, albumin, CBC, glucose, and acetone as necessary. • Obtain stool for culture and sensitivity (C&S), ova and parasites (O&P), *Cryptosporidium,* and acid-fast bacilli *to detect Mycobacterium avium-intracellulare (MAI).* **THERAPEUTIC INTERVENTIONS** • Provide dietary planning to encourage intake of high-calorie, high-protein foods. *Fatigue/weakness may prevent child from eating frequent feedings.* • Administer dietary supplements/total parenteral nutrition (TPN) as ordered. *Despite supplements, HIV may cause wasting syndrome.* • Administer antimonilial medication as ordered. *Oral and esophageal candidiasis can cause sore throat, may cause lack of appetite.* • Refer to food assistance program in community. • Administer antibiotics for GI pathogens. • Administer lactose-free diet.	Optimal nutritional support will be maintained.
High Risk for Fluid Volume Deficit **RELATED TO** Diarrhea Altered nutritional status Altered temperature regulation **DEFINING CHARACTERISTICS** Output > intake Sudden weight loss Decreased urine output Increased urine specific gravity Increased serum sodium Dry mucous membranes Change in vital signs: increased heart rate, hypotension	**ONGOING ASSESSMENT** • Assess hydration status (see Defining Characteristics). • Monitor I&O every shift. • Record daily weight. • Monitor electrolytes, serum and urine osmolarity, and specific gravity. • Monitor and document vital signs; report abnormalities. • Obtain stool cultures. **THERAPEUTIC INTERVENTIONS** • Encourage oral fluid intake. • Administer parenteral fluids as ordered. *Tachypnea, pain, nausea, and esophageal candidiasis may prevent oral intake. Vomiting, diarrhea, and night sweats may increase output.* • Administer antidiarrheal medication as ordered. • Administer antiparasitic medication as ordered.	Adequate fluid volume and electrolyte balance will be maintained.
Ineffective Breathing Pattern **RELATED TO** Inflammatory process Decreased lung expansion	**ONGOING ASSESSMENT** • Assess for presence of Defining Characteristics. • Monitor ABGs; note changes. **THERAPEUTIC INTERVENTIONS** • Position child with proper body alignment for optimal breathing pattern. *Sitting position improves lung excursion and chest expansion.*	Optimal respiratory status within limits of the disease will be achieved.

Continued.

Acquired immunodeficiency syndrome (AIDS) cont'd

NURSING DIAGNOSES/ DEFINING CHARACTERISTICS	NURSING INTERVENTIONS / *RATIONALES*	EXPECTED OUTCOMES
Ineffective Breathing Pattern cont'd Tracheobronchial obstruction Anxiety Decreased energy; fatigue **DEFINING CHARACTERISTICS** Dyspnea Shortness of breath Tachypnea Fremitus Cyanosis Cough Nasal flaring Respiratory depth changes Altered chest excursion Use of accessory muscles Pursed-lip breathing/ prolonged expiratory phase Increased anteroposterior chest diameter Clubbed digits Generalized lymphadenopathy	**THERAPEUTIC INTERVENTIONS cont'd** • Administer antiinfectives as prophylaxis. • Continue antiinfectives as prophylaxis. *When administering IV pentamidine, mix with D_5W and infuse over 1 hour. Watch for hypoglycemia, hypotension, and interstitial nephritis.* • Administer primary phencyclidine hydrochloride prophylaxis (for children <1 year old with CD_4 <1500, and for older children with CD_4 <400). • Maintain mechanical ventilation if needed. • Administer humidified oxygen. *Children with LIP (lymphocytic interstitial pneumonitis), a chronic lung syndrome, receive steroids and oxygen to decrease inflammation and dypsnea.*	
Altered Growth and Development **RELATED TO** HIV infection Prenatal exposure to illicit drugs Central nervous system infection **DEFINING CHARACTERISTICS** Loss of developmental milestones Lack of alertness Seizures Positive Kernig's sign Hypertonicity or hypotonicity Neck stiffness Irritability Lethargy	**ONGOING ASSESSMENT** • Assess for presence of Defining Characteristics. • Obtain maternal drug history. • Monitor CT or MRI scans. • Assist with spinal tap for culture and sensitivity (C&S). **THERAPEUTIC INTERVENTIONS** • Administer antibiotics as ordered. • Refer to developmental specialist. • Provide assistive devices while encouraging as much self-care and independence as comfortable *to limit developmental decline/deficits.*	Potential abilities will be maximized.

NURSING DIAGNOSES/ DEFINING CHARACTERISTICS	NURSING INTERVENTIONS / *RATIONALES*	EXPECTED OUTCOMES

Knowledge Deficit RELATED TO New condition **DEFINING CHARACTERISTICS** Multiple questions Lack of questions Confusion about disease, complications	**ONGOING ASSESSMENT**
	• Assess parental knowledge of disease, routes of transmission, complications, treatment, and modalities.
	
	THERAPEUTIC INTERVENTIONS
	• Instruct parent in dose, schedule, and side effects of antiviral, fungalstatic, prophylactic medication, and immunizations.
	• Instruct parent regarding schedule of outpatient appointments and treatments.
	• Instruct parent in signs/symptoms of disease, opportunistic infections, and neoplasms and person to whom information should be reported.
	• Instruct parent in routes of HIV transmission. *Parent may need to establish own HIV status.*
	• Instruct parent in methods of preventing HIV transmission:
	  Safe sex:
	    Kissing
	    Touching
	    Mutual masturbation
	    Vaginal or anal intercourse with latex condom and spermicidal lubricant
	  Nonoxyl-9 spermicide inactivates HIV in vitro; efficacy and side effects in vivo untested. Properly used, latex condom reduces HIV transmission risk for both partners.
	  Unsafe sex:
	    Vaginal or anal intercourse without condom
	    Sexual activities that cause bleeding
	• Instruct adolescent to avoid pregnancy. Instruct in birth control methods, including condom use.
	• Encourage use of clean IV equipment with recreational drugs. *HIV is quickly killed by 10% hypochlorite solution.* Flush syringe and needles with household bleach diluted ninefold with water; rinse with tap water. Refer to drug rehabilitation program.
	• Refrain from donating blood, semen, or organs if HIV positive.
	• Do not share razors, toothbrushes.
	• Clean blood or excreta containing blood with 10% hypochlorite solution. *Not necessary to use bleach to wash patient's dishes, clothes, or personal items.*
	• Avoid contact with people who have infectious diseases, especially children with chickenpox or other common childhood diseases. *HIV testing is inconclusive for first 15 months of life. Maternal antibody is acquired in utero. Infant's antibody formation may be delayed. HIV culture results are inconclusive unless positive.*
		Parent will verbalize understanding of disease process, transmission, complications, and treatment modalities.

High Risk for Infection To Health Care Provider RELATED TO Accidental contact with HIV	**ONGOING ASSESSMENT**
	• Monitor CDC guidelines for prevention of spread/protection.
	
	THERAPEUTIC INTERVENTIONS
	• Use universal precautions to prevent HIV spread:
	  Avoid unprotected contact with blood, semen, vaginal secretions, blood-tinged body fluids, wound drainage, breast milk, and fluids derived from blood (e.g., amniotic fluid, pericardial effusion). *These body fluids harbor HIV in quantities that may cause infection.*
	  Wear gloves when exposed to potentially infectious fluids. *Latex gloves provide effective barrier against HIV.*
		Health care worker will not become infected with HIV through patient exposure.

Continued.

Acquired immunodeficiency syndrome (AIDS) cont'd

NURSING DIAGNOSES/ DEFINING CHARACTERISTICS	NURSING INTERVENTIONS / *RATIONALES*	EXPECTED OUTCOMES
DEFINING CHARACTERISTICS History of exposure to HIV-positive blood, amniotic fluid, wound drainage, blood-tinged body fluids, or fluids derived from blood	**THERAPEUTIC INTERVENTIONS cont'd** Wear gloves when handling specimens. Wear gown when soiling is anticipated. Wear mask and goggles when potentially infectious body fluids may spray. Keep disposable Ambu bag and mask at bedside. Immediately clean spills of potentially infectious fluids with sodium hypochlorite (bleach) solution. *Bleach, cleaning solutions labeled tuberculocidal will kill HIV.* Prevent injury with needles or other sharp instruments. *Although most needle-stick injuries do not result in infection, risk exists.* Do not recap needles, resheath instruments. *Recapping needles most common cause of needle-stick injuries.* Dispose of sharps in rigid plastic container. Keep needle disposal container in child's room. Obtain assistance to restrain confused or uncooperative child during venipuncture or other invasive procedure. Take care to avoid needle-stick injuries during arrests/other emergencies. If needle-stick injury occurs, complete incident report; notify employee health service.	

Jeff Zurlinden, RN, MS

Aplastic anemia

Aplastic anemia (AA) is a disorder in which all blood cell structures are decreased as a result of the replacement of red marrow (cell-producing) with yellow marrow (fat) in the bone. Aplastic anemia can be congenital, acquired, or idiopathic. Congenital aplastic anemia is one of a number of anomalies seen in children with Fanconi's syndrome. Acquired aplastic anemia is caused by drug or chemotherapy, irradiation, ingested/inhaled toxic chemicals (benzene), infections, and myeloprolific disorders such as leukemia or lymphoma. Prognosis for congenital and acquired AA is fair. Idiopathic AA has no known or identifiable cause and prognosis is poor; it is usually a fatal condition.

NURSING DIAGNOSES/ DEFINING CHARACTERISTICS	NURSING INTERVENTIONS / *RATIONALES*	EXPECTED OUTCOMES
High Risk for Hemorrhage **Related To** Platelets <20,000/ mm³ Diminished cell production **Defining Characteristics** Extensive ecchymoses Oral bleeding Increased bleeding times	**Ongoing Assessment** ▪ Assess age and developmental level. ▪ Assess for areas of bruising/ecchymoses. ▪ Assess for obvious bleeding. ▪ Monitor stool and urine for occult blood. ▪ Monitor CBC with differential counts. ▪ Obtain type/crossmatch. ▪ Observe for febrile reaction to platelet transfusions. **Therapeutic Interventions** ▪ Protect child from injury by controlling environment and use of safety precautions: Do not take temperature rectally; axillary is preferred *to decrease risk of tissue trauma and bleeding.* Provide very soft toothbrush. Limit child's activities to safe play (i.e., no body contact sports, no gymnastics, no bicycle riding, use of safety scissors). ▪ Report increasing ecchymosis or active bleeding immediately. ▪ Administer platelet transfusion as ordered *to control bleeding.* ▪ Administer antipyretics as ordered. *Minor febrile reactions to platelet transfusions are common.*	Risk of hemorrhagic injury will be reduced.
Activity Intolerance **Related To** Anemia Diminished erythropoiesis **Defining Characteristics** Fatigue Decreased PO_2 Tachycardia Hypertension or hypotension	**Ongoing Assessment** ▪ Assess current activity level and activity level before illness. ▪ Interview for: Possible causes of diminished tolerance Known risks to cause aplastic anemia ▪ Assess for complaints of fatigue or irritability in young child. ▪ Assess CBC, pulse oximetry. ▪ Assess vital signs: respiratory and cardiac rates, BP. *Prolonged, severe anemia causes shock and cardiac failure.* **Therapeutic Interventions** ▪ Assist with diagnostic procedures, blood tests, bone marrow aspiration. Explain to child and parent before test occurs. ▪ Assist with ADL as needed, while allowing as much independence as possible. ▪ Pace activities to child's needs. ▪ Maintain IV access; may require central line or port. ▪ Administer medications (erythropoietin), transfusions (packed cells), and testosterone. *Testosterone enhances bone marrow production/cell growth.* ▪ Provide humidified oxygen as ordered *to saturate available circulating cells.*	Activity intolerance will be reduced.

Continued.

■ **Aplastic anemia cont'd**

NURSING DIAGNOSES/ DEFINING CHARACTERISTICS	NURSING INTERVENTIONS / *RATIONALES*	EXPECTED OUTCOMES
High Risk for Infection **RELATED TO** Pancytopenia **DEFINING CHARACTERISTICS** Fever Chills Rash Lethargy Pain Tachycardia Hypotension Cyanosis Mottling	**ONGOING ASSESSMENT** • Assess for Defining Characteristics. • Assess CBC with differential count. • Assess for recent platelet transfusion. *Febrile reaction may mimic infection.* • Assess for source of infection, recent contact with ill individuals, open wounds. • Monitor cultures: blood, urine, stool, and throat for bacteria and fungi. • Assess for impending septic shock; see Septic shock, p. 102. **THERAPEUTIC INTERVENTIONS** • Provide isolation (or private room) as needed. Screen visitors. • Assist with daily hygiene. Provide good mouth care. *Dental caries/poor hygiene can be major source of infection.* • Administer antibiotics/fungicides/steroids as needed. • Practice good handwashing.	Risks for infection will be reduced.
Body Image Disturbance **RELATED TO** Drug therapy Induced changes Activity intolerance **DEFINING CHARACTERISTICS** Verbal preoccupation with changes in body parts or function Refusal to discuss/ acknowledge change Actual change in structure/function Change in behavior (withdrawal, isolation, flamboyance)	**ONGOING ASSESSMENT** • Assess prescribed drug therapy for potential side effects. • Assess for actual body changes: Steroids cause moon face, weight gain. Testosterone causes virilization in both males and females, (i.e., deepened voice, hirsutism, growth of pubic hair, enlarged penis, flushed skin, and acne). Testosterone may also cause shortened stature if given without concurrent steroid therapy. **THERAPEUTIC INTERVENTIONS** • Discuss potential side effects with parent and child before drug regimen is implemented. • Plan for compensatory measures with clothes, facial hair removal. • Explain changes to friends/visitors *to decrease potential negative reactions toward child.* • Allow child to vent feelings or work through frustrations with play therapy. • Obtain social service or psychological consultation if necessary.	Body image disturbance will be reduced.
Knowledge Deficit **RELATED TO** New diagnosis Unfamiliar treatments Unfamiliar environment **DEFINING CHARACTERISTICS** Verbal expression of lack of knowledge or understanding Appearance of confusion Requests for information	**ONGOING ASSESSMENT** • Assess child's developmental level. • Assess parent and child for learning ability and style. • Assess for readiness. **THERAPEUTIC INTERVENTIONS** • Teach family to avoid causative agent, if known, *to prevent recurrence of acquired anemia.* • Provide ongoing information in manner that is understandable to learner. • Inform parent and child of necessary safety precautions and continuous medication in home setting. • Provide follow-up appointments and emergency numbers. • Provide information about community resources/self-help groups.	Parent and child will understand disorder and its treatment.

Michele Knoll Puzas, RNC, MHPE

Blood and blood product transfusion therapy

Homologous donated blood or autologous blood or blood components infused to achieve hemodynamic equilibrium.

WHOLE BLOOD; PACKED RBCs; PLATELET CONCENTRATION; GRANULOCYTES; FRESH FROZEN PLASMA; CRYOPRECIPITATION; ALBUMIN; FACTOR VIII CONCENTRATE

NURSING DIAGNOSES/ DEFINING CHARACTERISTICS	NURSING INTERVENTIONS / *RATIONALES*	EXPECTED OUTCOMES

High Risk for Injury: Anaphylactic Shock, Pulmonary Congestion, Circulatory Overload, Hyperkalemia, Hematoma, Hypothermia
 	
 RELATED TO
 	
 Hemolytic/allergic reaction to blood
 Volume overload
 Aged blood
 Inadequate IV access
 Cold blood
 	
 DEFINING CHARACTERISTICS
 	
 Chills
 Headache/nausea/ vomiting
 Urticaria/flushing
 Chest pain
 Flank pain
 Change in vital signs
 Change in mentation
 Hypothermia/hyperthermia
	ONGOING ASSESSMENT
	 ▪ Assess age and developmental level.
	 ▪ Assess medical history for recent trauma, clotting disorders, chemotherapy, bone marrow suppression, fluid shifts/imbalances.
	 ▪ Assess height/weight *to determine if volume and rate of blood ordered are appropriate.*
	 ▪ Assess for previous transfusions or reactions.
	 ▪ Assess adequacy of venous access.
	 ▪ Check appropriateness of component order; safety range of volume order; appropriate rate of transfusion.
	 ▪ Check for signed consent for blood transfusion. Infusion of blood product should begin within 30 minutes of receipt of blood on unit.
	 ▪ Check blood product and child's ID along with blood type and expiration date. *Any discrepancies must be resolved before product is administered.*
	 ▪ Assess child's cardiorespiratory status to determine amount and rate of infusion.
	 ▪ Take vital signs before therapy begins, then every 15 minutes for next hour, every hour thereafter.
	 ▪ Assess child for signs and symptoms of reaction to blood product.
	 ▪ If reaction occurs:
	    Continue to monitor vital signs.
	    Record I&O.
	    Obtain blood and urine specimen according to hospital policy; check for presence of hemoglobin, *which indicates intravascular hemolysis.*
	    Observe for signs of hemorrhage resulting from *intravascular coagulation.*
	
	 THERAPEUTIC INTERVENTIONS
	 ▪ Follow hospital policy for obtaining blood product from blood bank.
	 ▪ Prime blood tubing with normal saline solution, IV blood; connect to patient access. *Where fluid volume is strictly controlled, only 1 ml of normal saline solution necessary as barrier between IV maintenance solution and blood product to prevent hemolysis.*
	 ▪ If reaction occurs:
	    Stop transfusion and infuse normal saline solution.
	    Call physician.
	    Administer oxygen as ordered and monitor effectiveness. Position child to decrease respiratory distress.
	    Treat life-threatening reaction with Benadryl, epinephrine as ordered. *Epinephrine: adrenergic agent used to control allergic reactions and acute anaphylactic reactions. Benadryl: antihistamine used to prevent vasodilator effects of histamine, thus preventing edema, itching, bronchospasm if reaction occurs.*
	 ▪ If no reaction occurs:
	    Infuse total IV ordered blood; flush catheter with normal saline solution and reconnect maintenance solution.
	    Obtain posttransfusion vital signs.
	 ▪ Complete documentation of transfusion per hospital policy.
		Risk of transfusion reaction will be reduced.

Continued.

Blood and blood product transfusion therapy cont'd

NURSING DIAGNOSES/ DEFINING CHARACTERISTICS	NURSING INTERVENTIONS / *RATIONALES*	EXPECTED OUTCOMES
Knowledge Deficit **RELATED TO** Unfamiliarity with transfusion process Misinformation about risks of transfusion **DEFINING CHARACTERISTICS** Questioning Verbalized misconceptions Refusal to permit transfusion	**ONGOING ASSESSMENT** ▪ Assess child's/family's knowledge of transfusion process. ▪ Assess family's moral, ethical, and religious background as it relates to administration of blood. **THERAPEUTIC INTERVENTIONS** ▪ Reinforce physician's explanations; allow time for child/family to express concerns. ▪ Offer explanation of precautionary measures employed by blood bank *(blood tested for hepatitis B, non A-, non-B, and syphilis; also, tested for HIV antibody).* ▪ Acknowledge concerns. ▪ Explain procedure for administering blood *so child not concerned when vital signs are taken frequently, etc. Helps decrease fear of the unknown.*	Child/family will verbalize understanding of the need for a transfusion and the screening process performed before the transfusion begins.

Nedra Skale, RN, MS, CNA

Cancer and chemotherapy

Cancer *is a general term for a group of diseases characterized by uncontrolled, abnormal growth of cells. These abnormal cells can invade and destroy normal tissues. Cancer chemotherapy is the administration of cytotoxic drugs for the purpose of destroying malignant cells. The goal of chemotherapy may be curative, adjunctive, or palliative.*

NURSING DIAGNOSES/ DEFINING CHARACTERISTICS	NURSING INTERVENTIONS / *RATIONALES*	EXPECTED OUTCOMES
High Risk for Infection **RELATED TO** Neutropenia Immunosuppression Foreign object—central line catheter, implanted venous access port, Ommaya reservoir Myeloproliferative disorders (e.g., leukemia) **DEFINING CHARACTERISTICS** Fever Chills Lethargy/malaise Pain on urination Pain with bowel movements (i.e., perirectal pain) Cough Sore throat Rash Thrush	**ONGOING ASSESSMENT** ▪ Assess age and developmental level. ▪ Assess for Defining Characteristics. ▪ Evaluate frequent CBCs to measure absolute neutrophil count (ANC) (CBC/differential mandatory with incidence of fever). ▪ Assess for source of infection. ▪ Monitor blood, urine, stool, throat culture: Blood cultures for bacteria and fungus. *(Blood cultures should be drawn from central line [if applicable] and peripherally.)* ▪ Assess for impending septic shock: specifically tachycardia, hypotension, decreased LOC, cyanosis, or mottling. **THERAPEUTIC INTERVENTIONS** ▪ Administer IV antibiotics for fever, neutropenia as ordered. ▪ Educate parent to report fever and other defining characteristics. ▪ Isolate child from known infectious persons. ▪ Provide private room while in hospital. ▪ Administer varicella-zoster immune globulin (VZIG) for varicella exposure. ▪ Provide good oral hygiene. ▪ Practice good handwashing. ▪ Do not take temperatures rectally, administer no rectal medications, avoid dental work while neutropenic. ▪ Administer prophylactic antibiotics as ordered; co-trimoxazole (Bactrim) is given *to prevent pneumocystis pneumonia. Cancer patients with fever and neutropenia are at great risk for septic shock; their care should be considered urgent.*	Potential for infection will be reduced.

NURSING DIAGNOSES/ DEFINING CHARACTERISTICS	NURSING INTERVENTIONS / *RATIONALES*	EXPECTED OUTCOMES
DEFINING CHARACTERISTICS cont'd Tachycardia and hypotension Color changes (e.g., cyanosis, mottling)		
Body Image Disturbance **RELATED TO** Hair loss Weight loss Weight gain Skin changes Nail changes Abdominal distention Teasing from other children **DEFINING CHARACTERISTICS** Crying or sadness regarding physical changes Self-deprecating remarks Fear of others seeing "bald head" Self-isolation	**ONGOING ASSESSMENT** ▪ Assess for presence of Defining Characteristics. ▪ Observe for verbal/nonverbal cues *to note body image alteration.* **THERAPEUTIC INTERVENTIONS** ▪ Encourage use of caps, scarves, hats. ▪ Provide peer group with similar "problems" (e.g., camps, playroom activities). ▪ Encourage verbalization of feelings and concerns. ▪ Convey acceptance and understanding. ▪ Provide anticipatory guidance; prepare child for expected alteration in appearance; plan for agreed-upon coping mechanisms.	Coping mechanisms will be achieved.
Anxiety/Fear **RELATED TO** Developmental stage Fear of pain Fear of procedures Fear of side effects (i.e., anticipatory vomiting) Stranger anxiety Separation anxiety Lack of understanding because of age Prognosis **DEFINING CHARACTERISTICS** Crying, tantrums, acting out Anger Withdrawal/depression Anticipatory vomiting Regressive behavior: thumbsucking, decrease in toileting Demanding Nightmares	**ONGOING ASSESSMENT** ▪ Assess child's/family's anxiety/fear. ▪ Note verbal and nonverbal cues. **THERAPEUTIC INTERVENTIONS** ▪ Provide hospital and needle play *for desensitization.* ▪ Provide careful explanations in preparing for procedures. ▪ Allow to verbalize fears, anger. ▪ Allow child to act out. ▪ Encourage relaxation exercises and/or guided imagery as age appropriate. ▪ Correct misconceptions and fill knowledge gaps.	Anxiety/fear will be reduced.

Continued.

Cancer and chemotherapy cont'd

NURSING DIAGNOSES/ DEFINING CHARACTERISTICS	NURSING INTERVENTIONS / *RATIONALES*	EXPECTED OUTCOMES
Altered Nutrition: Less Than Body Requirements **RELATED TO** Vomiting/nausea/ diarrhea Mucositis, stomatitis, pain (mouth sores) Change in taste from chemotherapy Depression Disinterest in food **DEFINING CHARACTERISTICS** Documented inadequate caloric intake Weight loss Caloric intake not adequate to keep pace with disease state Irritability Weakness Fatigue	**ONGOING ASSESSMENT** ▪ Assess for Defining Characteristics. **THERAPEUTIC INTERVENTIONS** ▪ Provide good mouth care. ▪ Encourage use of oncology mouthwash or viscous lidocaine for mouth sores. *Controlling pain usually results in increased food intake.* ▪ Provide small, frequent meals of preferred foods. ▪ Minimize power struggles over food. ▪ Offer high-calorie food (e.g., milk shakes). ▪ Provide hyperalimentation/intralipids if child unable to take orally. ▪ Provide antiemetic medications.	Recommended body weight will be achieved/maintained.
Altered Oral Mucous Membranes **RELATED TO** Chemotherapy **DEFINING CHARACTERISTICS** Thrush Oral ulcerations Pain when drinking, chewing, swallowing Gagging/coughing caused by esophageal ulcerations or sloughing Reddened oral mucosa Weight loss/dehydration	**ONGOING ASSESSMENT** ▪ Assess for Defining Characteristics. **THERAPEUTIC INTERVENTIONS** ▪ Provide good oral hygiene/mouth care. ▪ Encourage use of oncology mouthwash, hydrogen peroxide rinse. ▪ Avoid spicy or acidic foods or beverages (i.e., *orange juice will sting*). ▪ Provide topical anesthetics (i.e., viscous lidocaine). ▪ Administer topical/oral antibiotics as ordered (Bactrim, Flagyl).	Skin integrity will be maintained.
High Risk for Injury: Bleeding **RELATED TO** Bone marrow suppression, thrombocytopenia Myeloproliferative disorders	**ONGOING ASSESSMENT** ▪ Assess for Defining Characteristics. ▪ Monitor CBC/platelet count frequently. **THERAPEUTIC INTERVENTIONS** ▪ Teach child/parent to assess for defining characteristics. ▪ Encourage use of soft toothbrush or cotton swabs for mouth care. ▪ Do not take temperatures rectally or give rectal medications. ▪ Prohibit aspirin products. ▪ Prohibit tampons (for teenagers). ▪ Avoid contact sports/motorcycle riding.	Potential for injury will be reduced.

NURSING DIAGNOSES/ DEFINING CHARACTERISTICS	NURSING INTERVENTIONS / *RATIONALES*	EXPECTED OUTCOMES
DEFINING CHARACTERISTICS Decreased platelet count Oozing from gums or nose Petechiae Bruising Hematemesis Hematuria Melena	**THERAPEUTIC INTERVENTIONS cont'd** • Instruct child not to take other medications without physician approval. *Some medications (including over-the-counter) cause platelet suppression.* • Administer platelet transfusions as needed. *Chemotherapy causes bone marrow suppression, and myeloproliferative disorders (leukemia) disrupt normal platelet production by replacing normal marrow elements with leukemic blast cells.*	

Anticipatory Grieving: Family
RELATED TO
Life-threatening illness
 	
DEFINING CHARACTERISTICS
Financial pressures
Marital/partner stress
Intermittent absence of child from home because of hospitalization
Work commitment conflicts
Sibling anxiety and grief
Sibling feeling of neglect
Possible loss of child
	ONGOING ASSESSMENT
	• Assess for identifying characteristics:
	   Change in sibling's grades or behavior
	   Change in parent's job performance
	   Sibling hostility to child
	   Depression in family members; *when cancer patient is child, family should be considered psychosocial unit of treatment.*
	
	THERAPEUTIC INTERVENTIONS
	• Inform family about cancer support groups such as Candlelighters.
	• Encourage sibling support groups.
	• Involve family in child's care.
	• Suggest parent take short vacations or long weekends.
	• Foster independence in sick child; encourage socialization.
		Grieving will not be debilitating.

Pain
RELATED TO
Procedures (i.e., venipunctures, lumbar punctures, access of implanted venous ports, access of Ommaya reservoir)
Chemotherapy side effects (i.e., mucositis, peripheral neuropathy [from vincristine])
Burn caused by extravasation of vesicant chemotherapy
Malignant process— "cancer pain"— may be related to tumor infiltration into bone, soft tissue, viscera, or nerves
	ONGOING ASSESSMENT
	• Assess for Defining Characteristics.
	• Use age-appropriate techniques to assess pain such as "color-your-pain" or "faces."
	
	THERAPEUTIC INTERVENTIONS
	• For vesicant burns: if extravasation suspected, apply ice for 24 hours and steroid tape. If blistering occurs, use Silvadene cream and sterile dressings.
	• For pain related to invasive procedures:
	   Use age-appropriate distraction techniques.
	   Prepare child for painful procedures.
	   Encourage child to participate in plan to manage pain.
	• Provide soothing and comfort techniques.
	• Administer pharmacological interventions, including local anesthetics (e.g., lidocaine), sedatives (e.g., Midazolam), opiods (e.g., morphine, meperidine). Oral analgesics such as acetaminophen, codeine, ibuprofen can also be administered for postprocedure pain.
	• Allow child to verbalize and/or act out painful procedures. *Young children have difficulty articulating pain and anger.* Use desensitization technique.
	• For pain from chemotherapy side effects:
	   See Oral ulceration intervention, p. 392.
	   Use oral or parenteral analgesics.
		Pain will be reduced.

Continued.

Hematologic/Oncologic/Immunologic Care Plans (Pediatric)

NURSING DIAGNOSES/ DEFINING CHARACTERISTICS	NURSING INTERVENTIONS / *RATIONALES*	EXPECTED OUTCOMES
DEFINING CHARACTERISTICS *Behavioral indicators:* Crying, fussing, withdrawal from social situations, reduction in play, decreased appetite, guarding, facial grimacing *Verbal indicators:* Crying out, grunting, verbalization of pain *Physical indicators:* Tachypnea, tachycardia, hypotension	**THERAPEUTIC INTERVENTIONS cont'd** ▪ For cancer pain: use nonpharmacological approaches as described above for Pain related to procedures. Use analgesic ladder *to provide analgesia appropriate to severity of pain.* ▪ Consider anesthetic approaches (i.e., nerve blocks *to manage side effects related to analgesics).*	
Diarrhea **RELATED TO** Side effect of chemotherapy **DEFINING CHARACTERISTICS** Loose or liquid stools Frequent loose stools Abdominal pain Cramping Hyperactive bowel sounds/sensations Signs of dehydration	**ONGOING ASSESSMENT** ▪ Assess for presence of Defining Characteristics. ▪ Assess effectiveness of present symptom control regimen. ▪ Check stool culture. **THERAPEUTIC INTERVENTIONS** ▪ Replace lost fluids orally or intravenously. ▪ Administer antidiarrheal medications. ▪ Provide good perineal care/cleaning. ▪ Apply topical perineal medications. *Many institutions have mixed preparations, including Desitin, nystatin cream, and Maalox.* ▪ Administer antibiotics as ordered *to treat diarrhea caused by infection.*	Normal bowel movements will be maintained.
Constipation **RELATED TO** Side effects of chemotherapy Decreased oral intake, poor nutrition **DEFINING CHARACTERISTICS** Distended abdomen Hypoactive bowel sounds Abdominal pain Radiological evidence	**ONGOING ASSESSMENT** ▪ Assess usual bowel pattern and changes. ▪ Assess for Defining Characteristics. **THERAPEUTIC INTERVENTIONS** ▪ Administer stool softeners. ▪ Encourage fluids by mouth. ▪ Decrease dose or change medications causing severe constipation. *Pain medications sometimes cause constipation.* ▪ Encourage fruit juices and high-fiber foods.	Constipation will be eliminated.
Knowledge Deficit: Family **RELATED TO** New diagnosis New procedures Unfamiliarity with hospital and treatment	**ONGOING ASSESSMENT** ▪ Assess family's preconception of childhood cancer/chemotherapy: "What is your experience/knowledge of cancer/chemotherapy?" ▪ Assess knowledge of diagnosis and treatment. ▪ Assess family's learning capabilities, including willingness/readiness to learn. ▪ Assess family resources; assess potential for noncompliance.	Understanding will be verbalized.

Cancer and chemotherapy cont'd

NURSING DIAGNOSES/ DEFINING CHARACTERISTICS	NURSING INTERVENTIONS / *RATIONALES*	EXPECTED OUTCOMES
DEFINING CHARACTERISTICS Asking many questions Apparent uncertainty or confusion Hesitancy to participate in child's care	**THERAPEUTIC INTERVENTIONS** ▪ Incorporate family into plan of care from time of diagnosis. ▪ Let family know their knowledge and participation is valued by health care team. *Parent sometimes feels inadequate to care for child or that health caregivers have usurped parent's role.* ▪ Educate family regarding treatment plan or protocol. Provide appropriate teaching materials. ▪ Instruct family on chemotherapy side effects. ▪ Teach family members new skills as needed, *so they can be active in child's care.* ▪ Provide discharge planning and follow-up as required.	
High Risk for Activity Intolerance **RELATED TO** Anemia Bone marrow suppression secondary to chemotherapy and/or myeloproliferative disorders (e.g., leukemia) Blood drawing Poor nutrition Chronic illness **DEFINING CHARACTERISTICS** Hgb <10 g Hct <30% Fatigue Headaches Pallor Shortness of breath	**ONGOING ASSESSMENT** ▪ Assess for Defining Characteristics. ▪ Monitor CBC. ▪ Rule out other possible causes for defining characteristics. **THERAPEUTIC INTERVENTIONS** ▪ Administer transfusion of irradiated leucocyte-poor packed RBCs (10-15 ml/kg) for Hgb <10, Hct <30%. ▪ Obtain frequent CBC, especially when patient at nadir. ▪ Encourage rest until transfusion can be given.	Activity intolerance will be reduced.
Ineffective Airway Clearance **RELATED TO** Mediastinal mass with impending airway obstruction **DEFINING CHARACTERISTICS** Cough Dyspnea Orthopnea Cyanosis when lying Dullness on chest percussion Pleural effusion	**ONGOING ASSESSMENT** ▪ Assess for Defining Characteristics. ▪ Obtain stat chest x-ray as indicated. ▪ Evaluate laboratory results: CBC, urine, electrolytes, Ca, Mg, uric acid, BUN, creatinine. **THERAPEUTIC INTERVENTIONS** ▪ Place emergency/resuscitation equipment and medications near bedside. ▪ Keep child calm and quiet. ▪ Assist with diagnostic procedures (i.e., pleural tap). ▪ Assist with emergency treatment (i.e., radiation or steroids). ▪ Discuss with physician possible need to transfer child to pediatric ICU.	Optimal respiratory status will be maintained.
High Risk for Fluid Volume Deficit **RELATED TO** Vomiting or diarrhea Poor oral intake	**ONGOING ASSESSMENT** ▪ Assess for Defining Characteristics. ▪ Assess history of I&O from child and/or family or hospital staff. Monitor I&O carefully. ▪ Assess weight frequently. ▪ Monitor laboratory values. ▪ Monitor vital signs, including orthostatic BP and pulse. *Orthostatic changes may indicate impending hypovolemic shock.*	Adequate fluid volume will be maintained.

Continued.

Cancer and chemotherapy cont'd

NURSING DIAGNOSES/ DEFINING CHARACTERISTICS	NURSING INTERVENTIONS / *RATIONALES*	EXPECTED OUTCOMES
DEFINING CHARACTERISTICS Dry lips, mouth, tongue Poor skin turgor Sunken eyes Decrease in urine output Weight loss Lethargy, listlessness Orthostatic changes Tachycardia Elevated BUN, creatinine Electrolyte imbalance No tears when crying	**THERAPEUTIC INTERVENTIONS** • Educate child/family on signs and symptoms of fluid volume deficit. • Administer antiemetic as ordered. *Antiemetics are most effective when given "around-the-clock" instead of prn.* • Offer food and fluids in small, frequent amounts. • Do not force food or fluids. • Maintain IV access if needed and provide IV fluids as ordered *to prevent dehydration. In some cases, IV hydration is initiated before administration of chemotherapy to offset potential complications of drug and to ensure adequate hydration.*	

Dinah Parmuth, RN, BSN

Disseminated intravascular coagulation

CONSUMPTION COAGULOPATHY; DEFIBRINATION SYNDROME; DIC

Inappropriate, accelerated consumption of coagulation factors resulting in hemorrhage. Disseminated intravascular coagulation (DIC) always occurs secondary to some other pathology and is associated with infection, neoplastic disorders, tissue trauma, and burns.

NURSING DIAGNOSES/ DEFINING CHARACTERISTICS	NURSING INTERVENTIONS / *RATIONALES*	EXPECTED OUTCOMES

Fluid Volume Deficit
RELATED TO
Blood loss
Depleted coagulation factors
 	
DEFINING CHARACTERISTICS
Prothrombin time (PT) >15 sec
Partial thromboplastin time (PTT) >25-35 sec
Hypofibrinogenemia
Thrombocytopenia
Elevated fibrin split products
Prolonged bleeding time
Oozing of blood from IV sites, drains, or wounds
Petechiae, purpura, hematomas
	ONGOING ASSESSMENT
	• Assess age and developmental level.
	• Examine skin surface for signs of bleeding; note:
	    Petechiae, purpura, hematomas
	    Oozing of blood from IV sites, drains, and wounds
	    Bleeding from mucous membranes
	• Observe for signs of bleeding from GI/GU tracts.
	• Note any hemoptysis or blood obtained during suctioning.
	• Observe for changes in mental status; institute neurological checklist.
	• Monitor vital signs.
	• Monitor coagulation profile.
	• Monitor Hct and Hgb.
	• Document amount and character of drainage on dressings; note frequency of dressing changes.
	• Observe for any increase in bleeding after initiating heparin therapy. If bleeding increased, notify physician for possible need to decrease drip.
	
	THERAPEUTIC INTERVENTIONS
	• Protect child from bleeding:
	    Eliminate pressure by turning child frequently.
	    If child is confused/agitated, pad side rails *to prevent bruising.*
	    Minimize IM/SC injections; apply pressure to injection site if puncture unavoidable.
	    Prevent stable clots from dislodging; if clot dislodges, apply pressure and cold compress.
		Optimal fluid balance will be maintained.

NURSING DIAGNOSES/ DEFINING CHARACTERISTICS	NURSING INTERVENTIONS / *RATIONALES*	EXPECTED OUTCOMES
DEFINING CHARACTERISTICS cont'd Bleeding from mucous membranes Hematuria, hemoptysis, blood in stools Cardiovascular changes (hypotension, dysrhythmias) CNS changes (decreased mental status, possible cerebral hemorrhage)	**THERAPEUTIC INTERVENTIONS** cont'd 　Apply pressure to any oozing site. 　Prevent trauma to catheters/tubes by proper taping; minimize pulling. 　Minimize number of cuff BPs; maintain arterial line. 　Use gentle suctioning *to prevent trauma to respiratory mucosa.* ▪ Administer fluids as ordered. ▪ Administer blood products as ordered; monitor child's response (observe for transfusion reaction). ▪ Administer heparin therapy as ordered *to interrupt abnormal accelerated coagulation. Heparin interferes with thrombin production, which is necessary for clot formation.* 　Infuse continuous heparin drip on infusion device. 　Maintain PTT at 2 times normal. 　Consider dosage alteration in child with hepatic or renal failure. ▪ See Fluid volume deficit, p. 19.	
Anxiety/Fear **RELATED TO** Presenting symptoms of DIC and/or staff reaction to disease process **DEFINING CHARACTERISTICS** Restlessness Increased awareness Increased questioning Crying	**ONGOING ASSESSMENT** ▪ Assess anxiety/fear level. ▪ Assess normal coping patterns. **THERAPEUTIC INTERVENTIONS** ▪ Inform parent of child's prognosis; prepare them for child's appearance. *Bleeding site and/or clots must be left undisturbed, result in sometimes shocking appearance.* ▪ Minimize staff conversations at bedside. ▪ Use calm approach with child. ▪ See Anxiety, p. 4/Fear, p. 18.	Anxiety/fear will be reduced.
High Risk for Injury **RELATED TO** Excess heparin Insufficient heparin *Note that heparin aborts clotting process by blocking production of thrombin.* **DEFINING CHARACTERISTICS** *Excess heparin:* Bleeding from IV sites, drains, wounds Petechiae, purpura, hematomas Bleeding from mucous membranes GI, GU bleeding Bleeding from respiratory tract PTT >2½ times normal	**ONGOING ASSESSMENT** ▪ Note adverse effects of heparin therapy: 　Any increase in bleeding from IV sites, GI/GU tracts, respiratory tract, wounds. 　Development of new purpura, petechiae, or hematomas. **THERAPEUTIC INTERVENTIONS** ▪ Maintain constant, uninterrupted infusion of heparin titrated to lab values and clinical situation. *As clinical situation improves, need for heparin decreases. Challenge lies in differentiating blood loss as an untoward effect of heparin therapy from worsening of DIC.*	Side effects of heparin therapy will be reduced.

Continued.

Disseminated intravascular coagulation cont'd

NURSING DIAGNOSES/ DEFINING CHARACTERISTICS	NURSING INTERVENTIONS / *RATIONALES*	EXPECTED OUTCOMES
DEFINING CHARACTERISTICS cont'd *Insufficient heparin:* Continued evidence of further clot formation (e.g., newly developed signs of pulmonary emboli or peripheral thromboemboli) Continued evidence of bleeding from DIC (abnormal clotting) PTT < twice normal		

Impaired Gas Exchange
 RELATED TO
 	
 Inappropriate coagulation
 Possible blood loss
 Decreased Hct and Hgb
 Acidosis
 Decreased circulation
 Poor oxygen exchange at cellular level
 Generalized systemic microvascular clot formation
 	
 DEFINING CHARACTERISTICS
 	
 Dyspnea
 Poor capillary refill
 Acral cyanosis
 Changes in mental status (confusion)
 Decreased PO_2 or decreased oxygen saturation
 Decreased Hgb
 Increased PCO_2
 Blood pH <7.3
 Acidic urine pH <4.5
	ONGOING ASSESSMENT
	 • Observe for signs of dyspnea, respiratory distress, poor capillary refill, acral cyanosis.
	 • Assess for confusion.
	 • Monitor vital signs.
	 • Monitor ABGs.
	
	 THERAPEUTIC INTERVENTIONS
	 • Maintain airway:
	   Encourage coughing.
	   Use suction as needed.
	   Elevate head of bed >45 degrees for dyspnea.
	 • Administer oxygen as ordered.
	 • Correct acid base imbalances.
	 • See Mechanical ventilation, p. 155, if appropriate.
		Gas exchange will be adequate.

Knowledge Deficit **RELATED TO** Lack of familiarity with procedures Unfamiliar environment **DEFINING CHARACTERISTICS** Increased questioning Lack of questions	**ONGOING ASSESSMENT** • Assess knowledge and readiness to learn. **THERAPEUTIC INTERVENTIONS** • Instruct child/parent to notify nurse of bleeding from wounds, IV sites, etc. • Instruct child to inform nurse of fatigue or dizziness. • Instruct child to try to avoid trauma, *which could precipitate further bleeding.* • Explain purpose of drug/transfusion therapy. • Explain rationale for therapy to parent and encourage parent and other visitors to remain calm while visiting.	Child/parent will verbalize basic understanding of DIC and its management (as appropriate for age).

Audrey Klopp, RN, PhD, CS, ET

Hemophilia

BLEEDERS

An inherited disorder of the clotting mechanism caused by diminished or absent factors necessary to the formation of prothrombin activator (the catalyst to clot formation). Classic hemophilia (type A) is caused by the lack of factor VIII; it is the most common and usually most severe type of hemophilia. Type B (Christmas disease) and type C hemophilia are caused by the lack of factors IX and XI, respectively. Symptom severity is directly proportional to the plasma levels of available clotting factors; depending on these levels, the disease is classified as mild, moderate, or severe. Patients with close to normal factor levels may only experience frequent bruising and slightly prolonged bleeding times. This care plan addresses the more severe symptoms of hemophilia.

NURSING DIAGNOSES/ DEFINING CHARACTERISTICS	NURSING INTERVENTIONS / *RATIONALES*	EXPECTED OUTCOMES
Injury: Hemorrhage **RELATED TO** Decreased concentration of clotting factors circulating in the blood: identified as factor VII, factor IX, or factor XI **DEFINING CHARACTERISTICS** Prolonged bleeding Petechiae Joint pain, swelling GI bleed Hematuria	**ONGOING ASSESSMENT** • Assess age and developmental level. • Assess bleeding. • Assess for type and severity of disease. • Perform physical assessment to determine sites of bruising and bleeding. • Assess for pain and swelling; *may indicate internal bleeding.* • Monitor vital signs, Hgb, and Hct. • Observe for reaction to blood product transfusion. **THERAPEUTIC INTERVENTIONS** • Apply sterile dressing to wounds. *Counting soaked dressings may help determine blood loss.* Apply pressure to bleeding site. • Anticipate need for blood replacement. *Volume expanders and O-negative blood should be immediately available in event of life-threatening hemorrhage.* • If bleeding is in joint (hemarthrosis), elevate and immobilize affected limb. Apply ice packs. • Control hemorrhage by administering cryoprecipitate or concentrated factor. • Document blood product transfusion per hospital policy. • Maintain universal precautions. *Hemophiliacs who received blood products before 1985 are at risk for becoming HIV positive.*	Risk of injury caused by hemorrhage will be reduced.
Pain **RELATED TO** Hemarthrosis Open wound Nerve compression caused by bleeding and swelling **DEFINING CHARACTERISTICS** Verbalized pain Crying Irritability	**ONGOING ASSESSMENT** • Assess pain and monitor for changes: Headache *may indicate intracranial bleeding.* Joint pain *may indicate hemarthrosis.* Abdominal pain *may indicate trauma and bleeding of major organ.* • Assess for permanent damage to limb: Paresthesia Joint changes, contractures **THERAPEUTIC INTERVENTIONS** • Provide analgesia or sedation if needed (*may not be allowed if head trauma is suspected*). • Immobilize affected limbs/joints. • Apply ice packs to painful joints. • Provide care in gentle, careful manner.	Pain will be relieved.

Continued.

399

Hemophilia cont'd

NURSING DIAGNOSES/ DEFINING CHARACTERISTICS	NURSING INTERVENTIONS / *RATIONALES*	EXPECTED OUTCOMES
High Risk for Ineffective Airway Clearance **RELATED TO** Bleeding in or around airway, neck, nose, pharynx, esophagus (blood may or may not be seen depending on site) Obstruction caused by tissue swelling **DEFINING CHARACTERISTICS** Dyspnea Abnormal breath sounds Verbalized difficulty in breathing	**ONGOING ASSESSMENT** • Assess trauma sites. • Observe for bleeding in or around airway. • Monitor vital signs, especially respiratory rate and breath sounds. **THERAPEUTIC INTERVENTIONS** • If neck or pharyngeal injury is suspected: Keep an oral airway and suction apparatus nearby. Keep tracheostomy setup available. Prepare for intubation. Administer required clotting factors *to stop bleeding in or around the airway.*	Risk of ineffective airway clearance will be reduced.
High Risk for Altered Level of Consciousness **RELATED TO** Intracranial bleeding **DEFINING CHARACTERISTICS** Headache Nausea, vomiting Inappropriate affect Impaired judgment or thought processes Impaired memory Dizziness Pupil changes Lethargy Coma	**ONGOING ASSESSMENT** • Assess for trauma sites. *Child may not remember head trauma; bruising may be hidden under hair.* • Perform neurological assessment and maintain neurological flow sheet for serial documentation and reference. **THERAPEUTIC INTERVENTIONS** • Notify physician immediately of signs of neurological compromise (see Defining Characteristics). • Administer clotting factors as ordered. • Prepare for surgical intervention. *Intracranial bleeding is life-threatening complication.*	Risk of neurological injury will be reduced.
High Risk for Impaired Physical Mobility **RELATED TO** Hemarthrosis Joint degeneration **DEFINING CHARACTERISTICS** Joint pain, swelling, discoloration Limited ROM	**ONGOING ASSESSMENT** • Assess current limitations. *Patients who are actively bleeding should have restricted mobility.* • When bleeding is controlled, assess for limited ROM, contractures, and bony changes in joints. *Repeated joint bleeds cause bone destruction, permanent deformities, and crippling.* **THERAPEUTIC INTERVENTIONS** • Provide gentle, passive ROM exercise when stable. • Encourage progression to active exercise as tolerated. • Provide assistive devices when needed. • Refer for physical therapy/occupational therapy and orthopedic consultations as required. • Instruct child/parent on preventive measures, including administration of factor products and application of protective gear. *Prevention of injury and hemarthrosis is best method of maintaining joint/limb mobility and use.*	Risk of impaired physical mobility will be reduced.

NURSING DIAGNOSES/ DEFINING CHARACTERISTICS	NURSING INTERVENTIONS / *RATIONALES*	EXPECTED OUTCOMES
Body Image/Self-Concept Disturbance **RELATED TO** Limited activity Deformities Scarring Presence of ambulatory aids or protective devices Medication administration Hospitalization Bruising Bleeding **DEFINING CHARACTERISTICS** Withdrawn or flat affect Self-deprecating remarks	**ONGOING ASSESSMENT** • Assess current perceptions of self-concept and body image. *Self-perceptions will differ depending on age and severity of illness. Example: a toddler, whose world consists of self and immediate family, will have less difficulty compared with adolescent, who places great emphasis on peer expectations.* • Assess attitude toward assistive/protective devices, limitations, and required medications. **THERAPEUTIC INTERVENTIONS** • Allow verbalization of feelings. • Correct misconceptions. • Provide alternatives to current protective devices; *may require creativity on both nurse's and parent's parts.* • Encourage participation in safe activities (i.e., *swimming may be an acceptable sport as opposed to football or wrestling*). • Provide positive feedback.	Self-concept/body image disturbance will be reduced.
Ineffective Individual Coping: Parent/Mother **RELATED TO** Hereditary cause of child's illness **DEFINING CHARACTERISTICS** Tearful Anxious Withdrawn Demanding Overcautious Agitated	**ONGOING ASSESSMENT** • Assess child's mother for signs of ineffective coping. *Hemophilia is genetic disorder transmitted by female carrier to children, primarily male children. Associated guilt feelings may interfere with usual coping behaviors.* • Assess available family structure and support systems. **THERAPEUTIC INTERVENTIONS** • Acknowledge mother's feelings and the normalcy of her reactions. • Correct misconceptions. • Provide psychological or social work referrals if needed. • Initiate contact with other hemophilia families. Contact National Hemophilia Foundation for information about parent groups. • Allow unlimited visiting. • Explain procedures, keep informed of progress.	Effective coping behaviors will be observed.
Anxiety/Fear **RELATED TO** Potential trauma Death AIDS **DEFINING CHARACTERISTICS** Agitated Tearful Unexplained fears Verbalized fear of death, hemorrhage, AIDS	**ONGOING ASSESSMENT** • Assess level of anxiety/fear. • Identify fears if possible; assess odds of occurrence. • Assess available supportive relationships. **THERAPEUTIC INTERVENTIONS** • Allow expression of fears, anger, and other feelings. • Discuss actual fears, likelihood of occurrence, preventive measures if available. • Provide psychiatric referral if necessary. *Hemophiliac may need help in controlling fears and anxiety. Fear of AIDS is especially destructive; assistance may be needed to prevent fear from controlling life.*	Anxiety/fears will be reduced.
Knowledge Deficit **RELATED TO** New diagnosis Emergency situation Surgical/dental needs	**ONGOING ASSESSMENT** • Assess current knowledge and physical abilities. • Assess cognitive abilities and readiness to learn.	Child and/or parent will understand hemophilia, its treatment, and home care.

Continued.

Hemophilia cont'd

NURSING DIAGNOSES/ DEFINING CHARACTERISTICS	NURSING INTERVENTIONS / *RATIONALES*	EXPECTED OUTCOMES

DEFINING CHARACTERISTICS
Questioning
Verbalized lack of understanding
	THERAPEUTIC INTERVENTIONS
	• Provide information concerning disease type, treatment, and progression.
	• Explain genetic transference to those of childbearing age. Refer for genetic counseling if needed.
	• When stable:
	 Discuss safety and prevention:
	  Safe toys, environment, and protective devices available for infants and young children (i.e., helmets, padding)
	  Safe activities for older child
	  Avoidance of aspirin products
	  Emergency care
	 Discuss prophylactic treatment with factors or cryoprecipitate *to prevent bleeding during dental or surgical procedures.*
	 Provide instruction on self-administration of IV factors, if applicable.
	 Provide follow-up appointments and emergency numbers.	

Michele Knoll Puzas, RNC, MHPE

Idiopathic thrombocytopenic purpura

Idiopathic thrombocytopenic purpura (ITP) is an acquired blood disorder that is characterized by increased destruction of circulating platelets. The cause is unknown. The pathophysiology includes platelets becoming coated with antiplatelet antibody. As a consequence, the platelets are recognized as foreign material and destroyed by the spleen. Signs and symptoms of ITP include the sudden onset of easy bruising with petechiae and ecchymosis distributed randomly over the entire body. Epistaxis or bleeding from other mucous membranes is common. The child may have a positive history of a recent febrile illness; usually an upper respiratory infection, rubella, or rubeolla have also been implicated. Caregivers must perform a careful assessment to differentiate the bruising of ITP from that of child abuse. The majority of children recover spontaneously in 6 to 12 months. In severe cases, or with lack of recovery, a splenectomy is sometimes performed.

NURSING DIAGNOSES/ DEFINING CHARACTERISTICS	NURSING INTERVENTIONS / *RATIONALES*	EXPECTED OUTCOMES
High Risk for Injury: Easy Bruising and Bleeding **RELATED TO** Autoimmune destruction of platelets	**ONGOING ASSESSMENT** • Assess age and developmental level. • Assess skin for appearance of new petechiae and ecchymosis. • Observe for bleeding from mucous membranes. • Monitor vital signs with BP every 4 hours. • Monitor daily lab values (i.e., CBC, platelet count). • Dipstick urine, guaiac or hematest stools every shift *to determine presence of blood.*	Risk for injury will be reduced.

NURSING DIAGNOSES/ DEFINING CHARACTERISTICS	NURSING INTERVENTIONS / *RATIONALES*	EXPECTED OUTCOMES
DEFINING CHARACTERISTICS History of easy bruising Random petechiae and ecchymosis all over body Bleeding from mucous membranes Reduced platelet count: <20,000 to 30,000 mm³/dl Higher than normal levels of megakaryocytes (parent cell of platelet) on bone marrow aspiration Prolonged bleeding time	**THERAPEUTIC INTERVENTIONS** • Protect child from accidental or therapeutically induced trauma *to limit new petechiae and areas of ecchymosis and prevent prolonged bleeding. Invasive procedures (i.e., intramuscular injections, suctioning, catheterization, or venipuncture) must be performed by experienced, skilled clinicians.* • Do not use aspirin or aspirin-containing products; *these products inhibit platelet aggregation.* • Administer one of possible treatment drugs for ITP, as ordered: steroids, high-dose gamma globulin. *These substances are used to elevate platelet count.*	

Altered Tissue Perfusion
RELATED TO
Hemorrhage
 	
DEFINING CHARACTERISTICS
Reduced platelet count <20,000-30,000 mm³/dl
Vital sign changes:
  Tachycardia
  Hypotension
Cool extremities
Pallor
Decreased central venous pressure (<3-5 mm Hg)
	ONGOING ASSESSMENT
	• Monitor vital signs and central venous pressure every 4 hours and as necessary.
	• Assess peripheral perfusion every 4 hours and prn.
	• Monitor daily lab values (i.e., CBC, platelet count, Hgb, Hct).
	• Observe for bleeding from mucous membranes and body orifices.
	• Assess for neurological changes.
	• Measure abdominal circumference every shift.
	• Perform Hematest or guaiac stool test, emesis, and nasogastric secretions.
	
	THERAPEUTIC INTERVENTIONS
	• Administer platelets or colloids as ordered *to maintain intravascular oncotic pressure.* Monitor for evidence of transfusion reaction.
	• If bleeding occurs, notify physician; administer therapy as ordered, including fresh whole blood, packed RBCs. Monitor for transfusion reaction.
		Adequate tissue perfusion will be maintained.

Anxiety/Fear: Parent/Child **RELATED TO** Concerns that child may have life-threatening illness Frightened to discover child covered with bruises Fearful of child "bleeding to death" if bleeding from mucous membranes Difficulty accepting that "no treatment" may be acceptable treatment	**ONGOING ASSESSMENT** • Assess parent's/child's level of anxiety/fear. • Assess parent's/child's knowledge level regarding diagnosis, treatment, and prognosis of ITP. • Identify parent's/child's effective coping mechanisms. **THERAPEUTIC INTERVENTIONS** • Reassure parent/child about progress of disease and treatment. • Answer all questions or refer to appropriate persons. • Assist family to identify and use effective coping mechanisms.	Parent/child anxiety/fear will be reduced.

Continued.

Idiopathic thrombocytopenic purpura cont'd

NURSING DIAGNOSES/ DEFINING CHARACTERISTICS	NURSING INTERVENTIONS / *RATIONALES*	EXPECTED OUTCOMES
DEFINING CHARACTERISTICS Restlessness Crying, tantrums, acting out Anger Withdrawal, depression Demanding		

Knowledge Deficit **RELATED TO** Home management of ITP **DEFINING CHARACTERISTICS** Verbalized lack of understanding of home management of ITP Multiple questions and concerns	**ONGOING ASSESSMENT** - Assess child's/parent's level of knowledge of disease and prognosis. - Assess child's/parent's ability to learn home management of ITP. - Determine child's/parent's readiness to learn. - Determine child's/parent's level of motivation to maintain home treatment program. **THERAPEUTIC INTERVENTIONS** - Instruct parent/child to avoid injury: 　Avoid rough, injury-prone activities such as contact sports, climbing trees, riding motorcycles. 　Move furniture with sharp edges and remove throw rugs for duration of illness. 　Use soft toothbrush to brush teeth. 　Monitor child when using scissors or other sharp objects. 　NOTE: Normal toppling and frequent falls of toddler are not dangerous. - Caution parents to avoid giving child aspirin or aspirin-containing products. - Instruct parents to assess child for bruising and bleeding. - Caution child not to blow nose forcefully and not to sneeze with nose and mouth closed. - Instruct parent to avoid constipation in child; ensure adequate fluids, fiber, and exercise. Avoid enemas. - Avoid taking temperatures rectally. - Instruct parent on emergency procedure for increased bleeding or serious injury: 　Notify health center immediately. 　Observe for symptoms of central nervous system bleeding (i.e., headaches, diplopia, projectile vomiting, lethargy, sensorium changes). - Instruct parent on signs and symptoms of hemorrhage—pale, diaphoretic skin, decreased urine output, confusion. - Emphasize need for close follow-up by physician. 　Platelet counts will be measured every 1 to 2 weeks. - Instruct parent/child on treatment drugs (i.e., dose, side effects). - Initiate referrals with public health nurse or other agency that can assist in overall management.	An understanding of ITP and home management will be achieved.

Sandra N. Roberts, RN, MSN

Sickle cell pain crisis

VASOOCCLUSIVE CRISIS; SICKLE CELL ANEMIA

Severe pain, usually in the extremities, caused by the occlusion of small blood vessels by the sickle-shaped red cells seen in sickle cell anemia. Abdominal pain, back pain, and central nervous system changes indicate occlusion, ischemia, and possible infarction in the spleen, lung, liver, and brain. This chronic disease causes impaired kidney, liver, and spleen function; strokes; blindness; increased susceptibility to infection; and ultimately a decreased life span.

NURSING DIAGNOSES/ DEFINING CHARACTERISTICS	NURSING INTERVENTIONS / *RATIONALES*	EXPECTED OUTCOMES

Pain
 RELATED TO
 Vasooclusive crisis hypoxia, which causes cells to become rigid and elongated, thus forming crescent shape
 Stasis of RBCs
 	
 DEFINING CHARACTERISTICS
 Complaint of generalized or localized pain
 Tenderness on palpation
 Inability to move affected joint
 Swelling to area
 Deformity to joint
 Warmth, discoloration
	ONGOING ASSESSMENT
	 • Assess age and developmental level.
	 • Assess pain every 2-4 hours using age-appropriate scale (see Pain, p. 35).
	 • Check laboratory values (e.g., Hgb electrophoresis for amount of sickling and RBC count). *Severe decrease in functioning RBCs may indicate need for transfusion.*
	
	 THERAPEUTIC INTERVENTIONS
	 • Administer medications according to sickle cell pain protocol:
	     Administer IM injections (meperidine [Demerol] or morphine sulfate) every 3 hours for first 48 hours.
	     Use antiinflammatory agent simultaneously with IM injections every 3 hours (Ascriptin or aspirin).
	     Start oral analgesic 48 hours after admission (Tylenol No. 3, Empirin, Percodan, Darvocet-N, or Darvon).
	     Use PCA morphine or Demerol for older child. *PCA allows child some control over amount and frequency of IV pain medications in a 1-hour period.*
	 • Use additional comfort measures:
	     Changing environment
	     Distractional devices/toys/videos
	     Relaxation techniques
	 • Obtain child life specialist consultation.
	 • Provide rest periods *to facilitate comfort, sleep, and relaxation.*
		Pain will be reduced.

Impaired Gas Exchange **RELATED TO** Stasis of sickled RBCs Vasooclusion Lung infarctions **DEFINING CHARACTERISTICS** Restlessness Irritability Hypoxia Diminished breath sounds Dyspnea Chest pain	**ONGOING ASSESSMENT** • Assess respirations. • Assess breath sounds. • Assess for chest pain. • Assess orientation and behavior. • Monitor ABGs and pulse oximetry. **THERAPEUTIC INTERVENTIONS** • Provide humidified oxygen. • Position for comfort and ease of respiratory effort. • Maintain IV fluids and prophylactic antibiotics if ordered. • Medicate for pain; *decreasing pain will allow for greater chest/lung expansion.* • Stay with anxious child. • Prepare for intubation/mechanical ventilation. • See Impaired gas exchange, p. 23.	Optimal gas exchange will be maintained.

Continued.

Sickle cell pain crisis cont'd

NURSING DIAGNOSES/ DEFINING CHARACTERISTICS	NURSING INTERVENTIONS / *RATIONALES*	EXPECTED OUTCOMES
High Risk for Altered Nutrition: Less Than Body Requirements **RELATED TO** Nutrient resources expended in response to illness Poor appetite **DEFINING CHARACTERISTICS** Loss of weight with or without adequate caloric intake Current weight 10% or more under ideal body weight Caloric intake inadequate to keep pace with abnormal disease/metabolic state	**ONGOING ASSESSMENT** • Document child's actual weight on admission. • Obtain nutritional history as appropriate. • Document appetite and I&O; encourage child's participation (daily log). **THERAPEUTIC INTERVENTIONS** • Assist child with meals as needed. • Consult dietitian when appropriate *to determine ideal weight, implement steps to ensure intake required to meet demands placed on body during illness as well as growth.* • If inadequate nutrition noted, see Altered nutrition: less than body requirements, p. 33.	Adequate nutrition will be maintained.

High Risk for Fluid Volume Deficit **RELATED TO** Inability to take fluids by mouth Pain **DEFINING CHARACTERISTICS** Decreased urine output Concentrated urine Output greater than intake Sudden weight loss Decreased skin turgor Increased thirst Dry mucous membranes Hypokalemia Hyponatremia	**ONGOING ASSESSMENT**
	 • Assess hydrational status:
	    Skin turgor
	    Mucous membranes
	    Daily weight
	 • Monitor strict I&O every 4-8 hours.
	 • Report urine output <30 ml/hr for 2 consecutive hours.
	 • Monitor serum/urine electrolytes and specific gravity.
	 • Monitor and document vital signs.
	 • Report abnormalities to physician.
	
	 THERAPEUTIC INTERVENTIONS
	 • Administer parenteral fluids as ordered:
	    $D_5W.2NS$ at 1½ times maintenance.
	    Maintain patent IV flow rate.
	    Continue IV fluids for 24-48 hours after oral pain management begins *to prevent dehydration and recurrence of pain crisis.*
	 • Encourage oral fluids as soon as possible.
	 • Provide desired fluids such as ice, tea, popsicles, milk.
		Fluid and electrolyte balance will be maintained.

Hyperthermia **RELATED TO** Infections of bone/ organ infarcts Splenic infarction causing spleen to lose ability to filter bacteria Decreased splenic production of phagocyte	**ONGOING ASSESSMENT** • Monitor vital signs every 2-4 hours. • Observe for chills *resulting from body's attempt to fight off fever.* • Observe for profuse diaphoresis. • Assess joints for redness, warmth, and swelling. • Observe skin for any wounds with drainage. • Review x-ray films and results with physician.	Normal temperature will be maintained.

Sickle cell pain crisis cont'd

NURSING DIAGNOSES/ DEFINING CHARACTERISTICS	NURSING INTERVENTIONS / *RATIONALES*	EXPECTED OUTCOMES
DEFINING CHARACTERISTICS Persistent rise in body temperature to >38.3° C (101° F) for 24-48 hours Positive blood, urine, or sputum cultures Positive x-rays for bony infarcts	**THERAPEUTIC INTERVENTIONS** • Administer antipyretics as ordered *to control fever.* • Provide cool sponge baths. • Keep child's body and linen clean and dry. • Administer antibiotics as ordered *to destroy invading bacteria.* • Push fluids as appropriate.	

High Risk for Ineffective Coping: Child/Family
RELATED TO
Repeated hospitalizations; chronic status of disease
 	
DEFINING CHARACTERISTICS
Poor school attendance
Poor performance
Withdrawal
Poor self-image
Tearful
Anxious
Demanding
	ONGOING ASSESSMENT
	• Assess child's ability to openly express feelings about disease.
	• Assess family involvement with patient care.
	
	THERAPEUTIC INTERVENTIONS
	• Provide primary nurse relationship.
	• Set aside talk times when pain is controlled. *Child in pain is not able to communicate concerns effectively.*
	• Identify needs/provide information on coping mechanisms for child and family:
	    Outside activities
	    Exercise programs (YMCA, health clubs)
	• Inform child/family of support systems available (e.g., National Association of Sickle Cell Anemia, in-house support group if available).
	• Use other resource persons:
	    Clinical specialists
	    Psychiatric liaison personnel
	    Social workers
		Coping strategies will be maximized.

Knowledge Deficit
RELATED TO
Unfamiliarity with disease process, treatment, complications
 	
DEFINING CHARACTERISTICS
Inability to define sickle cell disease
Inability to list signs and symptoms of crisis/infection
Lack of understanding of self-care preventive measures
	ONGOING ASSESSMENT
	• Assess level of understanding, developmental stage, and ability to learn.
	• Assess family involvement and readiness to learn.
	
	THERAPEUTIC INTERVENTIONS
	• Explain cause of sickle cell disease.
	• Instruct child and family on signs of impending crisis:
	    Verbal complaint of pain
	    Persistent low-grade temperature
	    Decreased appetite
	    Decreased fluid intake
	    Increased sleeping time
	    Swollen joints
	• Instruct on necessity of informing physician of signs of infection *that may lead to crisis.*
	• Instruct on importance of:
	    Pushing fluids, water, and juice
	    Food high in carbohydrates and protein; three balanced meals per day
	    Dressing appropriately for weather conditions. *Any added stress, such as severe cold weather, increases likelihood of crisis.*
	• Provide information concerning medications as ordered:
	    Pain medications
	    Antiinflammatory agents
	    Antibiotics
	• Stress importance of keeping clinic appointments and wearing Medic-Alert tag.
	• Inform child and family about support groups, and inform parents about importance of genetic counseling in planning families.
		Child and/or family will verbalize an understanding of sickle cell disease, prevention of crisis, and appropriate treatment.

Carol Boyd, RN, BSN; Michele Knoll Puzas, RNC, MHPE

Anemia in the growing premature infant

LOW BLOOD CELL COUNT

There is normally a 2- to 3-month delay after birth before erythropoiesis occurs in the premature infant. This delay is the result of the underproduction of red blood cells in relation to rapid growth in body mass. Anemia may result in varying degrees of compromise.

NURSING DIAGNOSES/ DEFINING CHARACTERISTICS	NURSING INTERVENTIONS / *RATIONALES*	EXPECTED OUTCOMES
High Risk for Injury: Decreased Oxygen Saturation Related to Decreased Oxygen-Carrying Capacity **RELATED TO** Insufficient number of RBCs secondary to: Frequent blood sampling Relative underproduction of RBCs compared to rapid somatic growth of premature infant **DEFINING CHARACTERISTICS** Hct below 40% (may vary based on age of infant) Suboptimal reticulocyte count Tachypnea Tachycardia Episodes of apnea and bradycardia Pallor Decreased perfusion Prolonged oxygen dependence in absence of bronchopulmonary dysplasia or other pulmonary pathology Respiratory compromise evidenced by grunting, flaring, retracting Lethargy Temperature instability Failure to gain weight despite adequate cal/kg/day	**ONGOING ASSESSMENT** • Assess Hct by heelstick every week or prn, as ordered. • If Hct <40%, monitor CBC and reticulocyte count. • Assess heart rate for tachycardia. *Rate >180/bpm indicates tachycardia.* • Assess respiratory status for: Grunting Nasal flaring Retractions Tachypnea • Record amount of blood drawn for laboratory sampling on I&O record; note daily total on 24-hour fluid balance sheet. • Calculate amount of blood drawn since last transfusion. • Notify physician if blood drawn ≥10% of normal circulating blood volume. • Assess infant's color for pallor. • Observe for decrease in infant's activity level; with oral feeding, note decreased ability to suck, increase in feeding time, cyanosis, or pallor with feeding. **THERAPEUTIC INTERVENTIONS** • Assist with packed RBC transfusion as ordered. • Use cardiorespiratory monitor *to detect tachycardia, bradycardia, or apneic episodes.* • Report abnormal blood gas findings to physician. • Provide supportive oxygen as ordered *to prevent tissue hypoxia.* • Decrease energy expenditure: Minimize handling of infant. Maintain neutral thermal environment. Initiate nasogastric feedings (until after transfusion) if infant compromised during oral feeding. • Consider supplementing formula with vitamins/iron drops *to increase erythropoietic activity.*	Injury from decreased oxygen-carrying capacity will be reduced.

Anemia in the growing premature infant cont'd

NURSING DIAGNOSES/ DEFINING CHARACTERISTICS	NURSING INTERVENTIONS / *RATIONALES*	EXPECTED OUTCOMES
Anxiety/Fear Regarding Blood Transfusion **RELATED TO** Religious beliefs (Jehovah's Witness) Fear of possibility of transfusion-transmitted disease (AIDS, cytomegalovirus, hepatitis) Previous association with transfusion signifying death/poor prognosis **DEFINING CHARACTERISTICS** Refusal to consent to transfusion Multiple questions Verbalization of anxiety/fear about transfusion-transmitted disease	**ONGOING ASSESSMENT** • Evaluate parent's understanding of infant's need for transfusion. • Determine parent's previous experience with blood transfusions. • Identify reason for fear and/or refusal to sign consent. • Assess family support systems. **THERAPEUTIC INTERVENTIONS** • Demonstrate nonjudgmental, supportive attitude toward parent. • If parental refusal results from religious beliefs, consult with attending physician, social worker, and legal affairs personnel to: Assist with arrangements for temporary guardianship. Inform parent of reasons for actions taken on child's behalf. • If refusal stems from fear of transfusion-transmitted disease, inform parent that he/she may, with blood bank guidelines, select known blood donor to reduce risk of transfusion-transmitted disease. *(Guidelines include: 17-65 years of age; in good health; not taking any medication except those approved by blood bank; no history of hepatitis, jaundice, malaria, syphilis. Contact blood bank for further restrictions.)* • Report to parent results of transfusion (improved color, increased Hct) as applicable after transfusion *to help alleviate parental anxiety.*	Anxiety/fear will be reduced.

Mary Lawson-Carney, RN; Herminia Inawat, RN

Care of the infant of a mother at risk for AIDS

HIV

Acquired immunodeficiency syndrome (AIDS) is an infectious disease caused by a human immunodeficiency virus (HIV). This retrovirus impairs the infant's immune system and weakens or destroys the body's ability to fight opportunistic infections. Infants may acquire this infection by intrauterine or perinatal route from an infected mother, or through blood transfusions given in the neonatal period.

NURSING DIAGNOSES/ DEFINING CHARACTERISTICS	NURSING INTERVENTIONS / *RATIONALES*	EXPECTED OUTCOMES
High Risk for Infection **RELATED TO** Human immunodeficiency virus (HIV) *Transmitted:* Antenatally: transplacental	**ONGOING ASSESSMENT** • Assess infant for risk of infection using Defining Characteristics. • Monitor for signs of respiratory distress. • Monitor vital signs and temperature every 2 hours. • Assess for unusual bleeding: Prolonged bleeding from venipuncture site Blood in: emesis, gastric aspirate, urine, stools • Monitor Hct, platelets, PT, and PTT as ordered *to detect blood loss and need for blood replacement therapy.*	Transmission of infection will be reduced as much as possible.

Continued.

Hematologic/Oncologic/Immunologic Care Plans (Neonatal)

NURSING DIAGNOSES/ DEFINING CHARACTERISTICS	NURSING INTERVENTIONS / *RATIONALES*	EXPECTED OUTCOMES

High Risk for Infection cont'd

Perinatally: contact with maternal blood during delivery

Postnatally: breast-feeding

Infants who may be at risk include:

Known maternal AIDS or ARC

Seropositive mother

Maternal IV drug abuser

Maternal blood product recipient

Recent Haitian immigrant

Mother whose sexual partner is: bisexual, hemophiliac, blood product recipient

DEFINING CHARACTERISTICS

Dyspnea

Tachypnea

Retractions

Cyanosis

Pneumocystis carinii pneumonia

CMV (cytomegalovirus)

Herpes simplex

Kaposi's sarcoma

Toxoplasmosis

Tachycardia

Temperature instability

Low birth weight

Diarrhea

Fever

Recurrent infections of otitis media

Craniofacial pattern:
Microcephaly
Prominent boxlike forehead
Flattened nasal bridge
Mild obligatory eyes
Patulous lips

Lymphadenopathy

Enlarged liver and spleen

ONGOING ASSESSMENT cont'd

- Monitor and repeat HIV testing in infant at 6 and 12 months of age. *Initial positive test at birth can result from passive transfer of antibiotics from mother.*

THERAPEUTIC INTERVENTIONS

- Provide ventilatory support as needed. *Respiratory infections are major cause of mortality.*
- Perform chest physical therapy (CPT) and suctioning *to maintain patent airway and maximize ventilation.*
- Transfuse with CMV-negative products from designated donors (family members or friends who have been screened), or a dedicated donor (same unit of blood from blood bank).
- Notify physician of low platelet count; *may be one of first signs of infection.*
- Use aseptic technique when caring for peripheral and central lines *because of increased susceptibility to bacterial, viral, and fungal infections.*
- Send serum to lab for HIV antibody testing.
- Use blood and secretion precautions as recommended by CDC.
- Counsel mothers who are HIV positive that breastfeeding should be discouraged, *since virus has been isolated in breast milk and could be mode of transmission.*

Care of the infant of a mother at risk for AIDS cont'd

NURSING DIAGNOSES/ DEFINING CHARACTERISTICS	NURSING INTERVENTIONS / *RATIONALES*	EXPECTED OUTCOMES
DEFINING CHARACTERISTICS cont'd Prolonged or unusual bleeding Recurrent bacterial sepsis Salivary gland enlargement Chronic eczema *Lab findings:* Anemia Thrombocytopenia (platelet count <150,000) High immunoglobin levels of IgB and IgA Decreased T_4 cells to T-suppressor cells (T_8) Decreased T lymphocytes		

Altered Nutrition: Less Than Body Requirements
RELATED TO
Enteral feeding intolerance
Malabsorption
Lactose intolerance
Emesis
Oral lesions
Diarrhea
Lethargy
 	
DEFINING CHARACTERISTICS
Weight loss
Documented inadequate caloric intake
	ONGOING ASSESSMENT
	▪ Assess for failure to thrive:
	  Monitor daily weights and head circumference.
	  Measure body length every week.
	▪ Assess for feeding intolerance:
	  Emesis
	  Residuals
	  Abdominal distention
	  Loose/frequent stools
	▪ Assess activity level.
	▪ Monitor serum electrolytes prn.
	
	THERAPEUTIC INTERVENTIONS
	▪ Allow adequate time for nipple feeding; *sucking and swallowing may be difficult because of oral herpes or thrush.*
	▪ Notify physician of signs of feeding intolerance identified in Assessment column.
	▪ Give soy formula as ordered. *Lactose intolerance can result from long-term antibiotic treatment and repeated GI infections. Formulas with lactose may also worsen diarrhea.*
	▪ Administer supplements *(to provide additional calories as needed for weight gain):*
	  MCT oil
	  Polycose
	  Total parental nutrition (TPN)
		Optimal weight gain will be achieved.

Impaired Skin Integrity
RELATED TO
Immunological deficit
Malnutrition
	ONGOING ASSESSMENT
	▪ Assess condition of skin:
	  Rashes
	  Lesions
	  Fissures
		Impaired skin integrity will be reduced.

Continued.

Hematologic/Oncologic/Immunologic Care Plans (Neonatal)

NURSING DIAGNOSES/ DEFINING CHARACTERISTICS	NURSING INTERVENTIONS / *RATIONALES*	EXPECTED OUTCOMES
DEFINING CHARACTERISTICS Interruption of skin surface Destruction of integumentary layers Pathogen invasion of body fluids Documented inadequate caloric intake	**ONGOING ASSESSMENT cont'd** • Assess for signs of impaired and/or infected skin: 　　Erythema 　　Edema 　　Dry, scaly skin 　　Abrasions 　　Bruised and pale areas • Weigh daily. **THERAPEUTIC INTERVENTIONS** • Report to physician any disruption to skin surface; *intact skin barrier is best defense against potential pathogens.* • Give daily bath and shampoo as tolerated; use mild soap *to reduce organisms on skin surface.* • Apply lotion to dry skin. • See High risk for impaired skin integrity, p. 41. • Provide sufficient ml/kg/day and cal/kg/day *to promote weight gain.*	
Altered Sensory Perception **RELATED TO** Lack of stimulation related to neonatal ICU environment Isolette **DEFINING CHARACTERISTICS** Irritability Delayed social smile Delayed tracking Avoiding eye contact Lack of attachment Hypotonia	**ONGOING ASSESSMENT** • Assess for developmental delays using Defining Characteristics. • Obtain baseline Denver Developmental Screen Test (DDST) *to determine fine and gross motor skills.* **THERAPEUTIC INTERVENTIONS** • Encourage parental visits and care participation *to promote parent-infant attachment.* • Place infant on sheepskin and use soft blanket rolls around infant *to provide tactile stimulation.* • Elevate head of bed *to promote vestibular stimulation.* • Place age-appropriate toys along sides of crib *to provide visual stimulation for infant who may spend much time with head turned to side.* • Place infant in swing as tolerated *to stimulate and improve motor growth.* • Hold infant in enface position while talking *to encourage eye contact and vocalization.* • Hold infant for feedings; *sitting position reduces hypotonicity.* • Play tape of parent's voice or use music box *to provide auditory stimulation.* • See Developmental enhancement, p. 66.	Altered sensory perception will be reduced.
Altered Physical Development **RELATED TO** *Encephalopathy:* Cortical atrophy Pyramidal tract involvement Calcification of basal ganglia **DEFINING CHARACTERISTICS** Hypotonia Hypertonia Poor coordination Loss of previously accomplished milestones	**ONGOING ASSESSMENT** • Assess for physical development using Defining Characteristics. • Repeat Denver Developmental Screen Test (DDST) at 1- to 2-month intervals *to determine developmental age-appropriateness.* **THERAPEUTIC INTERVENTIONS** • Encourage physical therapy/occupational therapy involvement *to maintain present physical function.* • Place infant in prone position *to increase use and strength of lower extremities.* • During feedings, hold infant in sitting position *to decrease hypotonicity.*	Optimal physical development will be achieved.

NURSING DIAGNOSES/ DEFINING CHARACTERISTICS	NURSING INTERVENTIONS / *RATIONALES*	EXPECTED OUTCOMES
High Risk for Impaired Home Maintenance/ Management **RELATED TO** Inadequate community resources Ill mother and infant with poor chance of survival **DEFINING CHARACTERISTICS** Social isolation Lack of confidence regarding ability to parent Parental expression of difficulty in preparing home for infant Loss of income Guilt Loss of control Low self-esteem	**ONGOING ASSESSMENT** • Assess parental ability to care for infant: Physically Emotionally Financially Support systems • Assess stability of family unit. • Assess other family members' reactions *to acceptance of and willingness to participate in infant's care.* **THERAPEUTIC INTERVENTIONS** • Have parent (as much as possible) assume total caretaking responsibilities before discharge. *Maximizing parental involvement will help ensure comfort level.* • Consult with support services before discharge *to ensure follow-up by multidisciplinary team.* • In conjunction with discharge planning, teach parent following care practices: Good handwashing *to protect infant from organisms* Enteric precautions, *especially when infant has diarrhea* How to take axillary temperature, *which will decrease risk of rectal fissure, a portal for pathogens* Common signs and symptoms of infection: Behavior change Loss of appetite Vomiting Fever Frequent sneezing and coughing Stress importance of follow-up care including immunization schedule; *prompt intervention important to prevention of additional complications.*	Appropriate home care activities will be demonstrated.

Cynthia R. Wilson, RN, BSN; Deborah Rickard, RN, BSN

Polycythemia

HYPERVISCOSITY

Venous hematocrit value greater than 65% or a venous hemoglobin greater than 22 mg% in the first week of life.

NURSING DIAGNOSES/ DEFINING CHARACTERISTICS	NURSING INTERVENTIONS / *RATIONALES*	EXPECTED OUTCOMES
High Risk for Injury: Altered Circulation **RELATED TO** Placental transfusions: Maternal-fetal transfusion Twin-twin transfusion Obstetrical manipulation (e.g., delayed cord clamping) Infants of diabetic mothers (increased erythropoiesis) Congenital adrenal hyperplasia Infants born to thyrotoxic mothers Small for gestational age infants Infants born at high altitudes	**ONGOING ASSESSMENT** • Observe infant's color. • Monitor capillary refill. • Monitor urine output. Report decreased urine output to physician. *Oliguria can be secondary to thromboembolic phenomena resulting in acute tubular necrosis.* • Assess for feeding intolerance. Report signs and symptoms of feeding intolerance to physician. *Thromboembolic pneumonia may result in necrotizing enterocolitis.* • Calculate fluid intake in ml/24 hr/kg of body weight *to ensure adequate hydration.* • Monitor Hct daily. • Monitor glucose levels. *As viscosity increases, plasma glucose decreases.* • If partial exchange needed, monitor vital signs every 15 to 30 minutes. **THERAPEUTIC INTERVENTIONS** • Warm heel of foot before drawing capillary Hct *to give better correlation with central venous Hct.* • Provide early feedings *to adequately hydrate, which decreases viscosity.* • Assist with partial exchange transfusion using fresh-frozen plasma *to replace calculated volumes of blood.* • See Necrotizing enterocolitis, p. 262.	Optimal circulation will be restored.
DEFINING CHARACTERISTICS Plethora Prolonged capillary refill Oliguria Thrombocytopenia Hypoglycemia Necrotizing enterocolitis		
High Risk for Ineffective Breathing Pattern **RELATED TO** Pulmonary venous congestion	**ONGOING ASSESSMENT** • Monitor vital signs and BP every 2 hours. • Note presence of respiratory distress symptoms as listed under defining characteristics. • Monitor continuous oxygenation (noninvasively). • Monitor ABGs; *acidotic state increases viscosity causing further impairment of tissue oxygenation.* **THERAPEUTIC INTERVENTIONS** • Administer oxygen as needed to maintain SaO_2 88%-92% *to ensure adequate cellular oxygenation and support aerobic metabolism.* • Place bed in semi-Fowler's position *to improve air exchange.*	Adequate breathing pattern is achieved.
DEFINING CHARACTERISTICS Central cyanosis Tachypnea Retractions Grunting Nasal flaring		

NURSING DIAGNOSES/ DEFINING CHARACTERISTICS	NURSING INTERVENTIONS / *RATIONALES*	EXPECTED OUTCOMES
High Risk for Injury: Altered Bilirubin Metabolism **RELATED TO** Increased number of hemolyzed cells, which will yield excessive amounts of bilirubin **DEFINING CHARACTERISTICS** Jaundice Pallor Central venous Hct >65 Hepatosplenomegaly Temperature elevations NPO status	**ONGOING ASSESSMENT** • Assess infant's color. • Monitor fractionated (total/direct) bilirubin levels and serial levels *to establish rate of bilirubin rise.* • Monitor temperature closely; *as infants in incubators or servo-controlled beds who receive phototherapy may become overheated.* • Weigh daily. • Monitor fluid balance closely. *Infants who receive phototherapy may have significant increase in insensible water loss.* **THERAPEUTIC INTERVENTIONS** • Initiate phototherapy as ordered *to prevent need for exchange transfusion.* • During phototherapy, patches should completely cover eyes *to prevent possible eye damage from light.* • Report to physician if infant develops "bronze baby syndrome," *caused by retention of bilirubin breakdown product produced by phototherapy.* • Provide early feedings as clinically tolerated *to stimulate peristalsis, which enhances bilirubin excretion via gut. Meconium stools contain large amounts of bilirubin.* • See Hyperbilirubinemia, p. 253.	Potential for kernicterus will be reduced.
High Risk for Injury: Neurological Status **RELATED TO** Suboptimal brain perfusion secondary to hyperviscosity **DEFINING CHARACTERISTICS** Lethargy Irritability Jitteriness Focal or generalized seizures Poor feeding	**ONGOING ASSESSMENT** • Closely monitor for signs and symptoms of altered neurological status as listed under Defining Characteristics. **THERAPEUTIC INTERVENTIONS** • If early feedings cannot be initiated, maintain IV rate to provide appropriate fluids and electrolyte requirements. • If signs and symptoms of neurological sequelae present, assist with partial exchange transfusion.	Risk for injury will be reduced.

Terry Griffin, RN, MS

Index